Food Allergy: Diagnosis and Management

Food Allergy: Diagnosis and Management

Editor: Kevin Parker

Callisto Reference
www.callistoreference.com

Callisto Reference,
118-35 Queens Blvd., Suite 400,
Forest Hills, NY 11375, USA

Visit us on the World Wide Web at:
www.callistoreference.com

ISBN: 978-1-63239-856-7 (Hardback)

The publisher's policy is to use permanent paper from mills that operate a sustainable forestry policy. Furthermore, the publisher ensures that the text paper and cover boards used have met acceptable environmental accreditation standards.

Printed in China.

Cataloging-in-publication Data

Food allergy : diagnosis and management / edited by Kevin Parker.
p. cm.
Includes bibliographical references and index.
ISBN 978-1-63239-856-7
1. Food allergy. 2. Food allergy--Diagnosis. 3. Food allergy--Prevention. 4. Food allergy--Prevention--Technological innovations. I. Parker, Kevin.
RC596 .F66 2017
616.975--dc23

Table of Contents

Preface

Hypersensitivity to certain food items causes food allergy. Certain foods such as peanuts, eggs and milk are the most common allergens. This book on food allergy deals with themes related to clinical manifestations of food allergy including its causes, diagnosis and effects. This book aims to shed light on some of the unexplored aspects of food allergy and the recent researches in this field. It is a compilation of chapters that discuss the most vital concepts and emerging trends in this field. It will serve as a valuable source of reference for graduate and post graduate students. This book with its detailed analysis and data, will prove immensely beneficial to professionals and experts involved in this area at various levels.

The main aim of this book is to educate learners and enhance their research focus by presenting diverse topics covering this vast field. This is an advanced book which compiles significant studies by distinguished experts. This book addresses successive solutions to the challenges arising in the area of application, along with it; the book provides scope for future developments.

It was a great honour to edit this book, though there were challenges, as it involved a lot of communication and networking between me and the editorial team. However, the end result was this all-inclusive book covering diverse themes in the field.

Finally, it is important to acknowledge the efforts of the contributors for their excellent chapters, through which a wide variety of issues have been addressed. I would also like to thank my colleagues for their valuable feedback during the making of this book.

Editor

1

Is Aboriginal Food Less Allergenic? Comparing IgE-Reactivity of Eggs from Modern and Ancient Chicken Breeds in a Cohort of Allergic Children

Matthias Egger[1], Claudia Alessandri[2], Michael Wallner[1], Peter Briza[3], Danila Zennaro[2], Adriano Mari[2], Fatima Ferreira[1], Gabriele Gadermaier[1]*

1 Christian Doppler Laboratory for Allergy Diagnosis and Therapy, University of Salzburg, Salzburg, Austria, **2** Center for Molecular Allergology, IDI-IRCCS, Rome, Italy, **3** Department of Molecular Biology, University of Salzburg, Salzburg, Austria

Abstract

Background: Hen's egg allergy ranks among the most frequent primary food allergies in children. We aimed to investigate sensitization profiles of egg allergic patients and compare *in vitro* IgE reactivities of eggs from ancient chicken breeds (Araucana and Maran) with those from conventional laying hen hybrids.

Methodology: Egg allergic children (n = 25) were subjected to skin prick test, double blind placebo controlled food challenge, and sensitization profiles to Gal d 1–5 were determined by allergen microarray. IgE binding and biological activity of eggs from different chicken breeds were investigated by immunoblot, ELISA, and mediator release assays.

Principal Findings: We found that Gal d 1 and Gal d 2 are generally major egg allergens, whereas Gal d 3–5 displayed high sensitization prevalence only in patients reacting to both, egg white and yolk. It seems that the onset of egg allergy is mediated by egg white allergens expanding to yolk sensitization in later stages of disease. Of note, egg white/yolk weight ratios were reduced in eggs from Auraucana and Maran chicken. As determined in IgE immunoblots and mass analysis, eggs from ancient chicken breeds did not differ in their protein composition. Similar IgE-binding was observed for all egg white preparations, while an elevated allergenicity was detected in egg yolk from Araucana chicken.

Conclusion/Significance: Our results on allergenicity and biological activity do not confirm the common assumption that aboriginal food might be less allergenic. Comprehensive diagnosis of egg allergy should distinguish between reactivity to hen's egg white and yolk fractions to avoid unnecessary dietary restrictions to improve life quality of the allergic child and its family.

Editor: Jacques Zimmer, Centre de Recherche Public de la Santé (CRP-Santé), Luxembourg

Funding: This work was supported by the Austrian Christian-Doppler Research Association, Biomay AG, Vienna, Austria, and the Italian Ministry of Health, Current Research Program 2009. The funders had no role in study design, data collection and analysis, decision to publish, or preparation of the manuscript.

Competing Interests: The authors have declared that no competing interests exist.

* E-mail: Gabriele.Gadermaier@sbg.ac.at

Introduction

Approximately 15% of the overall population suffers from IgE-mediated adverse reactions upon the ingestion of several kinds of food. According to the sensitization process, this disease can be divided into primary and secondary food allergies, affecting 9.4% and 5.5% of the population, respectively [1]. Adults often develop secondary food allergies as a consequence of primary sensitization through inhalant or contact allergens. Secondary food-induced symptoms are predominantly local and attributed to homologous molecules, which are recognized by cross-reactive IgE antibodies. In contrast, primary food allergy mainly affects children, is frequently characterized by severe symptoms, and the sensitization process, which takes place in the gastrointestinal tract, is mediated by the food allergen itself [2,3].

Allergic reactions to hen's egg represent one of the most frequent primary food allergies affecting around 1.6% of children below the age of three, but are in the majority of cases outgrown before school age [2,4]. So far, the official allergen list of the IUIS Allergen Nomenclature Subcommittee contains 6 chicken (*Gallus domesticus*) allergens while nine more IgE-binding egg proteins are listed in the Allergome database (www.allergome.org). Ovomucoid (Gal d 1), ovalbumin (Gal d 2), ovotransferrin (Gal d 3), and lysozyme (Gal d 4) constitute the most abundant proteins in the egg white fraction and have all been described as major allergens [5,6,7]. Gal d 1 is a highly glycosylated protein that is fairly resistant to heat and pepsin treatment and therefore, might cause severe allergic reactions upon consumption of cooked eggs [8,9]. Gal d 2 constitutes 54% (w/w) of the total egg white proteins but seems less stable to heat and gastric digestion [7,10]. Gal d 3 is an iron-binding heat-labile allergen that accounts for around 12% of the total egg white weight [11]. Sensitization to Gal d 4 can be exceedingly inconvenient, as it is commonly used as food preservative due to its antibacterial properties. Notably, egg white proteins are essential in the sweet cuisine constituting ingredients of many pastries and desserts [4,5,7]. Moreover, they have been revealed as occupational inhalant allergens in patients with baker's asthma [12,13].

Although to a lower frequency, allergic reactions to yolk have been reported [11,14]. Yolk represents an important emulsifier, and so far two allergens have been described at the molecular level. The first, alpha-livetin (Gal d 5), is partially heat-labile and belongs to the serum albumin protein family [6,13]. Besides eliciting egg allergy in children, Gal d 5 has been implicated in the development of secondary egg allergy in adults sensitized to avian inhalant antigens, a phenomenon termed "bird-egg syndrome" [15,16]. The second, vitellogenin (Gal d 6) has been identified recently and characterized as heat-resistant minor allergen in yolk [11].

Egg allergy has a significant effect on the quality of life and although symptoms are usually not life-threatening, severe anaphylactic reactions upon egg consumption have been reported [17]. As there is no efficient treatment for egg allergy so far, avoidance represents the only way to safely escape symptoms. However, as egg-derived components constitute ingredients of many cooked and manufactured food products, this approach is rather difficult and implies broad dietary restrictions [18]. The current tendency towards a deliberate, healthy, and balanced nutrition implicates a trend back to organic and natural foods. This heavily influenced food industry leading to customer-oriented changes in product development and marketing [19,20,21]. From the few hundred established chicken breeds only a small number is economically important as egg producers in poultry industry. Due to the worldwide demand, nowadays the majority of eggs is produced by high-performance laying hen hybrids [22]. Recently, eggs from ancient chicken breeds are getting promoted as aboriginal alternative trying to satisfy customer's requirements. Interestingly, the usage of laying hen hybrids in poultry industry since the 1950s is paralleled by a general increase in the prevalence of food allergy [23]. For this reason, we compared the allergenicity of eggs from conventional laying hen hybrids with those from ancient chicken breeds (Araucana and Maran). Within this study we investigated a cohort of 25 egg allergic children that were subjected to detailed *in vitro* and clinical allergy diagnosis.

Results

Egg allergic patients differ in their sensitization profiles

Studying a large cohort of 474 Italian subjects [24] displaying specific IgE to egg allergens revealed that egg sensitization predominantly affects male children (60%) in the age of 3 to 8 years (Figure 1A). For the present study we selected 25 patients displaying clinical symptoms upon egg consumption, which was confirmed by skin prick test (SPT) and double blind placebo controlled food challenge (DBPCFC) (Table 1). The average age of these children was 5.5 years and a stronger bias towards male gender was observed (20 male versus 5 female). The sensitization prevalence was highest for Gal d 1 (88%), Gal d 2 (76%), and Gal d 3 (48%), whereas reactivity to Gal d 4 and Gal d 5 were 24% and 28%, respectively (Table 1). As revealed by ELISA, 48% of egg allergic patients were sensitized to egg white and yolk (patients 1–12), whereas 52% displayed IgE antibodies with exclusive specificity for egg white components (patients 13–25). Notably, the concentration of egg white-specific IgE was significantly increased ($P = 0.015$) in the group of patients displaying additional sensitization to yolk (median 3.56 µg/ml versus 1.02 µg/ml). With 6.8±3.6 years (mean ± STD), the average age in this group was also slightly higher than for children belonging to the yolk-negative group (4.3±2.3 years). Moreover, the two groups differed in their allergen sensitization pattern (Figure 1B). In microarray experiments we found that Gal d 1 and Gal d 2 are relevant allergens in both patient groups, *i.e.* egg allergic children with and without yolk-specific IgE. By contrast, the sensitization prevalence to Gal d 3 and Gal d 4 was significantly higher in yolk-reactive patients (83% versus 15% and 42% versus 8%, respectively), even though those proteins are considered egg white allergens. As expected, IgE reactivity to Gal d 5 was exclusively detected in yolk-sensitized patients.

Clinical manifestation of egg allergy

As illustrated in Table 1, allergic children predominately displayed skin-related symptoms (90%), while 35 and 25% were recorded with angioedema and gastrointestinal symptoms after food challenge. Forty percent of patients suffered from more than a single clinical manifestation and two of those experienced anaphylaxis. Patients with gastrointestinal symptoms, angioedema, and/or anaphylactic symptoms were usually sensitized to both Gal d 1 and Gal d 2. Apart from that, we did not observe any correlation between clinical symptoms and sensitization to distinct allergens. A single patient experienced local oral allergy syndrome, 4 patients displayed airway symptoms, and conjunctivitis was reported by 3 patients.

Eggs of ancient chicken breeds display lower egg white to yolk weight ratios

Weights and pH values of eggs from Araucana, Maran, and laying hen hybrid chicken were determined in the laboratory

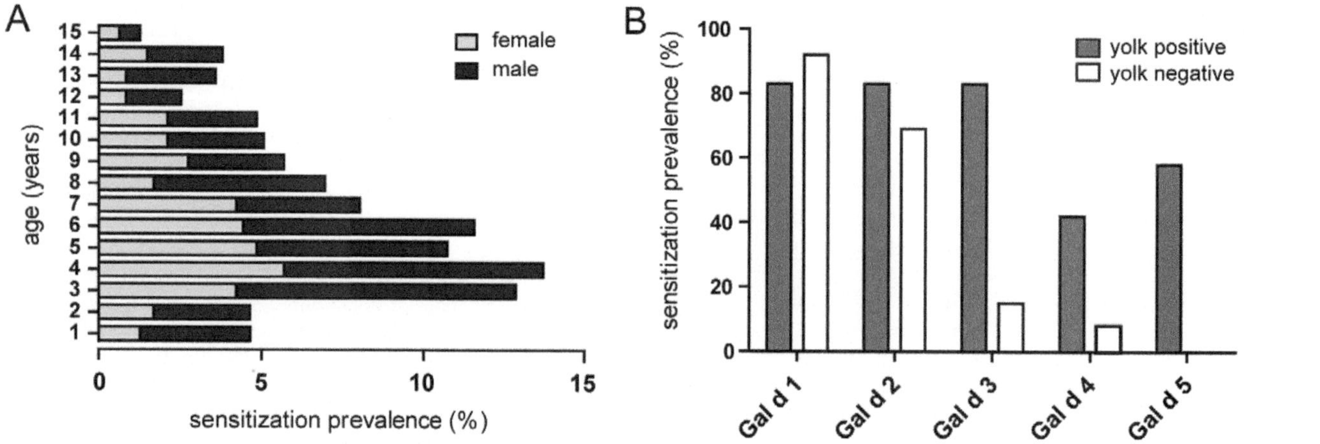

Figure 1. Age distribution and sensitization profile to hen's egg allergens. (A) Egg sensitized subjects (n = 474) were clustered according to age (1–15 years) and gender. (B) Sensitization prevalence to Gal d 1-5 of allergic patients reactive to egg white and yolk (P1–12) and those sensitized to egg white only (P13–25) are presented in grey (yolk positive) and white bars (yolk negative), respectively.

Table 1. Demographics and immunological characterization of hen's egg allergic patients.

Patient			SPT	ELISA				Symptoms recorded after DBPCFC	Reported Symptoms	ISAC				
#	gender	age		W	W^d	Y	Y^d			Gal d 1	Gal d 2	Gal d 3	Gal d 4	Gal d 5
1	m	10	19.3	6.92	4.54	5.57	5.61	AD, UR, AE	AD	5.28	5.58	4.65	7.31	10.18
2	m	11	43.1	1.20	1.40	1.39	1.48	AD, UR	AD	1.16	1.42	-	2.26	1.04
3	m	7	38.7	6.33	4.91	3.29	3.22	n.p.	GI, UR, AE, CO, RH, AS, AN	4.26	1.49	3.44	-	10.50
4	m	5	24.3	9.31	8.89	3.84	4.02	AD, GI	AD, GI	13.08	5.30	12.80	-	1.02
5	m	1	24.2	1.31	0.60	0.61	0.66	AD, UR	AD	2.81	2.73	6.48	4.09	-
6	m	7	22.4	1.98	1.61	0.33	0.53	n.p.	GI, UR, AE	26.50	9.38	5.34	1.82	-
7	m	3	17.3	1.40	-	0.60	0.51	AD, UR, AE	AD	-	1.35	3.93	-	0.64
8	m	9	22.4	4.76	4.84	1.88	2.10	AD, UR	AD	2.63	-	4.46	-	3.56
9	f	13	23.7	9.98	7.08	13.27	11.30	AD, UR	AD	2.73	-	11.69	-	21.28
10	m	4	24.1	2.35	2.72	0.67	0.73	AD, UR, AE	AD	2.40	4.02	1.14	-	-
11	m	7	21.5	7.36	5.00	3.16	3.46	GI	GI	2.47	1.68	1.25	-	-
12	m	4	15.8	0.63	0.71	0.45	0.39	UR	UR	-	1.62	-	0.83	-
13	f	7	14.9	0.91	0.77	-	-	AD, UR	AD	0.87	1.58	-	1.22	-
14	m	9	23.2	0.61	0.31	-	-	AD, GI	AD, GI	1.94	0.92	1.73	-	-
15	m	4	47.2	1.16	1.22	-	-	AD, UR	AD, UR	4.58	1.10	0.26	-	-
16	m	4	21.7	1.58	1.54	-	-	n.p.	GI, UR, AE, CO, AN	7.88	1.60	-	-	-
17	f	6	23.7	0.91	0.85	-	-	n.p.	GI, CO, RH, AS	2.50	1.36	-	-	-
18	m	4	26.7	1.02	1.35	-	-	AD, AE, UR	AD	1.11	1.54	-	-	-
19	m	1	45.7	4.64	3.21	-	-	AD, OAS, UR	AD, OAS	5.27	1.37	-	-	-
20	m	5	41.2	3.43	4.03	-	-	AD, GI, UR	AD, GI, UR	6.21	1.15	-	-	-
21	f	1	18.7	0.43	-	-	-	AD, AE	AD	-	0.13	-	-	-
22	m	3	8.1	0.45	0.26	-	-	n.p.	GI, UR	0.93	-	-	-	-
23	m	2	26.4	6.71	7.33	-	-	GI	GI	6.33	-	-	-	-
24	m	4	25.3	1.62	1.54	-	-	UR, AE	UR	5.55	-	-	-	-
25	f	6	27.3	0.76	0.74	-	-	AD, AE, UR	AD	3.07	-	-	-	-
mean	**f = 5 m = 20**	**5.5**	**25.9**	**3.11**	**2.62**	**1.40**	**1.36**	**AD = 16, UR = 15, AE = 7, GI = 5, OAS = 1**	**AD = 16, GI = 10, UR = 8, AE = 3, CO = 3, RH = 2, AS = 2, AN = 2,**	**4.38**	**1.81**	**2.38**	**0.79**	**2.01**

SPT were performed with commercially available egg white extracts and are presented as wheel area (mm^2). Specific IgE antibodies were measured by ELISA with coated native egg white (W), denatured egg white (W^d), native yolk (Y), and denatured yolk (Y^d) extracts; results are expressed as specific IgE concentrations in µg/ml. IgE reactivity to *Gallus domesticus* allergens were determined by microarray using Immuno solid-phase allergen chips (ISAC) and given in as kU$_A$/l. DBPCFC, double blind placebo controlled food challenge; AD, atopic dermatitis; AE, angioedema; AN, anaphylaxis; AS, asthma; CO, conjunctivitis; GI, gastrointestinal symptoms (including vomiting, diarrhea, and pain); n.p., not performed; OAS, oral allergy syndrome; RH, rhinitis; UR, generalized urticaria.

(Table 2). No significant differences in the pH of egg white and yolk fractions could be observed among different eggs. Noteworthy, eggs from chicken breeds with increased laying performance produced heavier eggs, a circumstance that is desired by food industry and deliberately created by the breeder. Eggs from laying hen hybrids primarily feature comparatively enlarged egg white and reduced yolk fractions. Average weight ratios of egg white/yolk were significantly different ($P<0.001$) constituting 1.7 and 2.4 for ancient chicken breeds and modern laying hens, respectively.

Eggs of different chicken breeds do not differ in their allergen composition

Egg white and yolk extracts from Araucana, Maran, and modern laying hen hybrids displayed similar protein composition and IgE-reactivity patterns as revealed by gel electrophoresis and IgE immunoblot analysis (Figure 2). Mass-spectrometry based identification of IgE-reactive bands demonstrated the presence of Gal d 1–4 in the egg white fractions from eggs of the three chicken breeds investigated. Noteworthy, we obtained only a single tryptic peptide derived from Gal d 1, presumably due to its enormous protein stability [25]. In the yolk fraction, Gal d 3, Gal d 5, and Gal d 6 were detected, and apart from the officially registered allergens, apolipoproteins were revealed as IgE-binding proteins.

Thermal treatment of egg white and yolk has no significant influence on IgE reactivity

ELISA experiments showed that thermal denaturation had only a minor impact on the IgE reactivity of egg extracts (Figure 3). No significant difference was observed between specific IgE concentrations

Table 2. Characteristics of ancient and modern hybrid chicken breeds.

Property of breed	Araucana	Maran	Laying hen hybrid
Age	before 1500	late 1800s	since the 1950s
Origin	Chile	France	USA
Laying performance	~180 per year	~200 per year	~320 per year
Egg shell color	green-white	dark brown	brown
Whole egg weight*	51.9±3.6 g	59.8±3.4 g	60.5±3.2 g
Egg white weight*	28.9±2.7 g	32.0±3.4 g	37.0±2.1 g
Yolk weight*	16.5±1.1 g	18.5±1.6 g	15.4±1.5 g
Ratio egg white/yolk (w/w)*	1.7±0.1	1.7±0.3	2.4±0.2
pH egg white	9.0	9.0	9.0
pH yolk	5.5	5.0	5.5

*Weights were determined and arithmetic means and standard deviations were calculated from 10 individual eggs.

to raw and heat treated egg white and to raw and thermally treated yolk of all eggs investigated. However, heat treatment abolished IgE reactivity to egg white extracts in 2 patients (patient 7 and 21), which were both negative for Gal d 1 (Table 1).

Eggs of different chicken breeds display comparable IgE binding and biological activity

ELISA experiments revealed similar levels of IgE reactivity of eggs from different breeds (Figure 3). Mean egg white-specific IgE titers were 3.09 μg/ml (Araucana), 3.17 μg/ml (Maran), and 3.11 μg/ml (laying hen hybrids); mean yolk-specific IgE titers 3.18 μg/ml (Araucana), 2.98 μg/ml (Maran), and 2.92 μg/ml (laying hen hybrids). Using the Wilcoxon signed rank test, we observed a difference for the IgE reactivity to egg yolk from Auraucana hen, which was evoked by 5/12 patients who demonstrated higher IgE values towards this breed. Similar IgE binding activities were reflected by a comparable mediator release capacity, with a slightly higher allergenic potential of egg yolk from Auraucana chicken (Figure 4). Highest degranulation values were observed at concentrations of 10 to 100 μg/ml for egg white and 100 to 10,000 μg/ml for yolk extracts. Thus, egg white seems to trigger a 100-fold stronger mediator release.

Discussion

Although in the majority of cases outgrown before school age, egg allergy can drastically decrease life quality due to the omnipresence of egg containing food products. Avoidance is usually difficult and implies broad dietary restrictions [7,17,18]. However, strongly limited diets are frequently unnecessary and even unfavorable for the patient [26]. For proper patient

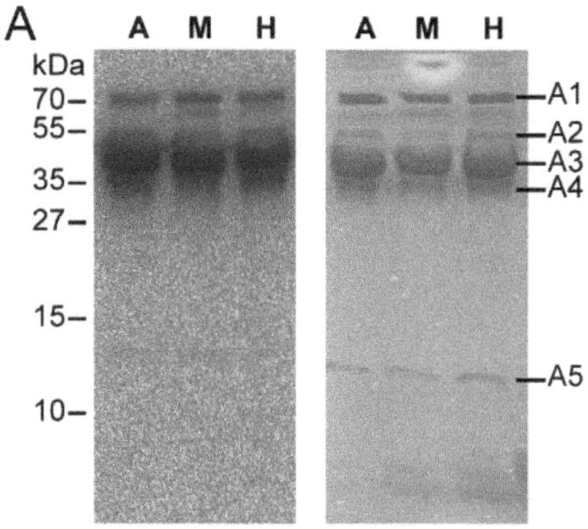

Band	Protein name	Allergen Name	MW [kDa]	SwissProt/TrEMBL
A1	Ovotransferrin	Gal d 3	77.8	Q4ADJ7
			77.8	P02789
			77.7	Q4ADJ6
A2	Ovalbumin	Gal d 2	43.8	P01014
			42.9	P01012
A3	Ovalbumin	Gal d 2	42.9	P01012
A4	Ovomucoid	Gal d 1	22.6	P01005
A5	Lysozyme	Gal d 4	16.2	B8YK79
			16.2	P00698
			14.3	P49663

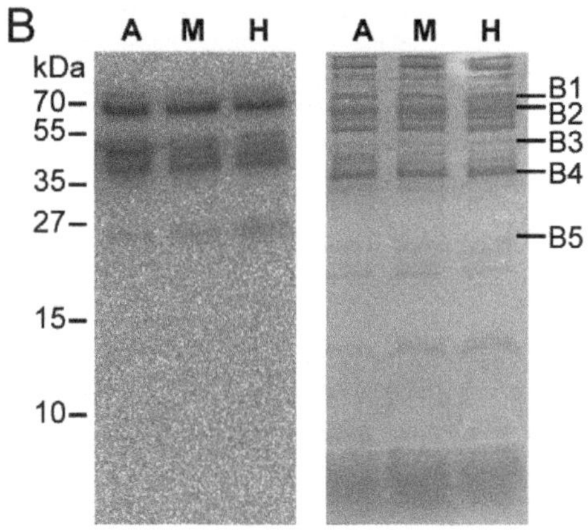

Band	Protein name	Allergen Name	MW [kDa]	SwissProt/TrEMBL
B1	Ovotransferrin	Gal d 3	77.8	Q4ADJ7
			77.7	P02789
B2	Livetin	Gal d 5	69.9	P19121
B3	Livetin	Gal d 5	69.9	P19121
	Apolipoprotein B	-	50.8	P11682
B4	Vitellogenin	Gal d 6	53.4	C35ZZ3
B5	Apolipoprotein A	-	30.6	P08250

Figure 2. Identification of allergenic egg components. IgE-reactive egg white (A) and yolk (B) extract components from Araucana (A), Maran (M), and conventional laying hen hybrid (H) breeds were detected by IgE immunoblotting (left charts). IgE-reactive bands (A1–5 and Y1–5) were excised from polyacrylamide gels (right charts), and subjected to mass spectrometry analysis. Corresponding proteins, their molecular weights (MW), and SwissProt/TrEMBL accession numbers are given in the tables.

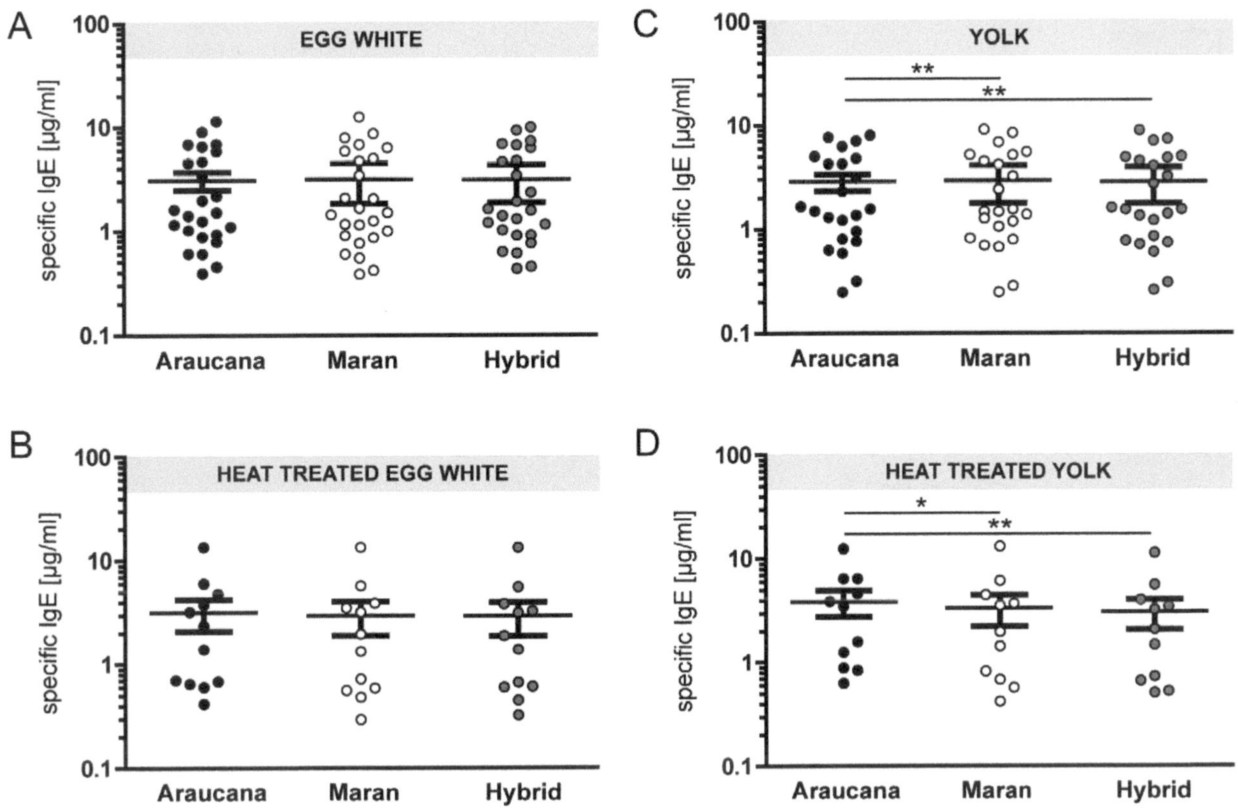

Figure 3. Allergenicity of egg white and yolk from different chicken breeds. Specific IgE levels to native and heat-treated egg white (A and B) and yolk (C and D) from Araucana (black circles), Maran (white circles), and conventional laying hen hybrid breeds (grey circles) were determined by ELISA. Circles represent values obtained from individual patients' sensitized to egg white (n = 25) and yolk (n = 12). Mean values are shown as solid line and whiskers indicate the standard error of the mean. Statistical analysis was performed using the Wilcoxon signed rank test. **<0.01; *<0.02.

management detailed diagnosis including molecule-based approaches [5,27] and/or food challenges [28,29,30] may assist the clinician to provide dietary advice. It is well known, that temperature and food matrix are important aspects determining the allergenicity of food proteins [31]. In this context, our data suggest that half of the children in the present study are likely to tolerate yolk and yolk-containing foodstuff. Moreover, two (8%) of our patients were negative for heated egg white in ELISA and able to consume cooked egg white without problems (Alessandri *et al*, unpublished). On the molecular level, our and recent data [9] clearly indicate that the risk for adverse reactions upon ingestion of cooked eggs is linked to Gal d 1 sensitization. Noteworthy, a previous study showed that more than 50% of egg allergic patients tolerated ingestion of extensively heated egg and continued intake was even beneficial for the patient [32]. Our results evidence that IgE reactivity to Gal d 5 serves as marker for yolk sensitization. Since not all of the yolk sensitized patients reacted to this allergen, other molecules, *e.g.* the recently identified Gal d 6 [11] or apolipoproteins [33], could play a role in yolk allergy.

Although eggs from different birds contain cross-reactive allergens, the development of egg allergy seems to be restricted to distinct avian species [34,35] and thus, some hen's egg allergic patients might tolerate consumption of eggs from duck or goose. Moreover, eggs from different chicken breeds might vary regarding their allergenicity. In fact, diverse apple cultivars have been demonstrated to differ in both, their allergen content and allergenic potential [36,37]. Thus, aboriginal eggs from ancient chicken breeds might be favorable for the allergic patient. Accordingly, we compared the allergenic properties of eggs from conventional laying hen hybrids with those from Araucana and Maran ancient chicken breeds.

We did not find major dissimilarities regarding IgE reactivity or biological activity between eggs from modern and ancient chicken breeds. Noteworthy, egg yolk from Auraucana chicken even showed a slightly elevated allergenic potential. Based on these clear *in vitro* data showing no advantage of eggs from ancient breeds, food challenges with Auraucana and Maran eggs were considered of minor scientific benefit. Moreover, it has previously been shown that continuous egg intake boosts systemic IgE responses in allergic patients [38]. Hence, repeated food challenges would be ethically irresponsible as they bear unnecessary risks for the allergic children. Of note, differences in the nutritional composition of Araucana eggs, *i.e.* higher cholesterol and lower protein content, have been previously shown [39] and might have an impact on predisposed patients. Eggs from ancient breeds varied regarding their significantly decreased egg white/yolk weight ratio. Hence, for a minority of patients decreased exposure to egg white allergens and/or non-allergological factors that were out of scope of this study might deliver a possible explanation for better tolerability. Taken together, the fact that hen's egg allergy was rising in the last century might be explained by environmental factors rather than by consumption of eggs from novel high performance laying hen breeds that were not available in the past.

So which then came first, the chicken or the egg? From the allergological point of view this intriguing question might be answered as follows: Although representing a putative sensitizer in

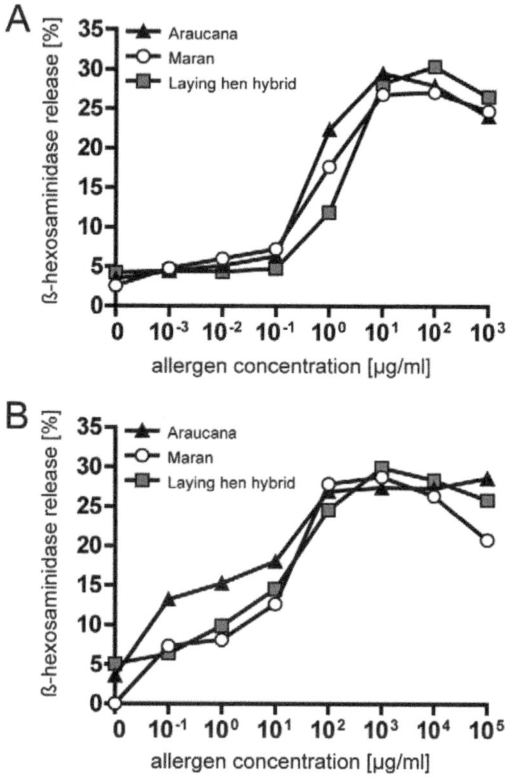

Figure 4. Biological activities of egg white and yolk from different chicken breeds. Transfected RBL-2H3 cells were passively sensitized with a serum pool of 8 patients. Mediator release was triggered with increasing concentrations of egg white (A) and yolk (B) extract.

the "bird-egg syndrome" [14] and more rarely in children with meat allergy [35,40], the chicken *per se* contributes little to primary egg allergy. By contrast, it seems that the egg, and in particular sensitization to egg white proteins, comes first. A picture is emerging in which the development of egg allergy seems to start with sensitization to Gal d 1 and Gal d 2. In the course of disease children raise additional IgE antibodies against other egg white (Gal d 3 and Gal d 4) and finally yolk allergens. This hypothesis is supported by our allergen profiling data and the fact that yolk-negative patients were by trend younger. Although additional yolk sensitization does not seem to cause more severe symptoms, it may worsen life quality because it enlarges dietary restrictions.

In summary, eggs from ancient chicken breeds cannot be considered less allergenic but might be better tolerated by some not severely affected patients due to their smaller egg white fraction. There are strong variations regarding the number and type of egg-containing foods that an individual patient can eat without experiencing adverse reactions. Therefore, detailed and molecule-based diagnosis distinguishing between sensitization to egg white and yolk is essential for improved patient management.

Materials and Methods

Ethics Statement

The study was approved by the Institutional Review Board of Istituto Dermopatico dell'Immacolata – IDI-IRCCS, Rome, Italy (n. 106-CE-2005), and signed informed consents were obtained from legal guardians.

Patients and serology

Sera were obtained from the Center for Molecular Allergology at IDI-IRCCS in Rome, Italy. Egg allergic children were selected according to typical case history and positive skin reactivity. Skin prick tests (SPT) were performed as previously reported [41] and were recorded as wheal areas. Specific IgE levels to Gal d 1–5 were determined using the ISAC 89, VBC-Genomics, Vienna, Austria [42] according to previously reported protocols [24]. Diagnostic and clinical features have been recorded using an electronic allergy health record (InterAll, Allergy Data Laboratories s.c., Latina, Italy).

Double-blind placebo controlled food challenge

Children were admitted to the Clinical Center in a fasting state. Administration of antihistamines, if used, was stopped at least 7 days before provocation test and none of the patients was under steroid treatment. Food challenge was carried out with commercially available raw eggs from hybrid hens in two different days. Eggs were mixed with 50 ml of non-sparkling mineral water plus two teaspoons of cocoa (Cacao Amaro, Perugina, Italy) and one spoon of white sugar (verum). After administration of an initial dose of 0.1 ml, amounts were increased to 1 ml and 10 ml in 30 minute intervals. Residual egg preparations were given until objective symptoms developed or until the equivalent of one egg was ingested.

Egg characterization and sample preparation

Eggs from ancient chicken breeds, *i.e.* Araucana and Maran, were obtained from the Hölzl poultry hatchery in Moosburg, Germany. Medium-sized eggs from conventional laying hen hybrids were purchased at the local grocery. Average weights from whole egg, egg white, and yolk, as well as egg white to yolk weight ratios were determined for 10 individual eggs from each chicken breed. Moreover, pH values of egg white and yolk fractions were measured with Whatman pH indicator stripes. For preparations of allergen extracts, 3 ml samples of yolk and egg white fractions were taken from 10 individual cracked eggs. To avoid egg white contaminations, yolks were gently punctured with a syringe and samples were taken carefully. Pooled samples were extracted overnight at 4°C in PBS pH 7.4 containing 2% polyvinylpyrrolidone, 2 mM phenylmethanesulfonylfluoride, 2 mM benzamidine, and 2 mM ethylenediaminetetraacetic acid at a concentration of 1 g/ml. After centrifugation at 21,000 g and 4°C for 30 min, samples were sonicated, and filtered through a 0.45 µm filter unit (Millipore, Bedford, MA, USA). Protein concentrations were determined by the method of Bradford, and egg extracts were stored at 4°C.

Gel electrophoresis and IgE immunoblotting

Egg white and yolk extracts were separated by SDS-PAGE under reducing conditions and stained with GelCode® Blue Reagent (Thermo Scientific, Waltham, MA). For immunoblots, extracts were separated by gel electrophoresis and electroblotted onto nitrocellulose Protan membranes (Schleicher & Schuell, Dassel, Germany). After blocking unspecific binding sites with 25 mM Tris HCl, pH 7.5, 0.5% bovine serum albumin (w/v), 150 mM NaCl, and 0.05% Tween 20 (v/v), membranes were incubated with a serum pool ($n = 25$) diluted 1:10 in the blocking buffer. Bound IgE was detected using ^{125}I-labelled anti human IgE (BSM Diagnostika, Vienna, Austria). Radiographic signals were visualized by overnight exposure to imaging plates and subsequent evaluation using a BAS-1800II Phosphor Imager scanner (Fuji Film, Tokyo, Japan).

Mass-spectrometry based allergen identification

IgE-reactive bands were excised from polyacrylamide gels and subjected to in gel digestion using the ProteoExtract All-In-One Trypsin Digestion Kit (Calbiochem, Gibbston, NJ). Tryptic peptides were separated by capillary reversed phase high pressure liquid chromatography (rpHPLC) directly coupled to a Quadrupole-Time of Flight mass spectrometer (QTof Ultima Global, Waters, Milford, MA) equipped with a Nanoflow spray head. Obtained mass data were processed and analyzed using the software Protein Lynx Global Server version 2.2.5 (Waters, Milford, MA) and evaluated using the SwissProt/TrEMBL database.

Enzyme-linked immunosorbent assay

Maxisorp plates (Nalge Nunc, Rochester, NY) were coated with 250 ng of egg extracts in PBS pH 7.4 overnight at 4°C. To assess IgE reactivity to heat-denatured egg allergens, egg extracts were incubated for 15 minutes at 95°C before use. After blocking unspecific binding sites with Tris-buffered saline pH 7.4, 1% bovine serum albumin (w/v), and 0.05% Tween 20 (v/v), coated antigen was incubated with patient's sera overnight at 4°C. Bound IgE was detected with an alkaline phosphatase-conjugated monoclonal anti human IgE antibody (BD Biosciences, Franklin Lakes, NJ). Specific serum IgE levels were calculated based on a semi-quantitative ELISA using purified human IgE (Serotec, Raleigh, NC) as internal standard.

Mediator release assays

Rat basophil degranulation assays were performed as previously described [43]. Briefly, rat basophil leukemia (RBL)-2H3 cells transfected with the human high-affinity IgE receptor were passively sensitized with a serum pool from egg allergic patients ($n = 8$) reacting to both egg white and yolk. Basophil degranulation was triggered by addition of serial protein dilutions, and β-hexosaminidase release was measured by enzymatic cleavage of the fluorogenic substrate 4-methyl umbelliferyl-N-acteyl-β-glucosaminide (Sigma, St. Louis, MO). Results are expressed as percentage of total enzyme content of Triton X100-treated cells.

Statistical analyses

Statistical evaluation of paired samples was performed using the Wilcoxon signed rank test; Mann-Whitney rank sum test and *t*-test were used for non-paired samples. A value of $P<0.02$ was considered statistically significant.

Acknowledgments

We thank the Hölzl poultry hatchery, Moosburg, Germany and Toni's Freilandeier, Knittelfeld, Austria for providing eggs.

Author Contributions

Conceived and designed the experiments: GG ME FF AM. Performed the experiments: ME CA MW PB DZ. Analyzed the data: ME GG. Contributed reagents/materials/analysis tools: AM CA DZ. Wrote the paper: GG ME FF.

References

1. Osterballe M, Mortz CG, Hansen TK, Andersen KE, Bindslev-Jensen C (2009) The prevalence of food hypersensitivity in young adults. Pediatr Allergy Immunol 20: 686–692.
2. Osterballe M, Hansen TK, Mortz CG, Host A, Bindslev-Jensen C (2005) The prevalence of food hypersensitivity in an unselected population of children and adults. Pediatr Allergy Immunol 16: 567–573.
3. Sicherer SH, Sampson HA (2006) 9. Food allergy. J Allergy Clin Immunol 117: S470–475.
4. Zuidmeer L (2011) You Can't Unscramble an Egg. Or Can You? Int Arch Allergy Immunol 154: 1–2.
5. Everberg H, Brostedt P, Oman H, Bohman S, Moverare R (2011) Affinity Purification of Egg-White Allergens for Improved Component-Resolved Diagnostics. Int Arch Allergy Immunol 154: 33–41.
6. Jacobsen B, Hoffmann-Sommergruber K, Have TT, Foss N, Briza P, et al. (2008) The panel of egg allergens, Gal d 1–Gal d 5: Their improved purification and characterization. Mol Nutr Food Res 52 Suppl 2: S176–185.
7. Mine Y, Yang M (2008) Recent advances in the understanding of egg allergens: basic, industrial, and clinical perspectives. J Agric Food Chem 56: 4874–4900.
8. Matsuda T, Watanabe K, Nakamura R (1983) Immunochemical and physical properties of peptic-digested ovomucoid. J Agric Food Chem 31: 942–946.
9. Urisu A, Ando H, Morita Y, Wada E, Yasaki T, et al. (1997) Allergenic activity of heated and ovomucoid-depleted egg white. J Allergy Clin Immunol 100: 171–176.
10. Takagi K, Teshima R, Okunuki H, Sawada J (2003) Comparative study of in vitro digestibility of food proteins and effect of preheating on the digestion. Biol Pharm Bull 26: 969–973.
11. Amo A, Rodriguez-Perez R, Blanco J, Villota J, Juste S, et al. (2010) Gal d 6 is the second allergen characterized from egg yolk. J Agric Food Chem 58: 7453–7457.
12. Escudero C, Quirce S, Fernandez-Nieto M, Miguel J, Cuesta J, et al. (2003) Egg white proteins as inhalant allergens associated with baker's asthma. Allergy 58: 616–620.
13. Quirce S, Diez-Gomez ML, Eiras P, Cuevas M, Baz G, et al. (1998) Inhalant allergy to egg yolk and egg white proteins. Clin Exp Allergy 28: 478–485.
14. Nevot Falco S, Casas Ramisa R, Lleonart Bellfill R (2003) [Bird-egg syndrome in children]. Allergol Immunopathol (Madr) 31: 161–165.
15. Quirce S, Maranon F, Umpierrez A, de las Heras M, Fernandez-Caldas E, et al. (2001) Chicken serum albumin (Gal d 5*) is a partially heat-labile inhalant and food allergen implicated in the bird-egg syndrome. Allergy 56: 754–762.
16. Szepfalusi Z, Ebner C, Pandjaitan R, Orlicek F, Scheiner O, et al. (1994) Egg yolk alpha-livetin (chicken serum albumin) is a cross-reactive allergen in the bird-egg syndrome. J Allergy Clin Immunol 93: 932–942.
17. Allen CW, Campbell DE, Kemp AS (2007) Egg allergy: are all childhood food allergies the same? J Paediatr Child Health 43: 214–218.
18. Allen CW, Kemp AS, Campbell DE (2009) Dietary advice, dietary adherence and the acquisition of tolerance in egg-allergic children: a 5-yr follow-up. Pediatr Allergy Immunol 20: 213–218.
19. Guerrero L, Guardia MD, Xicola J, Verbeke W, Vanhonacker F, et al. (2009) Consumer-driven definition of traditional food products and innovation in traditional foods. A qualitative cross-cultural study. Appetite 52: 345–354.
20. Hjelmar U (2010) Consumers' purchase of organic food products: A matter of convenience and reflexive practices. Appetite.
21. Pieniak Z, Verbeke W, Vanhonacker F, Guerrero L, Hersleth M (2009) Association between traditional food consumption and motives for food choice in six European countries. Appetite 53: 101–108.
22. Ekarius C Storey's Illustrated Guide to Poultry Breeds: Storey Pub.
23. Cochrane S, Beyer K, Clausen M, Wjst M, Hiller R, et al. (2009) Factors influencing the incidence and prevalence of food allergy. Allergy 64: 1246–1255.
24. Scala E, Alessandri C, Bernardi ML, Ferrara R, Palazzo P, et al. (2010) Cross-sectional survey on immunoglobulin E reactivity in 23,077 subjects using an allergenic molecule-based microarray detection system. Clin Exp Allergy 40: 911–921.
25. Lee JY, Kim CJ (2010) Determination of allergenic egg proteins in food by protein-, mass spectrometry-, and DNA-based methods. J AOAC Int 93: 462–477.
26. Kim JS, Sicherer S (2010) Should avoidance of foods be strict in prevention and treatment of food allergy? Curr Opin Allergy Clin Immunol 10: 252–257.
27. D'Urbano LE, Pellegrino K, Artesani MC, Donnanno S, Luciano R, et al. (2010) Performance of a component-based allergen-microarray in the diagnosis of cow's milk and hen's egg allergy. Clin Exp Allergy 40: 1561–1570.
28. Kemp AS, Allen CW, Campbell DE (2009) Parental perceptions in egg allergy: does egg challenge make a difference? Pediatr Allergy Immunol 20: 648–653.
29. Waring G, Levy D (2010) Challenging adverse reactions in children with food allergies. Paediatr Nurs 22: 16–22.
30. Ahrens B, Lopes de Oliveira LC, Schulz G, Borres MP, Niggemann B, et al. (2010) The role of hen's egg-specific IgE, IgG and IgG4 in the diagnostic procedure of hen's egg allergy. Allergy 65: 1554–1557.
31. Nowak-Wegrzyn A, Fiocchi A (2009) Rare, medium, or well done? The effect of heating and food matrix on food protein allergenicity. Curr Opin Allergy Clin Immunol 9: 234–237.
32. Lemon-Mule H, Sampson HA, Sicherer SH, Shreffler WG, Noone S, et al. (2008) Immunologic changes in children with egg allergy ingesting extensively heated egg. J Allergy Clin Immunol 122: 977–983 e971.
33. Walsh BJ, Barnett D, Burley RW, Elliott C, Hill DJ, et al. (1988) New allergens from hen's egg white and egg yolk. In vitro study of ovomucin, apovitellenin I and VI, and phosvitin. Int Arch Allergy Appl Immunol 87: 81–86.
34. Anibarro B, Seoane FJ, Vila C, Lombardero M (2000) Allergy to eggs from duck and goose without sensitization to hen egg proteins. J Allergy Clin Immunol 105: 834–836.

35. Langeland T (1983) A clinical and immunological study of allergy to hen's egg white. VI. Occurrence of proteins cross-reacting with allergens in hen's egg white as studied in egg white from turkey, duck, goose, seagull, and in hen egg yolk, and hen and chicken sera and flesh. Allergy 38: 399–412.
36. Matthes A, Schmitz-Eiberger M (2009) Apple (Malus domestica L. Borkh.) allergen Mal d 1: effect of cultivar, cultivation system, and storage conditions. J Agric Food Chem 57: 10548–10553.
37. Vlieg-Boerstra BJ, Van De Weg WE, Van Der Heide S, Kerkhof M, Arens P, et al. (2010) Identification of low allergenic apple cultivars using skin prick tests and oral food challenges. Allergy.
38. Reininger R, Exner H, Kuderna C, Rumpold H, Balic N, et al. (2003) Possible modes of allergen-specific sensitization and boosting in an atopic child. Int Arch Allergy Immunol 130: 275–279.
39. Millet S, De Ceulaer K, Van Paemel M, Raes K, De Smet S, et al. (2006) Lipid profile in eggs of Araucana hens compared with Lohmann Selected Leghorn and ISA Brown hens given diets with different fat sources. Br Poult Sci 47: 294–300.
40. Martinez Alonso JC, Dominguez Ortega FJ, Fuentes Gonzalo MJ (2003) [Angioedema due to sensitization to chicken meat]. Allergol Immunopathol (Madr) 31: 50–52.
41. Bernardi ML, Picone D, Tuppo L, Giangrieco I, Petrella G, et al. (2010) Physico-chemical features of the environment affect the protein conformation and the immunoglobulin E reactivity of kiwellin (Act d 5). Clin Exp Allergy.
42. Harwanegg C, Hiller R (2005) Protein microarrays for the diagnosis of allergic diseases: state-of-the-art and future development. Clin Chem Lab Med 43: 1321–1326.
43. Vogel L, Luttkopf D, Hatahet L, Haustein D, Vieths S (2005) Development of a functional in vitro assay as a novel tool for the standardization of allergen extracts in the human system. Allergy 60: 1021–1028.

2

Genetic Variations in *IL28B* and Allergic Disease in Children

Silvana Gaudieri[1,2,3]*[¶], Michaela Lucas[3,4¶], Andrew Lucas[3], Elizabeth McKinnon[3], Hiba Albloushi[2], Andri Rauch[5], Julia di Iulio[6], David Martino[7], Susan L. Prescott[7], Meri K. Tulic[7]

1 School of Anatomy and Human Biology, University of Western Australia, Nedlands, Australia, **2** Centre for Forensic Science, University of Western Australia, Nedlands, Australia, **3** Institute for Immunology and Infectious Diseases, Murdoch University, Murdoch, Australia, **4** PathWest and Laboratory Medicine, University of Western Australia, Nedlands, Australia, **5** University Clinic of Infectious Diseases, University Hospital Bern and University of Bern, Bern, Switzerland, **6** Institute of Microbiology, University Hospital Centre and University of Lausanne, Lausanne, Switzerland, **7** School of Paediatrics and Child Health, University of Western Australia, Nedlands, Australia

Abstract

Environmental changes affecting the relationship between the developing immune system and microbial exposure have been implicated in the epidemic rise of allergic disease in developed countries. While early developmental differences in T cell function are well-recognised, there is now emerging evidence that this is related to developmental differences in innate immune function. In this study we sought to examine if differences associated with innate immunity contribute to the altered immune programming recognised in allergic children. Here, we describe for the first time, the association of carriage of the T allele of the tagging single nucleotide polymorphism rs12979860 3 kb upstream of *IL28B*, encoding the potent innate immune modulator type III interferon lambda (IFN-λ3), and allergy in children ($p = 0.004$; OR 4.56). Strikingly, the association between rs12979860 genotype and allergic disease is enhanced in girls. Furthermore, carriage of the T allele at rs12979860 correlates with differences in the pro-inflammatory profile during the first five years of life suggesting this contributes to the key differences in subsequent innate immune development in children who develop allergic disease. In the context of rising rates of disease, these immunologic differences already present at birth imply very early interaction between genetic predisposition and prenatal environmental influences.

Editor: Alan Landay, Rush University, United States of America

Funding: MKT is supported by an NHMRC Career Development Award and SLP is supported by NHMRC Practitioner Fellowship. ML has been funded from a Raine Medical Research Foundation Priming Grant. The funders had no role in study design, data collection and analysis, decision to publish, or preparation of the manuscript.

Competing Interests: The authors have declared that no competing interests exist.

* E-mail: silvana.gaudieri@uwa.edu.au

¶ These authors contributed equally to this work.

Introduction

The threat of premature death caused by infectious diseases in developed countries has largely past since the widespread introduction of antibiotics and improved standards of personal cleanliness, yet paradoxically contemporary communities are now beset by a dramatic increase in the burden of chronic inflammatory diseases. This clearly highlights the susceptibility of the immune system to modern environmental changes [1]. Not only allergic conditions such as asthma, allergic rhinoconjunctivitis, food allergies and eczema are on the rise but autoimmune disorders (such as type 1 diabetes and chronic inflammatory bowel disease) as well as neurodegenerative and cardiovascular diseases [1], are now following the same alarming trends [2]. While complex lifestyle changes are driving this surge in disease, genetic factors are critically important in determining the susceptibility to environmental changes that can enhance inflammatory responses, and the predisposition to these diverse inflammatory diseases [1]. Furthermore, the rising rates of allergic disease in infancy clearly indicates that early gene-environment interactions, even before birth, play an important role in determining susceptibility to inflammation and immune disease [3].

Prospective longitudinal case-control comparisons of immune development in well-characterized children provide opportunities to assess development of innate inflammatory responses in relationship to genetic and clinical phenotype. Using this approach, our initial studies [4,5] revealed striking differences in the biological responses (to microbial products) of children who develop allergic disease. These children show increased inflammatory (IL-6, IL-1β and TNFα) cytokine production at birth and during their neonatal period, compared to children that remain non-allergic [4,5] and this is associated with subsequent propensity for allergic Type 2 adaptive responses [5]. Plasmacytoid dendritic cells (pDC) from these allergic children express high levels of bacterial recognition receptor, toll like receptor (TLR)2, during their first year of life compared to non-allergic controls [5]. In the children with allergy high expression of $TLR2^{+}$ on pDCs was strongly associated with a distinct innate immune response and allergic disease phenotype.

This new evidence that susceptibility to allergy may be associated with an altered innate immune development from birth prompts more detailed examination of underlying candidate pathways. Given clues that pDC function, which is pivotal in translating distinct innate stimuli into robust type I and III interferon (IFN) production, is affected in allergic children, we hypothesised that an alteration in the biology of type I and/or type III IFN might also be affected.

The newly discovered type III IFN family is composed of three closely related molecules in humans: IFN-λ1 (IL29), IFN-λ2 (IL28A), and IFN-λ3 (IL28B) that exhibit anti-viral activity [6] *via* a similar but likely independent mechanism to type I IFNs. These molecules are likely to have an immunomodulatory function as studies have shown that IFN-λ1-treated human DCs can induce proliferation of suppressor T cells [7], inhibit *in vitro* naïve and memory IL-13 responses in human T cells [8,9], augment antigen-specific IFNγ release [10], and upregulate TLR expression and their response to ligands [11]. Support for the role of IFN-λ in allergic disease can be extrapolated from relatively few studies that have examined their role in allergic asthma. Contoli and colleagues have shown that deficient IFN-λ induction (IFN-λ1 and IFN-λ2/3) by viral (rhinovirus) and bacterial (lipopolysaccharide) stimuli was associated with severity of asthma exacerbations in allergic asthmatics [12]. A recent study clearly demonstrated that IFN-λ2 can effectively induce type 1 immunity and suppresses Th2 immunity and consequently allergic airway disease in a mouse model of allergic asthma *via* its action on DCs [13].

Furthermore, genetic variations in *IL28B* (IFN-λ3) have been linked with differential expression of interferon-stimulated genes (ISG) in patients with chronic Hepatitis C [14,15] and with their outcome of IFN-α therapy [16,17]. Although the IFN-λ family comprises of the three related members, IFN-λ3 is to date the only member with genetic variations associated with differential expression profiles for downstream genes involved in the immune response and outcome for a disease that exhibits symptoms of dysregulation of the immune response. Accordingly, in this study we set to examine the relationship between *IL28B* genetic variation and allergic disease in children.

Results

Genetic variation at the tagging SNP rs12979680 3 kb upstream of *IL28B* is associated with risk of allergic disease

We present data showing support for *IL28B* playing a role in allergic disease. We genotyped 70 children (35 allergic and 35 non-allergic; Cohort 1) for the tagging SNP rs12979860 that resides 3 kb upstream of *IL28B*. Carriage of the T allele at rs12979860 has previously been shown to be highly predictive of poor Hepatitis C virus (HCV) infection and treatment outcome [16–19]. Here, presence of the T allele at rs12979860 was over-represented in children with allergic disease ($p = 0.004$; OR = 4.56, CI 1.7–12.6) (Fig. 1a). Although the frequency of the C allele was lower in allergic children compared to non-allergic children (0.6 vs 0.8, respectively) the strongest predictor of allergic disease was carriage of the T allele. The odds ratio obtained for this relationship (OR = 4.6) is akin to what was observed in a recent study examining the relationship between *IL28B* and HCV infection outcome in a single source cohort of similar size (OR = 4.1) (Fig. 1b). The single source cohort comprises women who were exposed to HCV contaminated immunoglobulin D in Ireland in the 1970s and inherently controls for ascertainment bias, clinical, demographic and viral factors that allow the optimal platform to assess the *IL28B* genetic contribution to HCV outcome. In studies that cannot account for these factors, the odds ratios obtained for the association of *IL28B* variants and HCV outcome are much lower (OR = 3.0 vs OR 4.1 and 7.4) [20]. In this study, the strict criteria used to assess allergic and non-allergic (non-atopic) children removed several confounding factors that allowed a better assessment of host genetic contribution to allergic disease. As sensitisation against environmental allergens in the Australian population is highly prevalent, the criteria used to select non-allergic children is critical and in this cohort selection for non-atopic children was based on an extensive array of clinical tests over the first five years of life; a critical period of immune ontogeny. Conservative assessment of the phenotype definition can offset the value of larger sample size in disease gene association studies [21]. Accordingly, the robust relationship we find between *IL28B* and allergic disease in a relatively small sample size suggests that *IL28B* (and effects on IFNλ-3 levels) is likely to play a dominant role in the susceptibility and development of allergic disease. These results are comparable to what has been reported for HCV infection and treatment outcome in which it is well established that *IL28B* variants are the strongest host genetic contributor to HCV outcome.

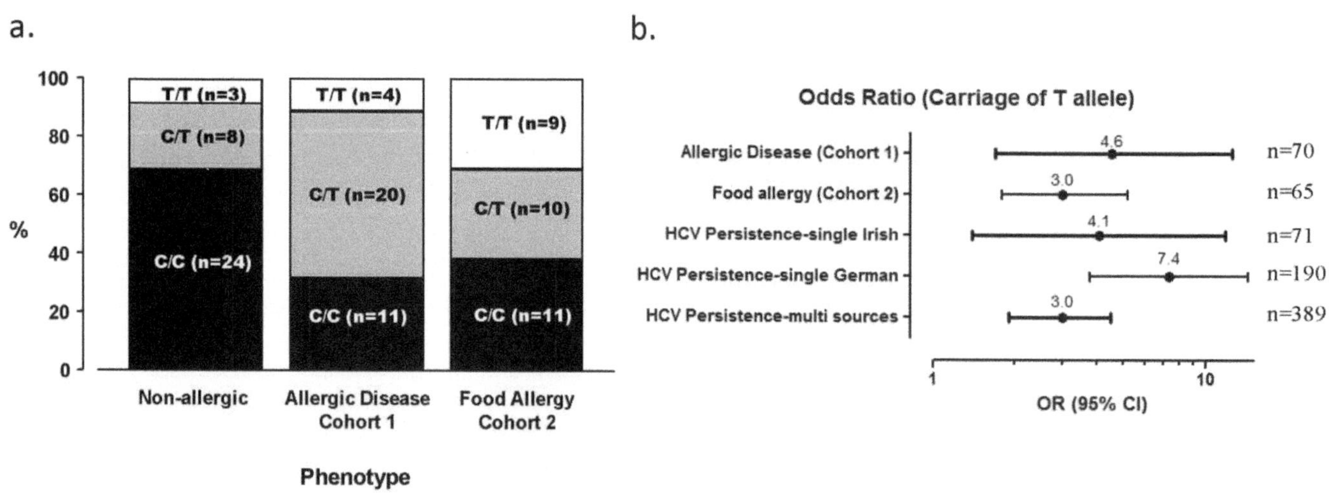

Figure 1. Variation at tagging SNP rs12979860 confers risk for allergic disease. a. Carriage of the T allele of rs12979860 is over-represented in children with allergic disease (cohort 1, n = 70) ($p = 0.004$). This relationship is also observed for children with IgE-mediated food allergy (Cohort 2, n = 60) ($p = 0.04$ dominant model). For both cohorts, the frequency of the different genotypes varies between disease and control subjects ($p = 0.02$; cohort 1 and cohort 2). **b.** Odds ratio (OR; 95% CI) for carriage of T allele of rs12979860 and allergic disease and for HCV persistence. Odds ratio values for HCV cohorts are from di Iulio et al [20] and Tillman et al [28]. ORs for allergic disease and food allergy adjusted for gender. ORs for HCV cohorts adjusted for HBV co-infection in all cohorts and gender in the multiple source cohort.

Association between rs12979860 genotype and food allergy: Validation of genetic association in food allergic cohort

We then extended our analysis between allergic phenotype and carriage of the T allele at rs12979860 to a second paediatric cohort (n = 30; Cohort 2) in which subjects were defined as clinically food allergic. These subjects were recruited from the same clinic and therefore have similar demographic characteristics as Cohort 1. When we compared these subjects to the screened non-allergic subjects (controls) as described above we found that carriage of the T allele at rs12979860 is also associated with food allergy (p = 0.04; OR = 3.0, CI 1.8–5.2) (Fig. 1b). Interestingly for Cohort 2 but not Cohort 1, the frequency of the homozygote T/T genotype was higher than observed in the non-allergic children (Fig. 1a). Accordingly, all subsequent analyses performed on Cohort 1 examined the influence of carriage of the T "risk" allele.

Association of rs12979860 genotype with allergic disease increases with age

In order to assess the impact of *IL28B* on early allergic phenotype, we examined the association of rs12979860 genotype with allergic outcome during early childhood using subjects in Cohort 1, as detailed clinical data on these subjects had been collected from follow-up visits during the first five years of life. There is a clear association between carriage of the T allele of rs12979860 and development of early allergic disease, particularly for sensitization against environmental antigens and IgE-mediated food allergy (Fig. 2). In the case of atopic dermatitis, there is a trend for discrimination between the rs12979860 genotype during the first year of life and this becomes significant from 2.5 years of age (Fig. 2). Clear diagnosis of asthma cannot be determined during the first year of life however carriage of the T allele is significantly associated with asthma diagnosis by age 5.

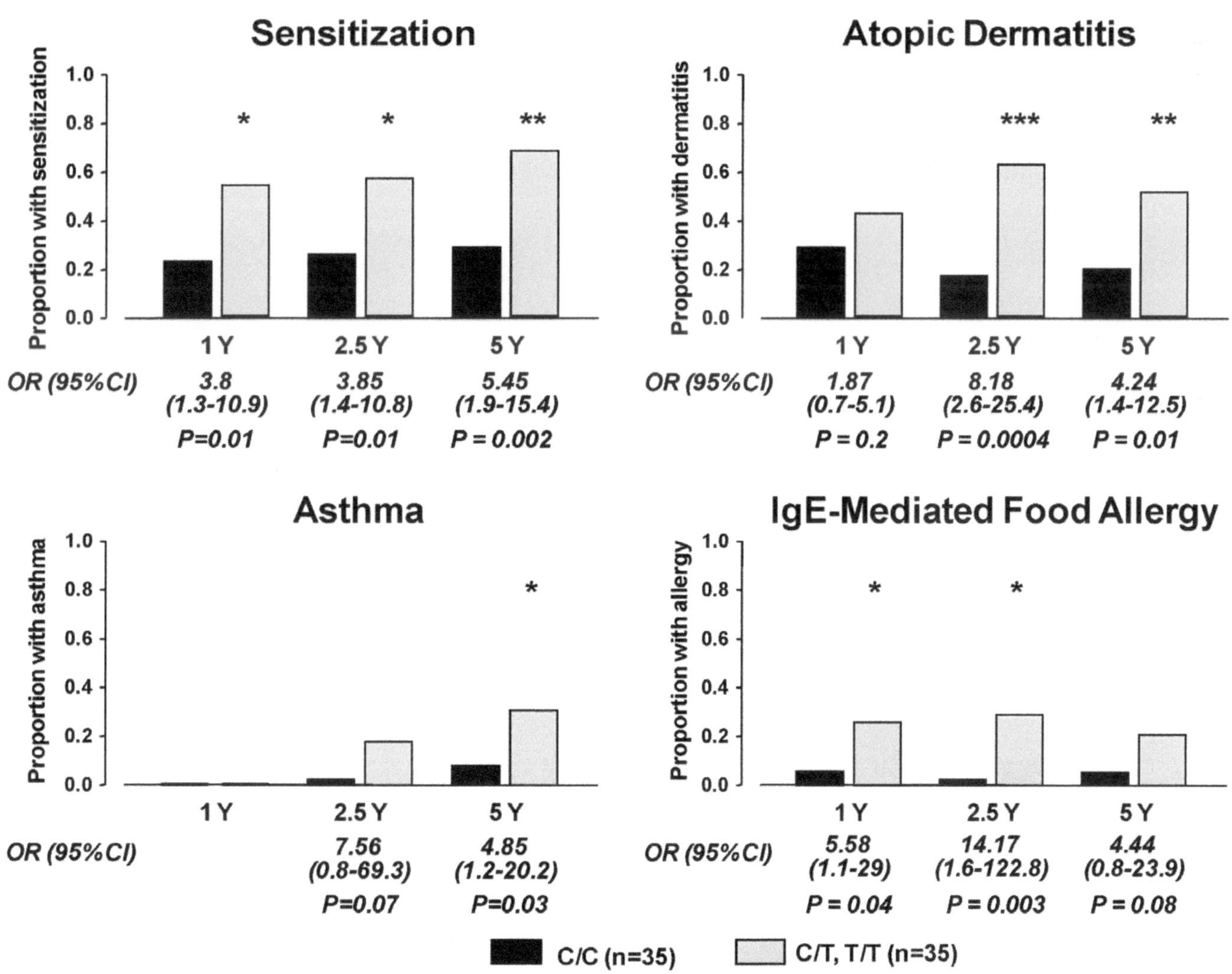

Figure 2. Carriage of the T allele of rs12979860 is associated with clinical presentation of allergic disease. Proportion of infants in cohort 1 that are sensitised, have doctor-diagnosed atopic dermatitis, asthma or IgE-mediated food allergy at 1, 2.5 or 5 years of age, with C/C (n = 35, black bars) or C/T, T/T (n = 35, grey bars) genotype. OR = odds-ratio. *P<0.05, **P<0.01 and ***P<0.001 versus age-matched C/C genotype.

Gender bias in the association of rs12979860 genotype with allergic disease

There is a significant interaction between gender and carriage of the T allele of rs12979860 for allergic disease (P = 0.04). The effect is particularly evident for sensitization (Fig. 3a top) and to a lesser extent for atopic dermatitis (Fig. 3a bottom) but not for asthma or IgE-mediated food allergy during early childhood (data not shown). Interestingly, it was only amongst females that we found differential trends in allergy status with age relative to rs12979860 genotype. Carriage of the T allele of rs12979860 in females but not males was associated with increased risk of sensitisation with age (P = 0.02; Fig. 3b). Conversely, amongst females with the C/C genotype we see a reduction in the proportion with atopic dermatitis with age (P = 0.04; Fig. 3b).

rs12979860 genotype correlates with innate immune function

We then examined the association between TLR-mediated innate immune function (namely IL-1B, TNF alpha cytokine production after TLR ligation with classical model ligands [5]) and rs12979860 genotype. We have previously shown a differential in the level of pro-inflammatory cytokine production after cord blood stimulation with select TLR ligands is associated with either allergic and non-allergic status in later life [5]. Briefly, children with allergic disease have higher levels of pro-inflammatory cytokines at birth (in cord blood) and during their early postnatal period, however this responsiveness declines with age and by pre-school age (5 years) is significantly depressed compared to age-matched non-allergic controls. In non-allergic children, TLR responses mature with age, which is necessary to elicit appropriate responses to pathogens. Here we show that this key difference in immune ontogeny is significantly associated with rs12979860 genotype and can be seen after the stimulation with the majority of TLR ligands (Fig. 4). In general, subjects with the C/C genotype (solid lines) are characterised by significantly lower levels of pro-inflammatory cytokine production at birth after TLR-dependent stimulation (exception being TLR8). For these individuals with the C/C genotype, a postnatal increase in IL-1β and TNF-α production following TLR stimulation (most pronounced for TLR2, 3, 4 and 7) is observed (Fig. 4). These findings are contrasted by the profile of TLR-dependent cytokine responses in children carrying the T "risk" allele (that is, C/T or T/T genotype; dashed lines) (Fig. 4), which shows high levels of pro-inflammatory cytokines at birth (in cord blood) in response to TLR ligation. Furthermore, TLR-induced pro-inflammatory cytokine responses in these children decline with age (in particular TNF production). These findings are consistent with our previous

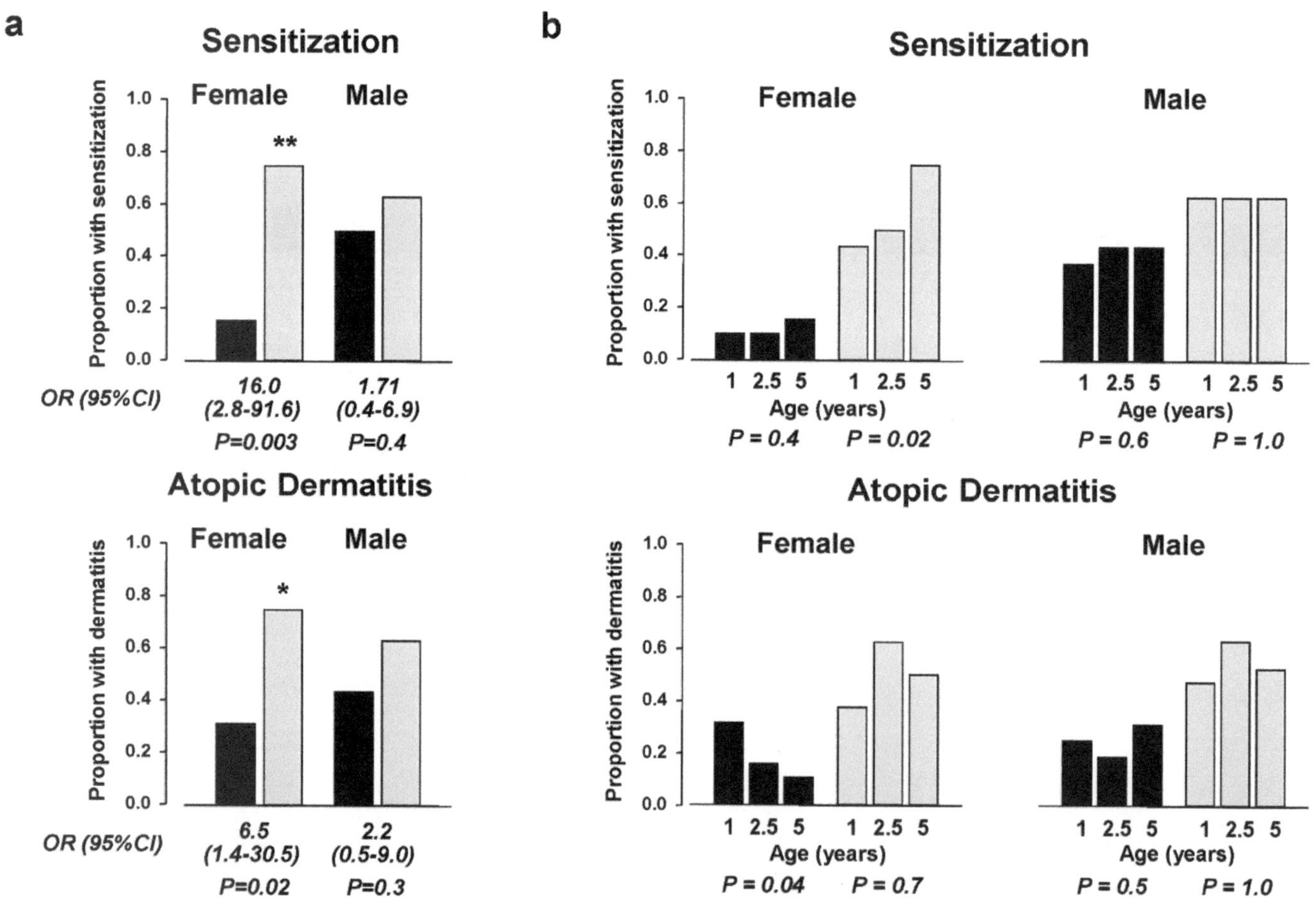

Figure 3. Gender differences in the association between carriage of the T allele of rs12979860 and allergic disease. a. Interaction between gender and carriage of the T allele of rs12979860 for sensitization (top panel) and atopic dermatitis (bottom panel) in cohort 1 in individuals with C/C (n = 35, black bars) or C/T,T/T (n = 35, grey bars) genotype. *P<0.05 and **P<0.001 versus females with C/C genotype. **b.** Trends in sensitization (top panel) and atopic dermatitis (bottom panel) levels with age relative to rs12979860 genotype. *P<0.05 versus proportion of sensitised females with C/C genotype and †P<0.05 versus C/T,T/T genotype in females with atopic dermatitis. OR = odds ratio.

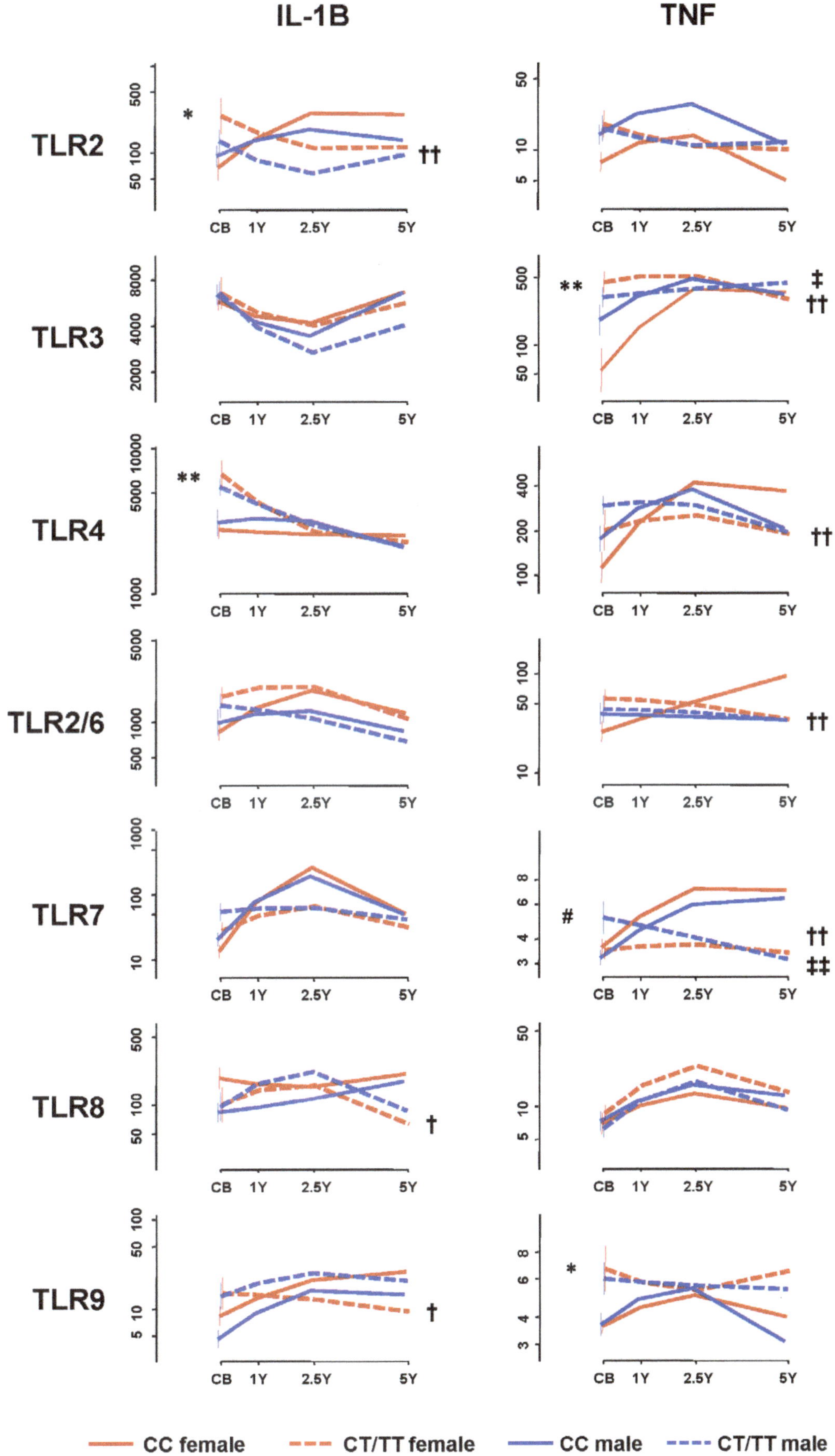

IL-1B
TNF
TLR2
TLR3
TLR4
TLR2/6
TLR7
TLR8
TLR9
CB 1Y 2.5Y 5Y
*
**
#
†
††
‡
‡‡
CC female
CT/TT female
CC male
CT/TT male

Figure 4. IL-1B and TNF cytokine production with age in peripheral blood mononuclear cells from individuals with C/C or C/T,T/T genotype stimulated with TLR agonists. Plots are scaled to span ~90% of the data range. Differences between groups with p-values<0.05 are annotated: CB measures of rs12979860 genotype C/T, T/T vs C/C amongst females (*: P≤0.01) and males (#: P≤0.01); average linear trend of profiles of C/T,T/T vs C/C amongst females (†: P≤0.01, ††: P≤0.001) and males (‡: P≤0.01, ‡‡: P<0.001).

observation in the same cohort showing a similar distinguishing pattern in cytokine profiles in allergic and non-allergic during the maturation of the immune system over the first five years of life [5]. Although this can be seen in male and female children, these trends are most pronounced in females with the C/C genotype (Fig. 4).

Discussion

Allergic disease is a complex trait with a substantial genetic contribution likely involving a number of different genes, gene-gene interactions and environmental influences. However, identifying the causative genes involved in the susceptibility and progression of allergic disease is hampered by heterogeneity in clinical phenotype, incomplete penetrance, typical modest or low genetic effect size of a single causative gene and the often immeasurable interaction between genes and the environment. Importantly, phenotypic definition is a critical factor to consider in association studies to optimise the ability to identify new genetic associations with disease [21]. In this study, the use of stringent criteria to define allergic and non-allergic children during the critical five-year follow-up from birth has resulted in a clinically well-differentiated disease and control group that should facilitate the identification of putative causative genes in allergic disease.

Our previous studies have clearly shown a different developmental trajectory for innate immune function between allergic and non-allergic children during early childhood [4,5]. Given the likely role of pDCs and IFNs in this framework, we investigated the role of genetic variations in *IL28B* in allergic disease. We show for the first time a strong association between genetic variations flanking and within *IL28B* and allergic disease. The effect of *IL28B* variations on atopy risk may be one of the strongest genetic predictors of allergic disease as most other candidate genes for allergic disease appear to have only a modest effect size. Interestingly, of more than a dozen genome-wide scans performed on atopic disease (including atopy, asthma and atopic dermatitis) none have highlighted this chromosomal region (www.genome.gov/gwastudies) as has been done for HCV infection and treatment outcome. This may be best explained by the clinical difficulty in phenotyping atopic and non-atopic subjects (particularly children) included in previous studies, given the high rate of atopy even in non-symptomatic subjects.

As an interesting analogy, HCV clearance (natural and treatment-induced) is associated with the C/C "protective" genotype of rs12979860 with a similar effect size. It currently remains speculative if the C/C genotype leads to higher or lower levels of IFN-λ (and specifically IFN-λ3) secretion (locally and systemically). Some studies have suggested that the C/C genotype is associated with diminished ISG expression (albeit mainly for liver and in HCV-infected subjects) [14,15]. Others have shown higher levels of IFN-λ in plasma in individuals who carry the C allele of rs12979860 (C/C and C/T subjects) [22]. Interestingly, subjects with autosomal dominant STAT3 deficiency (Hyper IgE syndrome) [23], which may lead to mutations in the IFN-λ signalling pathway, present with atopic dermatitis and high levels of IgE in serum. Thus, one could speculate that the C/T or T/T genotype in allergic children is associated with lower levels of IFN-λ secretion. Furthermore, IFN-λ is thought to suppress Th2-type immune responses, which are the hallmark of allergic disease. This is further supported by the recent study by Koltsida and colleagues who showed that IFN-λ can promote Th1 immunity and suppress Th2 responses in the mouse model of allergic asthma [13] initiating suggestions that IFN-λ could be used as a new treatment approach for allergic asthma [24]. In this study, we have demonstrated a relationship between higher levels of a pro-inflammatory cytokine profile at birth with diminished levels of these cytokines over time in children who carry the T allele of rs12979860 with an inverse relationship observed for children with the "protective" C/C genotype. However, levels of IFN-λ3 at relevant sites for atopic disease have not been established and the role of IFN-λ3 in IgE-mediated diseases and in the Th1/Th2 balance remains of great interest.

Frequencies of the rs12979860 alleles vary across populations with Africans having a higher frequency of the T "risk" allele than Caucasians and Asians [19]. In HCV infection and treatment outcome, frequency of the T allele of rs12979860 correlates with the known disparity in responses in different populations [19]. In allergic disease, it is known that there are differences in the prevalence and disease progression of allergic disease in populations [2] with African Americans shown to have much higher rates of death from asthma. A better link between *IL28B* allele frequencies and epidemiological studies may reveal how much *IL28B* variation contributes to ethnic disparities in the prevalence of atopic disease.

Here, we also clearly show a gender bias in the "protective" effect of the C/C genotype of rs12979860 in females compared to males in atopic disease. The gender bias extends to the relationship between rs12979860 and innate immune function. The reasons for this gender bias are not clear but may involve differential transcriptional control or hormonal responsiveness of relevant genes. Interestingly, female gender is also a predictor of favourable HCV infection outcome [25].

In view of the increasing burden of allergic disease in clinical practice, novel biomarkers that can be used for risk stratification of challenges, treatment and diet advice are invaluable. Definition of the *IL28B* genotype in children will allow the rapid identification of those children that are at risk of developing allergic disease and therefore management/intervention can be optimised accordingly. Overall, analysing the *IL28B* genotype is a simple cost-effective test that can be automated and already has been optimised for clinical practice as a predictive factor for outcome of HCV infection.

In conclusion, despite a proposed linkage between the level of environmental pathogenic exposure and allergy (hygiene hypothesis) no clear mechanistic linkage has been proposed that might explain the apparent enhanced susceptibility. Here for the first time we show that genetic variants in an innate microbial defence pathway (*IL28B*) are highly predictive of allergic disease with clear gender bias, and directly correlated with the innate immune function. These findings have broad-ranging implications for understanding the pathogenesis of not only allergic disease but many other inflammatory and autoimmune diseases.

Methods

Subjects

All children were recruited ante-natally from healthy pregnant mothers from obstetricians in Perth, Australia. Children were selected from 739 children enrolled in prospective birth cohorts designed to examine allergy pathogenesis. The first cohort (Cohort 1) consisted of 35 allergic and 35 non-allergic infants, which were followed from birth to age 5 years to assess their development of innate immune function and are described elsewhere [5]. Children were defined as non-allergic if they had no history of sensitisation or allergic disease at any age (based on at least 2 follow-up visits), or allergic if they have had a doctor-diagnosis of atopic dermatitis, allergic rhinitis, food allergy or asthma, *and* specific IgE to allergens as detected by a skin-prick test (SPT) at one or more clinic visits. Cohort 2 consisted of children with doctor-diagnosed food allergy (n = 30) recruited from the same research clinic as Cohort 1. IgE-mediated food-allergy was defined as a history of immediate symptoms after contact with food, ingestion of food, or both *and* a positive SPT to that food. Symptoms of acute food allergy included skin reactions (hives, rash, or swelling) and/or respiratory tract symptoms (cough, wheeze, or stridor) and/or gastrointestinal symptoms (abdominal pain, vomiting, or loose stools) and/or cardiovascular symptoms (collapse). In this cohort, 12/30 (40%) had severe food allergy (resulting in anaphylaxis). 27/30 (90%) had allergy to eggs, 13/30 (43%) allergy to nuts, 7/30 (23%) were allergic to house dust mite, 5/30 (17%) to cat dander and 20/30 (67%) reacted to multiple foods. Subjects in Cohort 1 and 2 were all of Caucasian ethnicity.

Ethics statement

Written, informed consent from the next of kin, carers or guardians on the behalf of the children participants was obtained for this study. Ethics approval was given by Princess Margaret Hospital Ethics Committee (EC07-74) and contributing Centres (EC2004/005). The protocol and the procedures of the study were conducted in conformity with the ethical guidelines of the Declaration of Helsinki.

IL28B Genotyping

Genotyping of the tagSNP rs12979860 upstream of *IL28B* on subjects in both cohorts was performed by TaqMan allelic discrimination using the Custom Assay designed by Ge and colleagues [16]. Typing of rs12979860 was performed by two independent laboratories blinded to the clinical phenotype with 100% concordance. There was no significant deviation from Hardy Weinberg equilibrium.

Further characterisation of the *IL28B* region was performed by examining an additional set of putative causal SNPs (rs8403219, rs28416813, rs8103142 and rs4803217) that reside within the promoter, coding and 3′ untranslated region of *IL28B* [20]. These SNPs are in strong linkage disequilibrium with rs12979860 and define the two main haplotypes of the block encompassing *IL28B*, with the type II haplotype containing the minor or "risk" allele(s) for at least one of the putative causal SNPs. As there was complete linkage disequilibrium between rs12979680 and the type II haplotype in all subjects, the p-value and OR were the same as for carriage of the T allele of rs12979860. Genotyping of the additional four SNPs within *IL28B* and another tagging SNP rs8099917 10 kb upstream of *IL28B* on subjects in Cohort 1 and 2 was performed by TaqMan allelic discrimination using Custom Assays and Assay on demand provided by Applied Biosystems as described by di Iulio *et al* [20].

Statistical analyses

Logistic regression was used to assess relative effects of genotype, gender and age on allergy status. Confidence intervals for odds ratios (OR) were obtained by exponentiating the 95% confidence interval for the log odds, estimated by the model coefficient, and p-values were determined by a Wald test. Multivariable models provided adjusted estimates and enabled assessment of variable interactions. Evaluation of trends in allergy status over age accommodated the within-individual correlations by assuming an autoregressive structure within a generalized estimating equation framework.

Cytokine measures were log-transformed prior to analysis to ensure approximate normality of residuals about mean values. Differences in baseline (cord blood) measures were assessed by standard linear regression. Mixed effect linear regression models were utilized for estimation of group-average changes in the measures over time since birth, and assessment of genotype and gender effects on the linear trend [26,27]. The models assumed an autoregressive correlation structure for accommodation of the within-individual dependencies. All statistical analyses were carried out using TIBCO Spotfire S+ 8.2 for Windows (TIBCO Spotfire Inc, Palo Alto 2010).

Author Contributions

Conceived and designed the experiments: SG ML MKT AL. Performed the experiments: HA SG MKT JdI. Analyzed the data: EM SG MKT ML AR. Contributed reagents/materials/analysis tools: SLP DM. Wrote the paper: SG ML MKT AL SLP.

References

1. Renz H, von Mutius E, Brandtzaeg P, Cookson WO, Autenrieth IB, et al. (2011) Gene-environment interactions in chronic inflammatory disease. Nat Immunol 12: 273–277.
2. Asher MI, Montefort S, Bjorksten B, Lai CK, Strachan DP, et al. (2006) Worldwide time trends in the prevalence of symptoms of asthma, allergic rhinoconjunctivitis, and eczema in childhood: ISAAC Phases One and Three repeat multicountry cross-sectional surveys. Lancet 368: 733–743.
3. Martino D, Prescott S (2011) Epigenetics and prenatal influences on asthma and allergic airways disease. Chest 139: 640–647.
4. Prescott SL, Noakes P, Chow BW, Breckler L, Thornton CA, et al. (2008) Presymptomatic differences in Toll-like receptor function in infants who have allergy. J Allergy Clin Immunol 122: 391–399.
5. Tulic MK, Hodder M, Forsberg A, McCarthy S, Richman T, et al. (2011) Differences in innate immune function between allergic and nonallergic children: New insights into immune ontogeny. J Allergy Clin Immunol 127: 470–478.
6. Sheppard P, Kindsvogel W, Xu W, Henderson K, Schlutsmeyer S, et al. (2003) IL-28, IL-29 and their class II cytokine receptor IL-28R. Nat Immunol 4: 63–68.
7. Mennechet FJ, Uze G (2006) Interferon-lambda-treated dendritic cells specifically induce proliferation of FOXP3-expressing suppressor T cells. Blood 107: 4417–4423.
8. Jordan WJ, Eskdale J, Srinivas S, Pekarek V, Kelner D, et al. (2007) Human interferon lambda-1 (IFN-lambda1/IL-29) modulates the Th1/Th2 response. Genes Immun 8: 254–261.
9. Srinivas S, Dai J, Eskdale J, Gallagher GE, Megjugorac NJ, et al. (2008) Interferon-lambda1 (interleukin-29) preferentially down-regulates interleukin-13 over other T helper type 2 cytokine responses in vitro. Immunology 125: 492–502.
10. Morrow MP, Pankhong P, Laddy DJ, Schoenly KA, Yan J, et al. (2009) Comparative ability of IL-12 and IL-28B to regulate Treg populations and enhance adaptive cellular immunity. Blood 113: 5868–5877.
11. Wolk K, Witte K, Witte E, Proesch S, Schulze-Tanzil G, et al. (2008) Maturing dendritic cells are an important source of IL-29 and IL-20 that may cooperatively increase the innate immunity of keratinocytes. J Leukoc Biol 83: 1181–1193.
12. Contoli M, Message SD, Laza-Stanca V, Edwards MR, Wark PA, et al. (2006) Role of deficient type III interferon-lambda production in asthma exacerbations. Nat Med 12: 1023–1026.
13. Koltsida O, Hausding M, Stavropoulos A, Koch S, Tzelepis G, et al. (2011) IL-28A (IFN-lambda2) modulates lung DC function to promote Th1 immune skewing and suppress allergic airway disease. EMBO Mol Med 3: 348–361.

14. Honda M, Sakai A, Yamashita T, Nakamoto Y, Mizukoshi E, et al. (2010) Hepatic ISG expression is associated with genetic variation in interleukin 28B and the outcome of IFN therapy for chronic hepatitis C. Gastroenterology 139: 499–509.
15. Urban TJ, Thompson AJ, Bradrick SS, Fellay J, Schuppan D, et al. (2010) IL28B genotype is associated with differential expression of intrahepatic interferon-stimulated genes in patients with chronic hepatitis C. Hepatology 52: 1888–1896.
16. Ge D, Fellay J, Thompson AJ, Simon JS, Shianna KV, et al. (2009) Genetic variation in IL28B predicts hepatitis C treatment-induced viral clearance. Nature 461: 399–401.
17. Suppiah V, Moldovan M, Ahlenstiel G, Berg T, Weltman M, et al. (2009) IL28B is associated with response to chronic hepatitis C interferon-alpha and ribavirin therapy. Nat Genet 41: 1100–1104.
18. Rauch A, Kutalik Z, Descombes P, Cai T, Di Iulio J, et al. (2010) Genetic variation in IL28B is associated with chronic hepatitis C and treatment failure: a genome-wide association study. Gastroenterology 138: 1338–1345.
19. Thomas DL, Thio CL, Martin MP, Qi Y, Ge D, et al. (2009) Genetic variation in IL28B and spontaneous clearance of hepatitis C virus. Nature 461: 798–801.
20. di Iulio J, Ciuffi A, Fitzmaurice K, Kelleher D, Rotger M, et al. (2011) Estimating the net contribution of interleukin-28B variation to spontaneous hepatitis C virus clearance. Hepatology 53: 1446–1454.
21. Evangelou E, Fellay J, Colombo S, Martinez-Picado J, Obel N, et al. (2011) Impact of phenotype definition on genome-wide association signals: empirical evaluation in human immunodeficiency virus type 1 infection. Am J Epidemiol 173: 1336–1342.
22. Langhans B, Kupfer B, Braunschweiger I, Arndt S, Schulte W, et al. (2011) Interferon-lambda serum levels in hepatitis C. J Hepatol 54: 859–865.
23. Tangye SG, Cook MC, Fulcher DA (2009) Insights into the role of STAT3 in human lymphocyte differentiation as revealed by the hyper-IgE syndrome. J Immunol 182: 21–28.
24. Edwards MR, Johnston SL (2011) Interferon-lambda as a new approach for treatment of allergic asthma? EMBO Mol Med 3: 306–308.
25. Thomas DL, Astemborski J, Rai RM, Anania FA, Schaeffer M, et al. (2000) The natural history of hepatitis C virus infection: host, viral, and environmental factors. JAMA 284: 450–456.
26. Liang KY, Zeger SL (1986) Longitudinal data analysis using generalized linear models. Biometrika 73: 13–22.
27. Zeger SL, Liang KY (1986) Longitudinal data analysis for discrete and continuous outcomes. Biometrics 42: 121–130.
28. Tillmann HL, Thompson AJ, Patel K, Wiese M, Tenckhoff H, et al. (2010) A polymorphism near IL28B is associated with spontaneous clearance of acute hepatitis C virus and jaundice. Gastroenterology 139: 1586–1592.

3

Prevention of Birch Pollen-Related Food Allergy by Mucosal Treatment with Multi-Allergen-Chimers in Mice

Elisabeth Hoflehner[1], Karin Hufnagl[1], Irma Schabussova[1], Joanna Jasinska[1], Karin Hoffmann-Sommergruber[2], Barbara Bohle[2], Rick M. Maizels[3], Ursula Wiedermann[1]*

1 Institute of Specific Prophylaxis and Tropical Medicine, Center for Pathophysiology, Infectiology and Immunology, Medical University of Vienna, Vienna, Austria,
2 Department of Pathophysiology and Allergy Research, Center for Pathophysiology, Infectiology and Immunology, Medical University of Vienna, Vienna, Austria,
3 Institute of Immunology and Infection Research, University of Edinburgh, Edinburgh, United Kingdom

Abstract

Background: Among birch pollen allergic patients up to 70% develop allergic reactions to Bet v 1-homologue food allergens such as Api g 1 (celery) or Dau c 1 (carrot), termed as birch pollen-related food allergy. In most cases, specific immunotherapy with birch pollen extracts does not reduce allergic symptoms to the homologue food allergens. We therefore genetically engineered a multi-allergen chimer and tested if mucosal treatment with this construct could represent a novel approach for prevention of birch pollen-related food allergy.

Methodology: BALB/c mice were poly-sensitized with a mixture of Bet v 1, Api g 1 and Dau c 1 followed by a sublingual challenge with carrot, celery and birch pollen extracts. For prevention of allergy sensitization an allergen chimer composed of immunodominant T cell epitopes of Api g 1 and Dau c 1 linked to the whole Bet v 1 allergen, was intranasally applied prior to sensitization.

Results: Intranasal pretreatment with the allergen chimer led to significantly decreased antigen-specific IgE-dependent β-hexosaminidase release, but enhanced allergen-specific IgG2a and IgA antibodies. Accordingly, IL-4 levels in spleen cell cultures and IL-5 levels in restimulated spleen and cervical lymph node cell cultures were markedly reduced, while IFN-γ levels were increased. Immunomodulation was associated with increased IL-10, TGF-β and Foxp3 mRNA levels in NALT and Foxp3 in oral mucosal tissues. Treatment with anti-TGF-β, anti-IL10R or anti-CD25 antibodies abrogated the suppression of allergic responses induced by the chimer.

Conclusion: Our results indicate that mucosal application of the allergen chimer led to decreased Th2 immune responses against Bet v 1 and its homologue food allergens Api g 1 and Dau c 1 by regulatory and Th1-biased immune responses. These data suggest that mucosal treatment with a multi-allergen vaccine could be a promising treatment strategy to prevent birch pollen-related food allergy.

Editor: Jacques Zimmer, Centre de Recherche Public de la Santé (CRP-Santé), Luxembourg

Funding: The work was funded by grants from the Austrian Science Fund (F01814, P14634-PAT, Y0784GEN, FWF T163). RMM is supported by a Wellcome Trust Programme Grant. The funders had no role in study design, data collection and analysis, decision to publish, or preparation of the manuscript.

Competing Interests: The authors have declared that no competing interests exist.

* E-mail: ursula.wiedermann@meduniwien.ac.at

Introduction

One of the most common type I pollionosis is caused by the airborne allergens of birch pollen (BP). In Europe, more than 70% of BP-allergic patients develop an immediate hypersensitivity reaction against pollen-related food allergens, termed as birch pollen-related food allergy (BPRFA) and clinically manifested as oral allergy syndrome (OAS). IgE antibodies specific for Bet v 1, the major BP allergen, cross-react with epitopes of homologous food allergens such as Mald1 (apple), Cora1 (hazelnut), Api g 1 (celery), or Dau c 1 (carrot) [1,2]. Due to this cross-reactivity, Bet v 1-specific IgE can induce hypersensitivity reactions towards these food allergens. The symptoms of the BPRFA are usually restricted to the oral cavity and can range from swelling and itching of lips, tongue, soft palate and pharynx to systemic reactions such as urticaria, asthma or even anaphylaxis [3,4]. Most of these patients also display food induced symptoms outside the BP season, indicating that homologous food allergens provide a perennial boost of BP-specific immune responses [5].

For BP mono-sensitized individuals common specific immunotherapy (SIT) is well established and is regarded as a successful therapy. However, for treatment of patients with multiple sensitivities or BPRFA, SIT has low efficacy and is associated with an increased risk of anaphylactic side-effects [1,6,7]. Improving this treatment could either be achieved by the application of well defined recombinant single allergens or a mixture thereof, or allergen peptides according to the patient T cell recognition pattern. Additionally, exploiting different routes of vaccination, e.g. changing the subcutaneous to a less invasive administration via the mucosa (i.e. oral, nasal, sublingual) could improve the efficacy of this treatment [8].

We previously demonstrated that mucosal administration of recombinant allergens prevented allergic sensitization in mono-sensitized mice [9]. In poly-sensitized mice, however, application of a mixture of recombinant antigens did not efficiently elicit protective effects [8,10]. More recently, we demonstrated that mucosal application of either a multi-peptide construct, covering the immunodominant T cell epitopes of the major birch and grass pollen allergens, or a multi-allergen chimer, consisting of the scaffold allergen Bet v 1 in its native conformation anchoring two or more immunodominant peptides from major grass pollen allergens, prevented multi-sensitization against these allergens [8,10].

In the current study we established a model of BPRFA in poly-sensitized mice to validate the protective effects of mucosal treatment with a respective chimer. For this purpose we designed a pollen-food-allergen chimer consisting of Bet v 1, acting as a potent tolerogen, fused with additional immunodominant peptides of its homologous food allergens Api g 1 from celery and Dau c 1 from carrot. Our data provide evidence for the efficacy and underlying mechanisms of mucosal treatment with this chimer in preventing local and systemic Th2 immune responses in poly-sensitized mice.

Methods

Animals

Female 7-week-old BALB/c mice (n = 12 per group) were obtained from Charles River (Sulzfeld, Germany). All experiments were repeated 3 times.

Ethics Statement

The animal studies were performed according to institutional guidelines for animal use and care. The study was approved by the Animal Experimentation Ethics Committee of the Medical University of Vienna and the Ministry of Science and Research (GZ 66.009/229-BrGT/2005; GZ 66.009/35-II/10b/2010).

Antigens and Antibodies

Recombinant Bet v 1.010, Api g 1.0101 and Dau c 1.0103 were obtained from Biomay AG (Vienna, Austria). Birch pollen (BP) from *Betula verrucosa* was purchased from Allergon (Välinge, Sweden), and protein extracts of BP, celery (*Apium graveolens) and* carrot (*Daucus carota*) were prepared as previously described [11,12].

Anti-TGF-β, anti-IL-10R and anti-CD25 blocking antibodies were produced in house at the University of Edinburgh, UK (and provided by R. Maizels). Rat IgG isotype control antibody was used (Sigma-Aldrich).

Epitope Mapping Studies

For T cell epitope mapping a panel of 48 peptides of Api g 1 and 48 peptides of Dau c 1 were used (provided by B. Bohle). Spleen cell suspensions from Api g 1 or Dau c 1 immunized mice were incubated with 5 μg/well of each of the peptides, which overlapped for three amino acids (neighbours sharing nine residues) spanning the whole amino acid sequence of the respective antigens. Proliferative responses were measured according to previous description [12].

Construction of the Birch Pollen–food–chimer Expression Plasmid

Complementary templates from Api g 1 (Genbank Access number: Z48967) and Dau c 1 (Genbank Access number: Z84376) respectively, were used to amplify the identified immunodominant encoding regions by PCR (cDNA templates were provided by K. Hoffmann-Sommergruber). Api g 1-T cell epitope specific primers were designed including *Nco*I and *Eco*RI restriction sites (Api g 1 fwd 5′-CATGCCATGGATGGAGTTAACAAGGAG-3′, Api g 1 rev 5′-ATGAATTCAACATGGTTTTCAATGGA-3′; restriction sites underlined); Dau c 1-T cell epitope specific primers were designed including *Hind*III and *Xho*I restriction sites (Dau c 1 fwd 5′-ACCAAGCTTGCCGTGGTTCCTGAAGAG-3′, Dau c 1 rev 5′-CCGCTCGAGTTAATTAGCAATGAGGTAGGC-3′).

For construction of the Api g 1-Bet v 1-Dau c 1-chimer we ligated the PCR amplicons of Api g 1 and Dau c 1 into the respective restriction sites on the 5′- and 3′-end of a pHis Parallel 2 - Bet v 1 plasmid, equipped with a hexahistidyl (6×His) affinity tag as previously described [8]. Subsequent DNA sequence analysis (GATC Biotech, Konstanz, Germany) verified correct sequences and the integrity of open reading frame.

Expression, Purification and Refolding of Recombinant Api g 1-Bet v 1-Dau c 1-chimer

The Api g 1-Bet v 1-Dau c 1-expression plasmid was transformed into electrocompetent BL 21(DE3)plysS *E. coli* cells (Invitrogen, NV Leek, Netherlands) and grown in LB/1 mM ampicillin medium at 37°C under vigorous shaking until an optical density (OD_{600}) of 0.7. Expression was induced by adding 0.001 mol/L isopropyl β-D-thiogalactopyranoside (IPTG) and incubation continued for additional 3 hours before harvesting.

6×His-tagged r Api g 1-Bet v 1-Dau c 1-chimeric protein was produced in inclusion bodies and therefore purified from *E. coli* lysate under denaturing conditions. Cells were solubilized in denaturating lysis buffer (8 mol/L urea, 0.1 mol/L NaH_2PO_4, 0.01 mol/L tris, pH 8.0) and purified by nickel nitrilotriacetic acid affinity column (GE Healthcare, Uppsala, Sweden).

Purified protein fractions were monitored by sodium dodecyl sulphate-polyacrylamide gel electrophoresis (SDS-PAGE), pooled and refolded by stepwise dialysis against 0.02 mol/L $NaPO_4$, pH 8.0 while gradually reducing urea concentration from 6 mol/L to 0 mol/L. After a final dialysis against 0.01 mol/L $NaPO_4$, pH 7.2, Api g 1-Bet v 1-Dau c 1-chimer was lyophilized and stored at −20°C.

Concentration of bacterial endotoxins was determined using the *Limulus amebocyte lysate* assay (QCL-1000, Cambrex, Walkersville, MD, USA) according to the users manual. Endotoxins were removed using the EndoTrap Blue affinity column (Profos, Regensburg, Germany) according to the manufacture's instructions. Protein concentration was determined using the bicinchronic acid protein assay (Pierce, Rockford, IL, USA).

Protein Analysis

Physiochemical identification and characterization of the recombinant construct was done by preparative HPLC and mass spectrometry (piCHEM, Graz, Austria), and secondary structure by far UV light circular dichroism spectroscopy (CD), as previously described [8].

Immunological characterization was done by immunoblot analysis using a monoclonal mouse anti-Bet v 1 IgG antibody (BIP1, 1/10), sera from 3 BP allergic patients with concomitant BPRFA containing Api g 1-, Dau c 1-, and Bet v 1-specific IgE (1/5) or mouse sera from a chimer-tolerized, poly-sensitized mouse (1/5). For detection secondary rat anti-mouse IgG1 antibody (1/500; BD Pharmingen, San Diego, CA, USA) followed by an alkaline phosphatise-conjugated goat anti-rat IgG (1/2000; Santa Cruz Biotechnology, Santa Cruz, CA, USA), or alkaline phosphatase-conjugated mouse anti-human IgE (1/1000; Pharmingen) antibodies and NBT/BCIP substrate mixture were used. Negative controls with sera from untreated mice and non-allergic patients, or buffer control were run in parallel.

Animal Treatment

Allergy prevention in mono-sensitized mice with either rBet v 1, rApi g 1 or rDau c 1. Mono-sensitization was performed by 3 intraperitoneal (i.p.) injections (day 22, 36, 50) of 5 µg per Bet v 1, Api g 1 or Dau c 1 adsorbed to aluminium hydroxide ($Al(OH)_3$; Serva, Heidelberg, Germany) in 14 day intervals, adapted from Hufnagl et al. [13]. For prevention of allergic sensitization 10 µg of either of the allergen Bet v 1, Api g 1 or Dau c 1 were intranasally (i.n.) applied in 30 µl of 0.9% NaCl 3 times in 7 day intervals (day 0, 7, 14), prior to mono-sensitization, adapted from Wiedermann et al. [12]. Samples were taken one week after the last treatment (day 57).

Allergy prevention in poly-sensitized mice with a mixture of all three allergens. Poly-sensitization was performed by applying a mixture of Bet v 1, Api g 1 and Dau c 1, 5 µg each adsorbed to $Al(OH)_3$ as described above. For prevention of poly-sensitization mice were i.n. pretreated with a mixture of 10 µg each of Bet v 1, Api g 1 and Dau c 1, in 30 µl of 0.9% NaCl. Allergy prevention and poly-sensitization protocols were adapted from Hufnagl et al. [10].

Allergy prevention with the birch pollen-food chimer in poly-sensitized mice. Intranasal pretreatment with the BP-food chimer was performed by using 15 µg of the chimer in 30 µl of 0.9% NaCl per application (adapted from Wild et al. [8]) as described above, prior to poly-sensitization. Control mice were i.n. sham-treated with 30 µl of 0.9% NaCl prior to poly-sensitization. One week after the last i.p. immunization, mice were sublingually (s.l.) challenged with a mixture of BP extract, carrot extract and celery extract, by applying 100 µg each in 15 µl of 0.9% NaCl with a pipette under the tongue of the mice. To prevent swallowing of the extracts mice were fixed in the scruff during and until 20 seconds after treatment. Mice were challenged on 3 consecutive days in 24 hour intervals (day 57, 58, 59). 24 hours after the last treatment mice were sacrificed (day 60) (Fig. 1).

In vivo application of neutralizing antibodies. In some experiments, i.n. chimer-pretreated and poly-sensitized mice were i.p. injected with 0.5 mg of blocking antibodies. Anti-CD25 was applied prior poly-sensitization (day 15) (adapted from Leech et al. and Wilson et al.) [14,15], anti-TGF-β before s.l. challenge (day 56) (adapted from Taher et al. [16]), and anti-IL-10R was injected before poly-sensitization (day 19) and before s.l. challenge (day 56) (adapted from Taher et al., Leech et al. and Wilson et al. [14,15,16]). Pretreated and poly-sensitized control mice were sham-treated with 0.5 mg isotype control antibodies.

Sampling

Blood samples were taken before treatment and on the day of sacrifice by tail bleeding. Sera were collected and stored at −20°C until analysis. On the day of sacrifice cell suspensions from spleen, cervical lymph nodes (CLN) and NALT were prepared as described [12,17,18]. Additionally, sublingual tissues (SLT) and buccal mucosa (BM) were prepared by excising the whole mandible from the head and dissecting the cheek skin and the tongue with the floor of the mouth (SLT). The cheek skin was stretched and mucosal tissue was scraped off with a scalpel and collected in RNA*later* buffer (Qiagen, Valencia, CA) for RNA isolation. SLT was separated from the tongue and stored in RNA*later* buffer as well [19].

Allergen-specific Antibody Levels and Total IgA in Serum

Microtiter plates (Nunc, Roskilde, Denmark) were coated with each of the recombinant allergens Bet v 1, Api g 1 or Dau c 1 (5 µg/mL) prior to incubation with sera in dilutions of 1/500 for antigen-specific IgG2a and 1/10 for antigen-specific IgA detection. Rat anti-mouse IgG2a or IgA antibodies (1/500, Pharmingen) were used, followed by peroxidase-conjugated mouse anti-rat IgG antibody (1/2000, Jackson Immuno Lab, West Grove, PA) [12]. Results show the OD values after subtraction of baseline levels from pre-immune sera.

For determination of total IgA levels in sera, microtiter plates (Nunc) were coated with rat anti-mouse IgA (1/250, clone C10-3, Pharmingen) and incubated with 1/100 diluted sera. For detection biotinylated anti-mouse IgA (1/1000, clone C 10-1, Pharmingen) antibody, streptavidin (1/10000) and ABTS substrate were used.

Results are shown in ng/mL after subtraction of baseline levels of pre-immune sera.

Rat Basophil Leukemia Cell Mediator Release Assay (RBL Assay)

For measurement of functional allergen-specific IgE, rat basophil leukemia (RBL) cells (RBL-2H3 cell line, ATCC, No. CRL-2256) were incubated with sera obtained from pretreated and poly-sensitized mice at dilutions of 1/10, 1/100 and 1/300. Degranulation of RBL cells was induced by adding 0.03 µg of Bet v 1, Api g 1 or Dau c 1 diluted in 100 µl Tyrodes buffer.

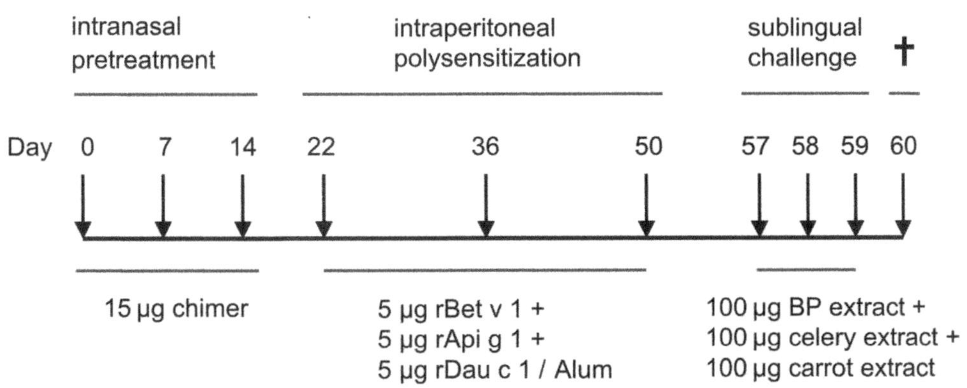

Figure 1. Experimental design. Mice were intranasally pretreated with either the chimer (chimer-treat) or sham-treated (poly-sens) 3 times in 7 days intervals followed by 3 intraperitoneal sensitizations with a mixture of rBet v 1, rApi g 1 and rDau c 1 in 2 weeks intervals. Thereafter, mice were sublingually challenged with a mixture of BP, celery and carrot extracts on 3 consecutive days.

Supernatants were analyzed for antigen-specific IgE-dependent β-hexosaminidase activity as previously described [13].

Cytokine Production

IL-4, IL-5, IFN-γ and TGF-β production was measured in spleen (5×10^6 cells/well), CLN (5×10^5 cells/well) and NALT suspensions (5×10^5 cells/well) incubated for 48 hours with each allergen (15 μg/well) as described [17]. Levels of IL-4, IL-5 and TGF-β were measured with ELISA kits (eBioscience, San Diego, CA, USA), IFN-γ levels were measured as previously described [20]. All cytokine levels are shown in pg/mL after subtraction of baseline levels of unstimulated cultures.

Magnetic Sorting of $CD4^+CD25^+$ Tregs and $CD4^+CD25^-$ T Effector Cells

$CD4^+CD25^-$ T effector cells (Teff) and $CD4^+CD25^+$ Treg cells were isolated from pooled spleen cells of chimer-pretreated or control poly-sensitized mice, with the MACS $CD4^+CD25^+$ Treg isolation kit (Miltenyi Biotec, Bergisch Gladbach, Germany), according to the manufacturer's protocol. The purity of sorted cells was acquired by flow cytometry using a BD FACSCalibur (BD Biosciences Pharmingen) and analysed by FlowJo software.

Treg Suppression Assay

$CD4^+CD25^-$ Teff cells (5×10^4) were cocultured in U-bottom 96-well plates with $CD4^+CD25^+$ Treg cells in various ratios (1/2, 1/8, 1/16). The cells were stimulated with 1 μg/mL anti-mouse CD3 (eBioscience) and 5×10^4 irradiated (3000 rad) splenocytes at 37°C for 3 days. For the last 16 hours of culture, cells were pulsed with 0.5 μCi ^{3}H-thymidine/well (Perkin-Elmer, Wellesley, MA, USA), harvested and proliferative responses were measured by scintillation counting (1450 Microbeta Liquid Scintillation and Luminescence counter, Perkin-Elmer). Results are expressed as absolute counts per minute (cpm). The percent suppression mediated by Treg cells was calculated by the following formula: [(cpm of Teff alone – cpm of Teff treated with Treg)/cpm of Teff cells alone]*100.

Quantification of mRNA Expression by Real-time RT-PCR

Total RNA from NALT was isolated from equal pooled cell suspensions. Total RNA extracted from RNA*later*-stabilized, pooled SLT and BM was homogenized in liquid nitrogen prior to purification by using RNeasy Minikit combined with DNase digestion (RNase-free DNase Set, Qiagen). The concentration of extracted RNA was measured by NanoDrop ND-1000 spectrophotometer (PeqLab, Erlangen, Germany), RNA probes were standardized and then reverse-transcribed into cDNA using iScript cDNA Synthesis Kit (Bio-Rad Laboratories, Hercules, CA, USA).

Gene expression was determined by quantitative real-time RT-PCR using LightCycler® FastStart kit with TaqMan® or CYBRGreen according to the manufacturer's instructions (Roche, Mannheim, Germany) on a LightCycler® instrument 1.2 (Roche). For quantification of TGF-β, IL-10 and Foxp3 mRNA, pre-designed TaqMan® assays were used. Data are presented as the relative ratio of the target genes to the housekeeping gene *5-aminolevulinic acid synthase 1* (*Alas1*) (Universal ProbeLibrary (UPL) probe #64, Roche) [21].

Statistics

Data are expressed as means ± SEMs from 3 independent experiments. For statistical analysis p values <0.05 were defined significant. Pair-wise comparison of sham-treated sensitized versus pretreated groups was performed by using the Mann-Whitney *U*-test and one-way ANOVA-test.

Results

Intranasal Pretreatment with Bet v 1, Api g 1 and Dau c 1 Alone or as a Mixture does not Suppress Immune Responses Against All 3 Allergens

Mucosal application of Bet v 1 prior to intraperitoneal polysensitization significantly reduced serum IgE responses as measured by IgE-induced basophil degranulation to Bet v 1, but not to Api g 1 or Dau c 1 (Fig. 2A). Similarly, mucosal application of Api g 1 or Dau c 1 prior to poly-sensitization showed significantly decreased IgE-induced β-hexosaminidase release only for the respective allergen (Fig. 2A).

In poly-sensitized mice, mucosal pretreatment with a mixture of all 3 allergens significantly reduced basophil degranulation to Bet v 1, but not to the homologous food allergens (Fig. 2B).

Construction and Characterization of the Birch Pollen-food Allergen Chimer

Based on previous T cell epitope mapping experiments with Api g 1 and Dau c 1 the immunodominant regions of these allergens were selected for designing the Bet v 1-food allergen chimer. In the case of Dau c 1 the immunodominant peptide detected in mice is also a major T cell epitope in allergic patients [22]. The immunodominant T cell epitope from Api g 1 (DGVNKEALTF-DYSVIDGDILLGFIESIENHV, peptide 27) including a 6×His-tag was inserted at the N-terminus of the Bet v 1.0101 encoding sequence. At the C-terminus the immunodominant T cell epitope of Dau c 1 (AVVPEENIKFADAQNTALFKAIEAYLIAN, peptide 47) was added (Fig.3A). Correct insertion of the templates was checked by sequence analysis.

After purification and refolding of the chimer with a theoretical mass of 27,6 kD, endotoxin levels of <0,05 EU/μg of purified protein were measured, which corresponds to baseline levels of commercially available proteins [9].

Secondary structure elements of the chimer, analyzed by CD spectra, were in good agreement with the spectra obtained from rBet v 1 [8]. Only minimal variations due to the added peptides (data not shown) were observed. Immunoblot analysis confirmed that the conformation of Bet v 1 remained unchanged after linkage of the peptides. The chimer was recognized by Bet v 1-specific monoclonal antibody (BIP1, lane 3) and by IgE from sera of 3 BP allergic patients with a BPRFA (lane 5, 6, 7) as well as IgE from sera of a chimer-treated poly-sensitized mouse (lane 1). Negative controls did not elicit any IgE binding to the chimer (lane 2, 8, 4, 9) (Fig. 3B).

Intranasal Pretreatment with the BP-food-chimer Suppressed Humoral and Cellular Immune Responses in Poly-sensitized Mice

Antibody responses. Intranasal pretreatment with the chimer significantly reduced IgE-mediated basophil degranulation to all three allergens in comparison to the untreated poly-sensitized group (Fig. 4A). Moreover, Api g 1-, Dau c 1- and Bet v 1-specific IgG2a antibody production was enhanced, indicating a shift towards Th1 responses (Fig. 4B). Additionally, pretreatment with the chimer increased serum levels of total and allergen-specific IgA antibodies in comparison to poly-sensitized controls (Fig. 4C).

Cytokine production. Pretreatment with the chimer significantly decreased IL-5 levels in supernatants of allergen restimulated spleen and CLN cell cultures (Fig. 5A). Additionally, the IgE

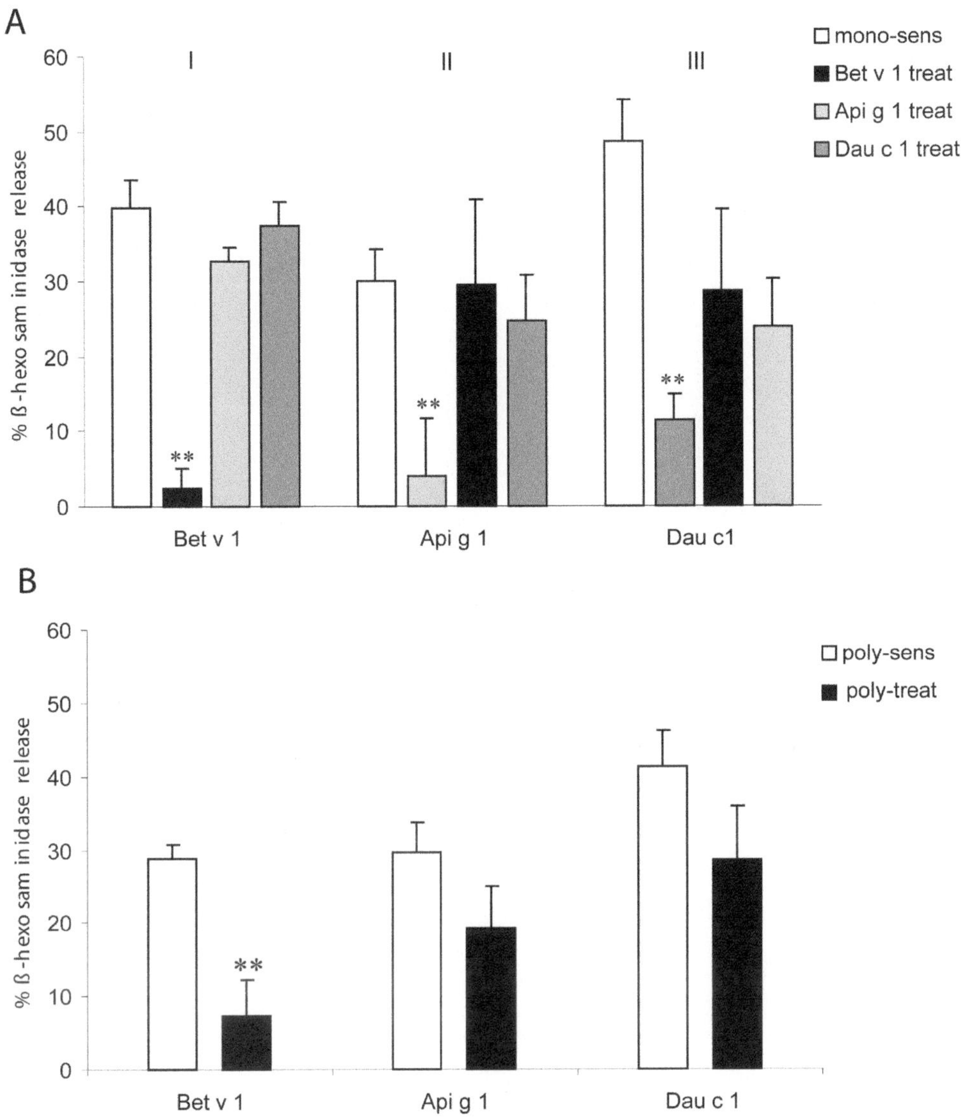

Figure 2. IgE-dependent allergen-specific basophil degranulation by sera. (**A**) ß-hexosaminidase release from (**I.**) rBet v 1-, (**II.**) Api g 1- or (**III.**) Dau c 1-sensitized mice; each group was i.n. pretreated with rBet v 1 (black bars), rApi g 1 (light-grey bars), rDau c 1 (dark-grey bars) or sham-treated (white bars). (**B**) ß-hexosaminidase release from mice i.n. pretreated with a mixture of rBet v 1/rApi g 1/rDau c 1 (black bars) compared with poly-sensitized controls (white bars). **p<0.01.

switching factor IL-4 was markedly reduced for all 3 allergens in spleen cell cultures of chimer treated mice compared to poly-sensitized controls: IL-4 (pg/mL): polysens: Bet v 1-restimulated: 14,35±22,60; Api g 1-restimulated: 43,92±53,84; Dau c 1-restimulated: 58,87±64,83; chimer-treat: Bet v 1-restimulated: 5,06±7,45; Api g 1-restimulated: 7,61±8,14**; Dau c 1-restimulated: 11,89±13,70**; **p<0,01.

IFN-γ production in spleen cell cultures was significantly enhanced after Bet v 1 - but not after Api g 1 or Dau c 1 - stimulations compared to poly-sensitized controls (Fig. 5B). However, in the CLN (Fig. 5B), and also in the NALT (data not shown) cultures, IFN-γ production was significantly increased in the pretreated mice after re-stimulation with all three allergens.

Prevention of Allergic Polysensitization with the Chimer is Associated with Regulatory Mechanisms

The mRNA expression of TGF-β, IL-10 and Foxp3 in NALT was enhanced in chimer-pretreated mice compared to poly-sensitized controls (Fig. 6A). Increased Foxp3 expression was detected in SLT and BM of chimer-pretreated mice (Fig. 6B).

Application of anti-TGF-β, anti-IL10R or anti-CD25 blocking antibodies significantly abrogated the suppression of IL-5 and IL-4 production in spleen cell cultures of chimer-treated mice (Fig. 7A). Furthermore anti-TGF-β treatment of chimer-treated mice led to diminished antigen-specific and total IgA levels in sera (Fig. 7B).

Treg cells isolated from chimer-treated mice exhibited stronger suppressive potential as Treg cells from poly-sensitized mice (Fig. 8). The percent suppression mediated by Treg cells isolated from chimer-treated mice was 4.8-fold higher (ratio 1/2) than Tregs derived from poly-sensitized mice.

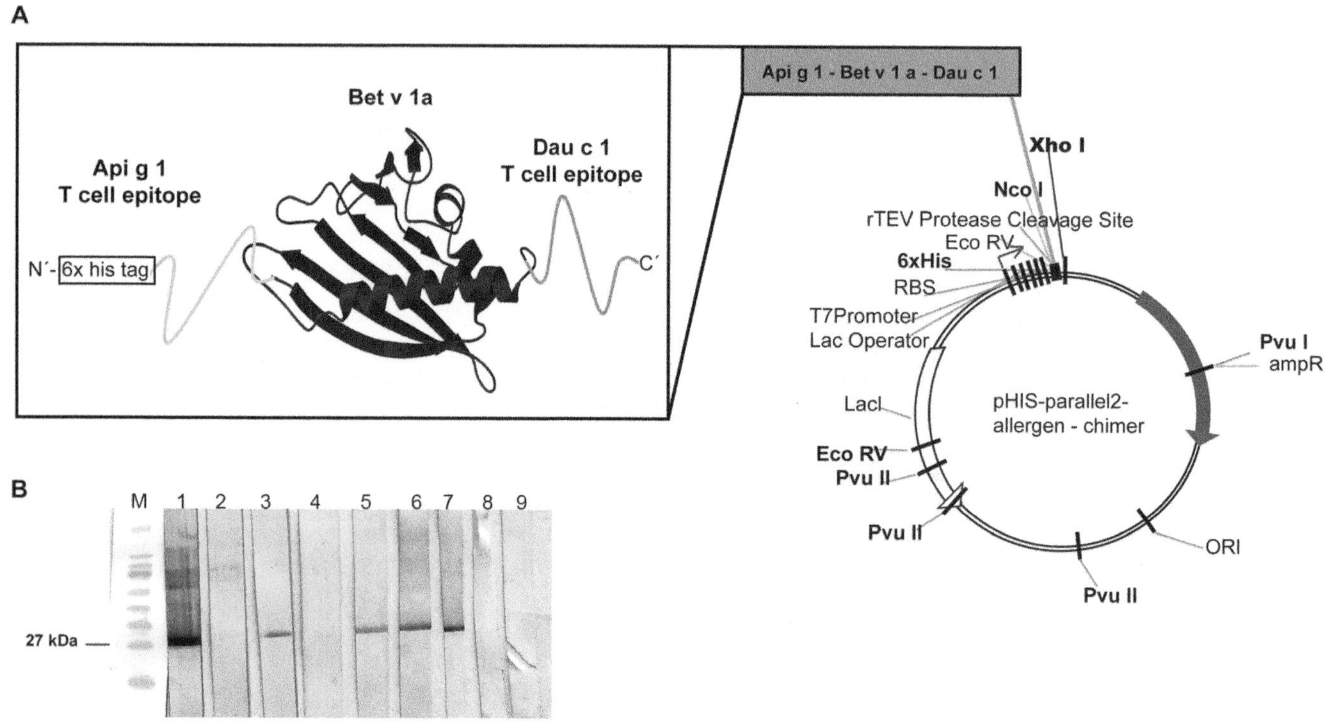

Figure 3. Construction and characterization of the pollen-food-chimer. (**A**) Design of the *pHis-parallel 2*-chimer composed of Bet v 1 protein, flanked by peptides from Api g 1 and Dau c 1. (**B**) Immunoblot: IgE binding to the chimer of sera from chimer-pretreated/poly-sensitized mice (lane 1) and of BP allergic patients with BPRFA (lane 5, 6, 7), and of Bet v 1 monoclonal antibody (lane 3). Negative controls sera from untreated mouse and non-allergic patient, or buffer control were run in parallel (lane 2, 4, 8. 9).

Discussion

Clinical data regarding the efficacy of specific immunotherapy (SIT) with BP against pollen-related food allergies provide controversial results: While it has been shown that SIT with BP extract could achieve good effects in mono-sensitized patients [23], SIT in multi-sensitized patients with BPRFA often provided only limited success on the food-related symptoms [6,7,24]. Bucher et al. attributed this observation to the reason that BPRFA is not only caused by Bet v 1-cross reactive allergens, but also due to other less well-defined cross-reactive food allergens, which are not included in BP extracts used for SIT [2]. Along these lines, Bohle et al. described the existence of exclusive food-specific T lymphocytes, additionally to BP-reactive T cells in pollen-food multi-sensitized patients and suggested this finding to be one of the reasons why allergic symptoms of pollen-related food allergens are not modulated by BP SIT [1].

Here we describe a murine model for BPRFA which enables us to study the role of both IgE and T cells responses in sensitization to Bet v 1 and Bet v 1-related food allergens as well as the efficacy of prevention of multi-sensitization using a novel allergen chimer covering the major T cell epitopes of Bet v 1, Dau c 1 and Api g 1 (Fig. 1, Fig. 3A).

In order to mimic the clinical situation of BPRFA with OAS, mice were challenged sublingually with pollen and food extracts. Our data show that the sensitization protocol led to systemic Th2-biased immune responses as well as local immune responses to Bet v 1, Api g 1 and Dau c 1. Similarly as seen in humans, we observed that mucosal application of the single allergens, in particular with Bet v 1, did not reduce the allergic responses to the related food allergens indicating that other than Bet v 1 epitopes are necessary for successful prevention of BPRFA (Fig. 2A). Furthermore, a mixture of the allergens also did not suppress the immune responses to all allergens (Fig. 2B). A similar negative interference between several protein allergens was previously described by us, when intranasally applying a mixture of birch and grass pollen allergens aiming to prevent allergic poly-sensitization to these allergens [8]. The failure to prevent allergic poly-sensitization with the allergen mixture pointed out the necessity for creating multi-allergen constructs.

Therefore, we engineered a pollen-food chimer, composed of the Bet v 1 protein as scaffold for linkage of the immunodominant T cell epitopes of Api g 1 and Dau c 1 (Fig. 3A). Of notice, these immunodominant T cell epitopes in mice are located in regions of the dominant T cell sequences of humans with BPRFA [22,25].

Mucosal application of the chimer led to a marked immuno-modulation characterized by a shift towards Th1 immune responses (increase in IgG2a) accompanied by a significant down-regulation of allergen-specific IgE to all three allergens (Fig. 4A/B). In accordance, reduced antigen-specific IL-4 and IL-5 levels versus significantly enhanced antigen-specific IFN-γ levels were observed in restimulated spleens and CLNs after chimer pretreatment (Fig. 5). These findings are in line with our previous studies in poly-sensitized mice using either poly-peptides, hybrid peptides or allergen chimers for prevention of poly-sensitization [8,10]. Additionally, intranasal pretreatment with the chimer increased IgA antibody levels primarily in sera (Fig. 4C) and less at the mucosal sites (data not shown). This might be explained by a matter of increased systemic circulation due to the highly vascularized tissue of the oral cavity, as it has been suggested in humans [26]. Studies by Pilette et al. showed that successful SIT positively correlates with increased serum IgA antibodies [27]. There is evidence that TGF-β plays a major role in IgA

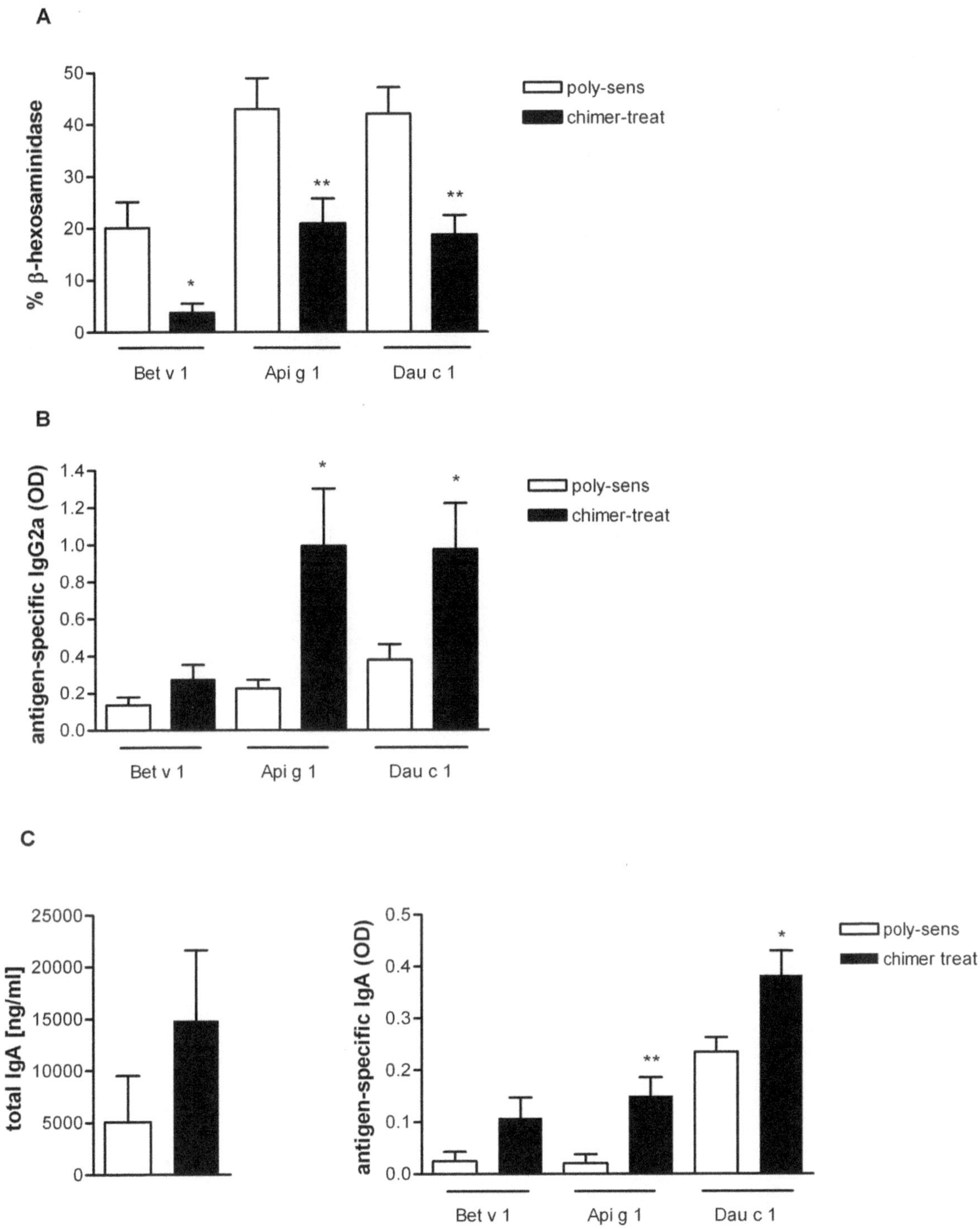

Figure 4. Antigen-specific cellular and humoral responses in mice pretreated with the chimer and poly-sensitized control mice. (A) IgE-mediated basophil degranulation. **(B)** Allergen-specific IgG2a antibodies in sera. **(C)** Total and antigen-specific IgA antibodies in sera. Chimer-pretreated mice (black bars); poly-sensitized control mice (white bars). $^{*}p<0.05$, $^{**}p<0.01$.

production [28,29]. Indeed, we have shown that the application of anti-TGF-β antibody to chimer-treated mice reduced IgA levels in sera (Fig. 7B).

Regarding the mechanisms of chimer-induced immunomodulation, we detected an upregulation of TGF-β, IL-10 and Foxp3 mRNA levels in the NALT (Fig. 6A). Additionally, increased Foxp3 mRNA expression occurred in sublingual tissue and the buccal mucosa (Fig. 6B). This is in line with our former data showing that immunomodulation with a grass-birch pollen chimer but also with Bet v 1 alone is mediated by Treg cells [8,9]. The clinical relevance of this finding is supported by human studies showing an increase of regulatory Foxp3-positive T cells in the nasal mucosa of patients after successful systemic as well as sublingual grass pollen SIT [30,31]. In the latter study it was suggested that regulatory T cells either migrate from draining lymph nodes to the sublingual tissue during SLIT or may be

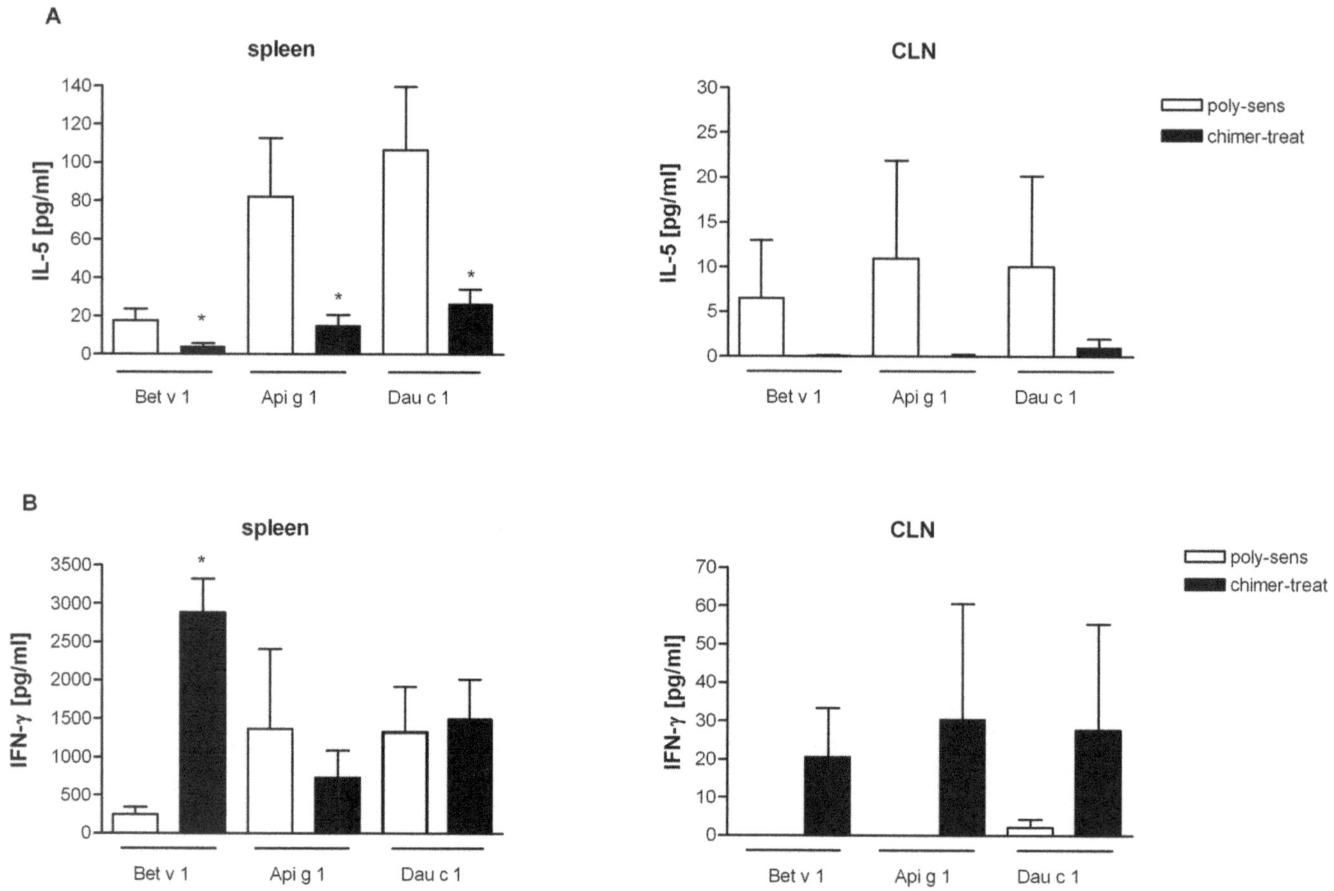

Figure 5. Antigen-specific cytokine production in mice pretreated with the chimer and poly-sensitized mice. (**A**) IL-5 levels and (**B**) IFN-γ levels in supernatants of spleen and cervical lymph nodes (CLN) cell cultures after antigen stimulation. Chimer-pretreated mice (black bars); poly-sensitized control mice (white bars). $^{*}p<0.05$, $^{**}p<0.01$.

induced by local dendritic cell-T cell interactions after repeated allergen exposure via the oral mucosa [31]. Furthermore, it was shown that sublingual treatment with allergens led to induction of IL-10 and TGF-β-releasing cells within the oral and nasal mucosa [31].

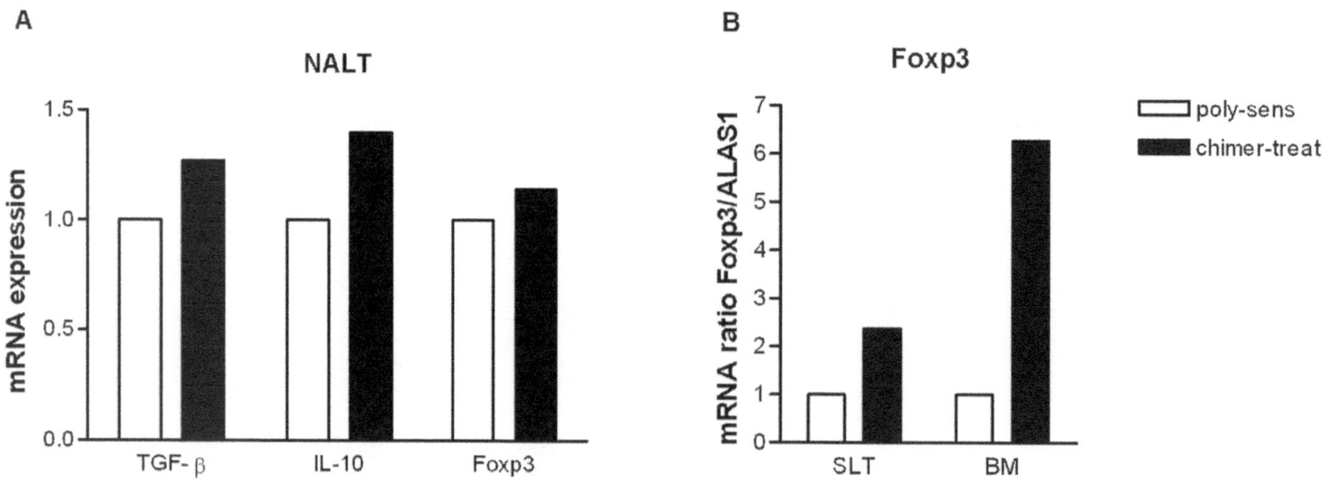

Figure 6. mRNA expression levels of regulatory markers on inductive and local effector sites. (**A**) TGF-β, IL-10 and Foxp3 mRNA expression in NALT, and (**B**) Foxp3 mRNA expression in SLT and BM of chimer-pretreated mice (black bars), shown as relative values in comparison with poly-sensitized controls (white bars). Data are presented as relative ratio of the target genes to the housekeeping gene *Alas1*.

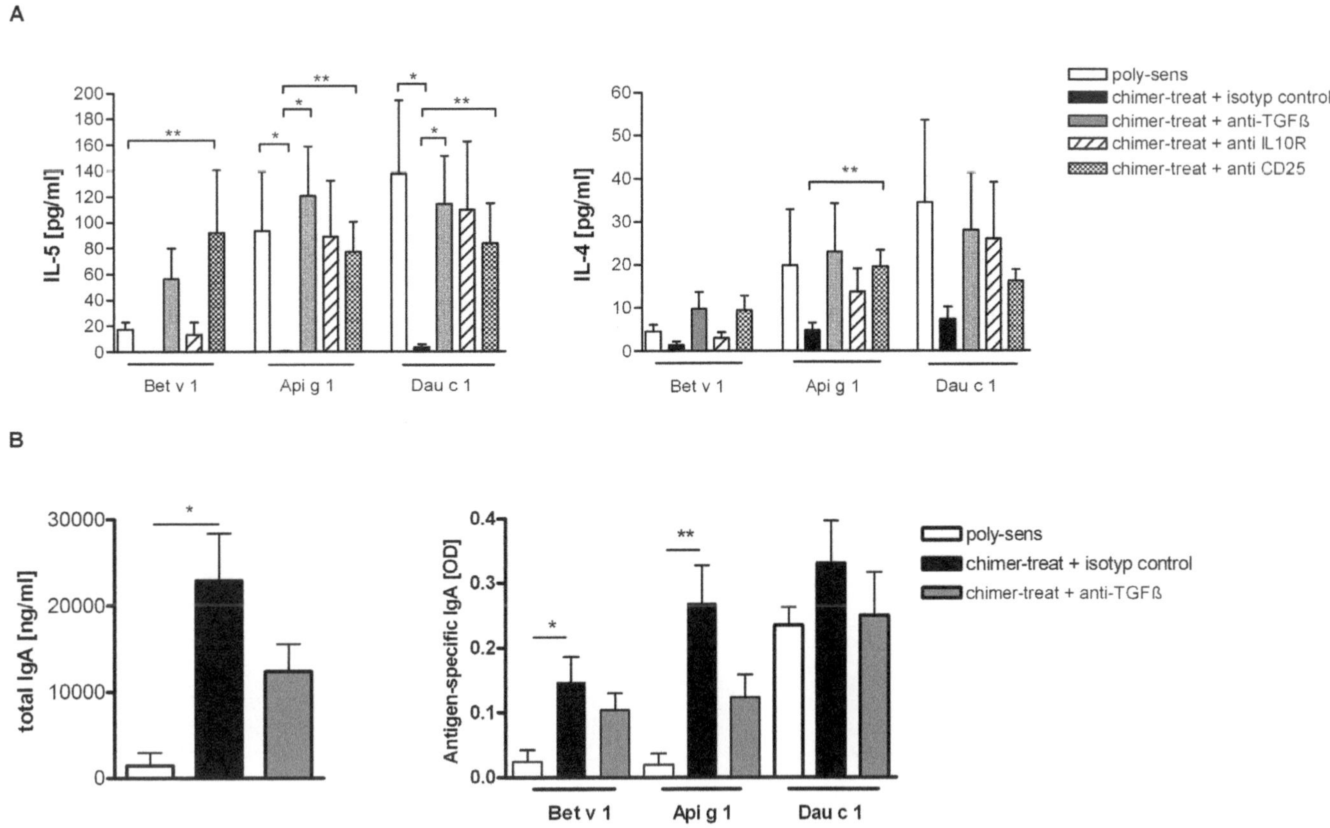

Figure 7. Effects of blocking antibodies. (**A**) Effects of anti-TGF-β, anti-IL-10R and anti-CD25 on levels of IL-5 and IL-4 in supernatants of antigen-stimulated spleen cell cultures. (**B**) Effects of anti-TGF-β on total and antigen-specific IgA production in sera. Chimer-pretreated mice treated with isotype control antibody (black bars) in comparison with chimer-pretreated and anti-TGF-β treated mice (grey bars), anti-IL10R treated mice (striped bars) and anti-CD25 treated mice (dotted bars). Poly-sensitized control group (white bars). *p<0.05, **p<0.01.

In order to investigate the immunosuppressive capacity of chimer-induced regulatory T cells in our BPRFA model, neutralizing antibodies against $CD25^+$ T cells, TGF-β and IL-10R were injected after mucosal application of the chimer and/or poly-sensitization in mice (Fig. 7A). Indeed, each of these antibodies significantly abrogated the suppressive effect of the chimer pretreatment, indicating that $CD25^+$-T cells, TGF-β as well as IL-10 play a potential role in immunomodulation for the prevention of BPRFA. Consistent with this, a study in house dust mite allergic patients showed that application of IL-10 and TGF-β blocking antibodies *in vitro* abrogated the immunosuppressive effects of $CD4^+CD25^+$-T cells induced by SIT [32].

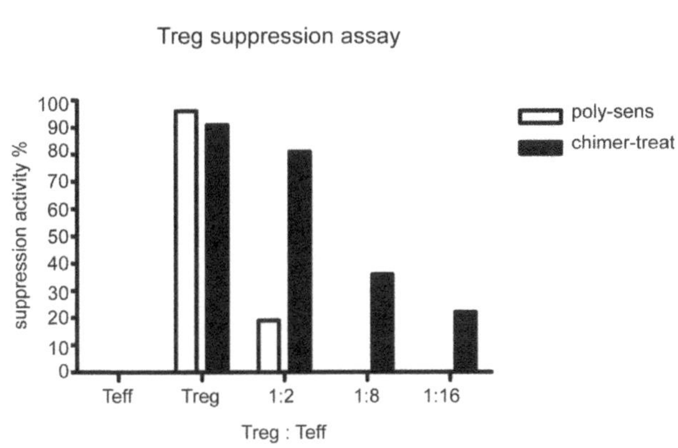

Proliferation [cpm]	Teff: Treg		
	1:2	1:8	1:16
poly-sens	6741 ± 407,32	9391 ± 810,86	9472 ± 1614,86
chimer-treat	392 ± 259,94***	1308 ± 645,97***	1595 ± 765,07***

*** *p* values < 0,001; using One-way-Anova test.

Figure 8. Characterization of Treg cells by Treg suppression assay. Suppressive activity of Treg cells derived from chimer-treated mice (black bars) and poly-sensitized controls (white bars). Purified $CD4^+CD25^-$ T effector cells (Teff) and $CD4^+CD25^+$ T regulatory cells (Treg) were obtained by cell sorting (MACS), then cultured alone or cocultured in three different ratios (Treg:Teff: 1:2, 1:8, 1:16) in combination with irradiated splenocytes and stimulated by anti-CD3 antibody, before pulsing with [^{3}H] thymidine. The percent suppression mediated by Treg cells is calculated by the following formula: [(cpm of Teff alone – cpm of Teff treated with Treg)/cpm of Teff cells alone]*100.

Allergic diseases have been linked with deficiency in function of Tregs [33]. Indeed we have shown that chimer-induced Tregs have higher suppression potential in comparison to Tregs derived from poly-sensitized mice (Fig. 8).

Taken together, we constructed an allergen-chimer for prevention of multiple sensitizations to pollen and pollen-related food allergens. We demonstrated that mucosally applied chimers covering important pollen and food-related epitopes can be used to down-regulate/prevent systemic and local allergic immune responses to all allergens, most likely by a combined induction of regulatory pathways and Th1-biased immune responses. Such mucosal allergen constructs might therefore provide promising new tools for mucosal intervention against different levels of multi-sensitization, including the birch pollen-related food allergy.

Acknowledgments

We thank our technical assistant Onisa Ul-haq for her support with all animal experiments; Gerlinde Hofstetter, who helped to prepare the food extracts; to Merima Bublin for her support with FPLC, to Sonja Gaier for her support with the CD, and to Birgit Wagner for her support with protein expression.

Author Contributions

Conceived and designed the experiments: UW. Performed the experiments: EH KH JJ IS. Analyzed the data: EH KH IS UW. Contributed reagents/materials/analysis tools: KHS BB RMM UW. Wrote the paper: EH UW.

References

1. Bohle B (2007) The impact of pollen-related food allergens on pollen allergy. Allergy 62: 3–10.
2. Bucher X, Pichler WJ, Dahinden CA, Helbling A (2004) Effect of tree pollen specific, subcutaneous immunotherapy on the oral allergy syndrome to apple and hazelnut. Allergy 59: 1272–1276.
3. Hoffmann-Sommergruber K (2000) Plant allergens and pathogenesis-related proteins. What do they have in common? Int Arch Allergy Immunol 122: 155–166.
4. Steinman H (2009) Oral allergy syndrome - whats new? Current Allergy & Clinical Immunology 22.
5. Geroldinger-Simic M, Zelniker T, Aberer W, Ebner C, Egger C, et al. (2011) Birch pollen-related food allergy: clinical aspects and the role of allergen-specific IgE and IgG4 antibodies. J Allergy Clin Immunol 127: 616–622 e611.
6. Hansen KS, Khinchi MS, Skov PS, Bindslev-Jensen C, Poulsen LK, et al. (2004) Food allergy to apple and specific immunotherapy with birch pollen. Mol Nutr Food Res 48: 441–448.
7. Mauro M, Russello M, Incorvaia C, Gazzola G, Frati F, et al. (2011) Birch-apple syndrome treated with birch pollen immunotherapy. Int Arch Allergy Immunol 156: 416–422.
8. Wild C, Wallner M, Hufnagl K, Fuchs H, Hoffmann-Sommergruber K, et al. (2007) A recombinant allergen chimer as novel mucosal vaccine candidate for prevention of multi-sensitivities. Allergy 62: 33–41.
9. Winkler B, Hufnagl K, Spittler A, Ploder M, Kallay E, et al. (2006) The role of Foxp3+ T cells in long-term efficacy of prophylactic and therapeutic mucosal tolerance induction in mice. Allergy 61: 173–180.
10. Hufnagl K, Winkler B, Focke M, Valenta R, Scheiner O, et al. (2005) Intranasal tolerance induction with polypeptides derived from 3 noncross-reactive major aeroallergens prevents allergic polysensitization in mice. J Allergy Clin Immunol 116: 370–376.
11. Bublin M, Radauer C, Wilson IB, Kraft D, Scheiner O, et al. (2003) Cross-reactive N-glycans of Api g 5, a high molecular weight glycoprotein allergen from celery, are required for immunoglobulin E binding and activation of effector cells from allergic patients. Faseb J 17: 1697–1699.
12. Wiedermann U, Jahn-Schmid B, Bohle B, Repa A, Renz H, et al. (1999) Suppression of antigen-specific T- and B-cell responses by intranasal or oral administration of recombinant bet v 1, the major birch pollen allergen, in a murine model of type I allergy. J Allergy Clin Immunol 103: 1202–1210.
13. Hufnagl K, Wagner B, Winkler B, Baier K, Hochreiter R, et al. (2003) Induction of mucosal tolerance with recombinant Hev b 1 and recombinant Hev b 3 for prevention of latex allergy in BALB/c mice. Clin Exp Immunol 133: 170–176.
14. Leech MD, Benson RA, De Vries A, Fitch PM, Howie SE (2007) Resolution of Der p1-induced allergic airway inflammation is dependent on CD4+CD25+Foxp3+ regulatory cells. J Immunol 179: 7050–7058.
15. Wilson MS, Taylor MD, Balic A, Finney CA, Lamb JR, et al. (2005) Suppression of allergic airway inflammation by helminth-induced regulatory T cells. J Exp Med 202: 1199–1212.
16. Taher YA, van Esch BC, Hofman GA, Henricks PA, van Oosterhout AJ (2008) 1alpha,25-dihydroxyvitamin D3 potentiates the beneficial effects of allergen immunotherapy in a mouse model of allergic asthma: role for IL-10 and TGF-beta. J Immunol 180: 5211–5221.
17. Wiedermann U, Herz U, Baier K, Vrtala S, Neuhaus-Steinmetz U, et al. (2001) Intranasal treatment with a recombinant hypoallergenic derivative of the major birch pollen allergen Bet v 1 prevents allergic sensitization and airway inflammation in mice. Int Arch Allergy Immunol 126: 68–77.
18. Asanuma H, Thompson AH, Iwasaki T, Sato Y, Inaba Y, et al. (1997) Isolation and characterization of mouse nasal-associated lymphoid tissue. J Immunol Methods 202: 123–131.
19. Cuburu N, Kweon MN, Song JH, Hervouet C, Luci C, et al. (2007) Sublingual immunization induces broad-based systemic and mucosal immune responses in mice. Vaccine 25: 8598–8610.
20. Winkler B, Baier K, Wagner S, Repa A, Eichler HG, et al. (2002) Mucosal tolerance as therapy of type I allergy: intranasal application of recombinant Bet v 1, the major birch pollen allergen, leads to the suppression of allergic immune responses and airway inflammation in sensitized mice. Clin Exp Allergy 32: 30–36.
21. Hufnagl K, Focke M, Gruber F, Hufnagl P, Loupal G, et al. (2008) Airway inflammation induced after allergic poly-sensitization can be prevented by mucosal but not by systemic administration of poly-peptides. Clin Exp Allergy 38: 1192–1202.
22. Jahn-Schmid B, Radakovics A, Luttkopf D, Scheurer S, Vieths S, et al. (2005) Bet v 1142–156 is the dominant T-cell epitope of the major birch pollen allergen and important for cross-reactivity with Bet v 1-related food allergens. J Allergy Clin Immunol 116: 213–219.
23. Asero R (1998) Effects of birch pollen-specific immunotherapy on apple allergy in birch pollen-hypersensitive patients. Clin Exp Allergy 28: 1368–1373.
24. Walker SM, Durham SR, Till SJ, Roberts G, Corrigan CJ, et al. (2011) Immunotherapy for allergic rhinitis. Clin Exp Allergy 41: 1177–1200.
25. Bohle B, Radakovics A, Jahn-Schmid B, Hoffmann-Sommergruber K, Fischer GF, et al. (2003) Bet v 1, the major birch pollen allergen, initiates sensitization to Api g 1, the major allergen in celery: evidence at the T cell level. Eur J Immunol 33: 3303–3310.
26. Moingeon P, Batard T, Fadel R, Frati F, Sieber J, et al. (2006) Immune mechanisms of allergen-specific sublingual immunotherapy. Allergy 61: 151–165.
27. Pilette C, Nouri-Aria KT, Jacobson MR, Wilcock LK, Detry B, et al. (2007) Grass pollen immunotherapy induces an allergen-specific IgA2 antibody response associated with mucosal TGF-beta expression. J Immunol 178: 4658–4666.
28. Sonoda E, Matsumoto R, Hitoshi Y, Ishii T, Sugimoto M, et al. (1989) Transforming growth factor beta induces IgA production and acts additively with interleukin 5 for IgA production. J Exp Med 170: 1415–1420.
29. Coffman RL, Lebman DA, Shrader B (1989) Transforming growth factor beta specifically enhances IgA production by lipopolysaccharide-stimulated murine B lymphocytes. J Exp Med 170: 1039–1044.
30. Radulovic S, Jacobson MR, Durham SR, Nouri-Aria KT (2008) Grass pollen immunotherapy induces Foxp3-expressing CD4+ CD25+ cells in the nasal mucosa. J Allergy Clin Immunol 121: 1467–1472, 1472 e1461.
31. Scadding GW, Shamji MH, Jacobson MR, Lee DI, Wilson D, et al. (2010) Sublingual grass pollen immunotherapy is associated with increases in sublingual Foxp3-expressing cells and elevated allergen-specific immunoglobulin G4, immunoglobulin A and serum inhibitory activity for immunoglobulin E-facilitated allergen binding to B cells. Clin Exp Allergy 40: 598–606.
32. Jutel M, Akdis M, Budak F, Aebischer-Casaulta C, Wrzyszcz M, et al. (2003) IL-10 and TGF-beta cooperate in the regulatory T cell response to mucosal allergens in normal immunity and specific immunotherapy. Eur J Immunol 33: 1205–1214.
33. Verhagen J, Akdis M, Traidl-Hoffmann C, Schmid-Grendelmeier P, Hijnen D, et al. (2006) Absence of T-regulatory cell expression and function in atopic dermatitis skin. J Allergy Clin Immunol 117: 176–183.

4

Effect of Heating and Glycation on the Allergenicity of 2S Albumins (Ara h 2/6) from Peanut

Yvonne M. Vissers[1,2]☯, Fany Blanc[3]☯, Per Stahl Skov[4], Phil E. Johnson[5], Neil M. Rigby[5], Laetitia Przybylski-Nicaise[3], Hervé Bernard[3], Jean-Michel Wal[3], Barbara Ballmer-Weber[6], Laurian Zuidmeer-Jongejan[7], Zsolt Szépfalusi[8], Janneke Ruinemans-Koerts[9], Ad P. H. Jansen[10], Huub F. J. Savelkoul[1], Harry J. Wichers[1,2,11], Alan R. Mackie[5], Clare E. N. Mills[5], Karine Adel-Patient[3]*

1 Cell Biology and Immunology Group, Wageningen University and Research Centre, Wageningen, The Netherlands, **2** Food Chemistry Group, Wageningen University and Research Centre, Wageningen, The Netherlands, **3** Unité d'Immuno-Allergie Alimentaire UR496, Département Alimentation Humaine, INRA, Jouy-en-Josas, France, **4** RefLab ApS, Copenhagen, Denmark, **5** Institute of Food Research, Norwich Research Park, Colney, Norwich, United Kingdom, **6** Allergy Unit, Department of Dermatology, University Hospital Zurich, Zurich, Switzerland, **7** Laboratory of Allergy Research, Department of Experimental Immunology, Academic Medical Centre, University of Amsterdam, Amsterdam, The Netherlands, **8** Department of Pediatrics, Medical University of Vienna, Vienna, Austria, **9** Department of Clinical Chemistry and Haematology, Rijnstate Hospital, Arnhem, The Netherlands, **10** Department of Otorhinolaryngology, Radboud University Nijmegen Medical Centre, Nijmegen, The Netherlands, **11** Food and Biobased Research, Wageningen University and Research Centre, Wageningen, The Netherlands

Abstract

Background: Peanut allergy is one of the most common and severe food allergies, and processing is known to influence the allergenicity of peanut proteins. We aimed to establish the effect of heating and glycation on the IgE-binding properties and biological activity of 2S albumins (Ara h 2/6) from peanut.

Methodology/Principal Findings: Native Ara h 2/6 was purified from raw peanuts and heated in solution (15 min, 110°C) in the presence or absence of glucose. Ara h 2 and 6 were also purified from roasted peanut. Using PBMC and sera from peanut-allergic patients, the cellular proliferative potency and IgE reactivity (reverse EAST inhibition) and functionality (basophil degranulation capacity) of allergens were assessed. Heating Ara h 2/6 at 110°C resulted in extensive denaturation, hydrolysis and aggregation of the protein, whilst Ara h 2 and 6 isolated from roasted peanut retained its native conformation. Allergen stimulation of PBMC induced proliferation and Th2 cytokine secretion which was unaffected by thermal processing. Conversely, IgE reactivity and functionality of Ara h 2/6 was decreased by heating. Whilst heating-glycation further reduced the IgE binding capacity of the proteins, it moderated their loss of histamine releasing capacity. Ara h 2 and 6 purified from roasted peanut demonstrated the same IgE reactivity as unheated, native Ara h 2/6.

Conclusions/Significance: Although no effect of processing on T-cell reactivity was observed, heat induced denaturation reduced the IgE reactivity and subsequent functionality of Ara h 2/6. Conversely, Ara h 2 and 6 purified from roasted peanut retained the structure and IgE reactivity/functionality of the native protein which may explain the allergenic potency of this protein. Through detailed molecular study and allergenicity assessment approaches, this work then gives new insights into the effect of thermal processing on structure/allergenicity of peanut proteins.

Editor: Jan-Hendrik Niess, Ulm University, Germany

Funding: The work described was carried out under the EU FP6 project "The Prevalence, Cost and Basis of Food Allergy Across Europe", EuroPrevall (Contract No. 51400). ENCM, PEJ and NR were also supported by the institute strategic programme grant to IFR from the Biological and Biotechnological Sciences Research Council in the UK. The funders had no role in study design, data collection and analysis, decision to publish, or preparation of the manuscript.

Competing Interests: The authors have declared that no competing interests exist. Per Stahl Skov is an employee of RefLab ApS, Copenhagen. There are no patents or products in development or marketed products to declare. This does not alter the authors' adherence to all the PLoS ONE policies on sharing data and materials, as detailed online in the guide for authors.

* E-mail: Karine.Adel-Patient@cea.fr

☯ These authors contributed equally to this work.

Introduction

Peanut allergy is relatively common in the USA and certain European countries with the prevalence of sensitization being estimated as 2% and clinical peanut allergy as 1.2% of 3–4 years old children in the UK [1]. Whilst the incidence appears to be stabilising in the UK [1], it is still rising in the USA [2]. The peanut 2S albumins Ara h 2 and Ara h 6 together with a third low abundance 2S albumin, Ara h 7 have been identified as major peanut allergens [3,4,5]. Ara h 2 and 6 comprise several isoforms of Mr 17 kDa and 15 kDa, respectively [6,7,8]. Produced as a single chain precursor they are proteolytically processed in peanut seeds into two subunits linked by intramolecular disulphide bonds [6,9]. Ara h 2, 6 and 7 are all members of the prolamin superfamily and share a characteristic cysteine skeleton with at least 8 conserved cysteine residues [9] and a three-dimensional structure comprising 5 α-helices arranged in a right-handed super helix. It appears this scaffold is stable to thermal processing and proteolysis [7,10,11].

Thermal processing of proteins can lead to alterations in their structure that can result in changes in their immunoreactivity/allergenicity. Typically, loss of tertiary structure is followed by reversible unfolding, while loss of secondary structure (70–80°C) leads to the formation of new intra/intermolecular interactions, rearrangements of disulfide bonds (80–90°C), and formation of aggregates (90–100°C) [12]. Heating in the presence of sugars found in the foods also leads to modification by the Maillard reaction (non-enzymatic browning). Free primary amino groups are attacked by carbonyl compounds during the Maillard reaction, leading to the formation of stable advanced glycation end products (AGE). Several studies have been performed to assess the IgE-binding capacity of purified allergens modified *in vitro* by heating and/or by Maillard reactions. In some cases, glycation of allergens enhanced their IgE binding capacity [13] or their T-cell immunogenicity [14,15] whereas in other studies, glycation had no effect or caused even decreased IgE-binding capacity [16,17]. Heating for 90 min at 100°C of recombinant refolded Ara h 2 led to a slight increase in its IgE binding capacity, which was further enhanced in the presence of glucose, maltose or ribose [18]. Heating native Ara h 2 for several days at 55°C in the presence of different sugars increased its IgE binding capacity compared to protein heated without sugar, which was related to the formation of AGE products [19]. Ara h 2 extracted from heat-processed peanut, such as roasting (140°C) was also found to enhance its IgE-binding capacity [20].

Although IgE binding capacities of modified allergens have been studied, sometimes with conflicting results, few data are available on the impact of heating on the protein structure and on the resultant biological activity of modified allergens compared to unmodified ones. In order to give new insights into the effect of thermal processing on structure/allergenicity of peanut proteins, we then purified and produced well-characterized native, heated and glycated Ara h 2/6, as well as corresponding protein from roasted peanut. Using a large panel of sera and peripheral blood mononuclear cells (PBMC) from well-characterized peanut-allergic patients recruited in different European countries, we then investigated the effect of thermal modifications on IgE reactivity of Ara h 2/6, but also on its biological activity, i.e. basophil activation, T-cell induced proliferation and cytokine production capacities.

Results

Effect of thermal processing on Ara h2/6 structure

Native Ara h 2/6 (N-Ara h 2/6) gave a far-UV CD spectrum typical of an α-helix rich protein (Figs 1A and 1B) consistent with previous studies [21] and was monomeric with a Mr of ~16 kDa (Fig. 1C) consistent with a mixed preparation of Ara h 2/6 [7]. After heating at 110°C for 5–10 min in the absence [H-Ara h 2/6, Fig. 1A] or presence [G-Ara h 2/6, Fig. 1B] of glucose secondary structure shifted toward an unordered state which dominated after 15 min heating, with a loss of both the maximum at 198 nm and the minima at 209 and 222 nm. Heating in the presence or absence of glucose also affected the aggregation state of the protein, with only ~20% of the protein remaining in its monomeric state (Fig. 1C). A broad peak eluting with a Mr ~28–30 kDa of aggregated protein, together with a smear of material of Mr 44–150 kDa corresponding to larger oligomers was observed. In addition, thermal treatment resulted in hydrolysis of the Ara h 2/6 to yield fragments of smaller size than the parent protein. Far-UV CD spectra obtained for Ara h 2 (data not shown) and Ara h 6 (Figure 1D) purified from roasted peanut were comparable and demonstrated the same α-helix rich protein structure as N-Ara h 2/6. Non-denaturating electrophoresis showed the proteins were mainly monomeric (data not shown).

In order to study the effect of heat-induced structural changes on allergenicity of 2S albumins, N-Ara h 2/6 was then further heated for 15 minutes at 110°C in the presence or absence of glucose.

Effect of thermal processing on PBMC induced proliferation and cytokine production capacity

No difference was observed between PBMC from PA or NA patients regarding differentiation markers, viability and cytokine secretion potency at the time of sampling and/or after polyclonal activation using αCD3/αCD28 antibodies (data not shown). The effect of thermal treatment on the capacity of Ara h 2/6 to stimulate T-cell proliferation and cytokine production by PBMC of peanut allergic patients was determined by culturing cells for 7 days in the presence or absence of native and thermally-modified Ara h2/6. Stimulation with Ara h 2/6 did not induce significant proliferation in the NA controls (Fig. 2A) and only three of the 12 PA subjects showed detectable numbers of Ki-67+ proliferating cells (10.5±4.8%) in the Ara h 2/6 stimulated cultures compared with medium alone (4.7±2.7). The CD4+CD25+ subset was the largest cell population present in the corresponding proliferating PBMC. Thermal treatment of N-Ara h 2/6 had no effect on its capacity to induce PBMC proliferation in the three subjects (Fig. 2B). PBMC cultures from NA subjects stimulated with the native and modified Ara h 2/6 did not show any cytokine induction for all five tested cytokines (Fig. 3 and data not shown). Conversely, IL-5 and IL-13 production was significantly and equally enhanced in PBMC cultures from 5 out of 12 PA subjects following stimulation with N-, H- or G-Ara h 2/6 (Figs 3A and 3B). Enhanced production of IL-10 and IFN-γ was observed in stimulated PBMC of PA subjects compared to NA subjects but was not significant for all stimuli tested (Figs 3C and 3D). IL-17 production was below 20 pg/ml for all tested conditions (data not shown).

Effect of thermal processing on the IgE binding capacity

Screening of the serum panel (n = 34, Table 1) showed variable levels of IgE specific to raw peanut extract and N-Ara h 2/6. Four sera with low specific IgE were excluded from subsequent analysis (sera #69, #76, #80 and #82). Effect of thermal treatment on the IgE binding capacity of Ara h 2/6 was then assessed using reverse inhibition. A typical inhibition curve for the reverse EAST assay obtained with serum #05-0209 is shown in Figure 4A and demonstrated that the thermal treatment of N-Ara h 2/6 at 110°C reduced its IgE binding capacity. Ara h 2/6 from roasted peanut (R-Ara h 2/6) had a similar albeit slightly reduced immunoreactivity to N-Ara h 2/6 from raw peanut. IC50 values calculated for the entire serum panel (n = 30) are consistent with this and show that extreme thermal processing did reduce the IgE binding capacity of Ara h 2/6 in a significant manner (Fig. 4B). The IC50 values for all tested sera increased 1.2 to 44-fold (mean = 9.6, n = 30) for H-Ara h 2/6 compared to N-Ara h 2/6 (Fig. 4 B). For 25 out the 30 tested patients, IC50 values for G-Ara h 2/6 were equivalent or 3.4-fold higher than those of H-Ara h 2/6 (mean = 1.7). For the last 5 patients, sampled in various countries, IC50 values were 1.2 to 1.7-fold lower for G-Ara h 2/6 compared to H-Ara h 2/6 (mean 1.4). These data show that for most patients glycation reduced the IgE reactivity of Ara h 2/6 still further compared with thermal treatment alone, and is consistent with the fact that IC50 values for G-Ara h 2/6 were 1.3 to 73-fold higher than that of N-Ara h 2/6 (mean = 14.5, n = 30). Ara h 2/6 from

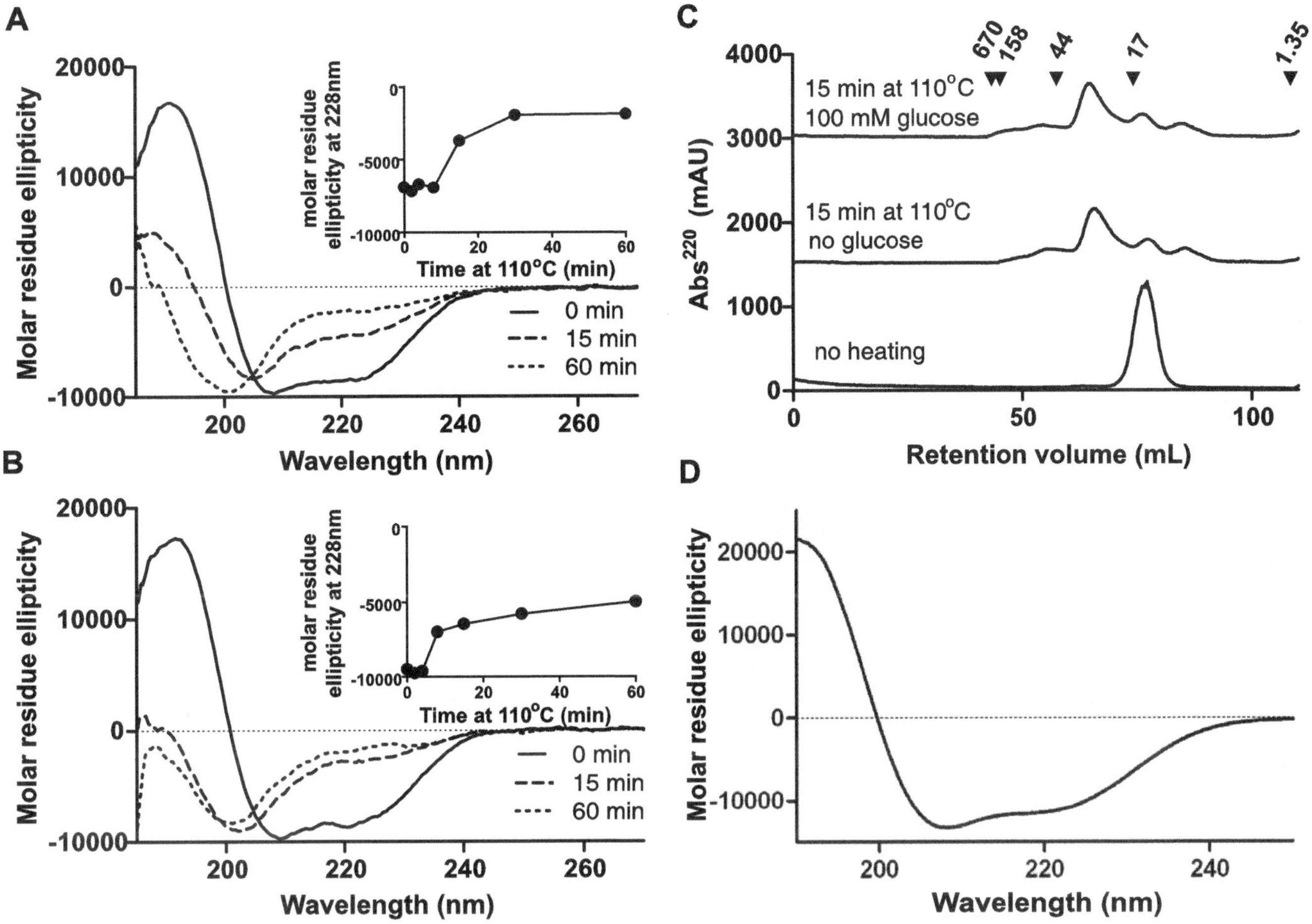

Figure 1. Effect of heating on secondary structure and oligomeric state of Ara h 2/6. Far-UV CD spectra of Ara h 2/6 heated alone (**A**, H-Ara h 2/6) or in the presence of 100 mM glucose (**B**, G-Ara h 2/6) before heating (N-Ara h 2/6, —) and for heated-cooled protein after heating to 110°C for 15 min (– – –) and 60 min (---). Inset graphs show change in molar residue ellipticity at 228 nm with heating time. Size exclusion chromatography profiles (**C**) are shown of the Ara h 2/6 before and after heating for 15 min at 110°C in the presence or absence of glucose. Retention volumes of molecular weight standards (size indicated in kDa) are shown by arrow heads. **D.** Far-UV CD spectra of Ara h 6 purified from roasted peanut.

roasted peanut (R-Ara h 2/6) had a similar albeit slightly reduced immunoreactivity to N-Ara h 2/6.

Effect of thermal processing on the mediator-releasing capacity

Subsequently an analysis of the effects of heating on the histamine releasing capacity of the Ara h 2/6 preparations was undertaken using human stripped basophils passively sensitized with 23 of the 34 peanut-allergic patients sera and compared with whole protein extract from raw or roasted peanut. No histamine release was induced by the different allergens when using a serum from patients not sensitized to peanut (data not shown), and the 23 sera from PA patients gave similar results. An example curve (serum #2305, Fig. 5A) shows significant histamine release for both extracts and purified allergens, the whole protein extract from raw and roasted peanut being comparable. As previously observed using RBL SX38 cells and Ara h 2 and Ara h 6 from roasted peanut [22], histamine release was induced at lower concentrations of these purified allergens when compared to peanut extracts. Heating reduced the biological potency of the Ara h 2/6, (Fig. 5A, $P<0.05$ when considering 23 sera), but intriguingly histamine release was induced at a lower concentration of heated-glycated than heated Ara h 2/6. The maximum histamine release induced by the purified allergens was only affected when comparing N-Ara h 2/6 to H-Ara h 2/6 ($P<0.05$ when considering the 23 sera).

Additionally, a mediator release assay using humanized Rat Basophilic Leukaemia cells was also performed using 6 individual sera. Figure 5B shows typical results of a representative serum (#70) and the inserted table represents the average protein concentrations needed to obtain 50% of the maximum mediator release induced by the native allergen (EC50). A 150 and 130 times increased EC50 value, corresponding to a decreased allergenic activity, was observed for H-Ara h 2/6 and G-Ara h 2/6, respectively, in comparison to N-Ara h 2/6. The EC50 value of G-Ara h 2/6 was lower compared to the EC50 value of H-Ara h 2/6; however, this was not tested to be significantly different.

Discussion

Boiled peanuts are consumed in many countries, from China to the Southern states of the USA. Boiling is performed for 2 to 7 hours, depending on the peanut source, and boiled peanut can be further canned, then involving further extensive heating (45 minutes at 120°C under 10 pounds pressure per square inch). Study of heat-induced structural changes and its impact on allergenicity of peanut allergens

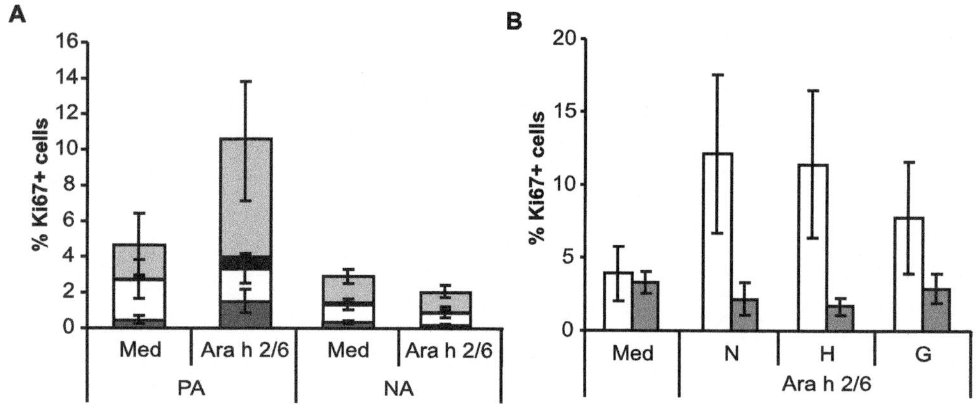

Figure 2. Effect of thermal treatment on subpopulation of proliferating cells. A. Fresh PBMC were left unstimulated (Med) or stimulated with N-Ara h 2/6 for 7 days. After harvesting, the cells were incubated with anti-CD4/CD25 antibody and afterwards stained for an anti-Ki-67 PE antibody. Data are mean percentage of Ki-67 positive cells ± SEM values for three (#65, #66 and #70) of the 12 PA subjects and seven NA controls. The percentage Ki-67+ cells was divided in the following subpopulations of cells: CD4-CD25- (dark grey bars), CD4+CD25- (white bars), CD4-CD25+ (black bars) and CD4+CD25+ (light grey) cells. **B.** Fresh PBMC were left unstimulated (Med) or stimulated with N-, H- or G-Ara h 2/6 for 7 days. Data are mean percentage of Ki-67 positive cells ± SEM values for three peanut-allergic patients (#65, #66 and #70) (white bars) and seven non-allergic controls (grey bars).

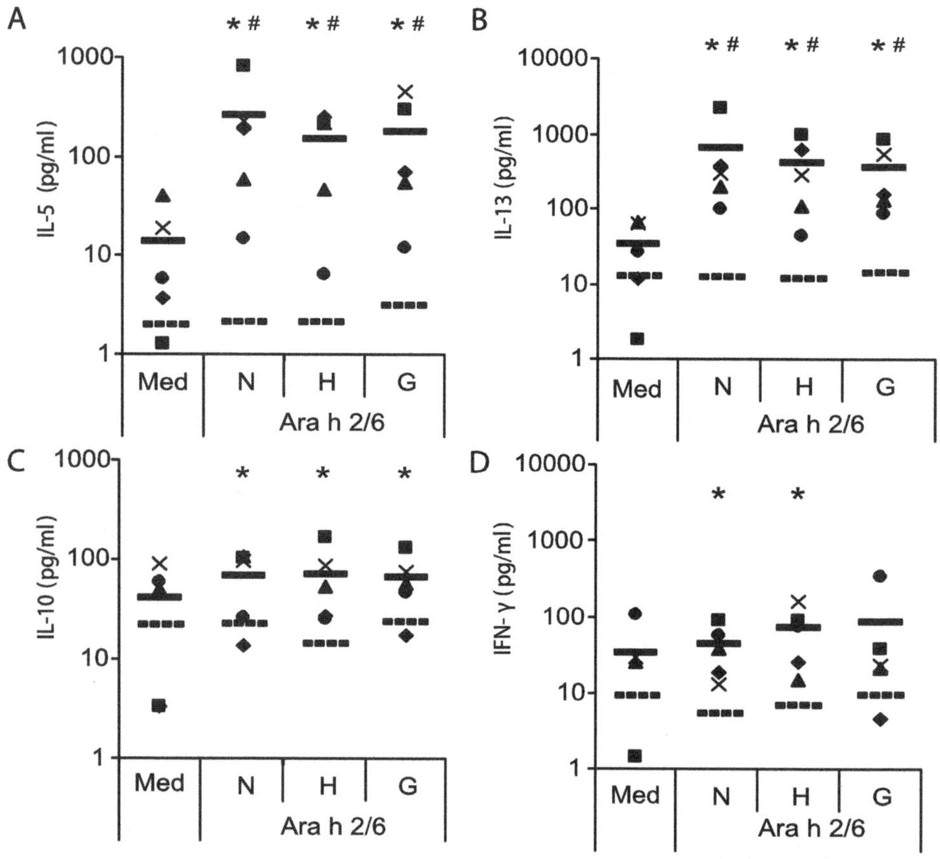

Figure 3. Effect of thermal treatment on cytokine induction capacity. Fresh PBMC were left unstimulated (Med) or stimulated with N-, H- or G-Ara h 2/6 and production of IL-5 (**A**), IL-13 (**B**), IL-10 (**C**) and IFN-γ (**D**) was measured after 7 days of culture. Symbols represent peanut-allergic patients #65 (■), #66 (♦), #70 (▲), #67 (●) and #73 (×). Horizontal bars represent the mean of the five PA responder subjects (solid) and the mean of 7 NA controls (dotted). Asterisks indicate statistically significant differences between the PA and the NA group and # indicate statistically significant differences between the medium and allergen-stimulated cultures for the PA group (*, #: $P<0.05$). No differences between the medium and allergen-stimulated cultures were observed for the NA group.

Table 1. Serological and clinical information for the 34 peanut allergic patients recruited in different European centres, within the Europrevall European project, used in EAST studies, basophil histamine release tests and/or PBMC proliferation tests.

Code	Gender (f/m)	Age	Peanut SPT (HEP index numbers)	Grade peanut allergy	Peanut RAST class	peanut CAP (IU/ml)	Anti-whole peanut IgE (IU/ml)	Anti-Ara h 2/6 IgE (IU/ml)	Other food allergies
2A	m	31	positive	3/4	5	51.7	43	31	
52A	m	41	nd	4	5	nd	166	62	
54A	f	11	2.2	1	6	>100	72	57	
55A	f	14	3.3	4	6	>100	363	137	
56A	m	16	1.5	2	6	>100	79	56	
58A	f	22	2.5	4	6	>100	171	110	Soy, lupine, pea
65	f	19	positive	3/4	6	>100	587	208	
66	m	18	positive	4	6	>100	290	71	
67	f	46	nd	3	5	54.4	95	35	Hazelnut, kiwi, cherries
68	f	20	positive	1	4	17.6	16	6	
69	m	21	positive	3/4	3	6.98	3.5	1.2	
70	f	21	positive	3/4	6	>100	224	76	Soy, pea, apple
73	f	22	positive	2/3	4	33.6	21	3.7	Hazelnut
76	m	23	positive	3	3	8.6	4.2	0.3	
77	m	25	positive	2	4	33.2	22	3.5	
78	f	24	positive	3	5	79.6	65	29	Hazelnut
80	m	27	positive	3	3	16	12	17	
82	f	18	positive	1/2	3	4.7	25	6.4	Kiwi, cherries
1682	m	33	nd	4	6	>100	13	10	
1691	m	22	nd	3	5	nd	50	54	
2207	m	28	nd	4	4	nd	38	26	Wheat, hazelnut, egg, almond
2209	f	27	nd	4	6	nd	75	51	Hazelnut, egg, wheat
2304	m	25	nd	3	6	nd	90	50	
2305	f	18	nd	4	nd	nd	52	36	
03-0043	f	20	1,54	3/4	6	>100	nd	852	Hazelnut, walnut, melon
03-0044	m	23	4,33	3	6	>100	nd	231	Egg, fish, shrimp, hazelnut, walnut, sesame, wheat, sunflower
03-0079	f	16	2,22	3	6	>100	nd	88	Pistachio, almond, brazil nut
05-0128	f	25	1,92	3	6	>100	nd	358	Soy, hazelnut, apple, peach
05-0165	f	18	0	3/4	6	>100	nd	429	Chickpea, bean, hazelnut, lentil
05-0195	m	31	2,13	3	5	63,5	nd	64	Soy
05-0209	m	20	99,98	4	5	70,2	nd	81	Pea, soy, bean
06-0010	m	19	2,2	3/4	5	67,4	nd	67	Fish
08-0069	m	17	2,08	1	6	>100	nd	139	Kiwi
12-0048	f	21	5,8	3/4	5	54,6	nd	88	Shrimp

HEP: histamine equivalent prick test; nd: not determined. Where known, other allergies of the subjects are indicated.
The origin of the sera is as follows: 2A: Zurich, 52A: Amsterdam, 54A-82: Arnhem, 1682-2305: Vienna; 03-0043 till 12-0048 EuroPrevall Serum Bank.
Grading is based on Brockow and Ring and on Sampson *et al.* [41,42]. Grade 1 = dermal symptoms; grade 2 = gastro-intestinal problems like nausea and or cramping; grade 3 = any of the former grades plus vomiting/diarrhoea and respiratory tract problems like throat pruritis or tightness, grade 4 = any of the former grades and respiratory arrest plus cardiovascular problems like hypotension.

after wet-thermal processing then appears of interest. Achieving model processing conditions to ensure that thermal modifications can be monitored by structural and immunological analysis is difficult since heating frequently renders much of the protein insoluble. This makes purification of proteins from cooked foods, such as roasted or boiled peanuts, cumbersome [23]. We then analyzed the effect of wet thermal processing on major peanut allergens, i.e. N-Ara h 2/6, previously purified from raw peanut. Like other members of the prolamin superfamily, the 2S albumin allergens of peanut appeared to be highly thermostable. The present detailed molecular study shows that these proteins only begin to unfold following heating at temperatures over 100°C, conditions which equate to boiling for extended times (longer than 15 min). After this time the protein adopts a random coil conformation and forms dimers and higher order oligomers, accompanied by hydrolysis of the peptide backbone. Such effects of thermal denaturation have been observed for other food

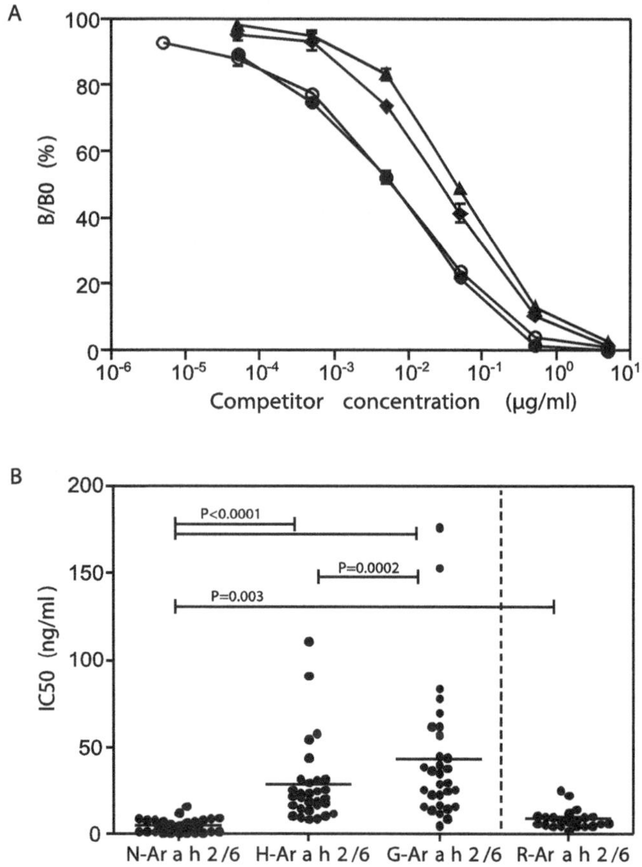

Figure 4. Effect of thermal treatment on the IgE binding capacity of Ara h 2/6. A. IgE capture inhibition curves obtained for sera #05-0209 with N-Ara h 2/6 (●), H-Ara h 2/6 (◆) or G-Ara h 2/6 (▲). IgE binding capacities of native and heated processed Ara h 2/6 was assessed by competitive assays in the IgE capture format. Inhibition was performed into microtiter plates coated with anti-IgE, and previously incubated with allergic patient sera at convenient dilution. Competition was then conducted by adding increasing concentrations of competitors at the same time as biotinylated N-Ara h 2/6. Competition obtained with Ara h 2/6 purified from roasted peanut is shown as a clear circle. **B**. Analysis of IC50 (ng/ml) values obtained using an IgE capture inhibition assay with native and heat processed Ara h 2/6 as competitors using 30 individual sera from peanut-allergic patients. Increase in IC50 value corresponds to a decrease in IgE-binding capacity. R-Ara h 2/6: mix of Ara h 2 and Ara h 6 purified from roasted peanut. Bars indicate a significant difference between the 2 corresponding treatments ($P<0.05$, non-parametric Wilcoxon signed rank test).

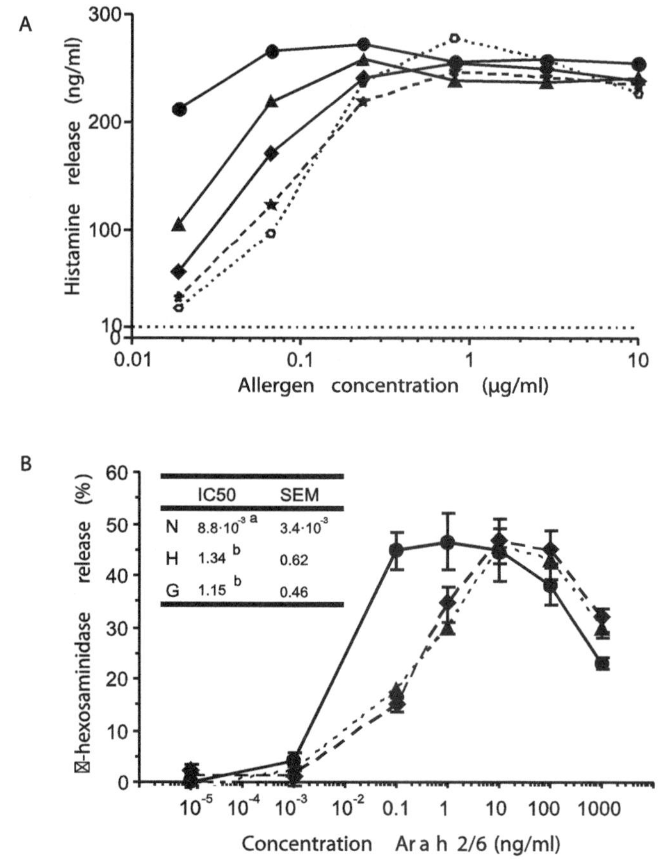

Figure 5. Effect of thermal treatment on the activation of effector cells induced by Ara h 2/6. (**A**) Human stripped basophils were passively sensitized with individual sera (#2305) and then incubated with increasing concentrations of N-Ara h 2/6 (●), H-Ara h 2/6 (◆), and G-Ara h 2/6 (▲), or whole peanut extract from raw (★) or roasted (○) peanut. Histamine release was assayed in corresponding supernatants. Twenty-three sera out of the 35 available corresponding to all sera from Zurich, Amsterdam, Vienna and EPSB, and sera 54A to 58A from Arnhem were used, giving similar results (not shown). No histamine release was induced by the different allergens when using a serum from patients not sensitized to peanut (data not shown). (**B**) Humanized RBL-2H3 cells were passively sensitized with sera from peanut-allergic patients (#70) and stimulated with increasing concentrations of native (N; –●–), heated (H; – –◆– –) or glycated (G; - - -▲- - -) Ara h 2/6. Error bars represent the SD of triplicate values. No β-hexosaminidase release was induced by the different allergens when using sera from non-allergic patients (data not shown). The table presented within the figure represents the average protein concentrations (ng/ml, n = 6) to obtain 50% of the maximum allergen release of the native allergen (EC50). Means without a common letter differ ($P<0.05$).

proteins, including the lipid transfer protein from barley which shares the same protein scaffold as the 2S albumins [24]. Interestingly, the Ara h 2 and 6 purified from roasted peanuts had retained the structural characteristics of the native protein purified from raw peanuts, as indicated by far-UV CD spectra and non-denaturing electrophoresis. In addition, proteins from roasted peanut have a similar IgE immunoreactivity as the unheated protein. These data thus demonstrate that the proportion of the protein in roasted peanut that was still soluble and then extractable had not been denatured by the roasting process, probably due to protection within the peanut seed.

In order to assess the effect of heat-induced structural changes on allergenicity of Ara h 2/6, the *in vitro* proliferation and cytokine production capacity of the native *vs* heated proteins were tested using PBMC from 12 peanut allergic (PA) and 12 control human donors. Out of the 12 PA, only 3 demonstrated significant proliferation, as assessed by Ki-67 labeling, and 5 demonstrated a significant cytokine production after *in vitro* stimulation. All of them had high levels of peanut specific IgE antibodies. This corroborates studies demonstrating a significant positive correlation between allergen-specific serum IgE levels and high numbers of IL-4-producing cells [25] or active proliferation of T cells and Th2 cytokine production [26]. However, it is worth noting that peanut-specific T-helper cells in PBMC of peanut allergic patients were found to be only 0.6% of the total CD4+ T cells [27], thus explaining the quite low rate of responders in our *ex vivo* stimulation assays. However this does not preclude that heat treatment of Ara h 2/6 did not influence cytokine production by PBMC from all of the 5 PA responders, regardless of the presence of glucose. Interestingly, internalization of glycated ovalbumin was recently studied in human dendritic cells and an increased uptake of glycated ovalbumin compared to the native protein was observed, which finally led to increased CD4+ T-cell immunogenicity of this protein [14,15]. However, in our study, monocytes are the primary antigen-presenting cell population, T cells are already primed by the proteins, and the used model allergens are different, which renders comparison difficult. Our results demonstrated that the hydrolysis, unfolding and aggregation of the Ara h 2/6 by intense heating, regardless of the presence of glucose, had no effect on stimulating the activity of PBMCs from PA-patients, as has been shown before for Bet v 1-related allergens [28,29]. This demonstrated that T-cell epitopes were still present in the modified proteins.

The IgE-binding capacity and the elicitation potency of the native *vs* heat-processed allergens were then studied using a large panel of sera from peanut allergic patients (n = 30 and 23, respectively). In fact, most of the studies aiming at analyzing the relationship between structure and allergenicity, and particularly the effect of processing on allergenicity of food proteins, generally use very few individual sera from allergic patients [18,23,30,31], even sometimes only one pool of such sera is available [11,19,32,33]. In the present study, a large population of peanut allergic patients from various European countries was involved leading to significant conclusions. Many studies have demonstrated that physicochemical modifications of proteins, e.g. resulting from processing, may impact on their IgE binding capacity. This includes denaturation or hydrolysis which may lead to the destruction of conformational epitopes, and thus to a decreased IgE binding capacity. Inversely, structural modifications may result in the unmasking of epitopes hidden in the tertiary structure of the molecule and that thus become available for IgE binding. The European Food Safety Authority opinion relating to the evaluation of allergenic foods for labelling purposes also acknowledged that the data available do not indicate whether and how food processing predictably influences allergenicity [34,35]. With regards to peanut 2S albumins, several linear epitopes have been identified for Ara h 2 [36,37,38,39] and some of them have been proposed as a marker of persistent peanut allergy [38]. However, the relative binding of IgE to the corresponding peptides *versus* to the native protein was not analyzed. Interestingly, Bernard and coworkers showed that the IgE binding capacity of Ara h 6 was decreased for all the peanut allergic patients in their study and even abolished for 25% of them when the molecule was denatured by reduction and carboxymethylation. This demonstrates the importance of conformation in the allergenicity of this protein and the presence of both conformational and linear epitopes, at least for 75% of their population [6]. In the present study, heat-induced denaturation, hydrolysis and aggregation of Ara h 2/6 result in a significant loss in IgE-binding capacity and ability of the protein to elicit histamine release for all tested sera. Altogether, these results suggest that IgE responses in peanut-allergic individuals are mainly directed towards the natively folded protein. Hydrolysis and oligomerisation observed after heating with or without glucose, may have led to further linear epitope degradation and masking. Thus, it appears that the sensitizing agent driving B-cell responses in this population was mainly native Ara h 2/6 which may have originated from either consumption of raw nuts, or more probably, represent the fraction of Ara h 2/6 that remains soluble and in its native state even after roasting. However, this also indicates that thermal processing can reduce the allergenic activity of peanut proteins, and may explain why processes such as boiling of peanuts, can reduce their allergenic activity [32].

This study showed that glycation in conjunction with thermal denaturation generally led to a further decrease of IgE binding capacity, rather than the increase found by others [18,40], although glycation did appear to preserve slightly more of the proteins mediator releasing capacity compared with heating alone. Some of these differences may relate to the wet-thermal processing procedures employed in this study. Further investigation using heat-denaturation of Ara h 2/6 under low moisture conditions will be required to explain these differences more fully.

In conclusion, heating to temperatures able to denature Ara h 2/6 caused a significant decrease in the proteins allergenicity whereas T cell stimulation was not affected which can render these modified proteins attractive for immunotherapy. It is evident that a soluble fraction of the Ara h 2/6 from roasted peanuts retains the conformation and allergenic activity of the native protein, explaining the allergenic potency of this protein.

Materials and Methods

Ethics statement

A written informed consent was obtained before the sample collection (serum or serum and PBMC) and the performed experiments were approved by the corresponding local ethical committees (Kantonale Ethikkommission Zürich, Medical ethical committee of the Amsterdam Medical Centre, Ethics Committee of Medical University of Vienna, Commissie Mensgebonden Onderzoek regio Arnhem-Nijmegen).

Patient characteristics

Thirty-four peanut-allergic (PA) patients (17 males and 17 females, mean age: 23 years) were recruited in Zurich, Amsterdam, Vienna and Arnhem, or were provided by the Europrevall Serum Bank (EPSB) (table 1). Peanut allergy was established using clinical history, physical examination, peanut specific IgE (ImmunoCAP and/or RAST (Phadia AB)) and/or objective clinical manifestations observed after peanut ingestion. Grading of food-induced anaphylaxis was according to severity of clinical symptoms [41,42]. Twelve PA subjects and 12 non-allergic (NA) controls, all recruited from the Allergology Practice Arnhem (APA, The Netherlands), donated cells for PBMC cultures.

Peanut 2S albumins (Ara h 2/6) preparations

Native 2S albumins containing both Ara h 2 and Ara h 6 (N-Ara h 2/6) were purified from unroasted redskin type peanut as described previously [21] and stored at −20°C prior to use. This purification involves ammonium sulphate fractionation and gel-filtration chromatography, avoiding the use of denaturing conditions such as reverse phase HPLC. Allergen identity was confirmed by in gel-trypsin digestion and MALDI mass spectrometry. Ara h 2 and Ara h 6 were purified from commercial roasted peanut as previously described [20] which involves anion exchange chromatography in 4 M urea followed by reverse phase HPLC, and then mixed (62% Ara h 2 and 38% Ara h 6) in proportions representative of proportions found in peanut [43] to provide a preparation further referred to as R-Ara h 2/6.

Proteins were standardized according to BCA kit from Pierce, following provider recommendations.

Heating and glycation treatments of peanut 2S albumins (Ara h 2/6)

Native Ara h 2/6 (N-Ara h 2/6, 4 mg/ml) in 32.5 mM phosphate buffer containing 100 mM NaCl, was heated for 15 min to 110°C alone (H-Ara h 2/6) or in the presence of 100 mM glucose (G-Ara h 2/6). Heating in the presence of glucose was undertaken to glycate the protein based on a previously used protocol [44]. Protein solutions were allowed to cool to room temperature prior to analysis.

Biochemical characterization of native and modified Ara h 2/6

Changes in Ara h 2/6 secondary structure were assessed using far-UV (190–260 nm) circular dichroism (CD) spectroscopy using either a J-710 or a JASCO-810 spectropolarimeter (Jasco Ltd., Japan) as previously described [7,21]. All data were calculated in terms of molar ellipticity. Aggregation state was monitored using size exclusion chromatography on a Superdex-75 column attached to an Äkta Basic FPLC (Amersham Biosciences, Little Chalfont, UK) [21], and calibrated with a set of gel filtration molecular weight standards (BioRad, Hertfordshire, UK).

Isolation, culture and stimulation of human peripheral blood mononuclear cells

PBMC were isolated and cultured as previously described [45]. Immunological phenotyping of freshly isolated PBMC was performed on a FACS Canto II (BD Pharmingen, San Diego, USA), using monoclonal antibodies and the procedure from BD Pharmingen (San Diego, USA). Stimuli were incubated for at least 30 min with polymyxin B (50 μg/ml, Sigma, Zwijndrecht, The Netherlands) to remove potential endotoxin activity prior to addition of the stimuli to the PBMC. PBMC were stimulated with αCD3/αCD28 (150 ng/ml αCD3, 100 ng/ml αCD28) or N-, H- or G-Ara h 2/6 (20 μg/ml) and supernatants harvested after 4 and 7 days of culture and stored at −80°C. The 20 μg/ml dose was determined as optimal in preliminary studies using doses ranging from 5 to 40 μg/ml (data not shown). The specificity of the proliferative and cytokine production capacities were assessed in a pilot study using PBMC from 5 peanut allergic patients with 2 control proteins (ovalbumin and purified 7S globulin from soy (Gly m 5), 20 μg/ml). No differences between the medium control and the control proteins with respect to cytokine induction and proliferation were observed. Early apoptosis and late apoptosis/necrosis was assessed on freshly prepared and 7 day cultured cells using double staining with APC-Annexin V and propidium iodide (PI) [46]. PBMC proliferation was studied on day 4 and day 7 by analysis of intracellular expression of the nuclear Ki-67 antigen (BD Pharmingen, San Diego, USA) [46] of PBMC previously stained with anti-CD4/CD25 antibody. Ki-67 expression by $CD4^+$ and $CD25^+$ cells was then determined by flow cytometry.

Cytokine analysis

Cytokine production by PBMC was analysed in supernatants of cells cultured for 4 and 7 days. The production of IL-5, IL-10, IL-13, IFN-γ and IL-17 by PBMC cultures was determined in harvested supernatants using Cytometric Bead Array (CBA, BD Biosciences, San Diego, CA) on a FACSCanto II cytometer and the procedure was performed according to the manufacturer's protocol. Preliminary experiments demonstrated low specific induction of IL-4 that correlated to higher specific induction of IL-5 and IL-13, all indicative of Th2 cellular responses. Therefore, IL-4 was not determined in the full experiments using PBMC from 12 NA and 12 PA donors. The detection limit was 1.1 pg/ml for IL-5, 0.13 pg/ml for IL-10, 0.6 pg/ml for IL-13, 1.8 pg/ml for IFN-γ and 0.3 pg/ml for IL-17.

IgE immunoreactivity

Concentrations of IgE specific to whole protein extract from raw peanut and to N-Ara h 2/6 were determined using enzyme allergosorbent tests (EAST) as previously described [3,20].

Reverse EAST inhibition was performed as described elsewhere [47] using anti-human IgE (mouse monoclonal, clone LE27) as a capture antibody, biotinylated N-Ara h 2/6 (200 ng/ml) as tracer and N-, H-, G- or R-Ara h 2/6 as inhibitors. N-Ara h 2/6 was labelled with biotin using EZ-link sulfo-NHS-LC biotin (Pierce, Rockford, IL). Assays were developed using streptavidin labelled with acetylcholine esterase (AChE) and Ellman's reagent. The absorbance of each well was measured at 414 nm and results expressed as $B/B0$, where $B0$ and B represent the amount of native Ara h 2/6 tracer bound to captured IgE in the absence or presence of a known concentration of inhibitor, respectively.

Effector cells activation by natural and modified allergens

Basophil histamine release (BHR) tests were performed as described in [49] using stripped basophils from fresh buffy coats (Blood Bank, National University Hospital of Copenhagen, Denmark) and reagents from RefLab (Copenhagen, Denmark). Twenty-three sera out of the 34 available were used individually in the BHR test, corresponding to all sera from Zurich, Amsterdam, Vienna and EPSB, and sera 54A to 58A from Wageningen.

RBL-2H3 cells expressing the α-chain of the human FcεRI receptor [49] were kindly provided by Drs. Vieths and Vogel (Paul-Ehrlich-Institut, Langen, Germany). RBL cells were cultured in MEM medium supplemented with 5% fetal calf serum and 1% glutamine (all from Gibco-BRL, Paisley, UK) at 37°C in a humidified atmosphere with 5% CO_2. Cells in stationary growth phase were harvested and plated in 96-well plates at 1.5×10^5 cell/well. Six sera from PA patients (#65, #66, #67, #70, #55A and #56A) at pre-determined convenient dilutions and two sera from non-allergic patients were added and incubated overnight to passively sensitize the cells. After washing, the cells were stimulated for 1 h with the allergens diluted in Tyrode's buffer containing 50% deuterium oxide [49]. The antigen-specific release was quantified by measuring β-hexosaminidase activity and expressed as percentage of the total β-hexosaminidase content that was obtained by lysing the cells with Triton-X100 (Sigma-Aldrich, Zwijndrecht, The Netherlands). The release data were fitted to four-parameter-logistic curves by non-linear regression using the SigmaPlot 10.0 software package, and EC50 values were calculated accordingly.

Statistical analysis

Statistical analysis was performed by using SPSS (v18.0, SPSS Inc., Chicago, USA) or GraphPad Prism v4.00 for Windows (GraphPad Software, San Diego, CA). Means and medians were analysed using Wilcoxon signed rank test for specific IgE levels and PBMC cytokine production and the Mann-Witney U test for comparing PBMC cytokine production between PA and the control patient groups. Differences were interpreted as significant when $P<0.05$.

Acknowledgments

We wish to thank Kurt Quartz for organization of the trial within Rijnstate Hospital, The Netherlands.

Author Contributions

Conceived and designed the experiments: YMV FB HFJS HJW ARM CENM KA-P. Performed the experiments: YMV FB PEJ NMR LP-N PSS HB KA-P. Analyzed the data: YMV FB HFJS CENM LP-N HB KA-P. Contributed reagents/materials/analysis tools: BB-W LZ-J ZS JR-K APHJ. Wrote the paper: YMV CENM KA-P. Contributed to final manuscript: J-MW HFJS HJW.

References

1. Venter C, Hasan Arshad S, Grundy J, Pereira B, Bernie Clayton C, et al. (2010) Time trends in the prevalence of peanut allergy: three cohorts of children from the same geographical location in the UK. Allergy 65: 103–108.
2. Sicherer SH, Munoz-Furlong A, Godbold JH, Sampson HA (2010) US prevalence of self-reported peanut, tree nut, and sesame allergy: 11-year follow-up. J Allergy Clin Immunol 125: 1322–1326.
3. Bernard H, Paty E, Mondoulet L, Burks AW, Bannon GA, et al. (2003) Serological characteristics of peanut allergy in children. Allergy 58: 1285–1292.
4. Flinterman AE, van Hoffen E, den Hartog Jager CF, Koppelman S, Pasmans SG, et al. (2007) Children with peanut allergy recognize predominantly Ara h 2 and Ara h 6, which remains stable over time. Clin Exp Allergy 37: 1221–1228.
5. Koppelman SJ, de Jong GA, Laaper-Ertmann M, Peeters KA, Knulst AC, et al. (2005) Purification and immunoglobulin E-binding properties of peanut allergen Ara h 6: evidence for cross-reactivity with Ara h 2. Clin Exp Allergy 35: 490–497.
6. Bernard H, Mondoulet L, Drumare MF, Paty E, Scheinmann P, et al. (2007) Identification of a new natural Ara h 6 isoform and of its proteolytic product as major allergens in peanut. J Agric Food Chem 55: 9663–9669.
7. Marsh J, Rigby N, Wellner K, Reese G, Knulst A, et al. (2008) Purification and characterisation of a panel of peanut allergens suitable for use in allergy diagnosis. Mol Nutr Food Res 52(Suppl 2): S272–285.
8. Suhr M, Wicklein D, Lepp U, Becker WM (2004) Isolation and characterization of natural Ara h 6: evidence for a further peanut allergen with putative clinical relevance based on resistance to pepsin digestion and heat. Mol Nutr Food Res 48: 390–399.
9. Shewry PR, Napier JA, Tatham AS (1995) Seed storage proteins: structures and biosynthesis. Plant Cell 7: 945–956.
10. Barre A, Borges JP, Culerrier R, Rouge P (2005) Homology modelling of the major peanut allergen Ara h 2 and surface mapping of IgE-binding epitopes. Immunol Lett 100: 153–158.
11. Lehmann K, Schweimer K, Reese G, Randow S, Suhr M, et al. (2006) Structure and stability of 2S albumin-type peanut allergens: implications for the severity of peanut allergic reactions. Biochem J 395: 463–472.
12. Davis PJ, Williams SC (1998) Protein modification by thermal processing. Allergy 53: 102–105.
13. Chung SY, Champagne ET (2001) Association of end-product adducts with increased IgE binding of roasted peanuts. J Agric Food Chem 49: 3911–3916.
14. Hilmenyuk T, Bellinghausen I, Heydenreich B, Ilchmann A, Toda M, et al. (2010) Effects of glycation of the model food allergen ovalbumin on antigen uptake and presentation by human dendritic cells. Immunology 129: 437–445.
15. Ilchmann A, Burgdorf S, Scheurer S, Waibler Z, Nagai R, et al. (2010) Glycation of a food allergen by the Maillard reaction enhances its T-cell immunogenicity: role of macrophage scavenger receptor class A type I and II. J Allergy Clin Immunol 125: 175–183.
16. Gruber P, Vieths S, Wangorsch A, Nerkamp J, Hofmann T (2004) Maillard reaction and enzymatic browning affect the allergenicity of Pru av 1, the major allergen from cherry (Prunus avium). J Agric Food Chem 52: 4002–4007.
17. Nakamura A, Sasaki F, Watanabe K, Ojima T, Ahn DH, et al. (2006) Changes in allergenicity and digestibility of squid tropomyosin during the Maillard reaction with ribose. J Agric Food Chem 54: 9529–9534.
18. Gruber P, Becker WM, Hofmann T (2005) Influence of the maillard reaction on the allergenicity of rAra h 2, a recombinant major allergen from peanut (Arachis hypogaea), its major epitopes, and peanut agglutinin. J Agric Food Chem 53: 2289–2296.
19. Maleki SJ, Chung SY, Champagne ET, Raufman JP (2000) The effects of roasting on the allergenic properties of peanut proteins. J Allergy Clin Immunol 106: 763–768.
20. Mondoulet L, Paty E, Drumare MF, Ah-Leung S, Scheinmann P, et al. (2005) Influence of thermal processing on the allergenicity of peanut proteins. J Agric Food Chem 53: 4547–4553.
21. Johnson PE, Van der Plancken I, Balasa A, Husband FA, Grauwet T, et al. (2010) High pressure, thermal and pulsed electric-field-induced structural changes in selected food allergens. Mol Nutr Food Res 54: 1701–1710.
22. Blanc F, Adel-Patient K, Drumare MF, Paty E, Wal JM, et al. (2009) Capacity of purified peanut allergens to induce degranulation in a functional in vitro assay: Ara h 2 and Ara h 6 are the most efficient elicitors. Clin Exp Allergy 39: 1277–1285.
23. Koppelman SJ, Bruijnzeel-Koomen CA, Hessing M, de Jongh HH (1999) Heat-induced conformational changes of Ara h 1, a major peanut allergen, do not affect its allergenic properties. J Biol Chem 274: 4770–4777.
24. Mills CEN, Gao C, Wilde PJ, Rigby NM, Wijesinha-Bettoni R, et al. (2009) Partially folded forms of barley lipid transfer protein are more surface active. Biochemistry 48: 12081–12088.
25. Gabrielsson S, Paulie S, Rak S, Lagging E, Van Hage-Hamsten M, et al. (1997) Specific induction of interleukin-4-producing cells in response to in vitro allergen stimulation in atopic individuals. Clin Exp Allergy 27: 808–815.
26. Turcanu V, Winterbotham M, Kelleher P, Lack G (2008) Peanut-specific B and T cell responses are correlated in peanut-allergic but not in non-allergic individuals. Clin Exp Allergy 38: 1132–1139.
27. Turcanu VH, Lack G (2005) Levels of circulating peanut-specific precursor T cells reflect peanut allergy status. J Allergy Clin Immunol 115: S62.
28. Bohle B (2006) T-cell epitopes of food allergens. Clin Rev Allergy Immunol 30: 97–108.
29. Schimek EM, Zwolfer B, Briza P, Jahn-Schmid B, Vogel L, et al. (2005) Gastrointestinal digestion of Bet v 1-homologous food allergens destroys their mediator-releasing, but not T cell-activating, capacity. J Allergy Clin Immunol 116: 1327–1333.
30. Scheurer S, Lauer I, Foetisch K, San Miguel Moncin M, Retzek M, et al. (2004) Strong allergenicity of Pru av 3, the lipid transfer protein from cherry, is related to high stability against thermal processing and digestion. J Allergy Clin Immunol 114: 900–907.
31. Morisawa Y, Kitamura A, Ujihara T, Zushi N, Kuzume K, et al. (2009) Effect of heat treatment and enzymatic digestion on the B cell epitopes of cow's milk proteins. Clin Exp Allergy 39: 918–925.
32. Beyer K, Morrow E, Li XM, Bardina L, Bannon GA, et al. (2001) Effects of cooking methods on peanut allergenicity. J Allergy Clin Immunol 107: 1077–1081.
33. Ehn BM, Ekstrand B, Bengtsson U, Ahlstedt S (2004) Modification of IgE Binding during Heat Processing of the Cow's Milk Allergen β-Lactoglobulin. J Agric Food Chem 52: 1398–1403.
34. EFSA (European Food Safety Authority) (2004) Opinion of the Scientific Panel on Dietetic Products, Nutrition and Allergies: Evaluation of allergenic foods for labelling purposes. EFSA journal 32: 1–197.
35. EFSA (European Food Safety Authority) (2010) Scientific Opinion on the assessment of allergenicity of GM plants and microorganisms and derived food and feed. EFSA journal 8: 1700.
36. Stanley JS, King N, Burks AW, Huang SK, Sampson H, et al. (1997) Identification and mutational analysis of the immunodominant IgE binding epitopes of the major peanut allergen Ara h 2. Arch Biochemistry Biophysics 342: 244–253.
37. Flinterman AE, Knol EF, Lencer DA, Bardina L, den Hartog Jager CF, et al. (2008) Peanut epitopes for IgE and IgG4 in peanut-sensitized children in relation to severity of peanut allergy. J Allergy Clin Immunol 121: 737–743.
38. Beyer K, Ellman-Grunther L, Jaärvinen KM, Wood RA, Hourihane J, et al. (2003) Measurement of peptide-specific IgE as an additional tool in identifying patients with clinical reactivity to peanuts. J Allergy Clin Immunol 112: 202–207.
39. Shreffler WG, Lencer DA, Bardina L, Sampson HA (2005) IgE and IgG4 epitope mapping by microarray immunoassay reveals the diversity of immune response to the peanut allergen, Ara h 2. J Allergy Clin Immunol 116: 893–899.
40. Maleki SJ, Kopper RA, Shin DS, Park CW, Compadre CM, et al. (2000) Structure of the major peanut allergen Ara h 1 may protect IgE-binding epitopes from degradation. J Immunol 164: 5844–5849.
41. Brockow K, Ring J (2009) Food anaphylaxis. Anal Bioanal Chem 395: 17–23.
42. Sampson HA (2003) Anaphylaxis and emergency treatment. Pediatrics 111: 1601–1608.
43. van Wijk F, Hartgring S, Koppelman SJ, Pieters R, Knippels LM (2004) Mixed antibody and T cell responses to peanut and the peanut allergens Ara h 1, Ara h 2, Ara h 3 and Ara h 6 in an oral sensitization model. Clin Exp Allergy 34: 1422–1428.
44. Sancho AI, Rigby NM, Zuidmeer L, Asero R, Mistrello G, et al. (2005) The effect of thermal processing on the IgE reactivity of the non-specific lipid transfer protein from apple, Mal d 3. Allergy 60: 1262–1268.
45. Jeurink PV, Vissers YM, Rappard B, Savelkoul HF (2008) T cell responses in fresh and cryopreserved peripheral blood mononuclear cells: kinetics of cell viability, cellular subsets, proliferation, and cytokine production. Cryobiology 57: 91–103.
46. Vissers YM, Snel J, Zuurendonk PF, Kleerebezem M, Wichers HJ, et al. (2011) Lactobacillus strains differentially modulate cytokine production by hPBMC from pollen-allergic patients. FEMS Immunology & Medical Microbiology 61: 28–40.
47. Bernard H, Drumare MF, Guillon B, Paty E, Scheinmann P, et al. (2009) Immunochemical characterisation of structure and allergenicity of peanut 2S albumins using different formats of immunoassays. Anal Bioanal Chem 395: 139–146.
48. Jensen LB, Pedersen MH, Skov PS, Poulsen LK, Bindslev-Jensen C, et al. (2008) Peanut cross-reacting allergens in seeds and sprouts of a range of legumes. Clin Exp Allergy 38: 1969–1977.
49. Vogel L, Luttkopf D, Hatahet L, Haustein D, Vieths S (2005) Development of a functional in vitro assay as a novel tool for the standardization of allergen extracts in the human system. Allergy 60: 1021–1028.

5

Ketamine Effects on Memory Reconsolidation Favor a Learning Model of Delusions

Philip R. Corlett[1]*[9], Victoria Cambridge[2][9], Jennifer M. Gardner[3], Jennifer S. Piggot[3], Danielle C. Turner[4], Jessica C. Everitt[4], Fernando Sergio Arana[2], Hannah L. Morgan[2], Amy L. Milton[4], Jonathan L. Lee[5], Michael R. F. Aitken[4], Anthony Dickinson[4], Barry J. Everitt[4], Anthony R. Absalom[6], Ram Adapa[7], Naresh Subramanian[2], Jane R. Taylor[1], John H. Krystal[1], Paul C. Fletcher[2,8]

1 Department of Psychiatry, Ribicoff Research Facility, Yale University, New Haven, Connecticut, United States of America, **2** Brain Mapping Unit, Department of Psychiatry, University of Cambridge, School of Clinical Medicine, Addenbrooke's Hospital, Cambridge, United Kingdom, **3** University of Cambridge, School of Clinical Medicine, Addenbrooke's Hospital, Cambridge, United Kingdom, **4** Department of Psychology, University of Cambridge, Cambridge, United Kingdom, **5** University of Birmingham, School of Psychology, Edgbaston, Birmingham, United Kingdom, **6** Department of Anesthesiology, University Medical Center Groningen, Groningen University, Groningen, The Netherlands, **7** Division of Anaesthesia, School of Clinical Medicine, University of Cambridge, Addenbrooke's Hospital, Cambridge, United Kingdom, **8** Cambridgeshire and Peterborough NHS Foundation Trust, Elizabeth House, Fulbourn Hospital, Cambridge, United Kingdom

Abstract

Delusions are the persistent and often bizarre beliefs that characterise psychosis. Previous studies have suggested that their emergence may be explained by disturbances in prediction error-dependent learning. Here we set up complementary studies in order to examine whether such a disturbance also modulates memory reconsolidation and hence explains their remarkable persistence. First, we quantified individual brain responses to prediction error in a causal learning task in 18 human subjects (8 female). Next, a placebo-controlled within-subjects study of the impact of ketamine was set up on the same individuals. We determined the influence of this NMDA receptor antagonist (previously shown to induce aberrant prediction error signal and lead to transient alterations in perception and belief) on the evolution of a fear memory over a 72 hour period: they initially underwent Pavlovian fear conditioning; 24 hours later, during ketamine or placebo administration, the conditioned stimulus (CS) was presented once, without reinforcement; memory strength was then tested again 24 hours later. Re-presentation of the CS under ketamine led to a stronger subsequent memory than under placebo. Moreover, the degree of strengthening correlated with individual vulnerability to ketamine's psychotogenic effects and with prediction error brain signal. This finding was partially replicated in an independent sample with an appetitive learning procedure (in 8 human subjects, 4 female). These results suggest a link between altered prediction error, memory strength and psychosis. They point to a core disruption that may explain not only the emergence of delusional beliefs but also their persistence.

Editor: Emmanuel Andreas Stamatakis, University of Cambridge, United Kingdom

Funding: This study was supported by the Wellcome Trust and the Bernard Wolfe Health Neuroscience fund. It was conducted at the Wellcome Trust Clinical Research Facility and the Wolfson Brain Imaging Centre (Addenbrooke's Hospital, Cambridge) and within the Behavioral and Clinical Neuroscience Institute supported by the Medical Research Council and the Wellcome Trust. The funders had no role in study design, data collection and analysis, decision to publish, or preparation of the manuscript.

Competing Interests: Philip Corlett reports receiving research support from AstraZeneca Pharmaceuticals, LP and consulting for Pfizer Pharmaceuticals. John Krystal reports consulting for AstraZeneca Pharmaceuticals, LP, Cypress Bioscience, Inc., HoustonPharma, Schering-Plough Research Institute, Shire Pharmaceuticals, and Pfizer Pharmaceuticals; Advisory Boards: Bristol-Myers Squibb, Eli Lilly and Co., Forest Laboratories, GlaxoSmithKline, Lohocla Research Corporation, Merz Pharmaceuticals, Takeda Industries, and Transcept Pharmaceuticals, Inc. Exercisable Warrant Options: Tetragenex Pharmaceuticals Inc.; Research Support: Janssen Research Foundation; Pending Patents: glutamatergic agents for psychiatric disorders (depression, OCD), antidepressant effects of oral ketamine, and oral ketamine for depression. Paul Fletcher has received consultancy fees from GlaxoSmithKline and an honorarium for a lecture from Astra Zeneca. This does not alter our adherence to all the PLOS ONE policies on sharing data and materials.

* E-mail: philip.corlett@yale.edu

[9] These authors contributed equally to this work.

Introduction

Associative learning forms the basis for belief formation [1]. It is driven by prediction error (PE) [1,2], and there is evidence that altered PE signal drives the formation of delusions, the abnormal beliefs that characterise mental illnesses like schizophrenia [3–5]. PE represents the mismatch between what we expect in a given situation and what we experience [6]. It guides learning directly; we form and strengthen explanatory associations (e.g. between causes and effects) by minimizing PE [6]. In addition, PE guides the allocation of attention [7]; we attend to and learn about stimuli with unpredictable consequences. PE is represented in a range of neural structures and circuits, most notably the midbrain dopamine cells in area A10, the striatum and the prefrontal cortex [8]. In addition to guiding learning about rewards, PEs are vital to social [9] and perceptual learning [10] as well as the formation of causal beliefs [1,2]. Based on these normative observations, we have proposed [3,11–13] that, if PE signals occur inappropriately, individuals would attend to and learn about stimuli, thoughts and percepts that others would ignore. As a consequence, they would develop beliefs that do not reflect the contingencies of the real world – delusions. There is growing evidence that this may be the case [3–5]: people with delusions exhibit inappropriate prediction error signals whose magnitude correlates with delusion severity.

This model accounts for why delusions emerge but not for why they persist. We argue [13–15] that disturbed PE, as well as leading to erroneous updating of beliefs (and, hence, the emergence of delusional ideas) may also be critical in their persistence [13–15]. While this may appear counter-intuitive, given that PE is associated with the flexible updating of learned expectations [6], latterly it has been demonstrated that PE-driven memory reconsolidation can strengthen memories in the absence of reinforcement: specifically, the surprising re-presentation of a retrieval cue can strengthen a memory [16]. Reconsolidation occurs when memories are recalled into a labile state, integrated with new information, and consolidated once more [17,18]. This process depends on PE [19], that is, surprising information returns related memories into a labile state [20]. Two competing processes are evoked [21]: on the one hand, there is extinction initiated by a negative PE signal, engendering competing learning [22] that overrides the original memory [23]. Extinction memories involve new learning, not simply forgetting of the old representation (as demonstrated by the fact that memories of the reinforced situation can recur spontaneously in rats and humans [23,24]). Negative PE

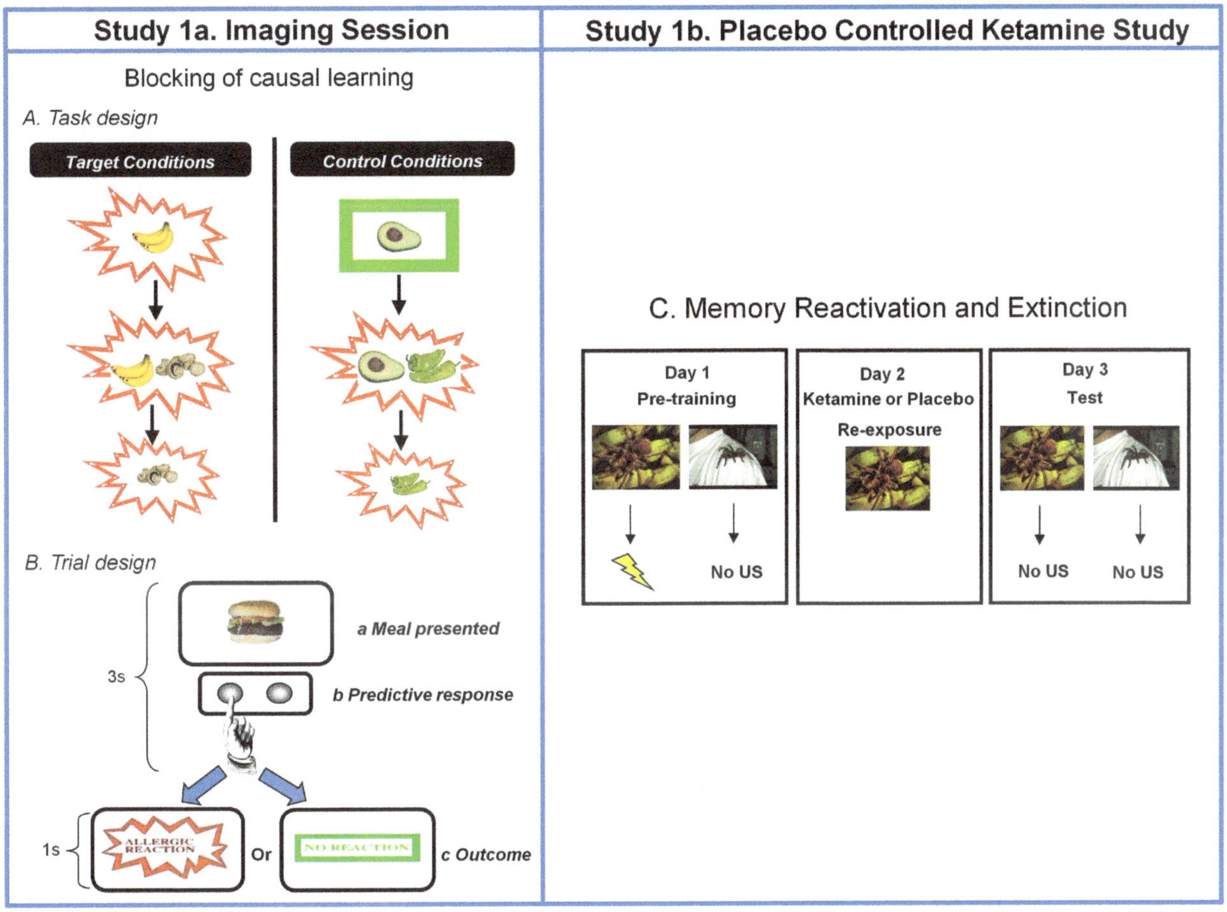

Figure 1. Study Design. *A. Task Design.* Target and control conditions for the food-allergy causal learning tasks. Subjects see that *bananas* cause an allergy in their patient. Subsequently they see that *bananas* and *mushrooms* cause the allergy. Their prior learning about bananas should block new learning about the mushrooms. In the final phase of training, subjects see the mushrooms causing the allergy; this violates any blocking that took place in the previous Stage. Blocking trials are compared to control events that are matched for the presence of allergy as well as novelty and familiarity (*Avocado and Chilies*). Likewise, at Stage 3, there are trials matched for novelty and familiarity that act as comparators for the blocking violation events. The figure depicts key trial types. Filler cues were also presented to control for the relative frequency of allergic reactions. Each trial type was presented 10 times for Stage 1 and 6 times for Stages 2 and 3 with the caveat that no trial type was repeated before all trial types had been presented. *B. Trial Design.* On each trial, subjects saw a meal that their patient had eaten for 3 seconds. During this time, they made a prediction response – pushing one button to predict an allergy and another to predict no allergy. They also held the button down for longer the more confident they were that they were making the right choice. Next they were shown the effect of that meal on their patient. If he suffered an allergy, they would see the words *Allergic Reaction* in red letters with a jagged border for 1 second. If there was no allergy, subjects saw the words *No Allergy* in green letters with a green rectangle around it for one second. *C. Memory Reactivation and Extinction Task.* In a follow up placebo-controlled behavioral study of ketamine, the same subjects from the scanning study attended the laboratory on three consecutive days twice (separated by at least one month). On Day 1, they learned that one visual stimulus predicted the delivery of a 90dB loud noise with 70% contingency and another cue never predicted load noise. The following day (Day 2) they saw the noise predicting cue whilst receiving an infusion of either ketamine or placebo. The next day (Day 3) they returned to the lab and observed the cues again in extinction. After 30 trials of extinction, they were reminded of the loud noise once more and observed a further five repetitions of each cue in extinction. We tracked skin conductance responses to the cues on Day 1 and Day 3. The subjects returned to repeat the procedure with different cues and received the other infusion the second time around.

signals guide this new learning [22]. On the other hand, the positive PE response to predictive cues [8,25,26] engages an expectation of reinforcement and leads to the reminder-based strengthening of the belief [21]. The precise balance between these processes is driven by the magnitude, sign and timing of the accompanying PE signal [19].

Given the growing evidence that the psychotic state is associated with aberrant PE [3,4,27–31], we have suggested that this extinction-reconsolidation balance may be fundamentally altered in delusions [14]. That is, altered PE signal leads patients to attend to and learn about events that healthy individuals would ignore [3,11–14,31,32]. This accounts for the emergence of delusions, which form as explanatory schemes [33]. But the same disturbance means that the delusion will be frequently reactivated, employed to explain subsequent experiences [34], and strengthened once more [13,14,35]. This strengthening may share a cognitive basis with the *illusory truth effect*, whereby judging the veracity of a statement enhances later belief in its truth [36]. Patients with delusions are more susceptible to the illusory truth effect, particularly for judgments related to their delusions [37]. We hypothesise that in psychosis, aberrant PE signal encourages inappropriate memory strengthening and delusion fixity, relative to extinction [14].

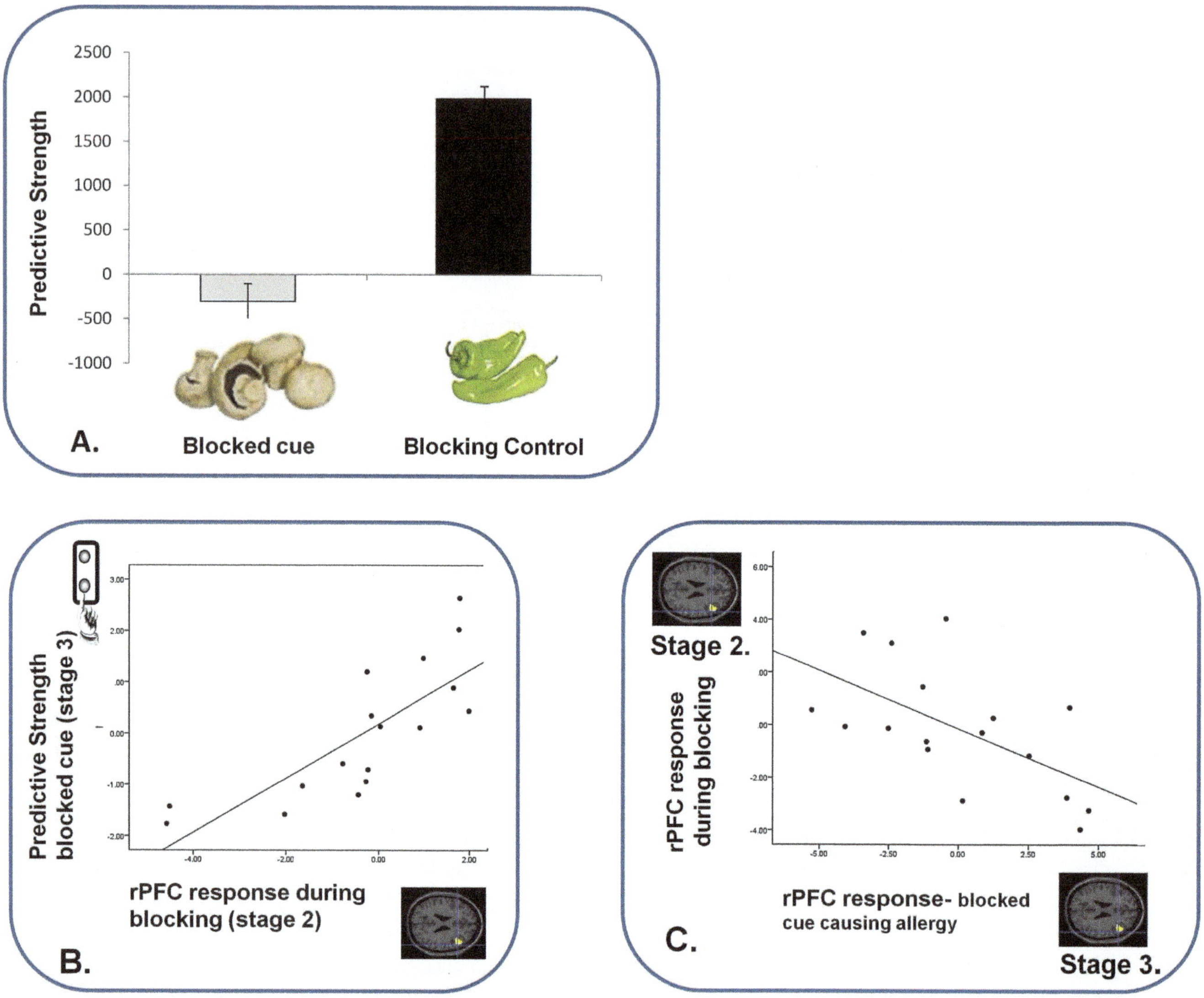

Figure 2. Blocking Behavior and its Relation to Brain Responses. *A. Behavioral Predictions For Blocked and Control Cues.* Subjects predicted with low confidence about the blocked cue, when exposed to it at Stage 3; confirming that blocking had taken place. Error bars represent SEM. Y-axis represents subjects' predictive strength; their degree of confidence (duration of predictive button push response) multiplied by correctness of their prediction. Hence lower scores reflect uncertain and unstable predictions, which we observed to blocked cues when compared with blocking control cues (whose causal association with the allergy is more robust). *B. Relating Predictions about the Blocked Cue (Stage 3) to Blocking Responses.* Subjects who showed the lowest confidence when predicting what would happen following the blocked cue had the most attenuated right DLPFC response during blocking trials. X-axis represents the right DLPFC parameter estimates extracted from a contrast image comparing blocking trials with blocking control trials. Y-axis represents subjects' behavioral predictions about the blocked cues prior to seeing their predictive outcomes at the first trials of Stage 3. *C. Relating Brain Responses During Blocking to those during Violation.* Subjects with the most attenuated DLPFC response during blocking showed the greatest right DLPFC response when that blocking contingency was subsequently violated. X-axis represents the right DLPFC response to observing the blocked cue causing the allergic response during Violation (Stage 3), compared with control event. Y-axis represents right DLPFC response to blocking trials compared with blocking-control trials.

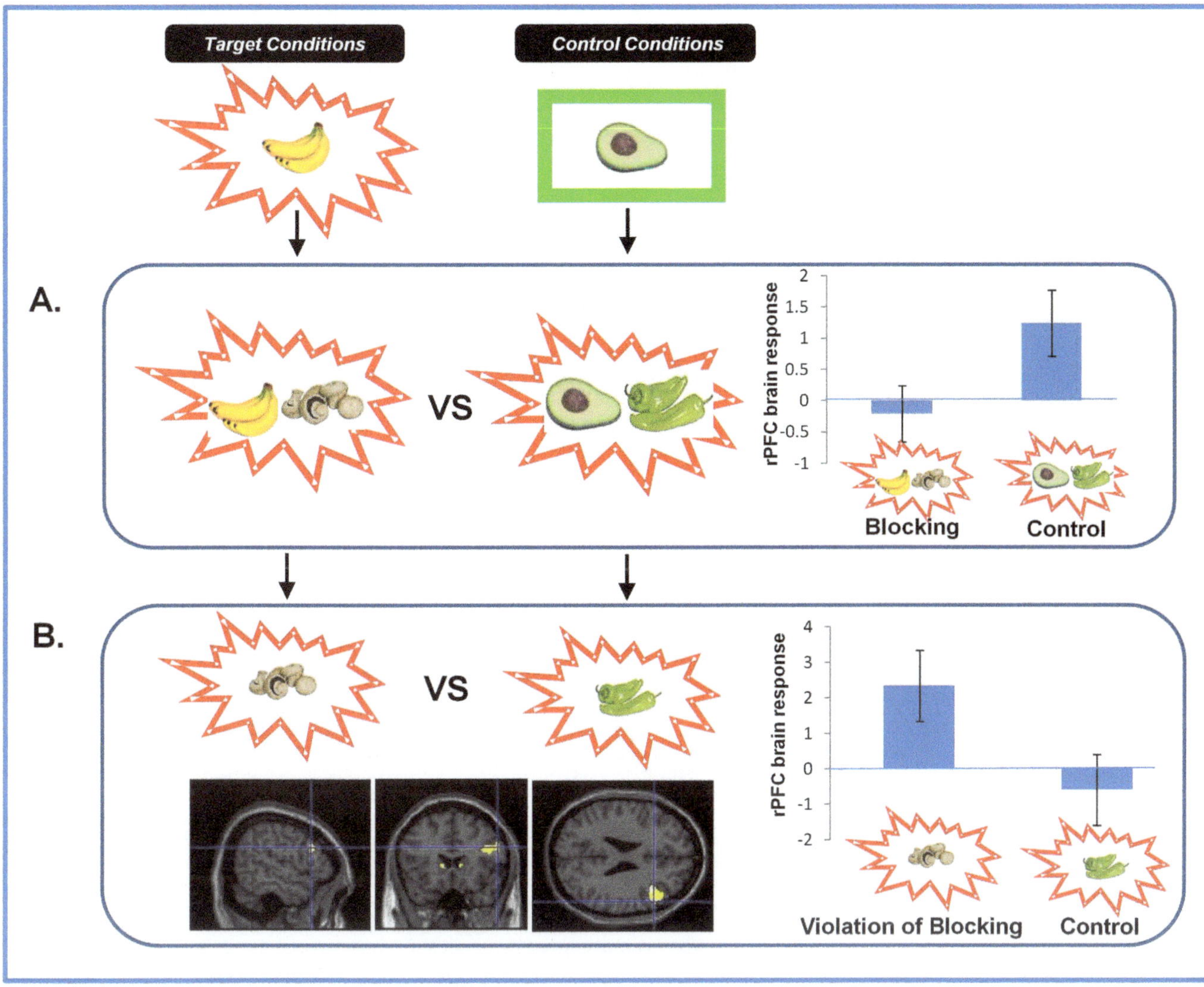

Figure 3. Brain Responses to Blocking and Violation of Blocking. *A. Brain responses to Blocking vs. Control Trials.* Right DLPFC responses to blocking trials were significantly attenuated compared with control trials. Parameter estimates extracted from SPM in arbitrary units. Error Bars represent standard error of the mean (SEM). *B. Brain Responses to the Violation of Blocking.* Violating the blocking at Stage 3 significantly engaged right DLPFC. Parameter estimates extracted from SPM in arbitrary units. Error bars represent SEM.

In short, we suggest that the same disturbance in PE may account for both the emergence and the persistence of delusions.

We tested this hypothesis using a drug model of psychosis [38,39]. In a previously published fMRI study, we quantified individual neural responses to PE [40]. The same participants were recruited to a placebo-controlled ketamine study, in which we assayed the psychotomimetic effects of ketamine as well as its impact upon the re-presentation of an aversive CS conditioned 24 hours previously (see Figure 1). We initially chose aversive learning and memory reconsolidation because, of the few reconsolidation studies in human subjects [20,41–44], none have previously examined appetitive memory. We hypothesized that, since ketamine engenders aberrant PE signal in response to unsurprising events [38], it should induce reactivation and strengthening of memories, and this effect should be directly relatable to individual variability in PE signal, measured using fMRI, as well as to the severity of ketamine-induced symptoms. Given that it could be argued that any effect of ketamine could be attributed to generalization of the unpleasant psychotomimetic experience to the reactivated cue, we conducted a follow-up behavioral study of appetitive conditioning (Study 2) in which an independent sample of subjects.

We carried out two studies: Study 1, in which we relate PE brain responses, Ketamine-induced psychopathology and ketamine effects on aversive memory reconsolidation, and Study 2, in which we examine ketamine effects on reactivated appetitive memories in a separate cohort of subjects. To be clear, the fMRI study (Study 1a) was not set up to characterize the neural correlates of memory reactivation or reconsolidation [44,45]. Rather it was conducted to capture individual differences in PE brain response. Those individual differences then formed the basis for exploring how variability in PE relates to the effects of ketamine on memory reconsolidation and the genesis of psychosis-like symptoms (Study 1b). A relationship between the neural marker for PE and reconsolidation across our studies would constitute evidence in favor of our hypothesis: PE disturbance is key to the formation and maintenance of delusions [14]. Study 2 aimed to clarify the interpretation of Study 1b.

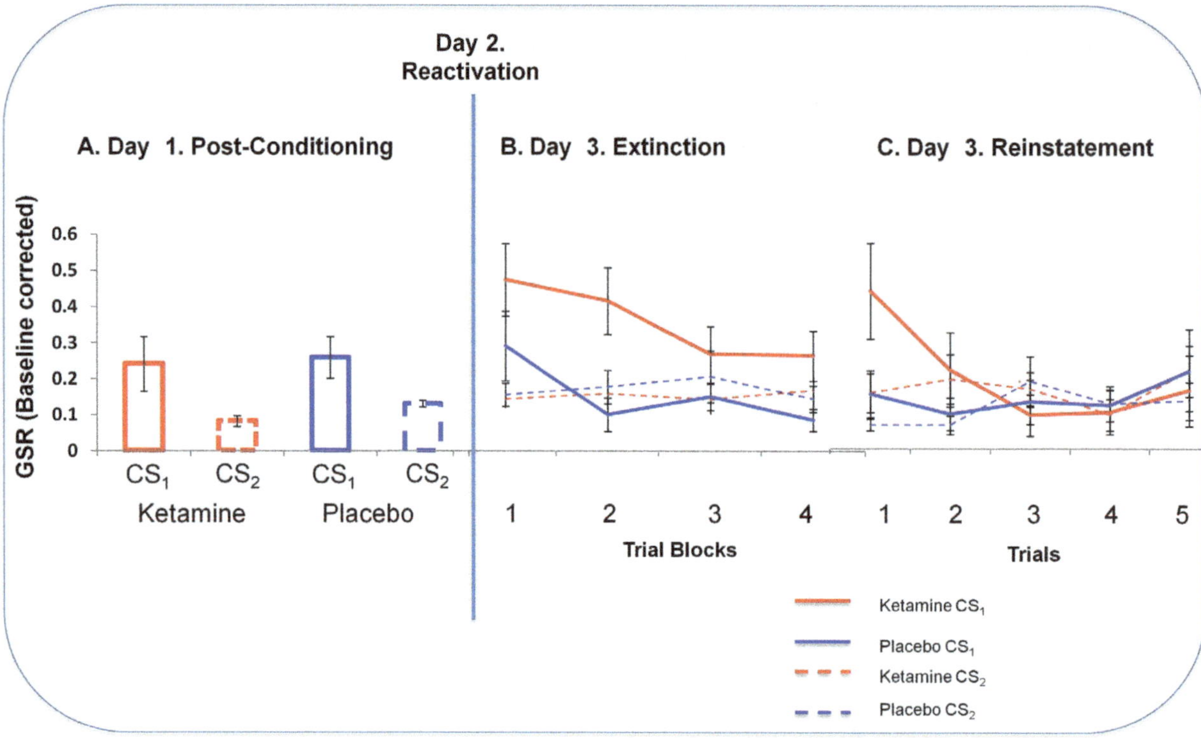

Figure 4. GSR Responses to Fear Cues Across Study Days. *A. Skin Conductance Responses to Cues after Initial Conditioning (Day 1).* Subjects means skin conductance responses to the final 3 trials at the end of initial conditioning on Day 1. Y-axis represents subjects Galvanic Skin Responses to the cues (ketamine in red, placebo in blue; solid lines represent the to be reactivated cues (CS_1) and dashed lines represent CS_2 (non-predictive and non-reactivated). Error bars represent SEM. *B. Skin Conductance Responses to Cues in Extinction (Day 3).* Subjects showed an elevated skin conductance response to the ketamine-reactivated cue compared with the cue reactivated under placebo. Error bars represent SEM. Line graph: Y-axis represents subjects GSR responses to blocks of four extinction trials to cues reactivated under ketamine and placebo. Ketamine data are shown in red, placebo in blue; solid lines represent the reactivated cues (CS_1) and dashed lines represent CS_2 (non-predictive and non-reactivated). Error bars represent SEM. *C. Skin Conductance Responses to Cues Following US reminder (Day 3, post extinction).* When subjects were re-exposed to the loud noise outcome and then presented with the cues 5 more times in extinction, responses to the ketamine reactivated cue returned most strongly. Y-axis represents galvanic skin conductance response. Ketamine data are shown in red, placebo in blue; solid lines represent the reactivated cues (CS_1) and dashed lines represent CS_2 (non-predictive and non-reactivated). Error bars represent SEM.

Methods

The study was approved by the Cambridge Local Research and Ethics Committee and was carried out in accordance with The Code of Ethics of the World Medical Association (Declaration of Helsinki). All subjects gave written informed consent.

Study 1 – Subjects

18 (8 female) right-handed, healthy volunteers (aged 19–28) were recruited through local advertisement. No subjects reported a history of psychiatric illness, drug abuse or contra-indications for MRI. We excluded subjects with any history of alcoholism as well as current smokers [46]. One subject was excluded upon discovery of a past history of psychiatric illness. Participants completed other cognitive tasks under ketamine (examining spatial learning and memory, bodily agency, instrumental agency and visual perception) [47,48]. Further observations will be reported elsewhere. For Stage 1 (fMRI), participants attended for testing on one occasion. For Stage 2, they attended on a total of six occasions (see below).

Study 1a comprised the fMRI study and 1b the placebo-controlled ketamine challenge. For each participant these were separated by a minimum of 4 weeks.

Study 1a – Functional Neuroimaging of PE signal. For Study 1, the fMRI stage (Study 1a) involved a Kamin blocking task [49] where initial causal learning blocked subsequent causal associations from forming to a contingent but redundant stimulus (see Figure 1). Blocking is a cornerstone of PE driven learning theories [8]; in the absence of PE, there is no learning about the blocked cue [50]. However, individuals with psychosis show attenuated blocking [51] as do healthy subjects treated with amphetamine [52], consistent with an aberrant PE account of psychosis [3,13,32,38]. Individuals showing weaker blocking have "inappropriate" PE, driving them to attend to and learn about the redundant blocked cue. This learning was captured behaviorally (the degree to which subjects made confident predictions about the blocked cue) and neurally (the magnitude of brain surprise response to trials that violate blocking). That is, subjects with stronger blocking should be more surprised to see the blocked cue predicting a salient outcome, while those with weaker blocking should be less surprised. The present procedure has some similarities with the unblocking effect, previously demonstrated in rodent conditioning [53] and human causal learning [54] and used recently in experimental animals to clarify the neural mechanisms of reward prediction and PE [55]. Although our task does not involve reward per se, it has previously been used to emphasize the importance of neural and behavioral PE mechanisms in the formation of causal beliefs about the world in the absence of explicit reward [1,2]. As in previous work, neural PE responses to events that violated what had previously been learned were used as a marker for the strength of previous learning [2].

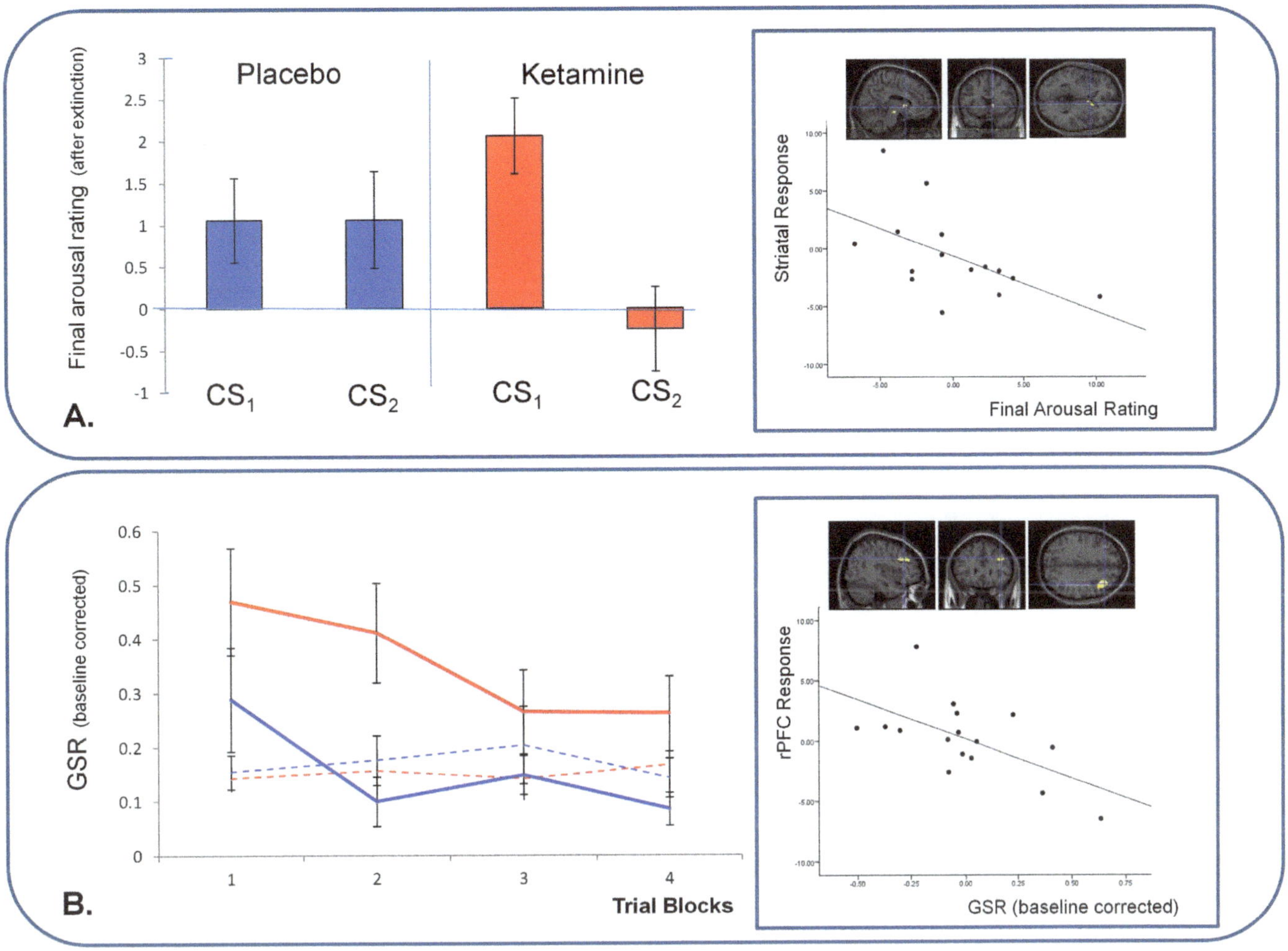

Figure 5. Responses to Fear Cues and their Relationship to PE Brain Responses. *A. Ratings of the Cues after Extinction and their relationship to Violation Responses.* Subjects rated the cue reactivated under ketamine as significantly more arousing than the cue reactivated under placebo. Those same subjects showed an aberrant striatal response during the violation of blocking indicative of inappropriate learning. Error bars represent SEM. Bar Graph: Y-axis represents subjects Final Arousal Ratings after the extinction trials, corrected by their initial ratings of the cues at baseline, such that residual ratings reflect conditioning. Scatterplot: X-axis represents those same Arousal ratings. Y-Axis represents parameter estimates extracted from right striatum from the contrast of blocking violation trials with their matched control events. *B. Skin Conductance Responses to Fear Cues and their relationship to violation Responses.* Subjects showed an elevated skin conductance response to the ketamine-reactivated cue compared with the cue reactivated under placebo. Subjects who showed the strongest skin conductance responses to cues reactivated under ketamine also showed the most inappropriate DLPFC response to the violation of blocking, indicating that they had learned inappropriately about the blocked cue. Error bars represent SEM. Line graph: Y-axis represents subjects GSR responses to blocks of four extinction trials to cues reactivated under ketamine and placebo. Scatterplot: X-axis represents the GSR to the first extinction trial (Ketamine minus placebo). Y-Axis represents parameter estimates extracted from right DLPFC from the contrast of blocking violation trials with their matched control events.

Furthermore, we assayed brain responses during blocking trials (compared with control events matched for novelty, familiarity and contingency with the outcome) as a further metric of aberrant PE – those subjects who imbue the redundant blocked cue with causal significance ought to have responses in PE-related regions during blocking trials – providing a neural metric of their aberrant PE at the time of the redundant trials.

We used an established causal learning approach, in which learned expectations are violated to produce a prediction error [2]. We examined Kamin blocking, in which prior learning interferes with what is subsequently acquired [49]. Subjects were asked to imagine themselves working as an allergist confronted with a new patient "*Mr. X*". Trials comprised presentation of a food picture (representing a meal eaten by Mr. X), a predictive button push response by the subject and, following this, an allergic-reaction or no reaction outcome. Subjects held the button down longer the more confident they felt in their prediction [2], providing a sensitive assay of learning as follows:

$$Predictivestrength = Rx(lengthofbuttonpush)$$

R is the predictive response (coded by +1 for prediction of an allergy and −1 for prediction of no allergy). The blocked cue induces a near zero score, since subjects should not learn about it.

Trial sequence. Training consisted of three phases: *Learning*; in which prior expectancies were developed, *Blocking*; in which those prior expectancies 'blocked' new learning, and *Violation*; which provided a metric for the strength of blocking. In brief, the key trials in Stage 1, *Learning*, comprised of single foods that caused or did not cause the allergy. There were also meals presented in this stage, which comprised of two different foods and were

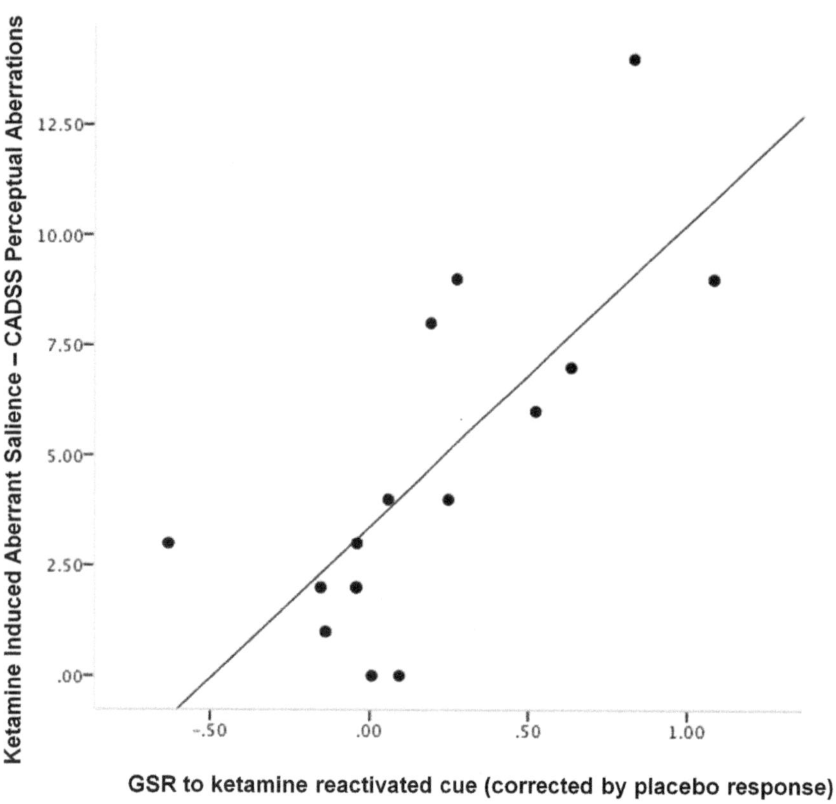

Figure 6. Relating Cue Responses to Psychotomimetic Response. *The relationship between ketamine induced aberrant salience and skin conductance responses to the cue reactivated under ketamine.* Subjects who experienced the most severe aberrant salience also showed the strongest skin conductance responses to the cue reactivated under ketamine. Plot features the difference in GSR response to the cue reactivated under ketamine from the cue reactivated under placebo on x-axis, CADSS perceptual subscale score (e.g., endorsing that background noises seemed louder, colors seem brighter, objects appeared to stick out from the background) on the y-axis.

employed as fillers such that subjects were not surprised by the appearance of meals of two foods during the subsequent blocking phase. In the *Blocking* phase, single items from Stage 1 were paired with novel food items. Having previously learned that a food from Stage 1 caused the allergy should block new learning to the novel food. Two separate blocking contingencies were presented, represented by different foods. In the blocking control condition, which served as a comparator in our imaging analysis (see below) a food that previously predicted no allergy was paired with a novel food and this compound caused the allergic reaction. In the final *Violation* phase, one blocked cue was shown causing the allergic reaction; responses to this cue were compared with those to the novel blocking control food leading to the allergic reaction (See Figure 1 for more information). In order to control for novelty, familiarity and contingency reversal, one of the cues subjected to blocking at Stage 2 was presented causing no allergy. Other filler cues were presented to balance for the presence and absence of an allergic reaction, across trials involving single foods and compounds of two foods. The food stimuli used were identical to those used in our prior work [2,3,38,56]. As in previous studies, the role played by the cues was randomized and counterbalanced across subjects such that variance in salience of the cues and their contingency with the outcomes were not confounded [2,3,38,56].

We focused our behavioral analyses on confirming that blocking did indeed occur in our subjects. To this end, we planned a paired t-test on subjects' prediction confidence for the first trial of Stage 3 on which they see the blocked cue alone (mushrooms in Figure 1) compared with their initial prediction the first time they saw the blocking control cue alone (chilies in Figure 1). Mean predictive confidence ratings were calculated such that subjects' responses to the initial presentations of blocking and control cues for both contingencies (confirmed and violated) both contributed to the behavioral analysis. This was legitimate because up until this point (i.e., before subjects saw the outcome at the first trial of Stage 3), the novelty, familiarity and contingency with the outcome of these parallel causal contingencies were identical.

fMRI Data Acquisition

We used a Siemens Trio scanner operating at 3 Tesla. 720 gradient echo T2*-weighted echo-planar images depicting blood oxygenation level-dependent contrast were acquired for each subject. The first seven images were discarded to avoid T1 equilibration effects. The remaining images covered the three task phases that ran continuously, in series; Stage 1 (Learning, 10 repetitions of each trial type) followed by Stage 2 (Blocking, 6 repetitions of each trial type) followed by Stage 3 (Violation, 6 repetitions of each trial type). Images were positioned parallel to the anterior commissure–posterior commissural line and comprised 35 slices, each of 2 mm with a 0.5 mm interslice gap. A repetition time of 1620 ms was used with an echo time of 30 ms and 90° flip angle. The scanner had a 192 mm field of view with a 64×64 data matrix.

fMRI Data Analysis

fMRI data were analyzed using SPM5 (Wellcome Department of Cognitive Neurology, London, UK; http://www.fil.ion.ucl.ac.

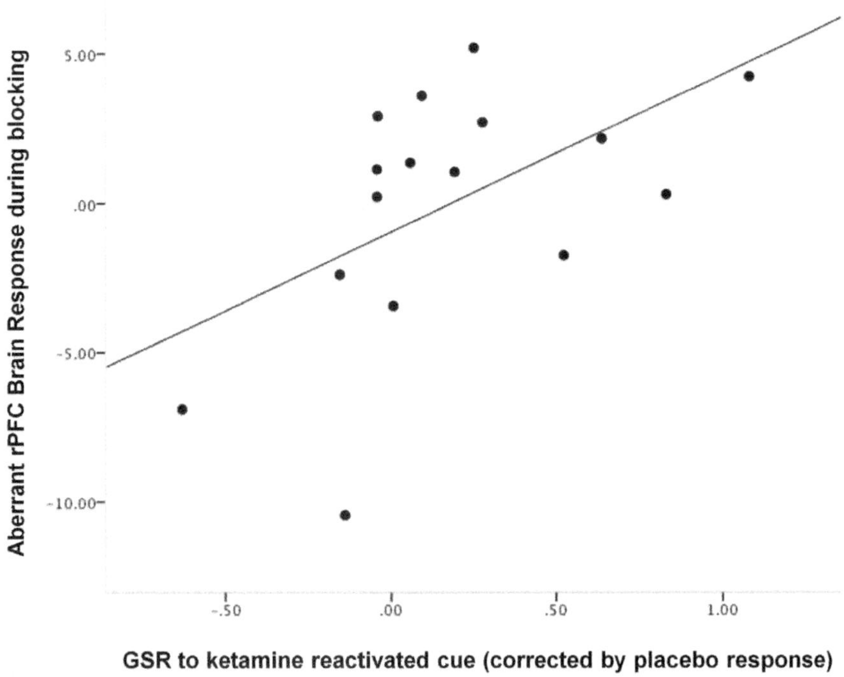

Figure 7. Relating Cue Responses to Aberrant PE During Blocking. The degree to which subjects inappropriately engage DLPFC during blocking trials correlated positively with their tendency to stronger GSR responses to ketamine-reactivated cues. This result is internally consistent with the Stage 3 finding – excessive responses during blocking and attenuated responses during its violation portend further memory strengthening in the context of ketamine. Plot features the difference in GSR response to the cue reactivated under ketamine from the cue reactivated under placebo on x-axis, rDLPFC responses during blocking trials (compared with control trials) on the y-axis.

uk/spm). Images were realigned, spatially normalized to a standard template and spatially smoothed with a Gaussian kernel (8 mm at full width half maximum). The time series in each session were high-pass filtered (to a maximum of 1/120 Hz) and serial autocorrelations were estimated using an AR(1) model. The average haemodynamic response to each event was designated at the presentation of the outcome. Trials were modeled using a canonical, synthetic haemodynamic response function used as a covariate in a general linear model. A parameter estimate was generated for each voxel for each event. Responses were parametrically modulated by the subjects' confidence in their prediction for that event. Individuals' contrast images, derived from the pair-wise comparisons between key events, were then entered into a second-level group analysis for each of the stages. Given our a priori hypotheses and prior work [3,38], we used the PickAtlas tool [57] to confine analyses to a single mask comprised of a series of regions of interest (ROI), total volume 1805 voxels: The five ROIs that comprised our mask were: right lateral prefrontal cortex (rPFC, a sphere of radius 10 mm centered on 50, 30, 28, the centroid generated by averaging across our prior studies of causal reasoning [2,38,56,58]), left and right striatum and left and right substantia nigra (defined anatomically using the tool [57]). Hence, responses and relationships in these regions were tested simultaneously by applying the mask.

Brain responses to events that violated blocking (i.e. events when the blocked cue was shown causing the allergy, *Mushrooms* in Figure 1) were compared with unsurprising control cues (*Chili* in figure 1). Subjects who blocked most should be most surprised by the blocked cue causing the allergy, indexed as more extensive frontostriatal activation in response to such trials.

We also identified brain responses to blocking trials (*banana* and *mushrooms*, Figure 1) relative to matched control events (*avocado* and *chilies*, Figure 1). This comparison revealed the brain regions engaged whilst blocking was taking place.

We aimed to determine the relevance of individual PE-responsiveness to the effects of ketamine on subsequent memory expression. Therefore, we computed correlations between phase 3 violation-related activation in the key ROIs (all 5 ROIs were combined into a single mask, volume 1805 voxels) and the effects of ketamine on subjective cognitive task performance applying small volume correction for multiple comparisons [59]. For each correlation we report the z-score in the particular regions implicated. All reported findings were associated with false discovery rate corrected p-values less than 0.05 [60] across the entire mask which comprised all ROIs. For illustrative purposes we plot the relationships between brain responses and behavioral ratings. We are aware of the potential for statistical non-independence or circularity in correlative analysis [61] and hence we do not re-compute Pearson's r-values for the relationship between the parameter estimates from our fMRI models and the cognitive measures of interest.

We computed the difference between the magnitude of ratings and Galvanic Skin Responses (GSR) to the cue reactivated under ketamine and its counterpart reactivated under placebo for each subject. Post-reactivation GSR responses were defined as the average response to the first block of 5 trials in extinction on Day 3. Ratings of valence and arousal were taken at the end of the extinction session and corrected by the ratings at the end of Day 1.

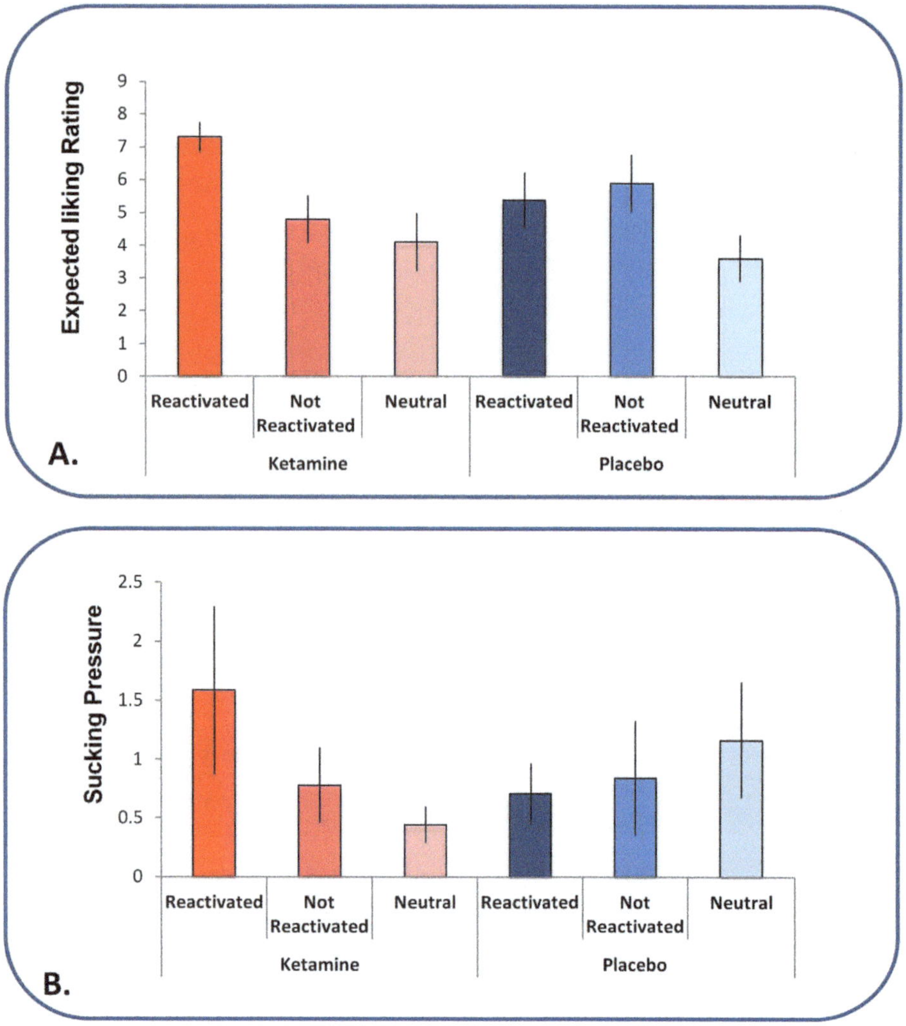

Figure 8. Appetitive Memory Reactivation. *A. Liking ratings of the liquid predicting cues.* Behavioral ratings of the cues on the first extinction trial (Day 3), following reactivation under ketamine or placebo (Day 2). Subjects liked the cue that had been reactivated under ketamine more than they liked the other cues and the cues from the placebo session. Error bars represent SEM. *B. Anticipatory sucking responses to the liquid predicting cues.* Anticipatory sucking in response to the first presentation of each cue type in extinction (Day 3) following reactivation under ketamine or placebo (Day 2). Subjects engaged in more anticipatory sucking prior to the cue that was reactivated under ketamine, the day after the ketamine session than the non-reactivated cues and the cues reactivated under placebo. Error bars represent SEM.

Study 1b – the effect of ketamine on memory reactivation

In the drug study (Study 1b, separated from Study 1a by at least 4 weeks), we employed ketamine as means of engendering psychotogenic aberrant PEs and we assayed the effects of reactivating a memory in the presence of such signals. As well as reporting their psychosis-like experiences (captured using a standard rating scale – see below), subjects completed a reconsolidation task involving initial Pavlovian conditioning of a picture stimulus as a predictor of an aversive auditory stimulus followed by re-presentation of the picture cue 24 hours later during ketamine or placebo infusion. The day after ketamine or placebo infusion, we tracked subjects' responses to the picture cue in extinction (i.e. in the absence of the aversive auditory stimulus).

The study was a double-blind, placebo controlled, randomized, within-subjects investigation of the effects of intravenous ketamine (the order of placebo and ketamine infusions was counterbalanced across subjects). An un-blinded clinician administered the infusions, however those administering cognitive tests and acquiring symptoms ratings remained blind. Subjects attended on two main study visits, once for drug, the other for placebo infusion. On the drug day, subjects received a computerized target controlled infusion of ketamine (200 ng/ml plasma) whilst they performed a series of cognitive tasks and a clinical interview exploring the presence, nature and severity of any psychotic symptoms. On the placebo day, a saline infusion was administered whilst subjects performed parallel versions of the cognitive tests and clinical interviews. There was a one-month washout period between drug and placebo visits to avoid effects related to activity of ketamine's metabolites.

Infusion protocol. Intra-venous catheters were inserted into the forearms, bilaterally, for ketamine infusion and serial blood sampling. Racemic ketamine (2 mg/ml) was administered by target-controlled infusion system using of a Graseby 3500 syringe driver pump (Graseby Medical Ltd, UK) under the control of Stanpump software (Freely available courtesy of Shafer S. http://opentci.org/doku.php?id=code:code). Steady state concentrations were implemented by administering a bolus, followed by

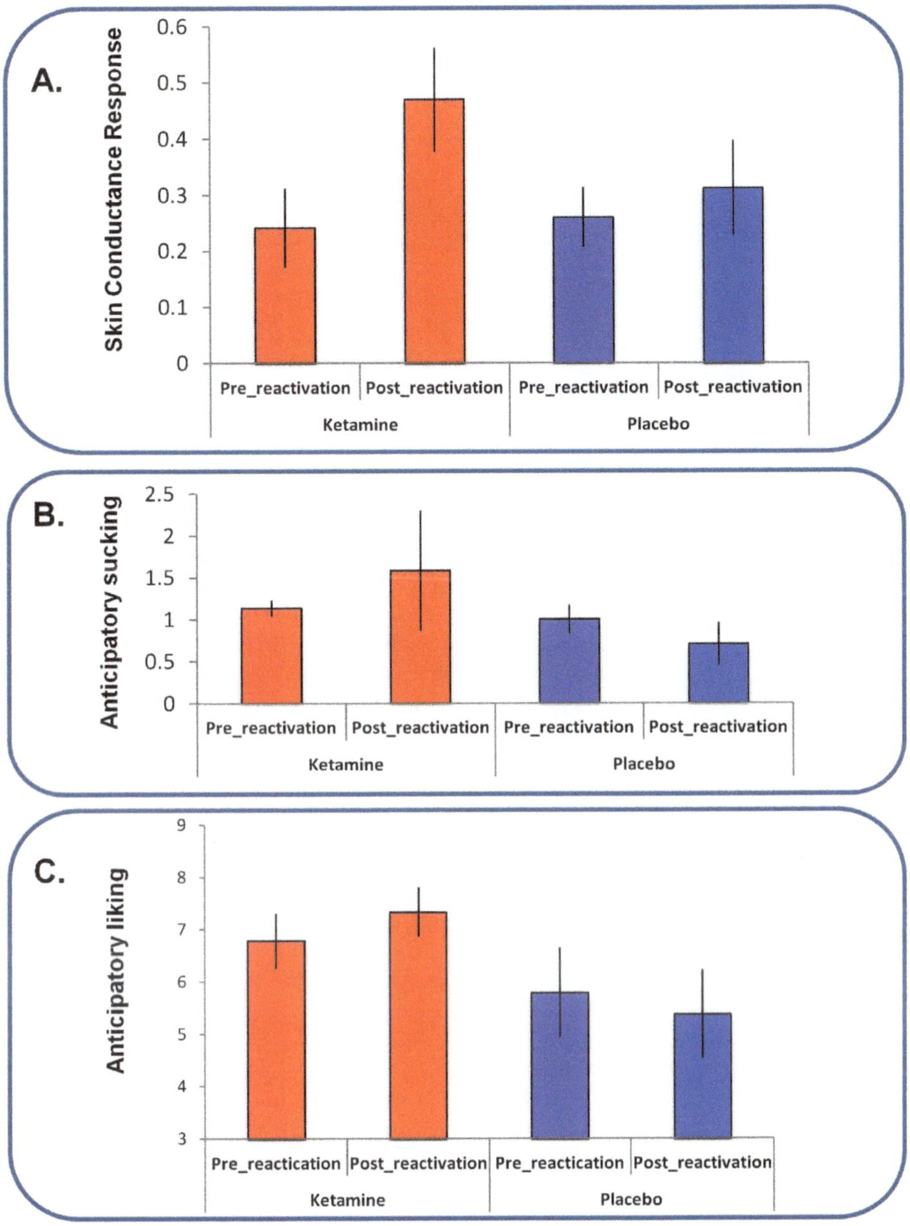

Figure 9. Memory Strengthening or Extinction Failure? *A. Skin Conductance Responses.* Skin conductance responses to the CS+ at the end of Day 1 (pre-reactivation, mean of final three trials) and the beginning of Day 3 (post reactivation, trial 1) for both the ketamine and placebo visits. Error bars represent SEM. *B. Sucking Pressure.* Anticipatory sucking to the cue predicting pleasant juice at the end of Day 1 (pre-reactivation) and the beginning of Day 3 (post-reactivation). Error bars represent SEM. *C. Expectancy Ratings.* Anticipatory liking ratings in response to the cue predicting pleasant juice at the end of Day 1 (pre-reactivation) and the beginning of Day 3 (post-reactivation). Error bars represent SEM.

an infusion whose rate was recalculated every 10 seconds; designed to replace drug removed by redistribution and metabolism. The infusion rates required for the bolus and maintenance infusion rates were determined by an algorithm in Stanpump, using a pharmacokinetic model for ketamine.

Fear conditioning, Reactivation and Extinction. This aspect of the procedure required six visits (three for placebo, three for ketamine). The day before the ketamine or placebo session (Figure 1, Day 1), subjects underwent aversive conditioning; learning about two visual conditioned stimuli (CS_1 and CS_2, each presented on 30 occasions). These were pictures of spiders, to which fear conditioning accrues readily [41,62,63].

On each trial, a cue appeared on screen for 4000 msec. CS_1 predicted the delivery of a 750 msec 90dB noise unconditioned stimulus (US) through noise canceling headphones on 70% of trials. CS_2 never predicted the US. We measured skin conductance responses from the non-dominant left hand. There was a mean inter-trial interval of 10 seconds. At the end of conditioning on experimental Day 1, subjects rated the two cues for valence and arousal.

On the drug or placebo infusion day (Figure 1, Day 2), subjects were fitted with the electrodes for recording skin conductance responses and the headphones for delivery of aversive USs. They were shown one single instance of CS_1. The aversive noise was not presented. Their skin conductance was not recorded during this single trial.

The day after the ketamine or placebo session (Figure 1, Day 3), CS_1 and CS_2 were presented a further 20 times, and neither cue predicted the US. Subsequently five un-cued USs were played and the cues were each presented again five times to quantify reinstatement of responding [41].

Since memory reconsolidation and extinction appear to be competing processes [14,21] and differentially sensitive to reminders of the unconditioned stimulus [41,42], we re-presented the aversive auditory stimulus followed by further extinction training through which we quantified the degree to which responding to the predictive cue could be re-evoked and re-extinguished, reasoning that reminders of the unconditioned stimulus should re-evoke responding to the conditioned stimulus [41]. If a memory cannot be reinstated, then we can be more confident that its reconsolidation has been blocked [41]. On the other hand, if responding is reinstated more strongly for the ketamine-reactivated cue than the placebo-reactivated cue, we can be more confident that we enhanced memory strength via reconsolidation [64].

At the end of the procedure, subjects rated the cues for valence and arousal.

Subjects' GSR responses were recorded using 9 mm Ag/AgCl electrodes filled with electrolyte paste and placed on the hypothenar surface and a BIOPAC MP150 system acquiring at a frequency of 50 Hz in concert with a PC running Acknowledge software (version 3.7).

We designated the 2 seconds prior to the onset of an event as a baseline and recorded the mean galvanic skin conductance response in microsiemen (μS). For each event, we identified an 8 second period following its onset and recorded the maximum skin conductance in μS [65]. We subtracted the baseline from the maximum response for each event thus identifying the skin conductance response to each event. To confirm acquisition of differential conditioning, we computed the mean GSR response to the final 5 CS_1 trials and the final 5 CS_2 trials on Day 1. For analysis of the 20-trial extinction session, we calculated a mean skin conductance score for 4 blocks of 5 trials comprising the 20 extinction trials. To examine reinstatement, we computed GSR responses to each of the final 5 non-reinforced CS_1 and CS_2 trials.

Clinical Interview. Subjects' symptoms were rated using the clinician administered dissociative states scale (CADSS) [66].

Planned analyses: Linking study 1a with study 1b

We sought to examine the relationship between the neural, behavioral and clinical datasets to test our hypothesis – that variation in prediction error signal would correlate with the effects of ketamine on memory reconsolidation and that subjects' behavioral responses following the reconsolidation manipulation would relate to the severity of their psychosis-like symptoms. Given that multiple experiments were conducted to examine this hypothesis, the potential for type-I error is high. We avoided this potential by focusing our correlational analyses on our *a-priori* predictions. First, our prior work related PE signal with the perceptual aberration sub-scale of the CADSS [38], hence, when relating imaging or behavioral findings to clinical data, we only examined this subscale. Next, our primary dependent variables coding the impact of ketamine during reactivation on reconsolidation were three-fold – subjects' GSR responses during initial extinction and their ratings of valence and arousal post-extinction. In order to limit our exposure to type-I error, we planned only to bring through the variables (of those 3) that were significantly impacted by ketamine to the regression analysis. We did not relate the reinstatement data to the neural or clinical data as they were gathered in order to confirm and inform upon any behavioral effects that we observed during extinction (i.e. whether or not we had modulated reconsolidation or blocked extinction). Finally, our plan was hierarchical; we related the neural and behavioral data (again, only those variables that were significantly impacted by ketamine), given any significant associations, we then explored the link between those behavioral variables and the clinical data (summarized by the perceptual subscale).

Therefore, the maximum number of potential regression analyses we could have computed was 6: three separate regressions of neural data on GSR, Valence and Arousal and three regressions of CADSS perceptual subscale on GSR, Valence and Arousal. In practice, given the results we obtained (see below), we computed four correlations: 2 between brain and behavioral data, and 2 between behavioral and clinical scales. These analyses harnessed the power of individual differences across subjects, constrained however, by our prior work [3,38] and hypotheses [14].

Study 2 – Ketamine's effects on reconsolidation of appetitive memory

As in Study 1b, this study employed a double-blind, placebo controlled, randomized, within-subjects design to assess the effects of intravenous ketamine on memory reactivation and subsequent reconsolidation, appetitive memory for juice rewards in this case. Subjects were 8 healthy volunteers who met the inclusion exclusion criteria for experiment 1 (4 female, aged 19–33).

As before, subjects attended on two main study sessions, once for ketamine, the other for placebo infusion. On the drug day, subjects received an infusion of ketamine (200 ng/ml plasma, administered by an un-blinded clinician exactly as in experiment 1) whilst they performed a series of cognitive tasks (to be reported elsewhere) and a clinical interview exploring the presence, nature and severity of any psychotic symptoms. On the placebo day, a saline infusion was administered whilst subjects performed parallel versions of the cognitive tests and clinical interviews. There was a one-month washout period between drug and placebo visits to avoid effects related to activity of ketamine's metabolites.

Reconsolidation of appetitive memories. The reconsolidation memory design followed the structure of experiment 1 closely. Subjects attended the laboratory on 6 occasions, 3 for the drug arm of the study and 3 for the placebo arm. Drug and placebo were administered in a randomized counterbalanced order.

On Day 1 the participant sat in front of a computer screen, holding four reward delivery tubes in their mouth. Three of these tubes, before reaching the mouth, converged on a 3 to 1 valve, allowing three different rewarding liquids to be received through one emerging tube that formed a mouthpiece and ensured the participant was comfortable during the task.

One of three visual stimuli (conditioned stimulus – CS) was presented on a computer screen, followed by the delivery of a liquid reward (unconditioned stimulus – US) corresponding to that CS. One of three NE-510 OEM High Pressure Syringe Pumps delivered 0.9 ml of liquid reward per infusion, through each delivery tube. Visual CS presentation and liquid US delivery were controlled using in-house computer software.

One cue predicted the delivery of blackcurrant juice drink, another the delivery of orange juice drink, and the third predicted water delivery. The first two cue-outcome pairings engendered positive associations between the previously neutral cues. The water US served as a neutral outcome. Each cue-outcome pairing was presented 25 times.

The final tube attached to the mouthpiece allowed monitoring of the pressure changes that occurred throughout the trial (to this end, participants are instructed to use their lips to form a tight seal round both tubes throughout the task). Pressure measurements were made with a Biopac^{TM} data acquisition system, which amplified and digitized the pressure signal that was then recorded using the 'Acknowledge^{TM} 3.9.0' software package.

During CS presentation, subjects anticipated how much they would like liquid they were about to receive by selecting a number between 1 and 9 on a computer keyboard, during presentation of the CS (1 = dislike, 9 = like very much).

On Day 2, whilst looking at the computer screen, the participant held the tubes in their mouth as per Day 1. However, just one trial occurs. The CS that predicted juice reward (either blackcurrant or orange randomized and counterbalanced across subjects) was presented and subjects made their anticipatory liking rating. Pressure changes were not measured.

On Day 3, participants held the tubes in their mouths and were presented with the CSs as per the learning phase. They were instructed to rate their anticipated liking of the liquid rewards, from 1 – 9, as they had in the learning phase. However, no liquids are delivered. Each CS was presented 15 times. Their anticipatory sucking during the CSs was also recorded.

Results

Study 1

Study 1a: Behavioral results. Subjects showed clear evidence of behavioral blocking. They were less likely to predict an allergy when confronted with the blocked cue, and their predictions were less confident ($t = 7.169$, 2-tailed, d.f. $= 16$, $p < 0.0001$ (Figure 2A).

Study 1a: fMRI results. Presenting the blocked cue causing the allergy engendered a PE response in rPFC ($x = 42$, $y = 18$, $z = 20$. z-score $= 2.50$. $p < 0.05$) and bilateral head of caudate ($x = -6$, $y = 16$, $z = 6$. z-score $= 2.99$, $p < 0.05$; $x = 4$, $y = 14$, $z = 6$. z-score $= 2.23$ $p < 0.05$), when compared with control trials (Figure 3B). Blocking trials were associated with an attenuated response in rPFC relative to control trials ($x = 42$, $y = 18$, $z = 20$. $p < 0.05$, Figure 3A). Subjects with the greatest reduction in rPFC response to blocking (Stage 2) showed the greatest subsequent evidence of blocking. That is, they showed a reduced tendency to predict an allergy in response to the blocked cue at Stage 3 ($z = 3.96$, $p < 0.05$, Figure 2B). As well as the rPFC response to blocking predicting subsequent behavior, it also predicted the magnitude of brain response to the subsequent violation of blocking ($z = 3.77$, $p < 0.05$ Figure 2C).

In brief, the behavioral and neural responses to blocking indicated the success of this experimental manipulation and were strongly consistent with our previous studies indicating a role for rPFC in error-dependent learning of causal associations. Having established this, the key question was whether variation across individuals in this PE response related to the effects of ketamine. From Study 1a we can extract a measure of variation PE driven belief formation between individuals. Study 1b had two aims: to assess the influence of ketamine administration upon processes related to belief persistence and to confirm that variation in ketamine effects was related to variation in the belief formation measure established in Study 1a.

Study 1b – within-subject placebo-controlled study of ketamine

Study 1b: Ketamine plasma levels. The mean ketamine plasma concentration across subjects was 259.8 +/−85.6 ng/ml.

Study 1b: Psychopathology. Compared to placebo, ketamine increased perceptual aberrations (CADSS perceptual subscale score, $t = 4.748$, d.f. $= 14$, $p < 0.0001$), which are associated with delusion-like ideation on ketamine [38,67], and phenomenologically similar to the delusional mood that portends delusion formation [33,68–71].

Study 1b: Cognitive effects of ketamine. Conditioning (Day 1) Subjects' skin conductance responses were consistent with differential conditioning to CS_1 versus CS_2 on the days prior to ketamine and placebo infusion. Focusing on mean responses to the last five trials in which each cue was presented, ANOVA revealed a main effect of cue (CS_1 vs. CS_2, $F_{(1,15)} = 9.273$, $p < 0.01$) but no difference between the cues that were to be reactivated under ketamine or placebo ($F_{(1,15)}$ =,0.557 $p > 0.4$) and the difference between CS_1 and CS_2 (i.e. learning) was equivalent for the cues that were to be reactivated under ketamine and those to be reactivated under placebo ($F_{(1,15)} = 0.111$, $p > 0.7$, Figure 4). Hence, any subsequent effects of drug administration on reactivated cues cannot be attributed to differential learning about the to-be-reactivated cues before they were reactivated.

Extinction and reinstatement of conditioned cues reactivated under ketamine or placebo

Post-Extinction Behavioral ratings. Note that all of these results relate to the third day of testing, i.e., 24 hours after the aversively trained cue had been re-presented under either ketamine or placebo. The difference reported between ketamine and placebo refers to changes in the impact of these cues arising from the manipulation 24 hours earlier.

Pleasantness. ANOVA revealed neither a significant main effect of ketamine, nor a significant drug by task interaction in terms of how unpleasant the subjects found the cues.

Arousal. ANOVA revealed no significant main effect of ketamine on arousal ratings. However, there was a significant drug by task interaction; subjects rated the cue that had been associated with delivery of the loud noise presented to them under ketamine as more arousing than an equivalent cue that they had been presented under placebo ($F_{(1,15)} = 4.69$, $p < 0.05$; Figure 5); reactivating an aversive memory under ketamine enhanced the salience of that memory.

Post reactivation Psychophysiology: Extinction, Reminder and Reinstatement

We compared GSRs to the cue reactivated under ketamine with those to its counterpart reactivated under placebo using within subjects ANOVA. There was a significant main effect of task ($F_{(3,45)} = 4.262$, $p < 0.05$); across blocks, responses extinguished. Crucially, there was a main effect of drug ($F_{(1,45)} = 10.87$, $p < 0.01$): Skin conductance responses to the cue reactivated under ketamine were significantly higher than those to the cue reactivated under placebo (Figure 4B).

There was no significant effect of ketamine on responses to the loud noise US-reminders or subsequent habituation (data not shown). That is, having ketamine 24 hours previous did not alter subjects' responses to un-cued loud noises.

Within-subjects ANOVA revealed stronger reinstatement to the cue reactivated under ketamine manifest as a significant drug by task interaction, $F_{(1,15)} = 2.113$, $p < 0.05$, Figure 4C).

Fear memory reactivation and prediction error. Subjects who rated the cue reactivated under ketamine as more arousing had a decreased PE response in the right striatum during the violation of blocking in the causal learning task, assayed 4-weeks earlier ($z = 2.84$, $p < 0.05$, Figure 5A).

Subjects with larger skin conductance responses to the ketamine-reactivated cue demonstrated an attenuated prefrontal response to the violation of blocking during causal learning assayed one month previously ($z = 2.86$, $p < 0.05$, Figure 5B).

Relating ketamine effects on memory reconsolidation to ketamine induced aberrant salience. Subjects who experienced most aberrant perceptual experiences (e.g., enhanced loudness of background noises) as measured by the perceptual subscale of the CADSS (related to aberrant PE in our prior work [38], and hence predicted to be involved *a priori*) showed the most ketamine-induced strengthening of their fear memories, manifest as an enhanced skin conductance to the re-presentation of the cue in extinction the day after the ketamine session (compared with placebo, $r = 0.741$, $p < 0.005$, Figure 6).

Post-hoc analysis: Relating Ketamine effects to brain responses during blocking

Our measure of aberrant PE involved the brain response to the violation of blocking. As a test of internal consistency, we assayed the correlation between the memory strengthening effect of memory reactivation under ketamine and responses during the blocking trials. Consistent with the aberrant PE learning interpretation, rDLPFC response to blocking events correlated positively with enhanced GSR in extinction ($z = 2.08$, $p < 0.05$, Figure 7).

The role of ketamine in enhancing persistence of memory for an aversive US in Study 1b might be due, in part or in full, to aversive aspects of the ketamine experience somehow enhancing the expression of CS-US knowledge, rather than the predicted influence on processes involved in extinction and reconsolidation.

Study 2 therefore was conducted to determine whether the effects of ketamine upon memory persistence would be observed for an appetitive US (consistent with a direct influence upon reconsolidation and extinction processes).

Study 2 – Appetitive learning (behavioral study only)

This follow-up study clarified the effects of ketamine on post-reactivation memory processing.

Subjects' anticipatory ratings of pleasantness reflected that by the end of conditioning on Day 1, they had learned the CS-US relationships. ANOVA revealed a main effect of cue ($F_{(2,14)} = 5.64$, $p < 0.05$), but no difference between the cues that were to be reactivated under ketamine compared to those that were to be reactivated under placebo 24 hours later ($F_{(1,7)} = 0.151$, $p > 0.7$) and the difference between CS_1 and CS_2 was equivalent for the cues to be reactivated under ketamine and those to be reactivated under placebo ($F_{(2,14)} = 0.88$, $p > 0.4$). In addition, the difference between anticipatory sucking pressure exerted to CS_1 and CS_2 was not significantly different across visits (paired sample t-test on difference in anticipatory sucking to CS_1 and CS_2, d.f. $= 7$, $t = 0.111$, $p > 0.9$), suggesting that this metric also indicated equivalent differential conditioning on Day 1 for ketamine and placebo.

Hence, subjects learned that the appetitive cues signified valued juices rather than neutral solution. Furthermore, they did so to an equivalent extent for cues associated with the ketamine session and those associated with the placebo visit. Any differences observed following reactivation could not be attributed to differences in prior conditioning.

Repeated measures ANOVA of the pleasantness ratings subjects gave for the cues revealed a trend toward a significant drug by cue interaction ($F_{(2,14)} = 2.715$, $p = 0.1$). When we examined exactly the same contrast we conducted in our aversive memory experiment, comparing ketamine reactivation to placebo reactivation, there was a significant interaction ($F_{(1,7)} = 6.377$, $p < 0.05$): cues reactivated under ketamine were rated as significantly more pleasant than those reactivated under placebo in extinction the following day (See Figure 8A). It is possible that association also retrieved the non-reactivated control cue during the re-activation on drug, hence the lack of significant interaction. However, the differences between ketamine and placebo reactivated positive cues are consistent with our findings from Study 1.

ANOVA revealed a significant drug by cue interaction ($F_{(2,14)} = 4.074$, $p < 0.05$). Subjects applied greater sucking pressure during the first exposure to the cue reactivated under ketamine than its placebo reactivated counterpart as well as the un-reactivated salient and neutral cues (Figure 8B).

Given the relatively small sample size, we did not examine individual difference regression analyses for Study 2.

Discussion

We observed that individual variability in the PE signal correlated with the strengthening of memories reactivated under ketamine and that this strengthening effect was correlated with the profundity of ketamine-induced perceptual disruptions. Furthermore, we partially replicated the strengthening effect in a new cohort of volunteers in whom appetitive memories were reactivated (there was only a trend towards drug by task interaction in the pleasantness ratings. The interaction was significant for the anticipatory sucking measures). Taken together, these findings support the hypothesized link between PE, retrieval-based memory modulation and psychopathology.

Our study demonstrated a clear blocking effect in human causal learning. During blocking trials, there was the expected [50] overall suppression of BOLD response in regions previously shown to be sensitive to PE [2,3,38,56,72]. When blocked cues were subsequently presented, group average predictive responses indicated that subjects had not learned to associate these cues with an outcome. Violation of that attenuated expectation was expressed neurally as a PE response in key frontostriatal regions [2]. Participants showing the lowest rPFC response during blocking trials showed the greatest subsequent behavioral evidence of blocking and the greatest subsequent neural "surprise" response when particular blocked cues proved unexpectedly to be predictors of an outcome (see Figure 2). More importantly, as we discuss below, variations in PE responding predicted individual vulnerability to the subsequent experiential and mnemonic impact of ketamine.

We determined the influence of ketamine on reactivated memories. Re-presentation of a pre-trained aversive cue under ketamine compared to placebo was associated with elevated ratings of unpleasantness and GSR when these were tested the following day. Crucially, individuals showing aberrant PE in the fMRI study were more susceptible to these enhanced effects. We argue that this underlines the importance of aberrant PE and subsequent memory processing in the pathophysiology of psychotic symptoms. Put simply, the failure of PFC to show an appropriate response to blocking (study 1a stage 2) and its ensuing violation (stage 3) are predictive of an enhanced vulnerability to the memory-altering effects of ketamine.

We considered the possibility that the strengthening of the reactivated cue occurred because the cue was associated with an aversive ketamine experience. However a similar (albeit weaker) effect in an appetitive conditioning in study 2 militates against this argument. For both aversive and appetitive reactivated cues, strength of responding (GSR and anticipatory sucking respectively) increased following ketamine. It is difficult to explain this observation in terms of attenuated extinction, since one would expect consistent responding from Day 1 to Day 3 for the ketamine reactivated cues and perhaps a decrease in responding for the placebo reactivated cue, which we did not observe.

It is perhaps surprising that ketamine (a non-competitive NMDA receptor antagonist with known amnestic effects [73]) appears to enhance reactivated memories. Initial pre-clinical studies of pharmacological effects on reconsolidation have demonstrated that NMDA receptor antagonism impairs or prevents memory reconsolidation. Importantly, however, only one rodent study employed ketamine as the NMDA blocking agent that perturbed drug-memory reconsolidation [74], others employ more potent NMDA receptor antagonists like MK-801 or PCP. The difference between our work and the rodent work may also have arisen because we are dealing with different response systems in human and rodent subjects [75,76]. Behavioral studies capture numerous measures of conditioning, ranging from subjective ratings, skin conductance measures and startle responses to conscious expectancies of subsequent outcomes. In the intact organism, these measures often cross-validate. However, in a reactivation-degradation procedure in human subjects, only some of these measures are disrupted whilst other remain intact [42]: startle responses are degraded whereas measures related to conscious awareness are not. Electrodermal conditioning reflects anticipatory arousal [77–79] and conscious awareness of contingent relationships seems critical for the expression of skin conductance responses [77–79]. These measures were the focus of our present research and we did not record startle responses (perhaps more akin to freezing in pre-clinical models). Furthermore, in considering the fact that a ketamine-induced memory strengthening is counter-intuitive, it is notable that, ketamine, when used as an anesthetic in accident victims, may enhance PTSD symptoms [80], perhaps suggesting that aversive memories are enhanced, although this claim is controversial [81]. Our data suggest that both appetitive and aversive memories may be enhanced, depending on what is brought to mind during the ketamine experience. This must give us pause for thought when we consider the increasing interest in using repeated ketamine as an anti-depressant.

Intriguingly, in Study 1b, subjective and objective measures of the strength of fear conditioning correlated with variability in different components of the PE circuit: variation in electrodermal response to a fear-cue reactivated under ketamine was correlated with aberrant prefrontal PE responding whereas variation in the lingering subjective arousal ratings of the fear-cue reactivated under ketamine correlated with aberrant striatal responding. These results are perhaps indicative of different roles for PE across different regions: striatal signals may compute predictive value or salience, whereas PFC PE may sculpt more complex global expectations [82]. This distinction echoes that between model-free and model-based reinforcement learning [83,84]. Both of these processes are driven by PE [82] and may be important for symptom generation and maintenance [3,12–15]. These data provide preliminary support for our model; aberrant PE drives delusion formation by imbuing stimuli, thoughts and percepts with a salience that demands explanation. Such an explanation requires rumination and memory reconsolidation, strengthening it inappropriately such that it eventually becomes impervious to contradictory evidence [14].

Another important point to take into account is that, as well as blocking NMDA receptors, ketamine engenders glutamate release [85], which may stimulate AMPA receptors [85] and engage intracellular signaling cascades that engender synaptogenesis [86]. For example, ketamine increases prefrontal extracellular signal regulated kinase (ERK) [87], a key regulator of the fate of reactivated memories [88]. Furthermore, memantine, an NMDA antagonist like ketamine, has been shown to facilitate aversive memory reconsolidation even when given two hours prior to memory reactivation in day-old chicks [89].

Prior work has shown that ketamine increases cortical excitability [90], increasing AMPA receptor stimulation [91]. Recently, transcranial direct current stimulation, which also increases cortical excitability, has been shown to enhance the strength of reactivated memories [92]. Rodent work has confirmed the crucial role of AMPA receptor mobilization in this post-reactivation strengthening effect [93]. Our own computational modeling work suggests that ketamine induces dis-inhibition of cortical microcircuits resulting in synaptic glutamate spillover [94,95]. In brain slices, this ketamine induced increase in glutamate release and EPSCs can be curtailed by propranolol [96], the beta-adrenergic receptor antagonist that has been shown to degrade reactivated memories across species [41]. Furthermore, the aberrant salience experiences and delusion-like ideas (that we presently relate to excessive PE driven memory reconsolidation) are ameliorated by lamotrigine, a drug that blocks presynaptic glutamate release and cortical excitability [97,98]. Taken together, these data suggest that ketamine-induced psychosis results from excessive glutamate release which engages aberrant prediction errors and hence excessive memory strengthening (even if those memories are false).

We should consider the possibility that ketamine is having a primary and deleterious effect on extinction, a pathophysiological process implicated in spontaneous confabulation, another delusion-like phenomenon [99,100], akin to the phenomenology of some ketamine experiences [12]. Indeed, extinction learning fails to consolidate in patients with schizophrenia [101]. While this is a reasonable consideration, a number of aspects of the experimental design and findings do not support this explanation (see Figure 9). First, day 1 entailed partial reinforcement and reactivation involved a brief single presentation of the conditioned stimulus. Both would shift the balance towards reconsolidation rather than extinction [19,21]. Second, there was no sign of an extinction effect for the placebo reactivation condition and, if anything, the cue appeared to exert a stronger effect at the beginning of the post-reactivation session (day 3) than it did at the end of learning on the pre-reactivation session (day 1), see Figure 9. In short, a simple explanation of these findings in terms of an attenuation of extinction is unlikely.

Although schizophrenia is associated with amnesia [102], patients do report hypermnesia for their symptom contents [103,104], and while these may be false memories [15,105], they may be vivid enough to engender post traumatic stress disorder (PTSD) symptoms [106]. It is notable that such delusional false memories can occur following long-term anesthesia that blocks NMDA receptors [106]. The present data raise the intriguing possibility that patients with schizophrenia rely on non-NMDA mediated forms of synaptic plasticity to represent their world. These learning mechanisms may produce less veridical but more robust representations hence the bizarreness and persistence of psychosis.

There are important caveats to the inferences we draw from these data and clearly, they warrant various follow-up studies. To begin with, the imaging effects we report are of small magnitude and the sample sizes, particularly in study 2, are small. Furthermore, future studies should include a non-reactivated control condition, which we included in study 2 but not study 1. It will be important to characterize PE and reconsolidation in patients with fixed delusions since an important difference from ketamine is that, though the latter induces psychotic percepts and delusion-like ideas, most subjects retain insight (although not always [67]). It would also be useful in future studies to examine the relationship between appetitive conditioning to primary reward and our causal learning PE signal and important, too, to assay the degree of arousal subjects report in future appetitive studies, since this was the dimension modulated by ketamine and related to striatal PE signal. Preclinical studies are underway in order to replicate and interrogate this strengthening effect of ketamine and its possible synaptic mechanisms. A more invasive approach will permit investigation at the synaptic level and circumvent the necessarily correlational approach adopted presently. Of course, correlation is not causation but it is a crucial first step in demonstrating that processes (in this case, PE, memory reconsolidation and delusions) are related [107] through shared variation with individual differences in neural PE signal [108].

Overall, while we can only speculate on the precise underlying mechanisms, the key observation here is that the same manipulation that can render an individual vulnerable to delusion-like ideas may also lead to memory persistence. These data are consistent with a theoretical model of delusions in which aberrations of a fundamental learning process, PE, can profoundly and persistently affect an individual's world view. Thus data thus provide an empirical basis for a mechanistic understanding of what has for a long time been considered '*ununderstandable*' [34]: the delusions that attend serious mental illnesses like schizophrenia. They demonstrate, moreover, the potential insights that clinical psychiatry may gain from developments in neuroscience.

Author Contributions

Conceived and designed the experiments: PRC VC PCF JRT JHK BJE AD MRFA JLL ALM. Performed the experiments: PRC VC JMG JSP DCT JCE FSA HLM ARA RA. Analyzed the data: PRC MRFA PCF NS ARA RA. Contributed reagents/materials/analysis tools: NS. Wrote the paper: PRC PCF JRT JHK JLL BJE ALM.

References

1. Dickinson A (2001) The 28th Bartlett Memorial Lecture. Causal learning: an associative analysis. Q J Exp Psychol B 54: 3–25.
2. Corlett PR, Aitken MR, Dickinson A, Shanks DR, Honey GD, et al. (2004) Prediction error during retrospective revaluation of causal associations in humans: fMRI evidence in favor of an associative model of learning. Neuron 44: 877–888.
3. Corlett PR, Murray GK, Honey GD, Aitken MR, Shanks DR, et al. (2007) Disrupted prediction-error signal in psychosis: evidence for an associative account of delusions. Brain 130: 2387–2400.
4. Schlagenhauf F, Sterzer P, Schmack K, Ballmaier M, Rapp M, et al. (2009) Reward feedback alterations in unmedicated schizophrenia patients: relevance for delusions. Biol Psychiatry 65: 1032–1039.
5. Romaniuk L, Honey GD, King JR, Whalley HC, McIntosh AM, et al. (2010) Midbrain activation during Pavlovian conditioning and delusional symptoms in schizophrenia. Archives of general psychiatry 67: 1246–1254.
6. Rescorla RA, Wagner AR (1972) A theory of Pavlovian conditioning: Variations in the effectiveness of reinforcement and non-reinforcement. In: Black AH, Prokasy, W.F., editor. Classical conditioning II: Current research and theory. New York: Appleton-Century-Crofts.
7. Pearce JM, Hall G (1980) A model for Pavlovian learning: variations in the effectiveness of conditioned but not of unconditioned stimuli. Psychol Rev 87: 532–552.
8. Schultz W, Dickinson A (2000) Neuronal coding of prediction errors. Annu Rev Neurosci 23: 473–500.
9. Behrens TE, Hunt LT, Woolrich MW, Rushworth MF (2008) Associative learning of social value. Nature 456: 245–249.
10. Rao RP, Ballard DH (1999) Predictive coding in the visual cortex: a functional interpretation of some extra-classical receptive-field effects. Nat Neurosci 2: 79–87.
11. Corlett PR, Frith CD, Fletcher PC (2009) From drugs to deprivation: a Bayesian framework for understanding models of psychosis. Psychopharmacology (Berl) 206: 515–530.
12. Corlett PR, Honey GD, Krystal JH, Fletcher PC (2010) Glutamatergic Model Psychoses: Prediction Error, Learning, and Inference. Neuropsychopharmacology.
13. Corlett PR, Taylor JR, Wang XJ, Fletcher PC, Krystal JH (2010) Toward a neurobiology of delusions. Prog Neurobiol.
14. Corlett PR, Krystal JH, Taylor JR, Fletcher PC (2009) Why do delusions persist? Front Hum Neurosci 3: 12.
15. Corlett PR, Simons JS, Pigott JS, Gardner JM, Murray GK, et al. (2009) Illusions and delusions: relating experimentally-induced false memories to anomalous experiences and ideas. Front Behav Neurosci 3: 53.
16. Lee JL (2008) Memory reconsolidation mediates the strengthening of memories by additional learning. Nat Neurosci 11: 1264–1266.
17. Misanin JR, Miller RR, Lewis DJ (1968) Retrograde amnesia produced by electroconvulsive shock after reactivation of a consolidated memory trace. Science 160: 554–555.
18. Nader K, Schafe GE, Le Doux JE (2000) Fear memories require protein synthesis in the amygdala for reconsolidation after retrieval. Nature 406: 722–726.
19. Pedreira ME, Perez-Cuesta LM, Maldonado H (2004) Mismatch between what is expected and what actually occurs triggers memory reconsolidation or extinction. Learn Mem 11: 579–585.
20. Sevenster D, Beckers T, Kindt M (2012) Retrieval per se is not sufficient to trigger reconsolidation of human fear memory. Neurobiology of learning and memory 97: 338–345.
21. Eisenhardt D, Menzel R (2007) Extinction learning, reconsolidation and the internal reinforcement hypothesis. Neurobiol Learn Mem 87: 167–173.
22. Pan WX, Schmidt R, Wickens JR, Hyland BI (2008) Tripartite mechanism of extinction suggested by dopamine neuron activity and temporal difference model. J Neurosci 28: 9619–9631.
23. Bouton ME (2000) A learning theory perspective on lapse, relapse, and the maintenance of behavior change. Health Psychol 19: 57–63.
24. Bouton ME (2002) Context, ambiguity, and unlearning: sources of relapse after behavioral extinction. Biol Psychiatry 52: 976–986.
25. Schultz W, Apicella P, Ljungberg T (1993) Responses of monkey dopamine neurons to reward and conditioned stimuli during successive steps of learning a delayed response task. J Neurosci 13: 900–913.
26. Schultz W, Dayan P, Montague PR (1997) A neural substrate of prediction and reward. Science 275: 1593–1599.
27. Freeman TP, Morgan CJ, Pepper F, Howes OD, Stone JM, et al. (2012) Associative blocking to reward-predicting cues is attenuated in ketamine users but can be modulated by images associated with drug use. Psychopharmacology.
28. Schmidt A, Bachmann R, Kometer M, Csomor PA, Stephan KE, et al. (2012) Mismatch negativity encoding of prediction errors predicts S-ketamine-induced cognitive impairments. Neuropsychopharmacology : official publication of the American College of Neuropsychopharmacology 37: 865–875.
29. Jensen J, Willeit M, Zipursky RB, Savina I, Smith AJ, et al. (2008) The formation of abnormal associations in schizophrenia: neural and behavioral evidence. Neuropsychopharmacology 33: 473–479.
30. Menon M, Jensen J, Vitcu I, Graff-Guerrero A, Crawley A, et al. (2007) Temporal difference modeling of the blood-oxygen level dependent response during aversive conditioning in humans: effects of dopaminergic modulation. Biol Psychiatry 62: 765–772.
31. Murray GK, Corlett PR, Clark L, Pessiglione M, Blackwell AD, et al. (2008) Substantia nigra/ventral tegmental reward prediction error disruption in psychosis. Mol Psychiatry 13: 239, 267–276.
32. Corlett PR, Honey GD, Fletcher PC (2007) From prediction error to psychosis: ketamine as a pharmacological model of delusions. J Psychopharmacol 21: 238–252.
33. Kapur S (2003) Psychosis as a state of aberrant salience: a framework linking biology, phenomenology, and pharmacology in schizophrenia. Am J Psychiatry 160: 13–23.
34. Jaspers K (1963) General Psychopathology: Manchester University Press.
35. Mishara AL, Corlett PR (2009) Are delusions biologically adaptive? Salvaging the doxastic shear pin. Behav Brain Sci 32: 530–531.
36. Begg IM, Anas A, Farinacci S (1992) Dissociation of Processes in Belief – Source Recollection, Statement Familiarity, and the Illusion of Truth. Journal of Experimental Psychology-General 121: 446–458.
37. Moritz S, Köther U, Woodward TS, Veckenstedt R, Dechêne A, Stahl C (2012) Repetition is good? An internet trial on the illusory truth effect in schizophrenia and nonclinical participants. Journal of Behavior Therapy and Experimental Psychiatry. E-pub.
38. Corlett PR, Honey GD, Aitken MR, Dickinson A, Shanks DR, et al. (2006) Frontal responses during learning predict vulnerability to the psychotogenic effects of ketamine: linking cognition, brain activity, and psychosis. Arch Gen Psychiatry 63: 611–621.
39. Honey GD, Corlett PR, Absalom AR, Lee M, Pomarol-Clotet E, et al. (2008) Individual differences in psychotic effects of ketamine are predicted by brain function measured under placebo. J Neurosci 28: 6295–6303.

40. Corlett PR, Fletcher PC (2012) The neurobiology of schizotypy: Fronto-striatal prediction error signal correlates with delusion-like beliefs in healthy people. Neuropsychologia 50: 3612–3620.
41. Kindt M, Soeter M, Vervliet B (2009) Beyond extinction: erasing human fear responses and preventing the return of fear. Nat Neurosci 12: 256–258.
42. Soeter M, Kindt M (2010) Dissociating response systems: erasing fear from memory. Neurobiol Learn Mem 94: 30–41.
43. Schiller D, Monfils MH, Raio CM, Johnson DC, Ledoux JE, et al. (2010) Preventing the return of fear in humans using reconsolidation update mechanisms. Nature 463: 49–53.
44. Agren T, Engman J, Frick A, Bjorkstrand J, Larsson EM, et al. (2012) Disruption of reconsolidation erases a fear memory trace in the human amygdala. Science 337: 1550–1552.
45. Schwabe L, Nader K, Wolf OT, Beaudry T, Pruessner JC (2012) Neural signature of reconsolidation impairments by propranolol in humans. Biological psychiatry 71: 380–386.
46. Petrakis IL, Limoncelli D, Gueorguieva R, Jatlow P, Boutros NN, et al. (2004) Altered NMDA glutamate receptor antagonist response in individuals with a family vulnerability to alcoholism. Am J Psychiatry 161: 1776–1782.
47. Morgan HL, Turner DC, Corlett PR, Absalom AR, Adapa R, et al. (2011) Exploring the impact of ketamine on the experience of illusory body ownership. Biological psychiatry 69: 35–41.
48. Moore JW, Turner DC, Corlett PR, Arana FS, Morgan HL, et al. (2011) Ketamine administration in healthy volunteers reproduces aberrant agency experiences associated with schizophrenia. Cognitive neuropsychiatry: 1–18.
49. Kamin L (1969) Predictability, surprise, attention, and conditioning. In: Campbell BA, Church, R.M., editor. Punishment and Aversive Behavior. New York: Appleton-Century-Crofts.
50. Waelti P, Dickinson A, Schultz W (2001) Dopamine responses comply with basic assumptions of formal learning theory. Nature 412: 43–48.
51. Moran PM, Al-Uzri MM, Watson J, Reveley MA (2003) Reduced Kamin blocking in non paranoid schizophrenia: associations with schizotypy. Journal of Psychiatric Research 37: 155–163.
52. O'Tuathaigh CM, Salum C, Young AM, Pickering AD, Joseph MH, et al. (2003) The effect of amphetamine on Kamin blocking and overshadowing. Behavioural pharmacology 14: 315–322.
53. Holland PC (1984) Unblocking in Pavlovian appetitive conditioning. Journal of experimental psychology Animal behavior processes 10: 476–497.
54. Le Pelley ME, Oakeshott SM, McLaren IP (2005) Blocking and unblocking in human causal learning. Journal of experimental psychology Animal behavior processes 31: 56–70.
55. McDannald MA, Lucantonio F, Burke KA, Niv Y, Schoenbaum G (2011) Ventral striatum and orbitofrontal cortex are both required for model-based, but not model-free, reinforcement learning. The Journal of neuroscience : the official journal of the Society for Neuroscience 31: 2700–2705.
56. Turner DC, Aitken MR, Shanks DR, Sahakian BJ, Robbins TW, et al. (2004) The role of the lateral frontal cortex in causal associative learning: exploring preventative and super-learning. Cereb Cortex 14: 872–880.
57. Maldjian JA, Laurienti PJ, Kraft RA, Burdette JH (2003) An automated method for neuroanatomic and cytoarchitectonic atlas-based interrogation of fMRI data sets. Neuroimage 19: 1233–1239.
58. Fletcher PC, Henson RN (2001) Frontal lobes and human memory: insights from functional neuroimaging. Brain 124: 849–881.
59. Worsley KJ, Marrett S, Neelin P, Vandal AC, Friston KJ, et al. (1996) A unified statistical approach for determining significant signals in images of cerebral activation. Hum Brain Mapp 4: 58–73.
60. Genovese CR, Lazar NA, Nichols T (2002) Thresholding of statistical maps in functional neuroimaging using the false discovery rate. Neuroimage 15: 870–878.
61. Vul E, Pashler H (2012) Voodoo and circularity errors. Neuroimage.
62. Ohman A, Mineka S (2001) Fears, phobias, and preparedness: toward an evolved module of fear and fear learning. Psychological review 108: 483–522.
63. Ohman A, Soares JJ (1998) Emotional conditioning to masked stimuli: expectancies for aversive outcomes following nonrecognized fear-relevant stimuli. Journal of experimental psychology General 127: 69–82.
64. Nomura H, Matsuki N (2008) Ethanol enhances reactivated fear memories. Neuropsychopharmacology : official publication of the American College of Neuropsychopharmacology 33: 2912–2921.
65. Orr SP, Metzger LJ, Lasko NB, Macklin ML, Peri T, et al. (2000) De novo conditioning in trauma-exposed individuals with and without posttraumatic stress disorder. Journal of Abnormal Psychology 109: 290–298.
66. Bremner JD, Krystal JH, Putnam FW, Southwick SM, Marmar C, et al. (1998) Measurement of dissociative states with the Clinician-Administered Dissociative States Scale (CADSS). J Trauma Stress 11: 125–136.
67. Pomarol-Clotet E, Honey GD, Murray GK, Corlett PR, Absalom AR, et al. (2006) Psychological effects of ketamine in healthy volunteers. Phenomenological study. Br J Psychiatry 189: 173–179.
68. Corlett PR, D'Souza DC, Krystal JH (2010) Capgras syndrome induced by ketamine in a healthy subject. Biol Psychiatry 68: e1–2.
69. Gross G, Huber G (1972) [Sensory disorders in schizophrenia]. Arch Psychiatr Nervenkr 216: 119–130.
70. Gray JA, Feldon J, Rawlins JNP, Hemsley D, Smith AD (1991) The Neuropsychology of Schizophrenia. Behav Brain Sci 14: 1–84.
71. McGhie A, Chapman J (1961) Disorders of attention and perception in early schizophrenia. Br J Med Psychol 34: 103–116.
72. Fletcher PC, Anderson JM, Shanks DR, Honey R, Carpenter TA, et al. (2001) Responses of human frontal cortex to surprising events are predicted by formal associative learning theory. Nat Neurosci 4: 1043–1048.
73. Fletcher PC, Honey GD (2006) Schizophrenia, ketamine and cannabis: evidence of overlapping memory deficits. Trends Cogn Sci 10: 167–174.
74. Zhai H, Wu P, Chen S, Li F, Liu Y, et al. (2008) Effects of scopolamine and ketamine on reconsolidation of morphine conditioned place preference in rats. Behavioural pharmacology 19: 211–216.
75. Hamm AO, Weike AI (2005) The neuropsychology of fear learning and fear regulation. Int J Psychophysiol 57: 5–14.
76. Weike AI, Schupp HT, Hamm AO (2007) Fear acquisition requires awareness in trace but not delay conditioning. Psychophysiology 44: 170–180.
77. Lovibond PF (2004) Cognitive processes in extinction. Learn Mem 11: 495–500.
78. Lovibond PF, Mitchell CJ, Minard E, Brady A, Menzies RG (2009) Safety behaviours preserve threat beliefs: Protection from extinction of human fear conditioning by an avoidance response. Behaviour research and therapy 47: 716–720.
79. Lovibond PF, Saunders JC, Weidemann G, Mitchell CJ (2008) Evidence for expectancy as a mediator of avoidance and anxiety in a laboratory model of human avoidance learning. Quarterly journal of experimental psychology 61: 1199–1216.
80. Schonenberg M, Reichwald U, Domes G, Badke A, Hautzinger M (2008) Ketamine aggravates symptoms of acute stress disorder in a naturalistic sample of accident victims. Journal of psychopharmacology 22: 493–497.
81. McGhee LL, Maani CV, Garza TH, Gaylord KM, Black IH (2008) The correlation between ketamine and posttraumatic stress disorder in burned service members. The Journal of trauma 64: S195–198; Discussion S197–198.
82. Daw ND, Niv Y, Dayan P (2005) Uncertainty-based competition between prefrontal and dorsolateral striatal systems for behavioral control. Nat Neurosci 8: 1704–1711.
83. Daw ND, Gershman SJ, Seymour B, Dayan P, Dolan RJ (2011) Model-based influences on humans' choices and striatal prediction errors. Neuron 69: 1204–1215.
84. Glascher J, Daw N, Dayan P, O'Doherty JP (2010) States versus rewards: dissociable neural prediction error signals underlying model-based and model-free reinforcement learning. Neuron 66: 585–595.
85. Moghaddam B, Adams B, Verma A, Daly D (1997) Activation of glutamatergic neurotransmission by ketamine: a novel step in the pathway from NMDA receptor blockade to dopaminergic and cognitive disruptions associated with the prefrontal cortex. J Neurosci 17: 2921–2927.
86. Li N, Lee B, Liu RJ, Banasr M, Dwyer JM, et al. (2010) mTOR-dependent synapse formation underlies the rapid antidepressant effects of NMDA antagonists. Science 329: 959–964.
87. Duman RS, Li N, Liu RJ, Duric V, Aghajanian G (2012) Signaling pathways underlying the rapid antidepressant actions of ketamine. Neuropharmacology 62: 35–41.
88. Duvarci S, Nader K, LeDoux JE (2005) Activation of extracellular signal-regulated kinase- mitogen-activated protein kinase cascade in the amygdala is required for memory reconsolidation of auditory fear conditioning. The European journal of neuroscience 21: 283–289.
89. Samartgis JR, Schachte L, Hazi A, Crowe SF (2012) Memantine facilitates memory consolidation and reconsolidation in the day-old chick. Neurobiology of learning and memory.
90. Hoffken O, Haussleiter IS, Westermann A, Lotsch J, Maier C, et al. (2012) Influence of (S)-ketamine on human motor cortex excitability. Experimental brain research Experimentelle Hirnforschung Experimentation cerebrale.
91. McNally JM, McCarley RW, McKenna JT, Yanagawa Y, Brown RE (2011) Complex receptor mediation of acute ketamine application on in vitro gamma oscillations in mouse prefrontal cortex: modeling gamma band oscillation abnormalities in schizophrenia. Neuroscience 199: 51–63.
92. Javadi AH, Cheng P (2012) Transcranial direct current stimulation (tDCS) enhances reconsolidation of long-term memory. Brain stimulation.
93. Rao-Ruiz P, Rotaru DC, van der Loo RJ, Mansvelder HD, Stiedl O, et al. (2011) Retrieval-specific endocytosis of GluA2-AMPARs underlies adaptive reconsolidation of contextual fear. Nature neuroscience 14: 1302–1308.
94. Murray JD, Anticevic A, Gancsos M, Ichinose M, Corlett PR, et al. (2012) Linking Microcircuit Dysfunction to Cognitive Impairment: Effects of Disinhibition Associated with Schizophrenia in a Cortical Working Memory Model. Cerebral cortex.
95. Anticevic A, Gancsos M, Murray JD, Repovs G, Driesen NR, et al. (2012) NMDA receptor function in large-scale anticorrelated neural systems with implications for cognition and schizophrenia. Proceedings of the National Academy of Sciences of the United States of America 109: 16720–16725.
96. Narimatsu E, Kawamata Y, Kawamata M, Fujimura N, Namiki A (2002) NMDA receptor-mediated mechanism of ketamine-induced facilitation of glutamatergic excitatory synaptic transmission. Brain research 953: 272–275.
97. Deakin JF, Lees J, McKie S, Hallak JE, Williams SR, et al. (2008) Glutamate and the neural basis of the subjective effects of ketamine: a pharmaco-magnetic resonance imaging study. Archives of General Psychiatry 65: 154–164.
98. Anand A, Charney DS, Oren DA, Berman RM, Hu XS, et al. (2000) Attenuation of the neuropsychiatric effects of ketamine with lamotrigine:

support for hyperglutamatergic effects of N-methyl-D-aspartate receptor antagonists. Arch Gen Psychiatry 57: 270–276.
99. Schnider A, Bonvallat J, Emond H, Leemann B (2005) Reality confusion in spontaneous confabulation. Neurology 65: 1117–1119.
100. Schnider A (2001) Spontaneous confabulation, reality monitoring, and the limbic system – a review. Brain Res Brain Res Rev 36: 150–160.
101. Holt DJ, Lebron-Milad K, Milad MR, Rauch SL, Pitman RK, et al. (2008) Extinction Memory Is Impaired in Schizophrenia. Biol Psychiatry.
102. Gold JM, Randolph C, Carpenter CJ, Goldberg TE, Weinberger DR (1992) Forms of memory failure in schizophrenia. Journal of Abnormal Psychology 101: 487–494.
103. Bleuler E (1908) Die Prognose der Dementia praecox (Schizophreniegruppe). Allgemeine Zeitschrift für Psychiatrie und psychischgerichtliche Medizin 65: 436–464.
104. Steinberg HR (1969) Hypermnesia and schizophrenia. Psychological Reports 25: 195–198.
105. Bhatt R, Laws KR, McKenna PJ (2010) False memory in schizophrenia patients with and without delusions. Psychiatry Research 178: 260–265.
106. Kiekkas P, Theodorakopoulou G, Spyratos F, Baltopoulos GI (2010) Psychological distress and delusional memories after critical care: a literature review. International nursing review 57: 288–296.
107. Underwood BJ (1975) Individual-Differences as a Crucible in Theory Construction. American Psychologist 30: 128–134.
108. Kosslyn SM, Cacioppo JT, Davidson R, Hughdahl K, Lovallo WR, Spiegel D, Rose R (2002) Bridging psychology and biology: The analysis of individuals in groups. American Psychologist 57: 341–351.

6

Allergies and Risk of Head and Neck Cancer: An Original Study plus Meta-Analysis

Jenn-Ren Hsiao[1]☯, Chun-Yen Ou[1]☯, Hung-I Lo[1], Cheng-Chih Huang[1], Wei-Ting Lee[1], Jehn-Shyun Huang[2], Ken-Chung Chen[2], Tung-Yiu Wong[2], Sen-Tien Tsai[1], Chia-Jui Yen[3], Yuan-Hua Wu[4], Wei-Ting Hsueh[4], Ming-Wei Yang[4], Shang-Yin Wu[3], Jang-Yang Chang[3,5], Kwang-Yu Chang[3,5], Chen-Lin Lin[6], Fang-Ting Wang[1], Yi-Hui Wang[5], Ya-Ling Weng[5], Han-Chien Yang[5], Jeffrey S. Chang[5]*

1 Department of Otolaryngology, National Cheng Kung University Hospital, College of Medicine, National Cheng Kung University, Tainan, Taiwan, **2** Department of Stomatology, National Cheng Kung University Hospital, College of Medicine, National Cheng Kung University, Tainan, Taiwan, **3** Division of Hematology/Oncology, Department of Internal Medicine, National Cheng Kung University Hospital, College of Medicine, National Cheng Kung University, Tainan, Taiwan, **4** Department of Radiation Oncology, National Cheng Kung University Hospital, College of Medicine, National Cheng Kung University, Tainan, Taiwan, **5** National Institute of Cancer Research, National Health Research Institutes, Tainan, Taiwan, **6** Department of Nursing, National Cheng Kung University Hospital, College of Medicine, National Cheng Kung University, Tainan, Taiwan

Abstract

Background: Although the relationship between allergy and cancer has been investigated extensively, the role of allergy in head and neck cancer (HNC) appears less consistent. It is not clear whether allergies can independently influence the risk of HNC in the presence of known strong environmental risk factors, including consumption of alcohol, betel quid, and cigarette.

Methods: The current paper reports results from: 1) an original hospital-based case-control study, which included 252 incident cases of HNC and 236 controls frequency-matched to cases on sex and age; and 2) a meta-analysis combining the results of the current case-control study and 13 previously published studies (9 cohort studies with 727,569 subjects and 550 HNC outcomes and 5 case-control studies with 4,017 HNC cases and 10,928 controls).

Results: In the original case-control study, we observed a strong inverse association between allergies and HNC [odds ratio = 0.41, 95% confidence interval (CI): 0.27–0.62]. The meta-analysis also indicated a statistically significant inverse association between HNC and allergies [meta-relative risk (RR) = 0.76, 95% CI: 0.63–0.91], particularly strong for allergic rhinitis (meta-RR = 0.55, 95% CI: 0.40–0.76). In addition, the inverse association between allergies and HNC was observed only among men (meta-RR = 0.67, 95% CI: 0.54–0.84) but not among women (meta-RR = 0.98, 95% CI: 0.81–1.18).

Conclusions: These findings suggest that immunity plays an influential role in the risk of HNC. Future studies investigating immune biomarkers, including cytokine profiles and genetic polymorphisms, are warranted to further delineate the relationship between allergies and HNC. Understanding the relationship between allergies and HNC may help devise effective strategies to reduce and treat HNC.

Editor: Michael Scheurer, Baylor College of Medicine, United States of America

Funding: This work was funded by the National Health Research Institutes (CA-101-PP-07), the National Research Program for Biopharmaceuticals (100CAP1015-6, NSC100-2325-B-400-013), the National Science Council (NSC99-2314-B-006-018-MY3, NSC101-2325-B-006-009) and the Establishment of Cancer Research System Excellence Program funded by the Department of Health, Executive Yuan (DOH101-TD-C-111-003, DOH101-TD-C-111-004), Taiwan. The funders had no role in study design, data collection and analysis, decision to publish, or preparation of the manuscript.

Competing Interests: The authors have declared that no competing interests exist.

* E-mail: jeffreychang@nhri.org.tw

☯ These authors contributed equally to this work.

Introduction

Head and neck cancer (HNC), including cancers of the oral cavity, oropharynx and larynx, is one of the leading cancers worldwide. Each year, approximately 400,000 cases of oral and oropharyngeal cancer and 160,000 cases of laryngeal cancer are diagnosed worldwide [1]. HNC is also a leading cancer among Taiwanese men, who have the second highest incidence of HNC in the world [2]. According to the Department of Health of Taiwan, HNC was the fourth most common cancer among Taiwanese men in 2009, with an annual incidence of 41 per 100,000 persons [3].

The occurrence of most HNC can be attributed to the consumption of alcohol, cigarette, and betel quid [4,5], although human papillomavirus infection also plays a role, particularly for oropharyngeal cancer [6]. Although alcohol, cigarette, and betel quid are the causes for the majority of the HNC cancer cases, most people who consume these three agents will not develop HNC in their lifetimes, which suggests the roles of other environmental and genetic factors [7,8]. Other potential risk factors for HNC include occupational exposures, poor oral hygiene, mouthwashes containing alcohol, and low fruit and vegetable intake [1,9]; however, there is insufficient knowledge regarding the pathogenesis of HNC.

Immune reactions manifested in the form of allergies have been extensively studied for their relationship with cancer risk [10–12]. Allergies usually result from an overactive immune response to substances in the environment among people with atopic tendency, who are genetically predisposed to produce immunoglobulin E (IgE) against common allergens [13–15]. The cross-linking of IgE on the surface of mast cells and basophils leads to a series of events resulting in allergic diseases, including allergic rhinitis, asthma, eczema, and food allergy [14].

Two hypotheses have been proposed to explain the inverse association between allergies and cancer, the "immunosurveillance hypothesis" and the "prophylaxis hypothesis" [11]. In the "immunosurveillance hypothesis", allergy does not play a direct role to reduce the risk of cancer but is merely a side effect of a more active immune function that effectively detects and eradicates malignant cells [11]. In contrast, allergy plays a direct role to reduce the risk of cancer in the "prophylaxis hypothesis" by expelling toxins or pathogens from the body [11]. A reduced risk associated with allergies has been consistently observed for glioma and pancreatic cancer [16,17], two cancers with largely unknown environmental risk factors. Compared to glioma and pancreatic cancer, the role of allergy in HNC appears less consistent. It is not clear whether allergies can independently influence the risk of HNC in the presence of known strong environmental risk factors, including alcohol, betel quid, and cigarette. In addition, only one previous study has examined the interaction between lifestyle factors (cigarette smoking and alcohol drinking) and allergies on the risk of HNC [18]. To this end, we conducted a hospital-based study to examine the association between allergies and HNC, including the interaction between allergies and alcohol, betel quid, or cigarette on the development of HNC. In addition, a comprehensive literature search was performed to conduct a meta-analysis, combining results from the published literature with the current study in order to explore the different aspects of the relationship between allergies and HNC and to generate new hypotheses for further investigations.

Materials and Methods

Original Study

This hospital-based case-control study was approved by the institutional review boards of the National Cheng Kung University Hospital and the National Health Research Institutes. All participants of the study signed a written informed consent.

Study subjects. All of the study subjects were recruited from the Department of Otolaryngology and the Department of Stomatology at the National Cheng Kung University Hospital from September 1, 2010 to June 30, 2012. The case subjects were patients newly diagnosed with HNC, including cancers of the oral cavity, oropharynx, and larynx, had no cancer history, aged 20 to 80 years, and had the ability to give informed consent. All HNC cases were pathologically confirmed squamous cell carcinoma. The controls subjects were patients who required surgery for non-cancerous diseases unrelated to cigarette smoking, alcohol drinking, or area nut/betel quid chewing, had no cancer history, had the ability to give informed consent, and frequency-matched to the cases on age (±5 years) and sex.

Data collection. In-person interview was conducted with each study subject by a trained interviewer using a standardized questionnaire. Demographic information, including sex, age, and educational level were collected. Detailed information (dose and duration) of the three major risk factors of HNC, including alcohol, betel quid, and cigarette, was ascertained. Study subjects were asked whether they had any of the five types of allergies, including allergic rhinitis, skin allergy, food allergy, drug allergy, and asthma. Those that responded positive were further asked about the age of onset for these allergies.

Statistical analysis. To assess for the differences in demographic variables and lifestyle habits (alcohol drinking, betel quid chewing, and cigarette smoking) between cases and controls, t-tests and chi-squared tests were performed for continuous variables and categorical variables, respectively. Multivariable unconditional logistic regression was performed to estimate the odds ratio (OR) and 95% confidence interval (CI) of HNC associated with allergies adjusted for age, sex, education, alcohol drinking (frequency), betel quid use (pack-years), and cigarette smoking (pack-years). Although, no pack-year definition has been established for betel-quid use, in order to adjust for the amount and the duration of betel quid use, a pack-year definition similar to the pack-year of cigarette of smoking was used, with 1 pack-year of betel quid use = 1 pack of betel quid (20 betel quids) use per day ×1 year. The analysis was first performed with all allergies combined (yes/no to any of the five allergies, number of allergies, duration of allergies, and age of allergic symptom onset). Subsequent analyses were performed to assess the association between HNC risk and individual types of allergies. To evaluate for the influence of allergy on the association between alcohol, betel quid, or cigarette and HNC, unconditional logistic regression was performed stratified by allergy status (yes/no). The heterogeneity of the association between alcohol, betel quid or cigarette and HNC risk by allergy status was assessed by the log-likelihood ratio test comparing the unconditional logistic regression model with the interaction term (allergy × alcohol, allergy × betel quid, or allergy × cigarette) to the model without the interaction term.

Meta-analysis

Literature search. A literature search was conducted until July 18, 2012 using the PubMed database and Thomson Reuters Web of Science with the search terms: "cancer AND ("allergies" OR "allergy" OR "atopy" OR "atopic" OR "asthma" OR "allergic rhinitis" OR "atopic dermatitis" OR "hive" OR "eczema") AND risk". A total of 1,463 articles were identified using the search terms (Figure 1). Articles were excluded if they had the following characteristics: 1) did not study allergy and cancer risk (n = 1,248); 2) commentary or response to commentary (n = 4); 3) review articles (n = 9); or 4) did not include HNC or did not report separate results for HNC (n = 191). Eleven articles were identified from this initial literature search.[18–28] No additional articles were identified by reviewing the reference lists of the 11 articles identified from the literature search. Two articles by Ericsson had overlapping information and only the most recent article was included in the current meta-analysis [21,22]. Three more articles [29–31] were identified by searching through the reference lists of four review articles [10–12,32]. Along with our original case-control study, a total of 14 studies (9 cohort studies with 727,569 subjects and 550 HNC outcomes and 5 case-control studies with 4,017 HNC cases and 10,928 controls) (Table S1) was included in the meta-analysis.

Data abstraction and calculation of summary statistics. The data extracted from each article included authors, year of publication, types of study (cohort or case-control

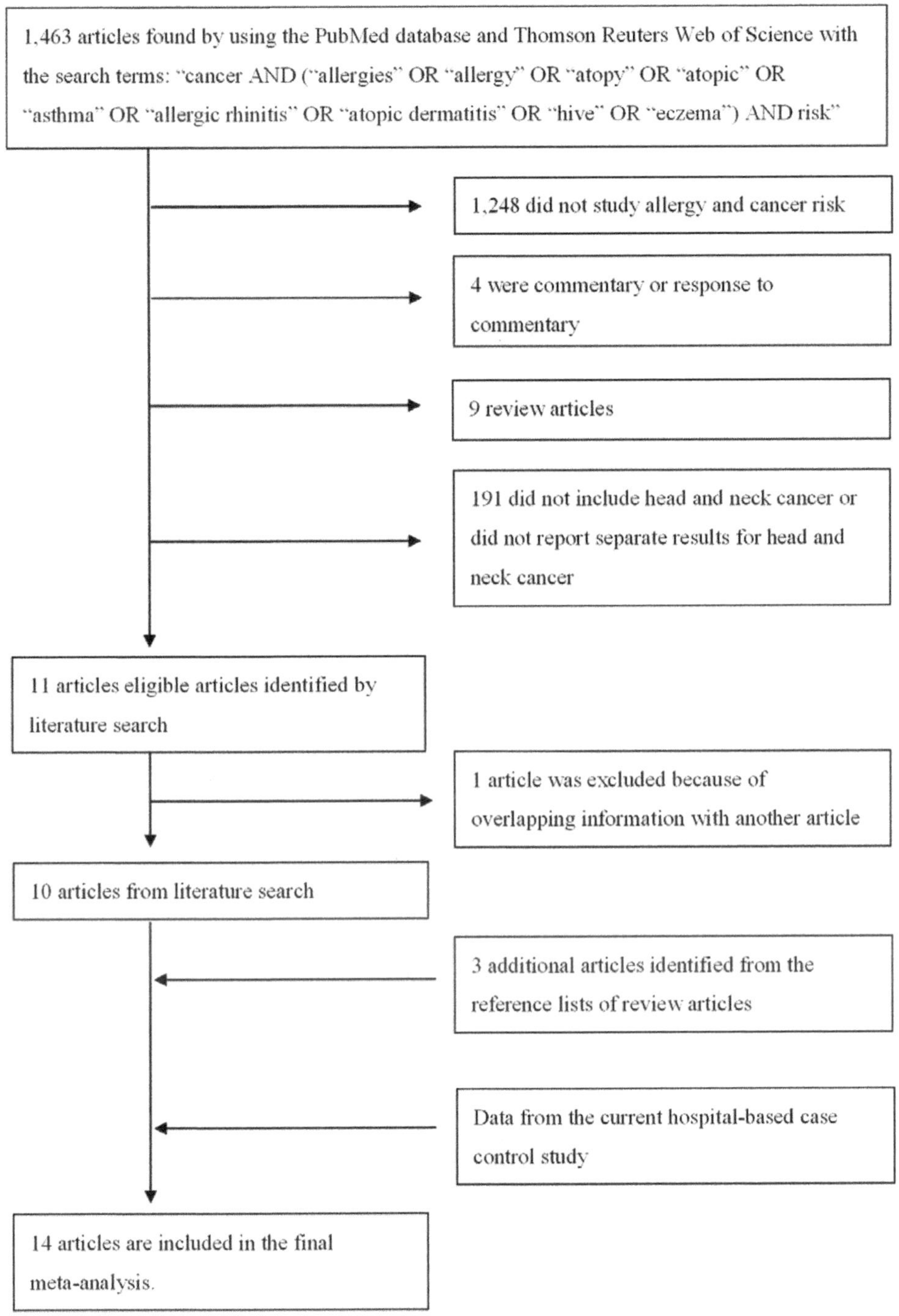

Figure 1. Process of article exclusion.

studies), number of study subjects, variables used for matching and for statistical adjustments, and relative risk (RR, which includes incidence ratio or standardize mortality ratio for cohort studies and odds ratio for case-control studies) with corresponding 95% CIs. For studies that presented only frequency data, RRs and 95% CIs were calculated using the exact method. If a study only reported RRs separately by gender, specific types of allergy or HNC sites, a meta-analysis with a fixed effects model was performed to combine stratum-specific RRs into an overall RR of HNC.

Statistical analysis. STATA software (version 11.0; Stata-Corp, College Station, TX, USA) was used to perform analyses of the current meta-analysis. Summary RRs (meta-RRs) was generated by the "metan" command [33]. The RRs of individual studies are displayed in a forest plot. I^2 statistic was used to evaluate inconsistencies between studies [34]. $I^2 = 0$–24.9%, 25–49.9%, and 50% or more represent low, moderate and high heterogeneity between studies, respectively. The summary RR was generated by a random effects model using the DerSimonian and Laird method if the heterogeneity was moderate to high ($I^2 \geq 25\%$) [35] and by a fixed effects model if the heterogeneity was low

Table 1. Demographic and lifestyle characteristics of the head and neck cancer patients and control subjects.

Characteristics	Cases N = 252 n (%)	Controls N = 236 n (%)	*P*
Age (years)			
Mean (SE)	55.3 (0.7)	53.5 (0.7)	0.05
Sex			
Male	238 (94.4)	220 (93.2)	0.57
Female	14 (5.6)	16 (6.8)	
Education			
≦ Elementary school	81 (32.1)	40 (16.9)	<0.0001
Junior high	77 (30.6)	42 (17.8)	
High school/Technical school	74 (29.4)	96 (40.7)	
Some college or more	20 (7.9)	58 (24.6)	
Alcohol			
Never+occasional	69 (27.4)	100 (42.4)	0.002
Former regular	49 (19.4)	33 (14.0)	
Current regular	134 (53.2)	103 (43.6)	
Never	62 (24.9)	85 (36.2)	<0.0001
1 drink per month	14 (5.6)	29 (12.3)	
1–2 drinks per week	10 (4.1)	14 (6.0)	
3–5 drinks per week	21 (8.4)	31 (13.2)	
Daily drinkers	142 (57.0)	76 (32.3)	
Betel quid			
Never	90 (35.7)	181 (76.7)	<0.0001
Former	103 (40.9)	36 (15.2)	
Current	59 (23.4)	19 (8.1)	
Pack-years (SE)	27.3 (2.9)	7.1 (1.3)	<0.0001
Cigarette			
Never	35 (13.9)	66 (28.0)	0.0001
Former	56 (22.2)	58 (24.6)	
Current	161 (63.9)	112 (47.4)	
Pack-years (SE)	35.1 (1.8)	23.5 (1.6)	<0.0001

Abbreviation: N, number; SE, standard error.

($I^2<25\%$). The analysis was first performed to generate an overall meta-RR measuring the association between all allergies combined and HNC risk. Additional analyses were performed by study design (cohort vs. case-control), by sex, by HNC sites, and by specific types of allergies (allergic rhinitis, skin allergy, or asthma). Sensitivity analysis was performed using the "metainf" command by excluding one study at a time to examine whether any individual study had a dominant effect on the summary RR. Publication bias was examined by viewing the funnel plot and by Egger's regression asymmetry test [36,37].

Results

Original Study

From September 1, 2010 to June 30, 2012, 252 HNC cases (166 oral cancers, 61 oropharyngeal cancers, and 25 laryngeal cancers) and 236 controls were successfully recruited with a participation of 74.3% and 86.5% for the cases and controls, respectively. The HNC cases were slightly older than controls (55.3 years vs. 53.5 years, $P = 0.05$) (Table 1). HNC cases and controls were similar in the distribution of sex (Table 1). Compared to controls, cases had lower educational levels (37% with ≥ high school education among cases vs. 65% with ≥ high school education among controls, $P<0.0001$) (Table 1). Cases had higher consumptions of alcohol, betel quid, and cigarette compared to controls in frequency, duration, and amount (Table 1).

Having any allergy was associated with a reduced risk of HNC (OR = 0.41, 95% CI: 0.27–0.62) (Table 2). This reduced risk was observed across all three HNC sites (oral cancer: OR = 0.36, 95% CI: 0.22–0.57; oropharyngeal cancer: OR = 0.49, 95% CI: 0.25–0.96; laryngeal cancer: OR = 0.48, 95% CI: 0.19–1.18). An inverse association between allergies and HNC was observed among both genders and was particularly strong for men (OR = 0.42, 95% CI: 0.27–0.64) but not statistically significant for women (OR = 0.67, 95 CI: 0.08–5.46), although the result for women was based on small numbers (14 cases and 16 controls). No clear trend in HNC risk was observed with the number of allergies or the duration of allergies (Table 2). In addition, the association between HNC risk and allergies did not differ by the age of allergy onset (<21 years vs. 21 years or older) (Table 2).

The most common type of allergy reported by the study subjects was allergic rhinitis (20% of cases and 41% of controls), which was

Table 2. The association between allergies and head and neck cancer.

Allergy	Head and neck cancer N = 252 n (%)	Control N = 236 n (%)	OR (95% CI)*	*P*
No	164 (65.1)	95 (40.3)	Referent	
Yes	88 (34.9)	135 (57.2)	0.41 (0.27–0.62)	<0.0001
Unknown	0 (1.2)	6 (2.5)	–	–
Number of allergies				
0	164 (65.1)	95 (40.2)	Referent	
1	54 (21.4)	80 (33.9)	0.39 (0.24–0.64)	0.0002
2	23 (9.1)	32 (13.6)	0.54 (0.28–1.02)	0.06
3 or more	10 (4.0)	17 (7.2)	0.40 (0.16–1.03)	0.06
unknown	1 (0.4)	12 (5.1)	–	–
Allergy duration				
No allergy	164 (65.1)	95 (40.3)	Referent	
<10 years	18 (7.1)	25 (10.6)	0.48 (0.23–0.99)	0.05
10–20 years	10 (4.0)	23 (9.7)	0.32 (0.14–0.75)	0.008
>20 years	48 (19.0)	67 (28.4)	0.45 (0.27–0.74)	0.002
Unknown	12 (4.8)	26 (11.0)	–	–
Age of allergy onset				
No allergy	164 (65.1)	95 (40.3)	Referent	
<21 years old	27 (10.7)	52 (22.0)	0.38 (0.21–0.68)	0.001
21 years or older	53 (21.0)	75 (31.8)	0.42 (0.26–0.69)	0.0005
Unknown	8 (3.2)	14 (5.9)	–	–

*OR was adjusted for age, sex, education, alcohol drinking (frequency), betel quid chewing (pack-years), and cigarette smoking (pack-years).
Abbreviations: CI, confidence interval; N, number; OR, odds ratio.

associated with a reduced risk of HNC (OR = 0.32, 95 CI: 0.20–0.52) (Table 3). A consistent reduction in the risk of HNC was seen with the other four types of allergies, including skin allergy, food allergy, drug allergy, and asthma.

The increased risk of HNC associated with alcohol drinking, betel quid chewing or cigarette smoking appeared stronger among those without history of allergies, although the tests for heterogeneity were not statistically significant (Table 4).

Meta-analysis (Table 5)

Combining the data from 14 studies (9 cohort and 5 case-control studies), the meta-analysis showed a reduced risk of HNC associated with having allergies (meta-RR = 0.76, 95% CI: 0.63–0.91, $I^2 = 76.5\%$) (Figure 2). Sensitivity analysis by dropping one study at a time did not indicate a dominant influence of any one individual study on the summary RR. The Egger's regression asymmetry test indicated no evidence of publication bias (p = 0.07). Funnel plot (Figure 3) showed that there may be minor evidence of publication bias with a slight over-representation of smaller studies (n = 2) [22,31] with a RR value greater than the meta-RR. However, the meta-analysis excluding those two smaller studies generated a result (meta-RR = 0.74, 95% CI: 0.62–0.90, $I^2 = 79.0\%$) that was nearly identical to the result that combined all 14 studies, which indicated that the possibility of publication bias was minimal.

The combined analysis of 9 cohort studies with 727,569 subjects with allergies and 550 HNC outcomes showed a 9% reduction in HNC risk associated with allergies, although not statistically significant (meta-RR = 0.91, 95% CI: 0.71–1.17, $I^2 = 74.0\%$). The combined analysis of 5 case-control studies with 4,017 HNC cases and 10,928 controls showed a statistically significant inverse association between allergies and HNC (meta-RR = 0.58, 95% CI: 0.44–0.78, $I^2 = 76.1\%$).

When stratified by sex, the inverse association between allergies and HNC was only observed among men (meta-RR = 0.67, 95% CI: 0.54–0.84, $I^2 = 68.2\%$) but not among women (meta-RR = 0.98, 95% CI: 0.81–1.18, $I^2 = 20.2\%$). In the analysis with specific types of allergies, the strongest reduced risk of HNC was observed for allergic rhinitis (meta-RR = 0.55, 95% CI: 0.40–0.76, $I^2 = 46.1\%$) and a weaker reduction in HNC risk was observed for skin allergy (meta-RR = 0.84, 95% CI: 0.62–1.14, $I^2 = 43.0\%$) and asthma (meta-RR = 0.86, 95% CI: 0.71–1.05, $I^2 = 63.1\%$). A reduced risk associated with allergies was observed across all three sites of HNC (meta-RR for oral cancer = 0.78, 95% CI: 0.61–1.00, $I^2 = 72.2\%$; meta-RR for oropharyngeal cancer = 0.69, 95% CI: 0.58–0.82, $I^2 = 33.6\%$; meta-RR for laryngeal cancer = 0.66, 95% CI: 0.47–0.92, $I^2 = 53.0\%$) (Table 5); however, similar to the results of all sites combined, the inverse association between allergies and subsites of HNC occurred predominantly among men.

Discussion

A statistically significant inverse association between allergies and HNC was observed in our hospital-based case-control study. Combining the results of our study and those from the 13 published studies, the meta-analysis also indicated a statistically significant inverse association between HNC and allergies, particularly for allergic rhinitis and predominantly among men.

The inverse association between allergies and cancer may be explained by two hypotheses, the "immunosurveillance hypothe-

Table 3. The association between head and neck cancer and specific types of allergies.

Allergies	Cases N = 252	Controls N = 236	OR (95% CI)*	P
Nasal allergy				
No allergy	164 (65.1)	95 (40.2)	Referent	
Yes	51 (20.2)	97 (41.1)	0.32 (0.20–0.52)	<0.0001
Other allergies	36 (14.3)	36 (15.3)	0.67 (0.37–1.20)	0.18
Unknown	1 (0.4)	8 (3.4)	–	–
Skin allergy				
No allergy	164 (65.1)	95 (40.2)	Referent	
Yes	39 (15.5)	40 (17.0)	0.67 (0.38–1.17)	0.16
Other allergies	49 (19.4)	92 (39.0)	0.32 (0.20–0.52)	<0.0001
Unknown	0 (0.0)	9 (3.8)	–	–
Food allergy				
No allergy	164 (65.1)	95 (40.2)	Referent	
Yes	20 (7.9)	23 (9.8)	0.63 (0.30–1.31)	0.21
Other allergies	68 (27.0)	112 (47.5)	0.38 (0.24–0.58)	<0.0001
Unknown	0 (0.0)	6 (2.5)	–	–
Drug Allergy				
No allergy	164 (65.1)	95 (40.2)	Referent	
Yes	16 (6.3)	29 (12.3)	0.44 (0.21–0.92)	0.03
Other allergies	72 (28.6)	105 (44.5)	0.41 (0.27–0.64)	<0.0001
Unknown	0 (0.0)	7 (3.0)	–	–
Asthma				
No allergy	164 (65.1)	95 (40.2)	Referent	
Yes	7 (2.8)	17 (7.2)	0.26 (0.09–0.73)	0.01
Other allergies	81 (32.1)	118 (50.0)	0.44 (0.29–0.67)	0.0001
Unknown	0 (0.0)	6 (2.6)	–	–

*OR was adjusted for age, sex, education, alcohol drinking (frequency), betel quid chewing (pack-years), and cigarette smoking (pack-years).
Abbreviations: CI, confidence interval; N, number; OR, odds ratio.

sis" and the "prophylaxis hypothesis" [11]. In the "immunosurveillance hypothesis", allergy is a side effect of an overactive immune function that effectively detects and eradicates malignant cells and does not play a direct role to reduce the risk of cancer [11]. In contrast, in the "prophylaxis hypothesis", allergy is directly involved in cancer prevention by expelling toxins or pathogens from the body [11]. A review by Sherman *et al.* observed that the inverse association between allergies and cancer was more commonly found among tissues or organ systems that interface with the external environment (*i.e.* glia, mouth and throat, colon and rectum, pancreas, skin, uterus and cervix, lung, bladder, and gastrointestinal tract) than among those that do not (*i.e.* ovaries, meninges, prostate, breast, and blood cells); this led them to conclude that the "prophylaxis hypothesis" may be the more appropriate explanation for the site-specific inverse association between allergies and certain cancers [11]. Although the results from our case-control study and meta-analysis appear to be consistent with the "prophylaxis hypothesis" because the three sites of HNC, oral cavity, oropharynx, and larynx, directly interface with the external environment, the role of "immunosurveillance hypothesis" cannot be ruled out by the evidence from this analysis. Further investigation is needed to delineate the underlying biological mechanism for the inverse association between allergies and HNC risk.

IgE plays a key role in most allergic reactions and evidence shows that IgE itself may possess anti-tumor activities [38]. An immunohistochemical study by Neuchrist *et al.* examined the distribution of immunoglobulins in squamous cell carcinoma of head and neck by comparing tumor and normal tissues [39]. They found that the distribution of IgE showed the largest difference, with significantly higher number of IgE-positive cells found in the tumor tissue compared to the normal tissue [39], which suggested that IgE may participate in tumor surveillance. In addition, IgE may also bind to cell surface IgE receptors, FcεRI and CD23, and engage several types of effector cells in antibody-dependent cellular cytotoxicity and antibody-dependent cellular phagocytosis against cancer cells [38]. Overall, the possible anti-tumor activities of IgE may partially explain the inverse association between allergies and cancer, including HNC.

In our original case-control study, there was a suggestion that allergies may attenuate the carcinogenic effect of alcohol, betel quid, or cigarette on the development of HNC risk, although the results were not statistically significant likely due to a sample size without sufficient statistical power. A possible explanation for the attenuating effect of allergies on HNC risk due to alcohol, betel quid, or cigarette may be a hyperactive immune function that can detect and destroy malignant cells before they have a chance to grow and expand. Alternatively, allergy-associated immune activities may rid body of the carcinogens before they have a chance to induce the oncogenic transformation of normal cells. However, in a previous study by Michaud *et al.* the association between allergies and HNC risk did not differ by smoking status (never smoker: OR = 0.75, 95% CI:0.54–1.04; former smoker: OR = 0.80, 95% CI: 0.62–1.02) or drinking status (less than 7 drinks per week: OR = 0.78, 95% CI: 0.60–1.01; greater than 25 drinks per week: OR = 0.59, 95% CI: 0.37–0.95) [18]. Unfortunately, among the studies to date, only Michaud *et al.* [18] and our study had examined the interaction between allergies and lifestyle factors (cigarette smoking, alcohol drinking, or betel quid chewing) on HNC risk, and thus, we were unable to explore this topic further in the meta-analysis.

The results from the meta-analysis showed that the inverse association between allergies and HNC was stronger among the case-control studies (meta-RR = 0.58, 95% CI: 0.44–0.78) compared to that among the cohort studies (meta-RR = 0.91, 95% CI: 0.71–1.17). All except one of the cohort studies on the association between allergies and HNC used data from medical records or clinical tests, whereas all of the case-control studies used self-reported data of allergies. Self-reported data might be more inaccurate due to recall errors associated with false memory or misinterpretation of non-allergic symptoms (*e.g.* common cold) as allergies. These recall errors were likely non-differential and would have biased the results toward the null; thus, the actual inverse association between allergies and HNC should be stronger in the absence of non-differential recall errors. Self-reported data in a case-control study can also be subject to differential recall bias. Usually, case subjects are more likely to ruminate about the possible causes of their diseases and may thus report more allergic symptoms, leading to a false positive association between allergies and HNC. However, the current meta-analysis indicated an inverse association between allergies and HNC for the case-control studies. In addition, the potential association between allergies and cancer is not well-known to the public; therefore, the inverse

Table 4. The association between lifestyle factors and head and neck cancer by allergy status.

Characteristics	Allergy = Yes OR (95% CI)*	Allergy = No OR (95% CI)*	Interaction *P*
Alcohol			
Never+non-daily drinkers	Referent	Referent	
Ever daily drinker	1.47 (0.76–2.85)	2.65 (1.37–5.13)	0.17
Never+non-daily drinkers	Referent	Referent	
Former daily drinker	1.18 (0.40–3.51)	2.23 (0.62–8.10)	
Current daily drinkers	1.56 (0.77–3.18)	2.73 (1.37–5.45)	0.39
Betel quid			
Never	Referent	Referent	
Ever	4.25 (2.14–8.42)	5.62 (2.84–11.12)	0.49
Never	Referent	Referent	
Former	3.82 (1.82–7.99)	6.31 (2.88–13.82)	0.49
Current	5.48 (2.08–14.45)	4.57 (1.80–11.59)	
Pack-years			
Never	Referent	Referent	
<20 pack-years	3.29 (1.44–7.49)	3.97 (1.66–9.50)	
≥20 pack-years	4.76 (2.04–11.09)	6.51 (2.84–14.95)	0.80
Cigarette			
Never	Referent	Referent	
Ever	0.98 (0.41–2.38)	2.63 (1.17–5.93)	0.09
Never	Referent	Referent	
Former	0.87 (0.31–2.41)	2.60 (1.05–6.42)	0.28
Current	1.05 (0.42–2.62)	2.66 (1.11–6.39)	
Pack-years			
Never	Referent	Referent	
<20 pack-years	0.62 (0.21–1.77)	3.17 (1.15–8.73)	0.11
≥20 pack-years	1.28 (0.51–3.22)	(1.04–5.62)	

*OR was adjusted for age, sex, education, alcohol drinking (frequency), betel quid chewing (pack-years), and cigarette smoking (pack-years).
Abbreviations: CI, confidence interval; OR, odds ratio.

association between allergies and HNC among the case-control studies is unlikely due to differential recall bias. Compared to the cohort studies, the case-control studies were more likely to suffer from reverse causality, since the information on allergies was ascertained after the diagnosis of HNC and the immune function might be affected by the oncogenic process. In our original hospital-based case-control study, even when we considered allergies occurring more than 10 years before the diagnosis of cancer (or before the interview date for the controls), a strong inverse association between allergies and HNC still existed. In a hospital-based case-control by Vena et al. which considered only allergies diagnosed five years before the hospital admission, a reduced risk of HNC associated with allergies was observed among men [26]. These indicate that reverse causality might not play a major role in the inverse relationship between allergies and HNC. Although cohort studies do not suffer from recall bias or reverse causality, they are not without limitations. A major limitation of cohort studies, especially when studying a rare disease or a disease with a long latency period (*e.g.* cancer), is that there may not be enough outcomes during the follow-up period to produce a precise effect estimate [40].

An alternative method to study the association between allergies and HNC is "Mendelian Randomization", which utilizes a functional genetic polymorphism as an instrumental variable to study the relationship between modifiable exposures and disease in observational studies [41]. Genetic polymorphisms are not subject to recall or selection biases and therefore may serve as a more objective marker. For example, interleukin-4 is a key cytokine that induces naïve T-helper cells to differentiate into T-helper 2 cells, which play a major role in the development of allergies [42]. The T allele of a promoter single nucleotide polymorphism of the interleukin-4 gene, C-589T (also known as C-590T or rs2243250), has been associated with a higher level of serum IgE and a higher risk of allergy [43]. To date, three studies have examined the relationship between rs2243250 and HNC, specifically oral cancer [44–46]. Two of the three studies showed an increased risk of oral cancer with either the C allele [45] or the CC genotype [46], consistent with an inverse association between allergies and HNC. However, one study reported an opposite finding with an increased risk of oral cancer associated with the TT genotype [44]. With more investigations of rs2243250 and other genetic polymorphisms associated with allergies, the true association and the underlying biological mechanism between allergies and HNC may be clarified.

The current meta-analysis suggests that the inverse association between allergies and HNC may be particularly strong for allergic rhinitis. It has been long observed that not all people with atopic tendency will develop allergic symptoms and those who develop

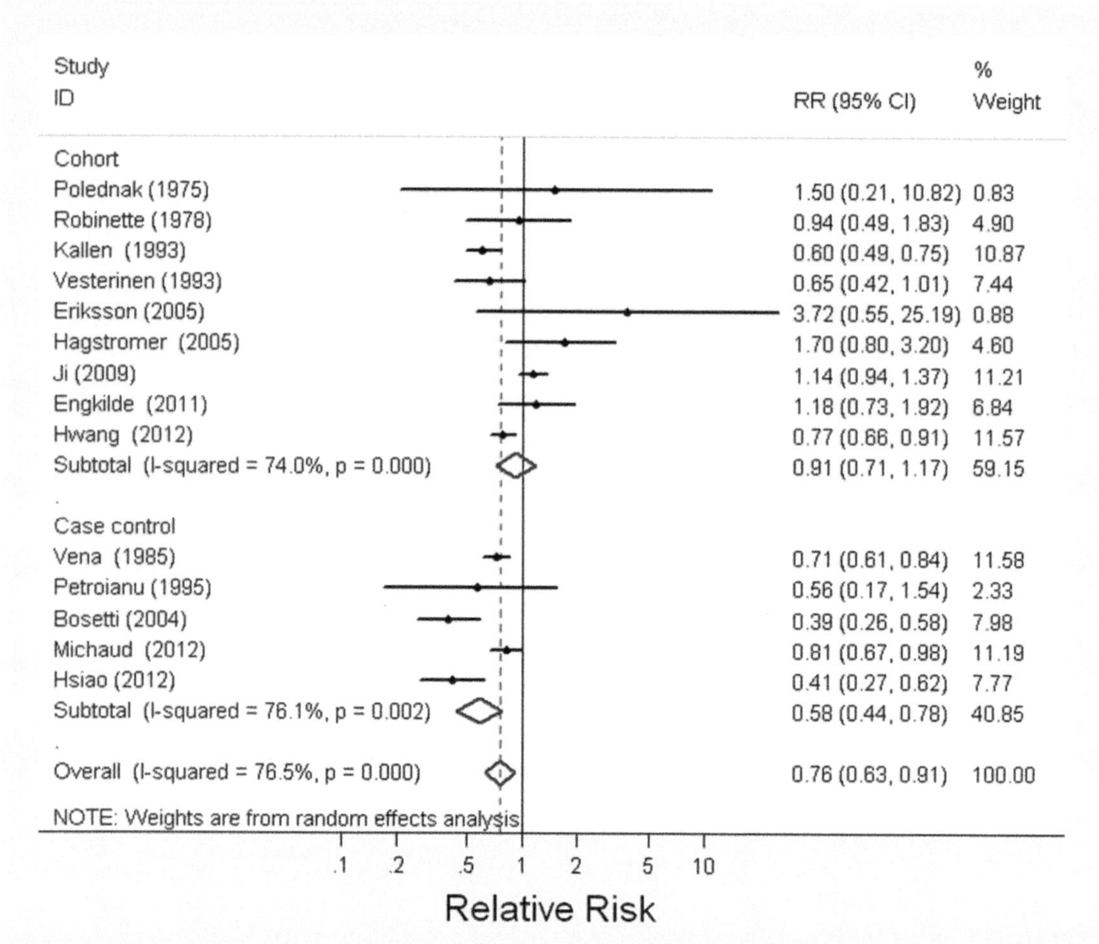

Figure 2. Meta-analysis assessing the association between allergies and head and neck cancer Risk.

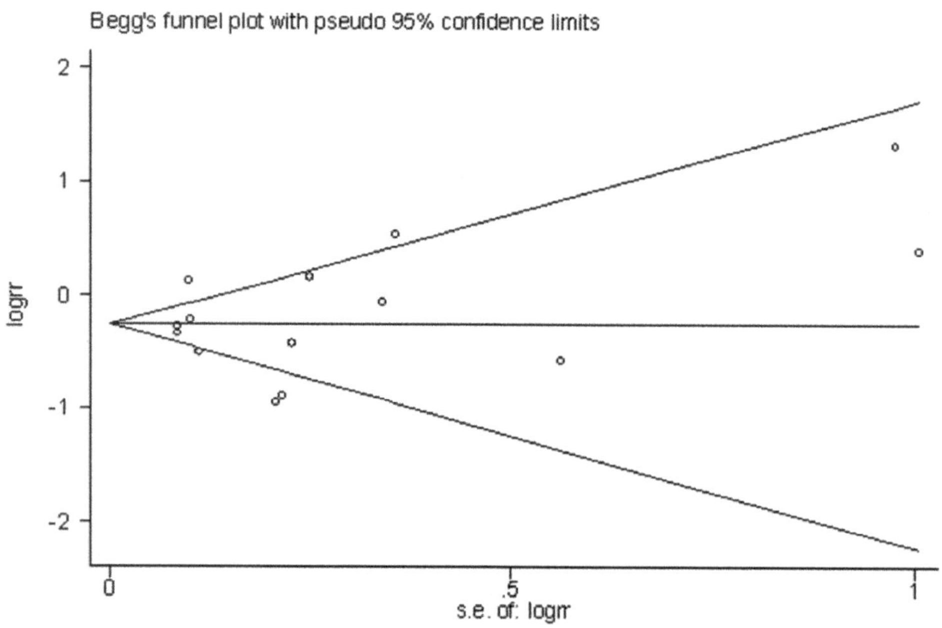

Figure 3. Funnel plot of the 14 studies assessing the association between allergies and head and neck cancer risk.

Table 5. Meta-analysis on the association between allergy and head and neck cancer.

	Both genders combined			Male			Female		
	n	Meta-RR (95% CI)*	I^2	n	Meta-RR (95% CI)*	I^2	n	Meta-RR (95% CI)*	I^2
Head and neck cancer									
All allergy combined	14	0.76 (0.63–0.91)	76.5	9	0.67 (0.54–0.84)	68.2	7	0.98 (0.81–1.18)	20.2
Study designs									
Cohort	9	0.91 (0.71–1.17)	74.0	5	0.80 (0.60–1.07)	34.7	3	0.89 (0.48–1.65)	47.2
Case–control	5	0.58 (0.44–0.78)	76.1	4	0.56 (0.39–0.81)	83.4	4	0.98 (0.79–1.21)	19.6
Allergic rhinitis	3	0.55 (0.40–0.76)	46.1	3	0.53 (0.42–0.66)	20.0	3	1.25 (0.77–2.04)	0.0
Skin allergy	5	0.84 (0.62–1.14)	43.0	4	0.82 (0.62–1.08)	0.0	3	0.78 (0.50–1.21)	0.0
Asthma	9	0.86 (0.71–1.05)	63.1	6	0.79 (0.61–1.02)	35.8	3	1.55 (1.02–2.38)	0.0
Oral cancer									
All allergy combined	9	0.78 (0.61–1.00)	72.2	7	0.64 (0.45–0.91)	69.1	4	1.06 (0.76–1.50)	33.7
Allergic rhinitis	3	0.56 (0.36–0.88)	66.6	3	0.48 (0.31–0.75)	48.8	2	1.31 (0.79–2.16)	0.0
Skin allergy	5	0.84 (0.52–1.34)	64.8	4	0.77 (0.48–1.25)	42.7	2	0.68 (0.42–1.12)	0.0
Asthma	6	0.88 (0.74–1.04)	0.0	5	0.76 (0.57–1.02)	0.0	2	1.59 (0.97–2.61)	0.0
Pharynx									
All allergy combined	10	0.69 (0.58–0.82)	33.6	7	0.67 (0.45–1.00)	61.4	4	1.12 (0.60–2.12)	49.5
Allergic rhinitis	3	0.43 (0.23–0.80)	37.1	3	0.49 (0.22–0.83)	41.7	0	–	–
Skin allergy	4	0.92 (0.65–1.30)	0.0	4	0.97 (0.62–1.50)	17.9	2	0.75 (0.33–1.74)	42.4
Asthma	7	0.67 (0.56–0.79)	0.0	5	0.79 (0.54–1.15)	0.0	2	2.06 (0.70–6.10)	0.0
Larynx									
All allergy combined	7	0.66 (0.47–0.92)	53.0	5	0.64 (0.42–0.96)	56.7	2	0.67 (0.22–2.04)	0.0
Allergic rhinitis	2	0.39 (0.13–1.13)	42.2	2	0.40 (0.15–1.08)	33.1	0	–	–
Skin allergy	2	1.07 (0.61–1.85)	0.0	2	1.10 (0.63–1.92)	0.0	0	–	–
Asthma	4	0.86 (0.58–1.28)	38.8	3	0.92 (0.48–1.74)	67.3	1	–	–

*The Meta-RR was generated by a random effects model using the DersSimonian and Laird method if the heterogeneity was high to moderate ($I^2 \geq 25\%$) and by a fixed effects model if the heterogeneity was low ($I^2 < 25\%$).
Abbreviations: CI, confidence interval; meta-RR, meta-relative risk; n, number of studies.

allergies can have different symptoms with some develop asthma while others develop allergic rhinitis or different combinations of symptoms [13,15]. Studies have detected IgE to specific allergens in the nasal washing among patients with allergic rhinitis regardless of their systemic allergy test status, suggesting the importance of local IgE production in the development of allergic rhinitis [15]. It is possible that allergic rhinitis may be an indicator for a more active local immunity in the upper aerodigestive tract against foreign substances, leading to a reduced HNC risk; however, this needs to be confirmed with further investigations.

The inverse association between allergies and HNC was present predominantly among men as indicated by the results of the current meta-analysis. While there is no obvious explanation for this observation, several HNC differences between men and women may provide clues. The incidence of HNC is higher among men than women, ranging from 1.6 times to 9.8 times higher depending on the anatomical sites and the regions of the world. Studies have shown that a higher proportion of HNC among men (74–82%) can be attributed to alcohol and cigarette compared to women (50–61%) [7,47,48], suggesting that HNC in women may have other causes that are less common among men. Although cigarette smoking may explain more of the HNC cases among men than among women, women appear to be more susceptible to the carcinogenic effect of cigarette. For those who smoked up to one cigarette pack per day, the HNC risk was higher in women (hazard ratio: 3.08, 95% CI: 1.77–5.36) than in men (hazard ratio: 1.26, 95% CI: 0.99–1.61) [49]. The possible differences in the causes of and the susceptibility to HNC between men and women may have contributed to their disparity in the association between allergies and HNC. More investigations on these gender differences may help establish the biological mechanism underlying the relationship between allergies and HNC.

Several limitations must be considered when interpreting the results of the current analysis. Because our case-control study is hospital-based, it is difficult to determine whether the cases and controls arise from the same source population. Our recruiting hospital is a major medical center in Southern Taiwan, and over 95% of our study subjects came from the county where the hospital is located. Even though we tried to exclude controls with diseases related to the use of alcohol, betel quid, and cigarette smoking, the possibility remains that our controls may not be representative of the background population for the cases. For the meta-analysis, studies were heterogeneous in design, patient population, disease sites, and types of allergies assessed. We explored the sources of heterogeneity by performing subgroup analyses by study design, disease sites, types of allergies, and gender. In addition, random-effect models were used to account for the heterogeneity across studies. Finally, the association between allergies and HNC was only assessed qualitatively with a binary status (yes vs. no) in the current analysis. More studies with quantitative measures of allergies (*e.g.* severity as indicated by the level of serum IgE, numbers of allergy-associated genetic variants, cytokine profiles) may provide a clearer picture to describe the relationship between allergies and HNC.

In summary, we observed an inverse association between allergies and HNC, particularly among men, in our original case-control study and meta-analysis. This suggests that immunity may play an important role to influence the risk of HNC. Future studies may investigate immune biomarkers, including cytokine profiles and genetic polymorphisms to further delineate the relationship between allergies and HNC. In addition, more studies are needed to determine whether allergies can reduce the risk HNC associated with alcohol, betel quid, or cigarette. Understanding the relationship between allergies and HNC may help devise effective strategies to reduce and treat HNC.

Supporting Information

Table S1 Fourteen studies (9 cohort studies and 5 case-control studies) included in the meta-analysis for the association between allergies and head and neck cancer.
(DOC)

Checklist S1 PRISMA Checklist.
(DOC)

Acknowledgments

We thank Dr. Neela Guha of the International Agency for Research on Cancer for her careful editing of the manuscript.

Author Contributions

Conceived and designed the experiments: JRH JSC. Performed the experiments: JRH JSC CLL FTW Y. Wang YLW HCY JSC. Analyzed the data: JRH CYO JSC. Contributed reagents/materials/analysis tools: JSC. Wrote the paper: JRH CYO JSC. Acquisition of data: JRH CYO HIL CCH WTL JSH KCC TYW STT CJY Y. Wu WTH MWY SYW JYC KYC CLL FTW Y. Wang YLW HCY JSC. Interpretation of data: JRH CYO HIL CCH WTL JSH KCC TYW STT CJY Y. Wu WTH MWY SYW JYC KYC CLL FTW Y. Wang YLW HCY JSC. Critically evaluated or revised the content of the manuscript: JRH CYO HIL CCH WTL JSH KCC TYW STT CJY Y. Wu WTH MWY SYW JYC KYC CLL FTW Y. Wang YLW HCY JSC. Approved the final manuscript: JRH CYO HIL CCH WTL JSH KCC TYW STT CJY Y. Wu WTH MWY SYW JYC KYC CLL FTW Y. Wang YLW HCY JSC.

References

1. Boyle P, Levin B, editors (2008) World Cancer Report. Lyon: International Agency for Research on Cancer.
2. International Agency for Research on Cancer. Globocan 2008. Available: http://globocan.iarc.fr/. Accessed 2012 Aug 1.
3. Department of Health, Taiwan, R.O.C. Annual Cancer Report, Year 2009. Available: http://www.bhp.doh.gov.tw. Accessed 2012 Aug 1.
4. Bouvard V, Baan R, Straif K, Grosse Y, Secretan B, et al. (2009) A review of human carcinogens–Part B: biological agents. Lancet Oncol 10: 321–322.
5. Secretan B, Straif K, Baan R, Grosse Y, El Ghissassi F, et al. (2009) A review of human carcinogens–Part E: tobacco, areca nut, alcohol, coal smoke, and salted fish. Lancet Oncol 10: 1033–1034.
6. Mehanna H, Beech T, Nicholson T, El-Hariry I, McConkey C, et al. (2012 Jan 20. doi: 10.1002/hed.22015. [Epub ahead of print]) Prevalence of human papillomavirus in oropharyngeal and nonoropharyngeal head and neck cancer-systematic review and meta-analysis of trends by time and region. Head Neck.
7. Hashibe M, Brennan P, Chuang SC, Boccia S, Castellsague X, et al. (2009) Interaction between tobacco and alcohol use and the risk of head and neck cancer: pooled analysis in the International Head and Neck Cancer Epidemiology Consortium. Cancer Epidemiol Biomarkers Prev 18: 541–550.
8. de Andrade M, Amos CI, Foulkes WD (1998) Segregation analysis of squamous cell carcinoma of the head and neck: evidence for a major gene determining risk. Ann Hum Genet 62: 505–510.
9. Guha N, Boffetta P, Wunsch Filho V, Eluf Neto J, Shangina O, et al. (2007) Oral health and risk of squamous cell carcinoma of the head and neck and esophagus: results of two multicentric case-control studies. Am J Epidemiol 166: 1159–1173.
10. Merrill RM, Isakson RT, Beck RE (2007) The association between allergies and cancer: what is currently known? Ann Allergy Asthma Immunol 99: 102–116; quiz 117–109, 150.
11. Sherman PW, Holland E, Sherman JS (2008) Allergies: their role in cancer prevention. Q Rev Biol 83: 339–362.
12. Turner MC, Chen Y, Krewski D, Ghadirian P (2006) An overview of the association between allergy and cancer. Int J Cancer 118: 3124–3132.
13. Kay AB (2000) Overview of 'allergy and allergic diseases: with a view to the future'. Br Med Bull 56: 843–864.
14. Durham SR, Smurthwaite L, Gould HJ (2000) Local IgE production. Am J Rhinol 14: 305–307.
15. Hoddeson EK, Pratt E, Harvey RJ, Wise SK (2010) Local and systemic IgE in the evaluation and treatment of allergy. Otolaryngol Clin North Am 43: 503–520, viii.
16. Linos E, Raine T, Alonso A, Michaud D (2007) Atopy and risk of brain tumors: a meta-analysis. J Natl Cancer Inst 99: 1544–1550.
17. Gandini S, Lowenfels AB, Jaffee EM, Armstrong TD, Maisonneuve P (2005) Allergies and the risk of pancreatic cancer: a meta-analysis with review of epidemiology and biological mechanisms. Cancer Epidemiol Biomarkers Prev 14: 1908–1916.
18. Michaud DS, Langevin SM, Eliot M, Nelson HH, McClean MD, et al. (2012) Allergies and risk of head and neck cancer. Cancer Causes Control 23: 1317–1322.
19. Bosetti C, Talamini R, Franceschi S, Negri E, Giacosa A, et al. (2004) Allergy and the risk of selected digestive and laryngeal neoplasms. Eur J Cancer Prev 13: 173–176.
20. Engkilde K, Thyssen JP, Menne T, Johansen JD (2011) Association between cancer and contact allergy: a linkage study. BMJ Open 1: e000084.
21. Eriksson NE, Holmen A, Hogstedt B, Mikoczy Z, Hagmar L (1995) A prospective study of cancer incidence in a cohort examined for allergy. Allergy 50: 718–722.
22. Eriksson NE, Mikoczy Z, Hagmar L (2005) Cancer incidence in 13811 patients skin tested for allergy. J Investig Allergol Clin Immunol 15: 161–166.
23. Hagstromer L, Ye W, Nyren O, Emtestam L (2005) Incidence of cancer among patients with atopic dermatitis. Arch Dermatol 141: 1123–1127.
24. Hwang CY, Chen YJ, Lin MW, Chen TJ, Chu SY, et al. (2012) Cancer risk in patients with allergic rhinitis, asthma and atopic dermatitis: a nationwide cohort study in Taiwan. Int J Cancer 130: 1160–1167.
25. Kallen B, Gunnarskog J, Conradson TB (1993) Cancer risk in asthmatic subjects selected from hospital discharge registry. Eur Respir J 6: 694–697.
26. Vena JE, Bona JR, Byers TE, Middleton E Jr, Swanson MK, et al. (1985) Allergy-related diseases and cancer: an inverse association. Am J Epidemiol 122: 66–74.
27. Vesterinen E, Pukkala E, Timonen T, Aromaa A (1993) Cancer incidence among 78,000 asthmatic patients. Int J Epidemiol 22: 976–982.
28. Ji J, Shu X, Li X, Sundquist K, Sundquist J, et al. (2009) Cancer risk in hospitalised asthma patients. Br J Cancer 100: 829–833.
29. Petroianu A, Chaves DN, De Oliveira O Jr (1995) Comparative incidence of allergy in the presence or absence of cancer. J Int Med Res 23: 358–363.
30. Robinette CD, Fraumeni JF Jr (1978) Asthma and subsequent mortality in World War II veterans. J Chronic Dis 31: 619–624.
31. Polednak AP (1975) Letter: Asthma and cancer mortality. Lancet 2: 1147–1148.
32. Wang H, Diepgen TL (2005) Is atopy a protective or a risk factor for cancer? A review of epidemiological studies. Allergy 60: 1098–1111.
33. Harris RJ, Bradburn MJ, Deeks JJ, Harbord RM, Altman DG, et al. (2008) Metan: fixed- and random-effects meta-analysis. The Stata Journal 8: 3–28.
34. Higgins JP, Thompson SG, Deeks JJ, Altman DG (2003) Measuring inconsistency in meta-analyses. Bmj 327: 557–560.
35. DerSimonian R, Laird N (1986) Meta-analysis in clinical trials. Control Clin Trials 7: 177–188.
36. Sterne JAC, Egger M, Smith GD (2005) Investigating and dealing with publication and other biases. In: Egger M, Smith GD, Altman DG, editors. Systematic Reviews in Health: Care Meta-Analysis Context. London: BMJ Books, 285–312.
37. Egger M, Davey Smith G, Schneider M, Minder C (1997) Bias in meta-analysis detected by a simple, graphical test. BMJ 315: 629–634.
38. Jensen-Jarolim E, Achatz G, Turner MC, Karagiannis S, Legrand F, et al. (2008) AllergoOncology: the role of IgE-mediated allergy in cancer. Allergy 63: 1255–1266.
39. Neuchrist C, Kornfehl J, Grasl M, Lassmann H, Kraft D, et al. (1994) Distribution of immunoglobulins in squamous cell carcinoma of the head and neck. Int Arch Allergy Immunol 104: 97–100.
40. Grimes DA, Schulz KF (2002) Cohort studies: marching towards outcomes. Lancet 359: 341–345.
41. Davey Smith G, Ebrahim S (2003) 'Mendelian randomization': can genetic epidemiology contribute to understanding environmental determinants of disease? Int J Epidemiol 32: 1–22.

42. Sokol CL, Barton GM, Farr AG, Medzhitov R (2008) A mechanism for the initiation of allergen-induced T helper type 2 responses. Nat Immunol 9: 310–318.
43. de Guia RM, Ramos JD (2010) The -590C/TIL4 single-nucleotide polymorphism as a genetic factor of atopic allergy. Int J Mol Epidemiol Genet 1: 67–73.
44. Vairaktaris E, Yannopoulos A, Vassiliou S, Serefoglou Z, Vylliotis A, et al. (2007) Strong association of interleukin-4 (−590 C/T) polymorphism with increased risk for oral squamous cell carcinoma in Europeans. Oral Surg Oral Med Oral Pathol Oral Radiol Endod 104: 796–802.
45. Gaur P, Mittal M, Mohanti B, Das S (2011) Functional variants of IL4 and IL6 genes and risk of tobacco-related oral carcinoma in high-risk Asian Indians. Oral Dis 17: 720–726.
46. Tsai MH, Chen WC, Tsai CH, Hang LW, Tsai FJ (2005) Interleukin-4 gene, but not the interleukin-1 beta gene polymorphism, is associated with oral cancer. J Clin Lab Anal 19: 93–98.
47. Anantharaman D, Marron M, Lagiou P, Samoli E, Ahrens W, et al. (2011) Population attributable risk of tobacco and alcohol for upper aerodigestive tract cancer. Oral Oncol 47: 725–731.
48. Blot WJ, McLaughlin JK, Winn DM, Austin DF, Greenberg RS, et al. (1988) Smoking and drinking in relation to oral and pharyngeal cancer. Cancer Res 48: 3282–3287.
49. Freedman ND, Abnet CC, Leitzmann MF, Hollenbeck AR, Schatzkin A (2007) Prospective investigation of the cigarette smoking-head and neck cancer association by sex. Cancer 110: 1593–1601.

7

Oral Peanut Challenge Identifies an Allergy but the Peanut Allergen Threshold Sensitivity Is Not Reproducible

Susanne Glaumann[1,2]*, Anna Nopp[3], S. G. O. Johansson[3], Magnus P. Borres[4,5], Caroline Nilsson[1,2]

1 Department of Clinical Science and Education, Södersjukhuset, Centre for Allergy Research, Karolinska Institutet, Stockholm, Sweden, 2 Sach's Children's Hospital, Södersjukhuset, Stockholm, Sweden, 3 Department of Medicine, Clinical Immunology and Allergy Unit, Karolinska Institutet, Stockholm, Sweden, 4 Thermo Fisher Scientific, Uppsala, Sweden, 5 Department of Pediatrics, Institute for Clinical Sciences, The Sahlgrenska Academy at the University of Gothenburg, Sweden

Abstract

Background: Double-blind placebo-controlled food challenge, DBPCFC, the gold standard for diagnosing food allergy, is time-consuming and potentially dangerous. A basophil allergen threshold sensitivity test, CD-sens, has shown promising results as a diagnostic tool in food allergy.

Objectives: To evaluate the reproducibility of oral peanut challenge and compare the outcome to CD-sens in peanut-sensitized children.

Methods: Twenty-seven children (4–19 years) underwent a DBPCFC followed by a single-blind oral food-challenge. The peanut challenges (1 mg to 5 g) were evaluated by severity scoring. Blood samples were drawn for CD-sens before the two first challenges.

Results: Thirteen children (48%) did not react at any of the challenges. Fourteen reacted at both peanut challenges but not to placebo. Only two of these children reacted at the same threshold dose and with the same severity score. All other children scored differently or reacted at different doses. For children with a positive challenge the geometric mean of the ratio of the doses was 1.834 ($p = 0.307$) and the arithmetic mean of the difference between the severity scores was 0.143 ($p = 0.952$). No association was obtained between the two peanut challenges regarding severity score ($r_s = 0.11$, $p = 0.71$) or threshold dose ($r_s = 0.35$, $p = 0.22$). Among the children positive in peanut challenge, 12 were positive in CD-sens. Two were low-responders and could not be evaluated. Geometric mean of the ratio of CD-sens values in children with a positive challenge was 1.035 ($p = 0.505$) but unlike for the severity score and the threshold dose the association between the two CD-sens values was strong ($r_s = 0.94$, $P < 0.001$).

Conclusions: For a positive/negative test the reproducibility is 100% for both peanut challenge and CD-sens. However, a comparison of the degree of allergen threshold sensitivity between the two tests is not possible since the threshold dose and severity scoring is not reproducible.

Editor: Anthony Peter Sampson, University of Southampton School of Medicine, United Kingdom

Funding: This work was supported in part by the Foundation "Mjölkdroppen", Sweden; Swedish Asthma and Allergy Associations Research Foundation, Sweden; Centre for Allergy Research, Karolinska Institutet, Sweden; Hesselman Foundation, Sweden; Foundation "Samariten", Sweden and Princess Lovisa's Association for Childrens Medical Care, Sweden. The funders had no role in study design, data collection and analysis, decision to publish, or preparation of the manuscript.

Competing Interests: MPB is employed at Thermo Fisher Scientific. This does not alter the authors' adherence to all the PLOS ONE policies on sharing data and materials. All other authors have declared they have no conflict of interest.

* E-mail: susanne.glaumann@sodersjukhuset.se

Introduction

Peanuts are one of the most common foods causing allergic reactions in children [1,2]. The severity of the reactions vary but can be life threatening [3] and lead to a decreased quality of life [4,5]. Peanut allergy is usually diagnosed by case history, skin prick test (SPT) and/or immunoglobulin E antibody (IgE-ab) determination. However, the diagnosis often needs to be confirmed by a food challenge. Double-blind placebo-controlled food challenge (DBPCFC) is considered the gold standard [6,7] and is an attempt to mimic real life exposure under standardized conditions. In addition, DBPCFC is the accepted reference test for food allergy when new diagnostic methods or therapies are evaluated [8]. However, DBPCFC is time consuming and associated with risks of severe allergic reactions. It is also difficult to objectively evaluate if a DBPCFC is positive or negative or to determine the severity of the allergy [9]. Besides, placebo reactions may occur in up to 13% of the DBPCFC [10].

The reproducibility of the severity of the reactions and the threshold doses at DBPCFC has to our knowledge so far not been properly documented. A score system for low dose DBPCFC for peanut integrating both symptoms and dose (<100 mg peanut protein) has earlier been published but the peanut challenges were

Table 1. Symptom score according to Astier [20] to evaluate clinical reactions in DBPCFC.

Symptom score	Symptoms
0	**no symptoms**
1	abdominal pain that resolved without medical treatment, rhino conjunctivitis or urticaria <10 paplers, rash
2	**one organ involved,** *abdominal pain requiring treatment, *generalized urticaria, *non laryngeal angioedema, *mild asthma (cough, fall of peak expiratory flow <20%)
3	**two organs involved** (of symptoms mentioned under 2)
4	**three organs involved** (of symptoms mentioned under 2) **or asthma** requiring treatment or laryngeal edema, or hypotension
5	**cardiac and respiratory symptoms requiring hospitalization in the intensive care unit**

not repeated to evaluate the reproducibility [11]. In addition there is no worldwide accepted score system available to evaluate both the severity of the reactions and threshold doses making it hard to compare the results from different studies.

New promising diagnostic tools like basophil allergen threshold sensitivity tests have been evaluated in allergy [12,13,14,15]. A basophil activation test represents the IgE-mediated inflammatory pathway of the allergic response [16,17]. In IgE-mediated allergy tissue mast cells and basophils in the blood are sensitized with IgE-ab against the allergen to which the individual reacts. By stimulating the basophils in vitro with decreasing doses of the allergen, the smallest amount of allergen stimulating the cells can be detected by determination of CD63 up-regulation by flow cytometry. This is designated as the basophil allergen threshold sensitivity, CD-sens [18] and the method has been shown to be an alternative to complex allergen in-vivo challenges. A good correlation has been found between CD-sens and SPT-titration [12] and allergen challenge tests in allergic rhino conjunctivitis [12] and allergic asthma [15] suggesting that CD-sens is a relevant marker of in vivo allergen sensitivity.

The aim of this study was to evaluate the reproducibility of oral peanut challenges for the determination of the allergen threshold sensitivity and to compare it to CD-sens to peanut.

Methods

Study Population

This study includes 27 children who were part of a previous study (n = 38) where peanut allergy was confirmed by double-blind placebo-controlled food challenge (DBPCFC) [13]. The children, aged 4–19 years old, were referred to Sach's Children's Hospital, Stockholm for an oral peanut challenge. All children had a suspected peanut allergy, IgE-ab to peanut (≥0.35 kU_A/L) in serum (ImmunoCAP®Thermo Fischer Scientific, Uppsala, Sweden) and/or a positive skin prick test (SPT) (≥3 mm) to peanut (Soluprick 1/20, ALK, Copenhagen, Denmark) at inclusion. Exclusion criteria were antihistamines or oral steroids taken 4 days prior to the challenge or a history of previous anaphylactic reactions to peanut. A DBPCFC followed by a single-blind oral food-challenge (SBOFC) was performed. The SBOFC was blinded for the child and the parents. In children reacting with severe allergic symptoms at the first peanut challenge the SBOFC was not performed due to ethical reasons. Thus, among 38 children 27 underwent two peanut and one placebo challenge and were included in the present study. All three challenges were planned to take place within one month. The median number of days between the two peanut challenges was 14 (range 7–126). For five children this interval was rather long due to common illness or for social reasons. Of these, three children were negative in both food challenges and CD-sens. For the other two the time between the challenges was 56 (patient J2) and 126 (patient J17) days, respectively.

Ethics Methods

The study was approved by the local ethics committee (Dnr 2008-1001-31/2) and the parents provided written consent.

Challenge Testing

The challenges were performed using a challenge medium with 11% peanut and 7% fat [19]. Increasing doses of peanut were given every 30 minutes in up to 5 steps from 1 mg to 5 g; dose 1 = 0.001 g, dose 2 = 0.01 g, dose 3 = 0.1 g, dose 4 = 1 g and dose 5 = 5 g. The smaller increase between dose 4 and 5 is based on the experiences from our routine DBPCFC because most children are unable to eat 91 g of the challenge medium, chocolate ball. A negative test was defined as no allergic symptoms during two hours after challenge completion. All children stayed at least 2 hours after the challenge and longer if needed. Symptoms were scored according to Astier et al. [20] (Table 1).

Blood Sampling

After preparation of the skin with local anaesthesia, a peripheral venous catheter was provided. Before the two first challenges a blood sample was drawn and stored at +4°C for a maximum of 24 hours for CD-sens analyses.

Basophil Analyses

Basophil allergen threshold sensitivity, CD-sens [12,18] was calculated by stimulating the cells with decreasing concentrations of peanut extract. The same batch of peanut raw material was used in all oral challenges and CD-sens analyses. The stock solution, 1/20 weight/volume, was further diluted 1/50 and designated 1 000 arbitrary units per mL (AU/mL). Each sample was tested with 0.1–1000 AU/mL. In summary, anti- FcεRI (Bühlmann Laboratories AG, Schönenbuch, Switzerland) and N-formyl-methionyl-leucyl-phenylalanin (fMLP) (Sigma Chemilcal Co, St. Louis, Missouri, US) were used as positive controls and RPMI as negative control. Leucocytes were stained with CD63 (Immunotech, Marseille, France) and CD203c (Immunotech) and counted in a Navios flow cytometer (Beckman Coulter, Inc., Fullerton, CA, USA). The cut-off determining a positive allergen test was set to 5% of CD63-positive basophils [12,18].

Individuals with basophils, which after anti-FcεRI stimulation, i.e. the positive control, responded with 0–5% CD63-upregulation were regarded as non-responders. For individuals with a response between 5–16% (low-responders) the results should be interpreted with caution. The cut off 16% was calculated from the positive

			1st peanut challenge			2nd peanut challenge		
Patient	sex	Age (years)	Symptoms	Severity score	peanut (g)	Symptoms	Severity score	Peanut (g)
J2	female	12.7	urticaria, stomach-ache mouth-itch	3	1.1	asthma, skin-itch, rhinitis, urticaria, stomach-ache	4	6.1
J8	male	15.4	stomach-ache mouth-itch	2	0.1	conjunctivitis, rhinitis, stomach-ache	2	1.1
J15	female	17.4	stomach-ache, mouth-itch	2	0.1	mouth-itch, stomach-ache, urticaria, rhinitis	3	1.1
J17	female	14.0	tiredness, mild asthma, mouth-itch	4	6.1	tiredness, stomach-ache, vomiting, conjunctivitis	2	6.1
J19	male	9.8	mouth-itch	1	0.01	mouth-itch, stomach-ache	1	3.6
J22	male	5.4	stomach-ache	1	4.1	conjunctivitis, stomach-ache, tiredness	2	6.1
J24	female	17.6	tiredness, vomiting, mouth- itch, stomach-ache	3	6.1	mouth-itch	1	1.1
J28	male	7.6	stomach-ache	1	6.1	erythema, stomach-ache, tiredness	1	6.1
J31	male	19.0	mouth-itch, urticaria, cough, stomach-ache, tiredness, erythema	4	1.1	mouth-itch	1	0.01
J33	female	12.2	mouth-itch	1	0.01	stomach-ache, tiredness	2	0.1
J36	male	18.4	mouth-itch, stomach-ache, tiredness	2	0.01	mouth-itch, stomach-ache	2	0.001
J38	female	7.9	cough, tiredness	2	0.01	hoarseness, cough, mouth-itch, conjunctivitis, rhinitis, vomiting, stomach-ache, tiredness, urticaria	4	6.1
J39	male	5.9	mouth-itch , stomach-ache tiredness	2	1.1	mouth-itch, asthma	4	1.1
J41	female	11.8	mouth-itch, stomach-ache, tiredness	2	0.1	mouth-itch, stomach-ache, tiredness	2	0.1

Figure 1. Age, sex, symptoms and Astier severity score [20] in children with two positive peanut challenges.

controls (mean 76%, −3SD) of an in-house reference material of 264 allergic children and adults [13].

Basophil allergen threshold sensitivity was measured as the lowest allergen concentration giving 50% (LC50) of maximum CD63 up regulation. CD-sens is defined as the inverted value for LC50 multiplied by 100 and describes the degree of the patient's allergen threshold sensitivity, that is a positive relation between the CD-sens value and the degree of the patient's allergen sensitivity. [18].

Statistics

In patients reacting at both challenges, Wilcoxon Signed Rank Test was used to test differences between the first and the second challenge for Astier score, threshold dose and CD-sens. The values for threshold dose and CD-sens were tested on log-transformed values, thus testing the relative change. The differences between the first and the second challenge are presented in Bland-Altman plots and the associations between first and second value were assessed with Spearman rank order correlation (r_s). No adjustment

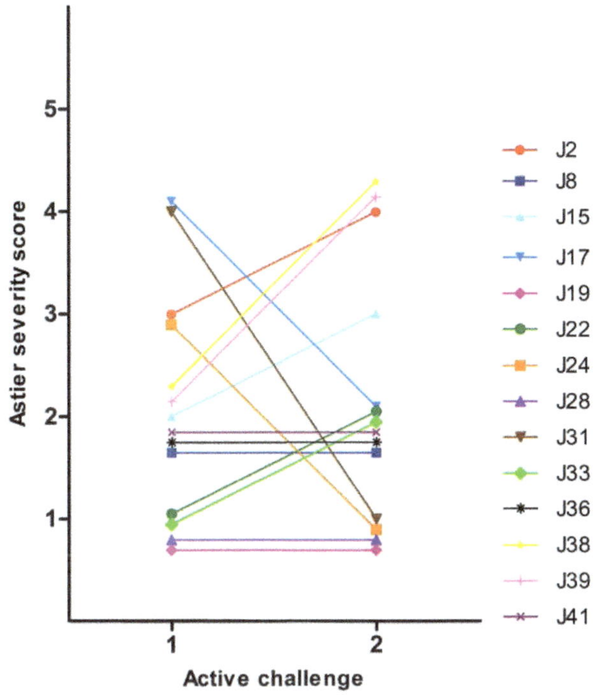

Figure 2. Severity scores according to Astier [20] in the same child at the two peanut challenges.

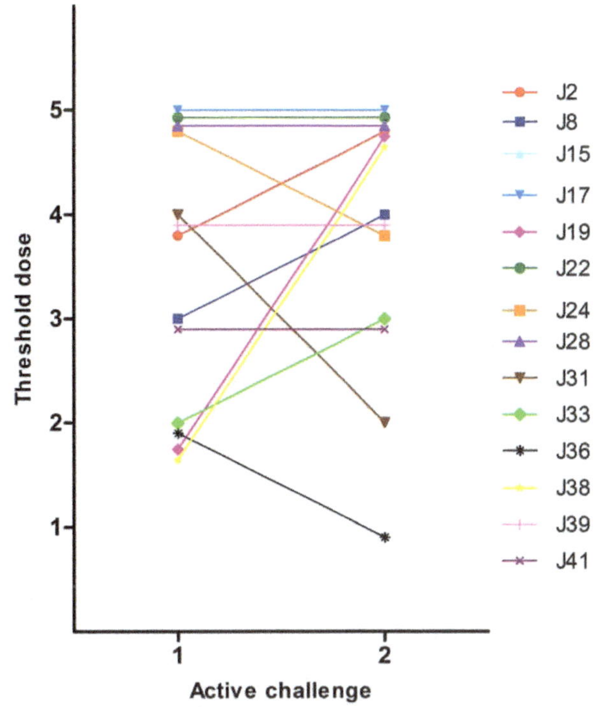

Figure 3. Threshold doses of peanut in the same child at the two peanut challenges. The amount peanut eaten were divided into 5 dose steps: Dose 1 = 0.001 g; Dose 2 = 0.01 g; Dose 3 = 0.1 g; Dose 4 = 1 g; Dose 5 = 3.6–5 g.

for multiple testing has been performed. Thus, significant results should be regarded as descriptive and explorative. Statistical analysis was carried out using IBM SPSS Statistic 20.0, Chicago, Ill, USA. A p-value <0.05 was considered significant.

Results

Patient Characteristics

The median age of the 27 children in the study was 12.2 years (range 5.4–19) and 48% were girls. All 27 children had a diagnosis of peanut allergy and where IgE-sensitized to peanut. Thirteen children had a clinical convincing history of peanut allergy and the other fourteen children were diagnosed with peanut allergy due to results of tests performed in routine clinical work-up.

Oral Food Challenge

The severity of the reactions was scored according to Astier et al. [20] (Table 1). Fourteen children (52%) reacted with allergic symptoms at both peanut challenges, but not on placebo, and were considered as positive (Figure 1). Two children (J28, J41) reacted at the same severity score and had the same threshold dose at the two peanut challenges while all other children (n = 12) scored differently or reacted at different threshold doses (Figure 2 and 3). Thirteen children (48%) did not react at any of the three challenges. All children negative in the challenges consumed full doses (6.1 g peanut). In children with a positive challenge the arithmetic mean of difference in the severity scores (challenge 2 - challenge 1) was 0.143 ($p = 0.952$) (Figure 4) and the geometric mean of the ratio of the doses (challenge 2/challenge 1) was 1.834 ($p = 0.307$) (Figure 5). No association was obtained between the first and the second peanut challenge regarding severity score ($r_s = 0.11$, $p = 0.71$) or threshold dose ($r_s = 0.35$, $p = 0.22$).

CD-sens

CD-sens was performed on blood drawn before the first and second challenges in all children (n = 26) except one. In this child, blood was collected at the second and third challenges due to a misunderstanding. All children with a positive CD-sens at the first challenge where also CD-sens positive at the second challenge. The peanut CD-sens values are presented in figure 6 and 7. Twelve of 14 children with positive challenges were positive in CD-sens to peanut. The remaining two could not be evaluated since they were low responders i.e. had a too low response to the

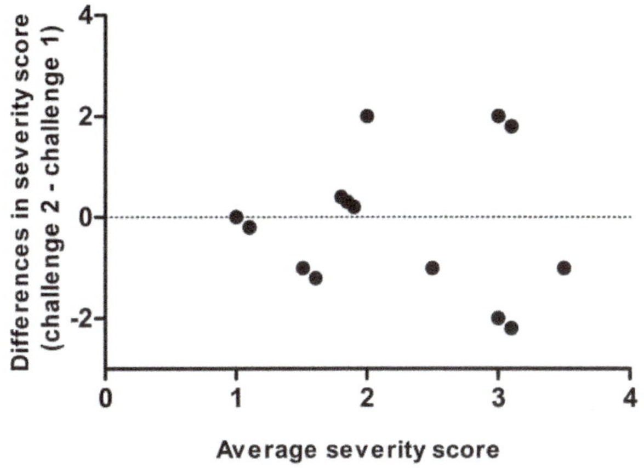

Figure 4. The differences in severity score (challenge 2–challenge 1) in each child with positive peanut challenges, presented as a Bland-Altman plot. The arithmetic mean of the difference between the severity scores was 0.143.

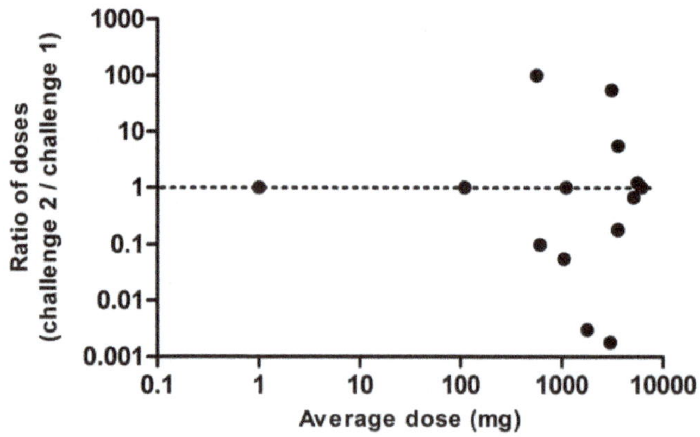

Figure 5. The differences in the ratio of the dose, mg (challenge 2/challenge 1) in each child with positive peanut challenges, presented as a Bland-Altman plot with logarithmically transformed data. The geometric mean of the ratio of the doses was 1.834.

positive control anti-FcεRI (<16%). Three children had slightly positive values in CD-sens (0.3–0.5) but were negative in challenge. However, all 10 children negative in CD-sens were also negative at both peanut challenges. The geometric mean of the ratio of CD-sens values (challenge 2/challenge 1) in children with a positive challenge was 1.035 ($p = 0.505$) (Figure 8) and the association between the two CD-sens values was strong ($r_s = 0.94$, $P < 0.001$).

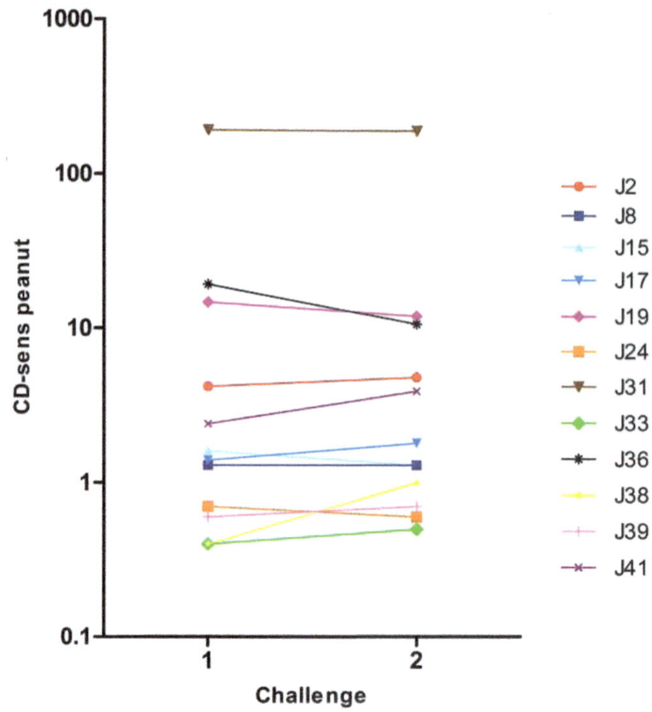

Figure 6. Peanut CD-sens values in the same child at the two peanut challenges.

Discussion

The aim of this study was to evaluate the reproducibility of oral peanut challenges (DBPCFC and SBOFC) for the determination of the allergen threshold sensitivity and to compare it to CD-sens to peanut. However, in contrast to CD-sens it was not possible to quantitatively estimate the allergen threshold sensitivity with oral peanut challenge in a reproducible way. Thus, a comparison of the degree of allergen threshold sensitivity obtained by oral peanut challenge with CD-sens, was not possible to achieve.

The DBPCFC is an attempt to mimic real life exposure under standardized conditions and is today the gold standard for the diagnosis of food allergy [21,22]. However, it is difficult to evaluate the reactions at DBPCFC [9] and each research group is using its own severity scores [11,23,24]. Besides, there are several factors affecting the outcome of a food challenge in addition to the amount of allergen given during challenge, for example aversion to the tested food and the evaluation of subjective symptoms [9]. Thus, reactions to placebo at the DBPCFC have been reported in a significant number [10]. This is in contrast to our study where no positive reactions to placebo occurred.

In the present study all children but two reacted with a different severity score or at another dose when the peanut challenge was repeated. Several studies have tried to determine the threshold dose in peanut allergic patients to predict the clinical sensitivity [24,25,26]. Van der Zee and colleagues [24] aimed to evaluate if the presence of risk factors for a severe allergic reaction to peanut is associated with the patient's clinical sensitivity by determine the eliciting dose of peanut in a DBPCFC and thereby predicting the severity of the allergic reaction. However, they were not able to find a relation between the threshold dose in DBPCFC and the severity of a previous reaction at home. Besides, Skirpak and colleagues [27] evaluated a 23 weeks oral immunotherapy to milk with DBPCFC before and after treatment. The outcome of the food challenge was based on the lowest dose causing a reaction and not from changes in the severity of the reactions. In that study 29% of the patients in the placebo group ($n = 7$) did not react at the same dose at the second DBPCFC. Although the numbers of patients in that study was low, the results indicate that food challenges can be difficult to reproduce [27]. These findings are in line with our observations showing that the severity of the clinical reaction of an oral peanut challenge is not reproducible.

A food challenge can tell you if a patient is allergic or not [13] but when we in this paper investigated the allergen threshold sensitivity and its reproducibility we could not demonstrate a reproducibility of the peanut challenges for determination of allergen sensitivity.

In CD-sens the correlation between the two CD-sens values was strong. A good correlation does not always mean that there is a high reproducibility, but with a high reproducibility there should be a good correlation. For the peanut challenge we could not demonstrate any statistical differences or correlations for doses or symptoms between the two challenges. Thus the low correlation support that the reproducibility was poor for dose and severity score. Difficulties to determine allergen thresholds doses at food challenges have also been noted by others [28]. This is in contrast to CD-sens where we did not find any significant differences but a significant and strong correlation between the two CD-sens occasions. This is supporting that CD-sens measured at different time-points strongly are associated.

Since the CD-sens value is directly related to the allergen concentration of the preparation used and since allergen extracts are not satisfactorily standardized the CD-sens values cannot be compared between different allergens [15]. In this study we used, for the CD-sens analyses, an extract of the same raw material used at the oral challenges. However, since we were not able to determine the patient's allergen threshold sensitivity by oral

	1st challenge		2nd challenge	
Patient	CD-sens Peanut	LC50 (AU/mL)	CD-sens Peanut	LC50 (AU/mL)
J2	4.2	23.6	4.8	21.1
J8	1.3	77.2	1.3	74.5
J15	1.6	62.4	1.3	78.4
J17	1.4	69.4	1.8	56.0
J19	14.8	6.8	12	8.3
J22	Low responder	Low responder	Low responder	Low responder
J24	0.7	149.7	0.6	166.4
J28	Low responder	Low responder	Low responder	Low responder
J31	192	0.5	188	0.52
J33	0.4	263.0	0.5	220.0
J36	19.2	5.2	10.6	9.4
J38	0.4	272.0	1.0	96.0
J39	0.6	162.0	0.7	136.0
J41	2.4	41.7	3.9	25.5

Figure 7. Peanut CD-sens values in children with two positive peanut challenges.

challenge we could not compare the severity of the peanut challenge reaction with CD-sens to peanut.

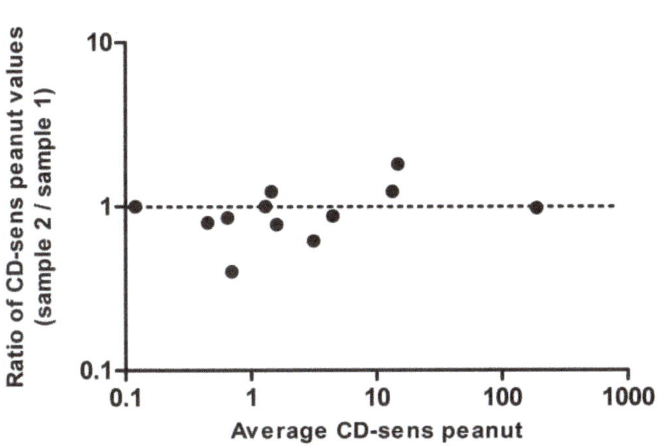

Figure 8. The differences in the ratio for peanut CD-sens values (challenge 2/challenge 1) in each child with positive peanut challenges, presented as a Bland-Altman plot with logarithmically transformed data. Geometric mean of the ratio of CD-sens values was 1.035.

CD-sens has previously been shown to have a good correlation with clinical tests of allergen sensitivity e.g. SPT-titration [12] and allergen challenge in rhino-conjunctivitis [12] and allergic asthma [15]. Interestingly, in allergic asthma there was an excellent correlation between CD-sens and the allergic inflammation behind the bronchial sensitivity but not between CD-sens and the non-specific bronchial hyper-reactivity [12]. Thus, we propose that CD-sens can be used in food allergy to predict the patient's basic allergen sensitivity. CD-sens allows evaluation and monitoring over time of the degree of allergen sensitivity with no risk for the patient. In addition, CD-sens is also, cost effective and time saving.

The strength of the present study is that all oral peanut challenges were performed in the same clinic with the same experienced senior physician grading the patient's clinical reaction and symptom score. An error introduced by performing the second peanut challenge as SBOFC, e.g. that the nurse performing the test was aware of the results of the first challenge, would have resulted in a falsely too good correlation. However, no correlation was found.

Since this is a rather small study the results should be interpreted with caution. Another limitation is that all children with severe anaphylactic reaction at the first peanut challenge were excluded for clinical and ethical reasons when the study was planned, we expected a severe reaction to re-occur. It should also be noted that the blood samples for CD-sens analyses were drawn at the first two challenges and not at the two peanut challenges.

To our knowledge there is no published study investigating the reproducibility of oral food challenge regarding both severity score and dose. Thus, clinical trials using DBPCFC for testing the outcomes of treatments [24,27] can only be correctly evaluated if the study includes information about the reproducibility of the challenges.

We conclude that we were not able to determine the severity of an allergic reaction to peanut since the children reacted at a different dose or with another severity score when the challenge was repeated. However, for a positive/negative test result, the concordance between the two CD-sens values and the two peanut challenges were 100% respectively, but comparison of the degree of allergen threshold sensitivity between the two tests was not possible to achieve since the threshold dose and severity scoring were not reproducible.

If DBPCFC should continue to be used as gold standard for the diagnosis of a food allergy and to predict the severity of a potential clinical reaction, its precision and reproducibility must be documented and improved. Besides, it is of great importance to develop a scoring system integrating both the symptom severity grade and the allergen dose and which can be used world-wide. CD-sens shows promising result with only small variations between the two test occasions but further studies of the role of CD-sens in food allergy diagnosis and treatment trials are most urgent.

Acknowledgments

We would like to thank all children and their parents for participating in the study. We are also very grateful to Ann-Charlotte Sundqvist and the nurses at the Allergy Department, Sachs' Children's Hospital for skilful participation in oral peanut challenges. We wish to acknowledge Åse Olerud and Justus Adédoyin for help with basophil analyses and serological tests and Magnus Rudengren for statistical help. Finally a special thanks to Gunnar Lilja and Malin Berthold for valuable advice in the writing process of the manuscript.

Author Contributions

Conceived and designed the experiments: AN SGOJ CN MPB. Performed the experiments: CN SG AN. Analyzed the data: SG AN. Contributed reagents/materials/analysis tools: SGOJ MPB CN. Wrote the paper: SCG CN AN SGOJ MPB.

References

1. Osborne NJ, Koplin JJ, Martin PE, Gurrin LC, Lowe AJ, et al. (2011) Prevalence of challenge-proven IgE-mediated food allergy using population-based sampling and predetermined challenge criteria in infants. J Allergy Clin Immunol 127: 668–676 e661–662.
2. Chafen JJ, Newberry SJ, Riedl MA, Bravata DM, Maglione M, et al. (2010) Diagnosing and managing common food allergies: a systematic review. JAMA 303: 1848–1856.
3. Sampson HA, Mendelson L, Rosen JP (1992) Fatal and near-fatal anaphylactic reactions to food in children and adolescents. N Engl J Med 327: 380–384.
4. Cummings AJ, Knibb RC, Erlewyn-Lajeunesse M, King RM, Roberts G, et al. (2010) Management of nut allergy influences quality of life and anxiety in children and their mothers. Pediatr Allergy Immunol 21: 586–594.
5. Ostblom E, Egmar AC, Gardulf A, Lilja G, Wickman M (2008) The impact of food hypersensitivity reported in 9-year-old children by their parents on health-related quality of life. Allergy 63: 211–218.
6. Bock SA, Sampson HA, Atkins FM, Zeiger RS, Lehrer S, et al. (1988) Double-blind, placebo-controlled food challenge (DBPCFC) as an office procedure: a manual. J Allergy Clin Immunol 82: 986–997.
7. Bock SA (2000) Evaluation of IgE-mediated food hypersensitivities. J Pediatr Gastroenterol Nutr 30 Suppl: S20–27.
8. Gellerstedt M, Bengtsson U, Niggemann B (2007) Methodological issues in the diagnostic work-up of food allergy: a real challenge. J Investig Allergol Clin Immunol 17: 350–356.
9. Niggemann B (2010) When is an oral food challenge positive? Allergy 65: 2–6.
10. Vlieg-Boerstra BJ, van der Heide S, Bijleveld CM, Kukler J, Duiverman EJ, et al. (2007) Placebo reactions in double-blind, placebo-controlled food challenges in children. Allergy 62: 905–912.
11. Hourihane JO, Grimshaw KE, Lewis SA, Briggs RA, Trewin JB, et al. (2005) Does severity of low-dose, double-blind, placebo-controlled food challenges reflect severity of allergic reactions to peanut in the community? Clin Exp Allergy 35: 1227–1233.
12. Nopp A, Johansson SG, Ankerst J, Bylin G, Cardell LO, et al. (2006) Basophil allergen threshold sensitivity: a useful approach to anti-IgE treatment efficacy evaluation. Allergy 61: 298–302.
13. Glaumann S, Nopp A, Johansson SG, Rudengren M, Borres MP, et al. (2012) Basophil allergen threshold sensitivity, CD-sens, IgE-sensitization and DBPCFC in peanut-sensitized children. Allergy 67: 242–247.
14. Rubio A, Vivinus-Nebot M, Bourrier T, Saggio B, Albertini M, et al. (2011) Benefit of the basophil activation test in deciding when to reintroduce cow's milk in allergic children. Allergy 66: 92–100.
15. Dahlen B, Nopp A, Johansson SG, Eduards M, Skedinger M, et al. (2011) Basophil allergen threshold sensitivity, CD-sens, is a measure of allergen sensitivity in asthma. Clin Exp Allergy 41: 1091–1097.
16. Sabato V, van Hengel AJ, De Knop KJ, Verweij MM, Hagendorens MM, et al. (2011) Human basophils: a unique biological instrument to detect the allergenicity of food. J Investig Allergol Clin Immunol 21: 179–184.
17. Shreffler WG (2006) Evaluation of basophil activation in food allergy: present and future applications. Curr Opin Allergy Clin Immunol 6: 226–233.
18. Johansson SG, Nopp A, van Hage M, Olofsson N, Lundahl J, et al. (2005) Passive IgE-sensitization by blood transfusion. Allergy 60: 1192–1199.
19. van Odijk J, Ahlstedt S, Bengtsson U, Borres MP, Hulthen L (2005) Double-blind placebo-controlled challenges for peanut allergy the efficiency of blinding procedures and the allergenic activity of peanut availability in the recipes. Allergy 60: 602–605.
20. Astier C, Morisset M, Roitel O, Codreanu F, Jacquenet S, et al. (2006) Predictive value of skin prick tests using recombinant allergens for diagnosis of peanut allergy. J Allergy Clin Immunol 118: 250–256.
21. Lieberman JA, Sicherer SH (2011) Diagnosis of food allergy: epicutaneous skin tests, in vitro tests, and oral food challenge. Curr Allergy Asthma Rep 11: 58–64.
22. Nowak-Węgrzyn A, Assa'ad AH, Bahna SL, Bock SA, Sicherer SH, et al. (2009) Work Group report: Oral food challenge testing. Journal of Allergy and Clinical Immunology 123: S365–S383.
23. Codreanu F, Collignon O, Roitel O, Thouvenot B, Sauvage C, et al. (2011) A novel immunoassay using recombinant allergens simplifies peanut allergy diagnosis. Int Arch Allergy Immunol 154: 216–226.
24. van der Zee T, Dubois A, Kerkhof M, van der Heide S, Vlieg-Boerstra B (2011) The eliciting dose of peanut in double-blind, placebo-controlled food challenges decreases with increasing age and specific IgE level in children and young adults. J Allergy Clin Immunol 128: 1031–1036.
25. Eller E, Hansen TK, Bindslev-Jensen C (2012) Clinical thresholds to egg, hazelnut, milk and peanut: results from a single-center study using standardized challenges. Ann Allergy Asthma Immunol 108: 332–336.
26. Flinterman AE, Pasmans SG, Hoekstra MO, Meijer Y, van Hoffen E, et al. (2006) Determination of no-observed-adverse-effect levels and eliciting doses in a representative group of peanut-sensitized children. J Allergy Clin Immunol 117: 448–454.
27. Skripak JM, Nash SD, Rowley H, Brereton NH, Oh S, et al. (2008) A randomized, double-blind, placebo-controlled study of milk oral immunotherapy for cow's milk allergy. J Allergy Clin Immunol 122: 1154–1160.
28. Assa'ad AH, Bahna SL (2012) Food allergy: diagnosis and beyond. Ann Allergy Asthma Immunol 108: 289–290.

8

High-Throughput NMR Assessment of the Tertiary Structure of Food Allergens

Stefano Alessandri[1], Ana Sancho[2¤a], Stefan Vieths[3], Clare E. N. Mills[2¤b], Jean-Michel Wal[4], Peter R. Shewry[5], Neil Rigby[2], Karin Hoffmann-Sommergruber[6]*

1 CERM, Centro di Ricerca di Risonanze Magnetiche and Department of Agricultural Biotechnology, University of Florence, Florence, Italy, **2** Institute of Food Research, Norwich, United Kingdom, **3** Paul-Ehrlich-Institut, Langen, Germany, **4** INRA, UR496 Immuno-Allergie Alimentaire, CEA/iBiTeC-S/SPI, CEA de Saclay, Gif sur Yvette, France, **5** Rothamsted Research, Harpenden, United Kingdom, **6** Department of Pathophysiology and Allergy Research, Medical University of Vienna, Vienna, Austria

Abstract

Background: *In vitro* component-resolved diagnosis of food allergy requires purified allergens that have to meet high standards of quality. These include the authentication of their conformation, which is relevant for the recognition by specific IgE antibodies from allergic patients. Therefore, highly sensitive and reliable screening methods for the analysis of proteins/allergens are required to assess their structural integrity. In the present study one-dimensional 1H Nuclear Magnetic Resonance (1D 1H-NMR) analysis was adopted for the assessment of overall structural and dynamic properties and authentication of a set of relevant food allergens, including non-specific lipid transfer proteins from apple, peach and hazelnut, 7/8S seed storage globulins from hazelnut and peanut, 11S seed storage globulins from hazelnut and peanut, caseins from cows' and goats' milk and tropomyosin from shrimp.

Methodology/Principal Findings: Two sets of 1D 1H-NMR experiments, using 700 MHz and 600 MHz instruments at 298 K were carried out to determine the presence and the extent of tertiary structure. Structural similarity among members of the individual allergen families was also assessed and changes under thermal stress investigated. The nuclear magnetic resonance (NMR) results were compared with structural information available either from the literature, Protein Data Bank entries, or derived from molecular models.

Conclusions/Significance: 1D ^{1}H-NMR analysis of food allergens allowed their classification into molecules with rigid, extended and ordered tertiary structures, molecules without a rigid tertiary structure and molecules which displayed both features. Differences in thermal stability were also detected. In summary, 1D ^{1}H-NMR gives insights into molecular fold of proteins and offers an independent method for assessing structural properties of proteins.

Editor: Vladimir N. Uversky, University of South Florida College of Medicine, United States of America

Funding: This work was funded by the EU through the EuroPrevall project (FOOD-CT-2005-514000). Rothamsted Research and the Institute of Food Research are funded by the Biotechnology and Biological Sciences Research Council (BBSRC) of the United Kingdom. KHS is supported by the Grant SFB-F46-B19 from the Austrian (FWF) Science Fund. The funders had no role in study design, data collection and analysis, decision to publish, or preparation of the manuscript.

Competing Interests: The authors have declared that no competing interests exist.

* E-mail: Karin.hoffmann@meduniwien.ac.at

¤a Current address: Department of Molecular Biology, University of Salzburg, Salzburg, Austria
¤b Current address: School of Translational Medicine, Manchester Academic Health Science Centre, Manchester Interdisciplinary Biocentre, University of Manchester, Manchester, United Kingdom

Introduction

IgE-mediated food allergies are caused by non-toxic dietary proteins of animal or plant origin. Once sensitized, predisposed individuals develop allergic symptoms upon intake. Clinical manifestations range from mild, local reactions to generalised severe, even life-threatening conditions. However, only a restricted number of proteins are capable of inducing allergic sensitization and elicitation [1].

Conventional *in vitro* allergy diagnosis is based on the detection of specific IgE antibodies directed against allergens present in total extracts of food materials. In the recent past the concept of component-resolved diagnosis, in which total extracts are replaced by panels of single allergens for each food, has been introduced aiming at improved sensitivity, reproducibility and specificity of the assay [2–4]. However, the quality of the test performance depends on the quality of the analytical tools used. Therefore, the concept of an allergen library was developed within the EuroPrevall project [5] which included purified members of the allergen families known as non-specific lipid transfer proteins (nsLTPs), 7S seed storage globulins, 11S seed storage globulins, caseins from cows' and goats' milk and tropomyosin from shrimp. State of the art methods for the purification of allergenic food proteins were collated and a catalogue of quality criteria was agreed, including the evaluation of analytical methods for their authentication [6].

IgE antibodies produced by allergic individuals to a food allergen display different specificities and may be directed against linear and conformational epitopes. Particularly for the conformational, discontinuous IgE epitopes a 3-dimensional structure of the purified allergen closely resembling that of the protein in its natural environment is mandatory for reliable *in vitro* diagnosis. Therefore, highly efficient methods to assess the structural integrity of these proteins are required. It is particularly important to confirm that individual batches of purified proteins resemble the naturally occurring protein in their structures and properties, displaying either rigid, intermediate or flexible tertiary structures the latter being important for allergens that may exist in partially-unfolded states induced by thermal processing [7,8].

Nuclear Magnetic Resonance (NMR) spectroscopy is one of the main techniques used to study the structural properties of native and processed proteins and is capable of atomic resolution in aqueous solutions. i.e. under conditions similar to the physiological state. It provides information on the positions, bonds and movements of specific atoms with nuclei which have a spins different from zero, primarily ^{1}H, and on their environment. Such information can be used for the characterization of a protein in terms of structural, chemical and dynamic properties [7,8]. However, 3D-structure determination may require isotopically-labelled protein to allow such highly resolved structures to be determined. In addition, the instrumental and human resources required for this type of NMR experiment, and the concentrations of proteins that are required, also make it impossible to currently define them as "high-throughput". An alternative is to use 1D NMR spectra as an initial screening tool, to differentiate between protein chains with rigid and ordered tertiary structures, from those that are randomly coiled and those proteins that are more mobile, disordered or flexible. 1D ^{1}H-NMR spectra already contain enough information to evaluate whether a protein has some tertiary structure, although the signals are not assigned and the determination of 1D ^{1}H-NMR spectra is much less time consuming than other kind of NMR experiment. Close inspection of one-dimensional ^{1}H spectra also provides information about the extent of tertiary structure in partially-structured proteins, about mixtures where only one fraction is structured or about mixture of conformers like molten globules [9]. Aggregation can be also detected by observing the line width of the signals because the width of the signals in a solution NMR spectrum is correlated with the size of the molecule. Such NMR screening is considered a useful tool for identifying targets which have a high probability of producing crystals of sufficient quality for x-ray diffraction studies or are amenable to structural analysis by NMR. 1D ^{1}H-NMR screening allows structural genomics and proteomics studies to be focused on the most promising targets and, therefore, significantly reduces the cost of production of novel 3D protein structures [10,11].

Several examples of the range of structural types that are represented by allergens were chosen, from totally unstructured molecules (caseins), to proteins belonging to families characterized by a rigid and ordered tertiary structure (non specific lipid transfer proteins, nsLTP), representing the most important plant food allergens families [12,13]. These included the nsLTPs as representatives of the prolamin superfamily and are identified as allergens in fruits, vegetables and nuts. In Rosaceae fruits they are major allergens accounting for severe allergic reactions in patients. Non specific lipid transfer proteins are stabilised by four disulfide bridges and typically resistant to thermal and enzymatic treatment [14]. The structure of Pru p 3, the major allergen from peach, was determined by X-ray crystallography [15] (PDB entries 2alg and 2b5s). Another dominant plant food allergen family are the cupins, to which seed storage proteins belong. These can be divided into two groups based on their sedimentation coefficients. These include the 7S vicilin-type globulins which are typically trimeric proteins [16] and the 11S legumin-type globulins, after post-translational processing, typically consist of six subunit pairs that interact noncovalently. Allergens from this protein family are identified from legumes, nuts and seeds. The 11S or 7S globulins can form both trimeric and hexameric structures: reversible aggregation into hexamers is possible, for 7S globulins, depending on the ionic strength and 11S globulins are assembled via a trimeric intermediate [16].

Representatives of the animal food allergen families were tropomyosins and caseins. Tropomyosins are known as major allergens in seafood and minor inhalant allergens in cockroaches and mites. Typically non vertebrate tropomyosin has a molecular mass of 33 kDa and is a homodimer of two parallel alpha helical molecules with a flexible coiled-coil structure each [17] that allows the tropomyosin to assemble around the actin filaments [18].

Caseins are typically unfolded proteins and account for the majority in the protein fraction of mammalian milk. Cow's milk casein is known as a major food allergen especially in young children. Whole caseins are mixtures of four different proteins: alpha-S1-casein (199 AA, 23.6 kDa), alpha-S2-casein (207 AA 25.2 kDa), beta-casein (209 AA, 24 kDa), k-casein (169 AA, 19 kDa; [19]). Bovine caseins consist of flexible disordered and mobile loops, with only few residues included in short portions that could be organised at the secondary level.

The aim of the current study was to apply 1D ^{1}H-NMR spectroscopy to structural analysis of a range of allergens from major allergen families and to assess its potential as an effective high throughput method. The structural characteristics of the allergens within a protein family and reversible and irreversible structural transitions due to temperature changes were also investigated.

Materials and Methods

Preparation of the allergens

Non-specific lipid transfer proteins were purified from apple (*Malus domestica*, Mal d 3), peach (*Prunus persica*, Pru p 3) and hazelnut (*Corylus avellana*, Cor a 8) as described previously [20–22]. 7S and 11S seed storage globulins were purified from hazelnut (*Corylus avellana*, Cor a 11, Cor a 9) and peanut (*Arachis hypogaea*, Ara h 1, Ara h 3) as described previously [22,23]. Caseins were purified from cows' (*Bos domesticus*, Bos d 8) and goats' milk (Whole caprine casein, WCC [24]). Tropomyosin, the major allergen from brown shrimp (*Penaeus aztecus*, Pen a 1) was produced as a recombinant protein and purified accordingly [17]. The natural and recombinant allergens were tested for their IgE-binding activity using allergic patients sera as previously described and their primary and secondary structures verified by N-terminal sequencing, MALDI-TOF-MS analysis and far-UV CD-spectroscopy [5]. An overview of the allergens used in this study, their acronyms and physicochemical parameters together with the experimental conditions of the NMR analyses are summarised in Table 1.

Nuclear magnetic resonance spectroscopy

Allergen solutions were prepared in H_2O/D_2O 9:1, (0.50 ml, with concentration ranging from 0.39 mM to 0.03 mM) in aqueous buffer systems (pH ranging from 7.0 to 7.8) as detailed in the legends for figures. The solutions were transferred into high-quality NMR tube with argon as headspace gas. Before and after the NMR experiments, the allergens were stored at 253 K (−20°C). Two High Resolution NMR experiments were carried out, using an Avance 700 spectrometer by Bruker, operating at a proton resonance frequency of 700 MHz (11.7 Tesla). The two experiments differed in the method of managing the water signal.

Table 1.

Protein family	Function	Allergen* designation	Source	Mol Mass	PDB ID**	1-D-^{1}H-NMR Analyses	
						Experimental conditions (protein conc.; buffer)	**Structure**
Plant Food Allergens							
Non specific lipid transfer proteins	Plant defence, transfer of lipids	Mal d 3	Apple *Malus domestica*	9 kDa	2alg (Peach)	0.08 mM; 20 mM phosphate; pH 7.4	folded
		Pru p 3	Peach *Prunus persica*	9 kDa	2alg, 2b5s	0.39 mM; 25 mM phosphate; pH 7.0	folded
		Cor a 8	Hazelnut *Corylus avellana*	9 kDa	2alg (Peach)	0.15 mM; 25 mM phosphate, 150 mM NaCl; pH 7.0	
Cupin superfamily							
Vicillin-type (7/8S globulin)	Seed storage	Cor a 11	Hazelnut *Corylus avellana*	48 kDa	2ea7 Chain A (Adzuki Bean)	0.04 mM; 50 mM phosphate, 150 mM NaCl; pH 7.5	folded
		Ara h 1	Peanut *Arachis hypogaea*	62 kDa	3fz3 (Almond)	0.03 mM; 50 mM MOPS, 20 mM NaCl pH 7.8	predominantely folded
Legumin-type (11S)	Seed storage	Cor a 9	Hazelnut *Corylus avellana*	60 kDa	3fz3 (Almond)	0.03 mM; 50 mM phosphate, 150 mM NaCl; pH 7.5	predominantely folded
		Ara h 3/4 Ara h 3.0101 Ara h 3.0201	Peanut *Arachis hypogaea*	60 kDa	3c3v (partial structure)	0.14 mM; 50 mM phosphate, 150 mM NaCl; pH 7.5	predominantely folded
Animal Food Allergens							
Casein	Ca^{2+} binding	Bos d 8	Cow's milk *Bos domesticus*	19–24 kDa		0.08 mM; 40 mM phosphate; pH 7.4	non folded
			Goat's milk *Capra hircus*	19–24 kDa		0.19 mM; 40 mM phosphate; pH 7.4	non folded
Tropomyosin	Regulator of muscle contraction	Pen a 1	Shrimp *Penaeus aztecus*	33 kDa	1c1g (Pig)	0.13 mM; 20 mM MOPS, 0.5 M NaCl; pH 7.6	non folded

*Allergen designations according to the IUIS Allergen nomenclature committee (www.allergen.org).
**Solved and available structures are listed, with their PDB entries. If models were generated then the respective template structure is given.

The pulse program of the first experiment included a 1D sequence with pre-saturation to minimize the water signal [25]. The second experiment is based on gradient-based water suppression by 1D excitation sculpting using 180° water-selective pulses [25]. It increases the overall sensitivity and decreases the distortion of the baseline, but some signal near the (suppressed) water peak can be suppressed. This can be checked by the pre-saturation experiment.

For each sample and for each experiment 256 scans at 298 K (25°C) were routinely programmed, due to the low sample concentration. More scans were required for proteins with higher molecular mass and more diluted protein solutions (Mal d 3, Ara h 3/4, Cor a 9, Ara h 1, Cor a 11) as specified in the legends of the corresponding figures, where variations in the number of scans and of the field strength are reported, with the molecular weights and the molarities of the samples and the buffer conditions. The spectra were initially evaluated considering the dispersion of the signals in the regions of the methyl protons (−0.5–1.5 ppm), alpha-protons (3.5–6.0 ppm), and amide protons (6.0–10.0 ppm).

The consistency of the allergen spectra with information available in the scientific literature and with structures either deposited into the Protein Data Bank (PDB) or supported by a publication, was routinely checked. If no experimental structure was available, the comparison with a modelled structure was performed [26–29] and its consistency with the NMR spectra checked.

Study of thermal stability

The stability of the nsLTPs (Mal d 3, Pru p 3 and Cor a 8) to thermal stress was studied using a 600 MHz spectrometer equipped with a probe suited to work at high temperature. A series of experiments was performed consisting of stepwise heating of each sample from 298 K (25°C) to a maximum 358 K (85°C), by 5 K intervals. After each step an NMR water pre-saturation (zgpr) experiment was launched and the spectrum evaluated. If significant structural changes were detectable, the sample was cooled to 298 K and scanned to verify whether the detected structural change was reversible. If the maximum temperature allowed by the probe had not been already reached, the sample was heated to the next threshold.

A minimum of 128 scans was programmed for each NMR experiment, extended to 512 for the most diluted samples (Mal d 3). A minimum of 20 minutes was required to reach the thermal equilibrium after each 5 K heating step. A minimum of 90 minutes was required after each cooling step and after each following heating step. All the experiments were conducted under near-neutral pH condition. The thermal stability of Pru p 3 was also studied in acidic solution (adjusting to pH 3 by addition of HCl).The pH was checked before and after the experiments.

Modelling of allergens

The modelled structures were obtained using the fully automated protein structure homology-modelling server SWISS-MODEL [25,27,28] and were selected based on the protein family of the template, the sequence identity between the target and the template, the modelled residue range of the target, the QMEAN Z-Score and the QMEAN4 global score of the model [26,30–32]. Models of low quality are expected to have strongly negative QMEAN Z-scores. The QMEAN describes the likelihood that a given model is of comparable quality to experimental structures. The QMEAN4 ranges between 0 and 1 with higher values indicating better models among alternative models of the same target.

Results and Discussion

NMR analysis

Since large chemical shift dispersions, especially in the methyl group region between 1.0 ppm and −1.0 ppm and in the amide region down-field of 8.5 ppm can be used as a reliable indicator for protein folding [10,33] this approach was taken to assessing the structural attributes of the selected allergens. Few broad peaks around 8.3 ppm are a good indicator of a protein without an ordered tertiary structure, because this is a region characteristic of backbone amides in random-coil configuration. By contrast, several peaks, possibly narrow and resolved, dispersed beyond 8.5 ppm (8.5–11 ppm) are the signature of a rigid and ordered tertiary structure. However, the signals of the amide protons can be broadened due to chemical exchange especially at non-acidic pH. This can be a drawback at protein concentrations close to the detection limit when amide signals are to be observed. Isolated methyl group signals upfield of 0.5 ppm can be more sensitive and reliable probes for folded protein as they are not affected by chemical exchange broadening. In addition, their signal intensities are higher because three equivalent protons contribute rather than one proton of the amide group. Therefore, a wide signal dispersion in the aliphatic region of the spectrum between 1.0 and −1.0 ppm, versus a steep flank of the dominant peak at approximately 1 ppm reliably discriminates rigid and ordered tertiary structures from random-coil or flexible structures. This is because the loss of high field methyl peaks indicates a reduction in tertiary side chain organization, which can be considered complete when the NMR spectrum is characterized by few, rather narrow, but poorly dispersed peaks that are indicative of extremely mobile residues. This condition can be usually achieved as a result of protein unfolding in strongly acidic condition usually in the presence of a high concentration of urea [34].

A thermodynamically distinct state of proteins showing properties of both native and denatured proteins is "molten globule" [35]. Molten globules are considered as intermediates on the protein folding/unfolding process but in some cases, molten globules exist as stable conformers, with rigid but different tertiary structure [9]. The NMR spectrum of a molten globule protein is characterized by few, extremely broad peaks, especially for most of the backbone amide groups.

Whilst spectral signals from certain allergens (Ara h 1, Cor a 9, Cor a 11, Mal d 3) were weak and spectra were dominated by buffer signals this did not affect the readability of the critical spectral regions.

All the spectra were consistent with the corresponding structures deposited in the PDB, or with structures that could be modelled starting from the sequence and anticipated on the basis of the proteins family membership. Analysis of the 1D ^{1}H-NMR spectra then allowed the classification of the allergens under study as follows.

Prolamin superfamily - nsLTPs

The NMR spectra of these nsLTPs (Fig. 1 and Fig. 2) show the unmistakable features of rigid and extended tertiary structures which is not affected by low pH environment and is in line with the 2D studies performed with Pru p 3 by Wijeshina-Bettoni et al [14]. There are many narrow and resolved peaks throughout the whole spectral window, notably in the methyl and amide-aromatic regions. The spectra of these allergens are very similar: for example, the extreme methyl region between 1 and 0 ppm and the aromatic region between 6 and 8 ppm. This fact gives experimental support to the similarity of the modelled structures of Mal d 3 and Cor a 8, and the experimental structure of Pru p 3 (Fig. 3), as expected from the high degree of sequence homology and conserved cysteine residues forming disulfide bridges. Thus Mal d 3 (Uni Prot entry: Q9M5X7), and Cor a 8 (Uni Prot entry: Q9ATH2), share 81.3% and 59% sequence identity with Pru p 3 (Uni Prot entry: P81402), respectively. The overall intact 3D structure is relevant for IgE-binding activity of Pru p 3 and is reduced when alkylation and reduction of the protein was performed [36]. Therefore, Pru p 3 was subjected to stepwise heat treatment to investigate whether heating processes have an impact on its overall structure.

During thermal treatment the spectra gradually change towards the denatured state. Under acidic conditions (Fig. 4, pH 3) the increasing loss of tertiary structure of Pru p 3 is apparent from the decreasing dispersion of peaks either in the methyl region (around 0 ppm) or in the amide-aromatic region (6–10 ppm). Irreversible denaturation is not detectable until 358 K (85°C) and the 298 K (25°C) spectra, scanned before and after heating, overlap perfectly. These data are in good agreement with the studies on heat resistance of barley LPT from Perrocheau et al. [37]. Under neutral conditions (Fig. 4, pH 7) two major differences can be observed during thermal denaturation of natural Pru p 3. The former is an irreversible structural transition occurring between 353 K (80°C) and 358 K (85°C): the final room temperature spectrum shows only a few broad and poorly dispersed peaks in the amide-aromatic and in the methyl region and the absence of resonances upfield and downfield. The latter represents the disappearance of amide resonances (7–9 ppm) as the temperature rises. This is due to proton exchange with the solvent, and depends on pH, temperature and accessibility of exchangeable protons, which increases with unfolding, and can be due to the transition to a molten-globule state. Native Mal d 3 shares the same behaviour as Pru p 3 when heated in neutral conditions (data not shown). Heating was stopped at 348 K (75°C) for Cor a 8 due to instrumental problems. The protein refolds to the 25°C tertiary structure after the heat-induced unfolding at the maximum tested temperature (data not shown).

Cupins – seed storage globulins

The higher molecular mass of globulins as compared to nsLTPs and their propensity to aggregate into more complex quaternary structures seriously limits the resolution of their NMR spectra (Fig. 5). This could be a particular problem for Cor a 9, due to the possible presence of the hexameric form. A series of signals, though basically unresolved, can be observed in the extreme methyl region of all the spectra (around 0.5 ppm) indicating regions of rigid tertiary structure. On the other hand, the presence of extended mobile regions must be considered, due to the few broad peaks that can be observed in the whole spectral window, notably in the HN region between 6 and 8 ppm. By contrast, the same region of the Cor a 11 spectrum is populated by several better resolved and narrow resonances that give a clear indication of rigid and ordered regions. Both, Cor a 9 and Cor a 11 show a noticeable signal broadening in the backbone NH region between 8.0 and 8.7 ppm, that could indicate the presence of a molten globule state. Narrow, weak signals are observed against a background of broad peaks in the Ara h 3/4 spectrum which could be due to the presence of both lighter monomers and more massive aggregations in the mixture (Fig. 5).

Up to now two sequences of 7/8S globulin Ara h 1, from peanut (63.5 kDa) (UniProt entries P43237 and P43238) were characterised [38]. Very recently, the structure from the Ara h 1 core region without the N-terminal extension and the C-terminal flexible region was determined [39]. Both isoforms could be modelled using the 7S globulin from adzuki bean [40] as a

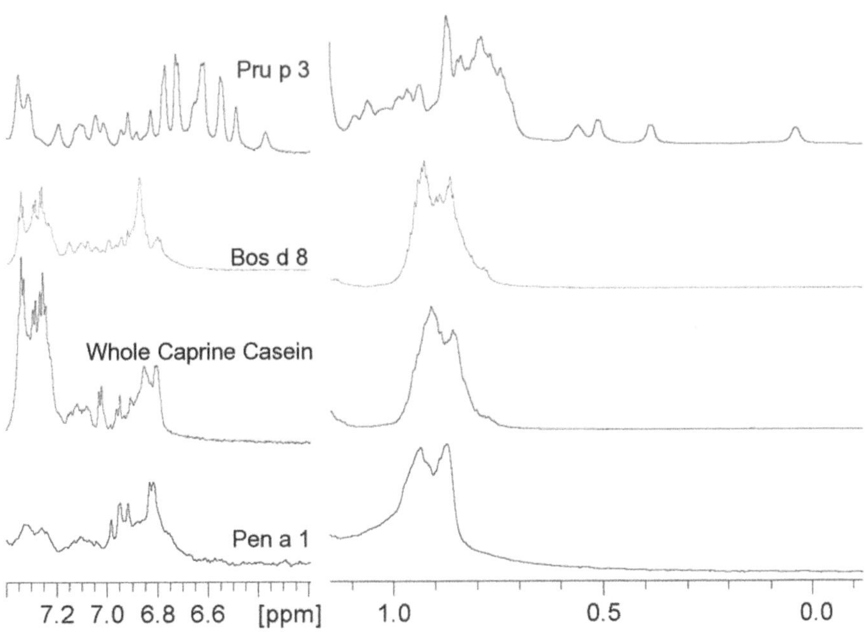

Figure 1. NMR spectra typical for allergens with random coil structure, compared with a spectrum of an allergen with rigid tertiary structure. Two enlarged regions of the spectra (gradient-based water suppression NMR experiment) of purified casein fraction from cow (Bos d 8, 0.08 mM, 900 MHz cryoprobe, 40 mM phosphate, pH 7.4), and goat (whole caprine casein, WCC, 0.19 mM; 40 mM phosphate pH 7.4), and of the recombinant tropomyosin from shrimp (Pen a 1, 0.13 mM, 36.4 kDa, MOPS 20 mM, NaCl 0.5 M, pH 7.6) are shown. The 0.3–1.2 ppm region includes the extreme methyl signals while the 6.2–7.4 ppm region includes the resonances of aromatic ring protons, side chain HN, and part of backbone HN; These spectra are typical of random coil structures, as indicated by the absence of signal upfield 6.6 ppm and 0.7 ppm. The same enlarged regions of the spectrum of Pru p 3 (0.39 mM, 91 AA, 9.2 kDa) are shown (top) to underline the difference between spectra of folded and unfolded proteins.

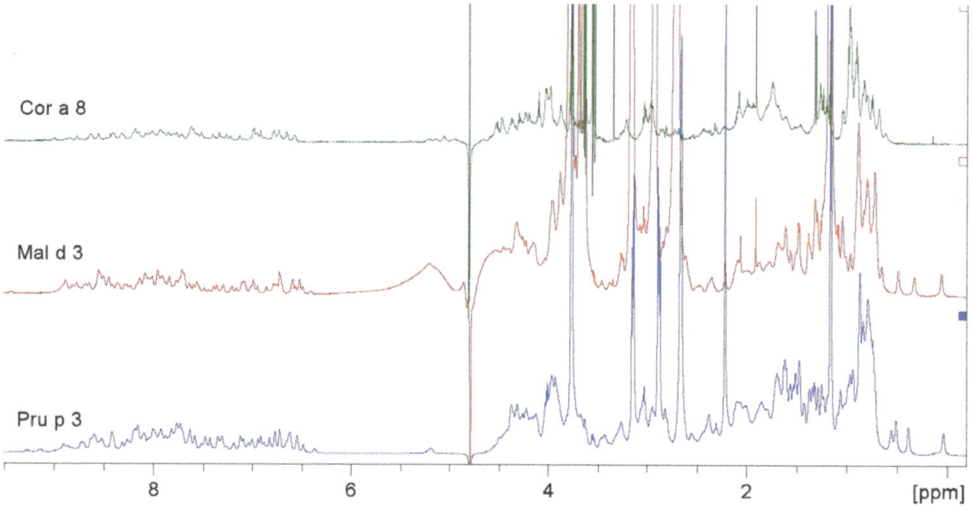

Figure 2. NMR Spectra of non specific lipid transfer protein, nsLTP, from peach (Pru p 3), apple (Mal d 3) and hazelnut (Cor a 8). The spectra (gradient-based water suppression NMR experiment) of nsLTPs from different sources are compared: Cor a 8 from hazelnut (115 AA, 11.8 kDa, 0.15 mM; 25 mM phosphate, NaCl 150 mM, pH 7.0), Mal d 3 from apple (115 AA, 11.4 kDa, 0.08 mM, 6504 scans; 20 mM phosphate, pH 7.4), Pru p 3 from peach (91 AA, 9.2 kDa, 0.39 mM; 25 mM phosphate, pH 7.0). These spectra indicate the presence of extended, rigid and ordered tertiary structure for all three molecules and display a high degree of similarity.

template (PDB accession 2ea7), with 48% of sequence identity (Fig. 6). The template and the modelled monomer can be divided into two similar modules (N- and C-terminal), each showing an extended loop domain. The models could be verified by the crystal based analysis of the Ara h 1 core fragment [39,41]. Already identified IgE epitopes, were mapped on the models and it became evident that some of these epitopes were only surface exposed when the trimer formation was disrupted [42].

A partially resolved structure (PDB entry 3c3v) has been reported as Ara h 3 (now designated: Ara h 3.0101; Swiss prot Entry: O82580) [43]. It consists of an N-terminal domain and a C-terminal domain. Three regions of the N-terminal domain and the tail of C-terminal domain are disordered (Fig. 7). Using this structure as a template a model was built of the isoform reported as Ara h 4 (now designated: Ara h 3.0201; Swiss Prot entry: Q9SQH7) [44]. The model which shares 75.5% sequence identity with "Ara h 3" (Fig. 7) was calculated including the unresolved regions of the experimental structure, and is consistent with the presence of extended, partially structured, mobile regions.

IgE epitopes were identified on the surface of Ara h 3, some of them specific for the peanut allergen and some of them shared with other legumin type allergens highlighting the molecular basis for cross-reactivity [45].

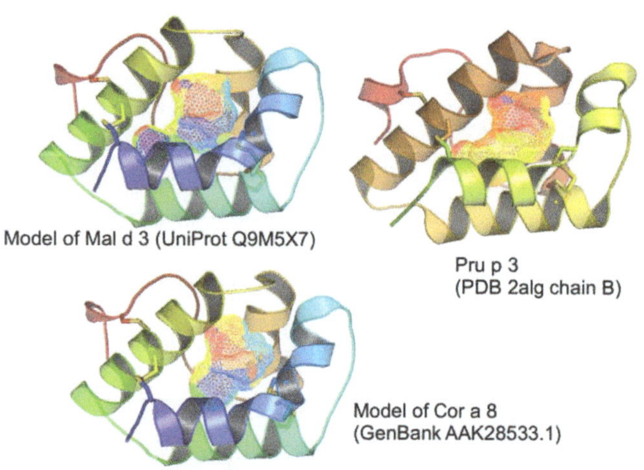

Figure 3. Modelled and experimental structures of nsLTPs from apple, peach and hazelnut. Models of Mal d 3 and Cor a 8 based on the experimental structure of Pru p 3 as template (PDB 2alg, chain B, 92 residues). Disulphide bonds are rendered as sticks and the internal hydrophobic cavity is rendered as a mesh surface. The modelled residue range is 25–115 for both models. QMEAN Z-score = −1.895 (Mal d 3) and −1.639 (Cor a 8).

No experimental structure of hazelnut globulins is known to date. Again a homology model was built (Fig. 6) using the Cor a 11 sequence [46] starting from its 48 kDa precursor sequence (Swiss Prot entry: Q8S4P9), with 32.5% of identity with the template PDB 2ea7, chain A, corresponding to the adzuki bean 7S globulin [40]. The model is trimeric, with each monomer formed by two very similar modules and each module containing an extended loop domain. Similarly a model was built using the Cor a 9 sequence (GenBank: AAL73404.1) which has 51.8% sequence identity to the almond globulin [47,48] (PDB 3fz3) (Fig. 8). The structure of this template, and of the derived model, shows similarities with the structure of the 11S globulin Ara h 3/4 (Ara h 3.0101 and Ara h 3.0201; Fig. 7 and Fig. 8).

Narrow, weak signals in are observed against a background of broad peaks in the Ara 3/4 spectrum which could be due to the presence of both lighter monomers and more massive aggregations in the mixture (Fig. 5).

The spectra of all of the globulins provide experimental support for their modelled structures and are consistent with our knowledge of the structural characteristics of this family of proteins including their tendency towards aggregation, the ubiquity of isoforms, and the presence of extended mobile regions in their tertiary structure.

Tropomyosin and Caseins

The NMR spectra of the sample of Pen a 1 under study and the spectra of caseins are very similar. These spectra (Fig. 1) show the

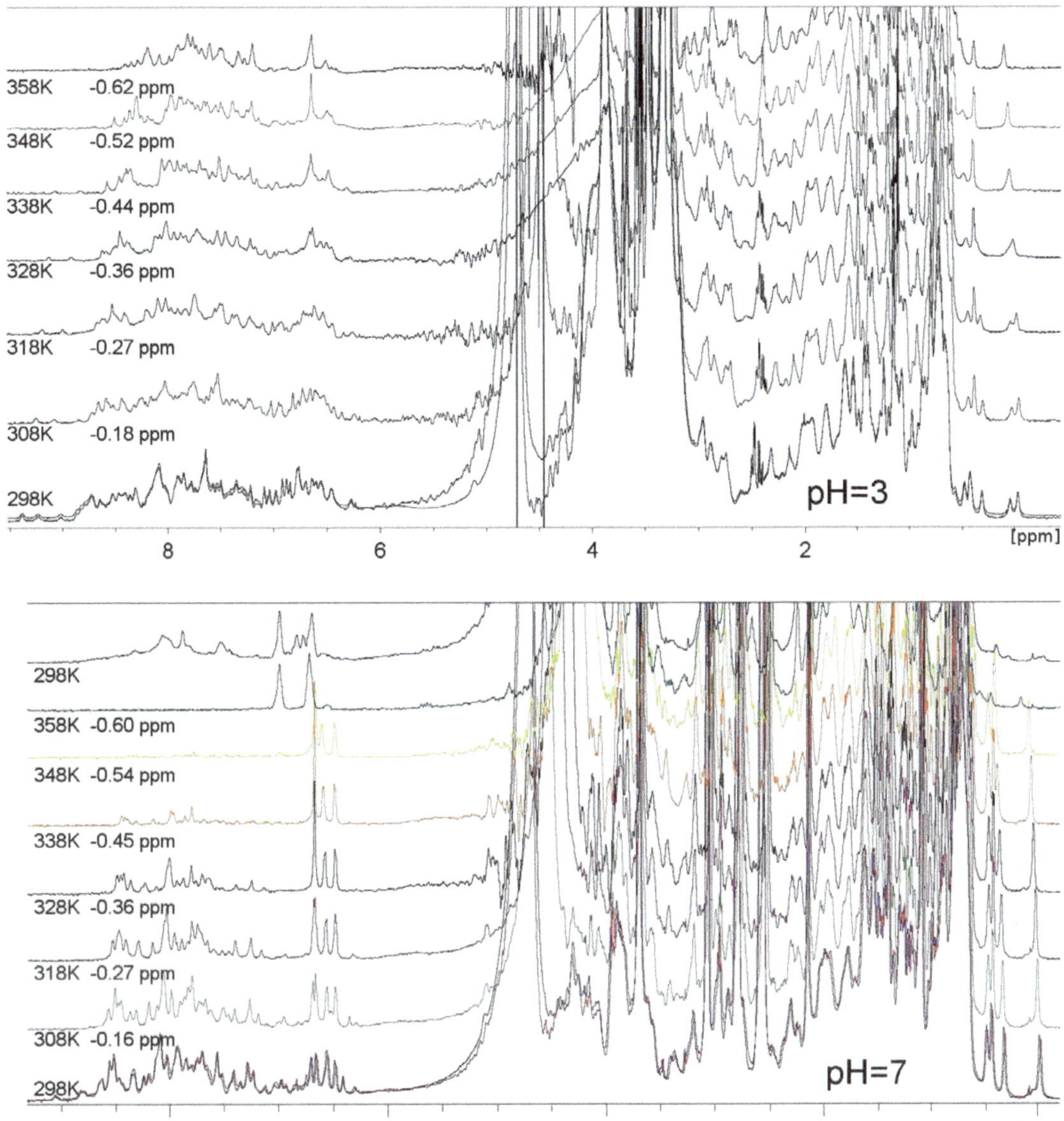

Figure 4. NMR spectra of nsLTP from peach, Pru p 3 under thermal treatment in acidic and near-neutral pH conditions. Heating of Pru p 3 (0.39 mM, 91 AA, 9.2 kDa) under acidic (pH 3.0) and neutral (pH 7.0) conditions; pre-saturation NMR experiments. To improve readability, the spectra at T>298 K are aligned with the reference spectrum at 298 K (25°C), by shifting them upfield as indicated after the temperature. pH 3.0 bottom: NMR spectra of Pru p 3 scanned at 298 K before and after heating up to 358 K (85°C). pH 7.0, bottom: NMR spectra of Pru p 3 scanned at 298 K before and after heating up to 358 K. top: spectrum scanned at 298 K after 358 K heating. In neutral conditions the protein undergoes irreversible denaturation, in the 80°C–85°C range of temperature.

typical characteristics of random coil structures with extended regions of the spectral window being devoid of signals and a few broad peaks at characteristic intervals. The dominant methyl peak at approximately 1 ppm is a distinctive signature of a random-coil or extremely flexible structure. Single narrow signals can be observed on the envelope of broad peaks which are not resolved to the baseline because they are confined in narrow spectral ranges, confirming the high mobility of the residues of these samples. A model was constructed of Pen a 1 (Accession No. DQ151457.1) [49] based on the structure of pig cardiac muscle tropomyosin [50] (PDB 1c1g, chain A) with which it shares 56.2% sequence identity (Fig. 9). This has a coiled-coil structure which can undergo a transition from a coiled coil to molten-like state before complete dissociation of the two chains, chains that are flexible and can be unfolded at physiological temperature [51]. This could explain the observation that the NMR spectrum is characteristic of a mobile, unfolded structure. Detailed studies on the epitope mapping of this major allergen identified linear IgE epitopes with increased antibody binding activity when grafted onto non allergenic tropomyosin [17].

The spectra of the caseins were similarly characterised by a lack of signals between 6.2 and 6.6 ppm and 0.0 and 0.7 ppm, respectively (Fig. 1) indicative of their highly mobile structure. The fact that unfractionated caseins are mixtures of four different molecules is not apparent because alpha-s1-casein, beta-casein, alpha-s2-casein and k-casein [19], all share similar molecular weight and lack secondary and tertiary structure, and therefore

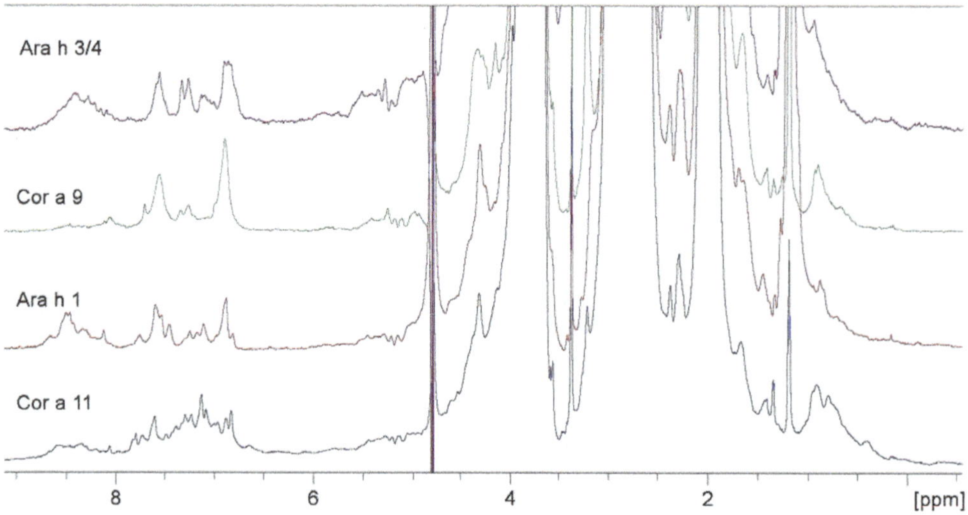

Figure 5. NMR Spectra of globulins from peanut and hazelnut. The spectra (gradient-based water suppression NMR experiment, 848 scans) of selected globulins from different sources are presented: Ara h 3/4 (mixture of isoforms of 11S globulins from peanut, 37.0 kDa, putative concentration 0.14 mM; 50 mM phosphate, NaCl 150 mM, pH 7.5), Cor a 9 (11S globulin from hazelnut, 40 kDa, 0.03 mM, 50 mM phosphate, NaCl 150 mM, pH 7.5), Ara h 1 (7/8 S globulin from peanut, 63.5 kDa, 0.03 mM, 50 mM MOPS, NaCl 200 mM, pH 7.8), Cor a 11 (7/8S globulin from hazelnut 48 kDa, 0.04 mM, phosphate 50 mM, NaCl 150 mM, pH 7.5), Signals, though basically unresolved due to high MW and possible aggregation, can be observed in the extreme methyl region of all the spectra (around 0.5 ppm) which indicate of regions of rigid tertiary structure. The presence of extended disordered regions must also be considered, due to the few broad peaks that can be observed in the whole spectral window, especially in the HN region between 6 and 8 ppm and especially for Cor a 9. On the contrary the same region of Cor a 11 is populated by several more resolved and narrow resonances, indicative of rigid and ordered regions. Both, Cor a 9 and Cor a 11 show a noticeable signal broadening in the backbone NH region (8.0–8.7 ppm), indicating the presence of the molten globule state in solution. In the Ara 3/4 spectrum, narrow, weak signals, can be observed on an envelope of broader peaks. They could be due to the lighter (non-aggregated) component of the mixture.

their residues share very similar structural environment as confirmed also by the great similarity of all these spectra.

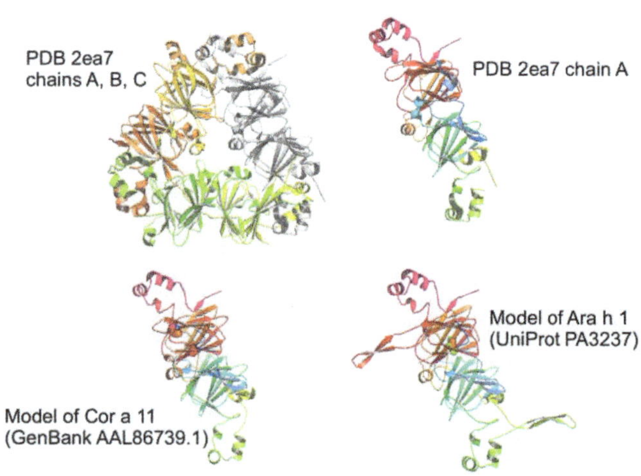

Figure 6. Modelled and experimental structures of 7/8S globulins from peanut, hazelnut and adzuki bean. Models of 7/8S globulins from peanut (Ara h 1, 614 residues) and hazelnut (Cor a 11, 448 residues), both based on 7S globulin from adzuki bean (PDB 2ea7 chain A) as template. Either the monomer (chain A) or the trimer (chain A rendered with the same orientation, in light gray) of the template are shown. The presence of mobile parts is indicated by the many extended loops of the models, corresponding to similar extended loops or to unresolved regions of the template. Modelled residue range: 161–583 (Ara h 1), 55–435 (Cor a 11). Sequence Identity [%]: 49 (Ara h 1), 32 (Cor a 11). QMEAN Z-score = −1.614 (Ara h 1), −0.956 (Cor a 11). QMEAN Z-score of Ara h 1 = 0.669 (0.600 if it is modelled on PDB 2cv6 chain A, corresponding to 8S globulins of mung bean).

Structural classification of allergens

On the basis of the NMR analysis the proteins could be classified into three groups. The first group included those molecules whose spectra showed the unquestionable signature of their tertiary structure: nsLTPs (Fig. 1 and Fig. 2) and the hazelnut 7/8S globulin, Cor a 11. However, the NMR data indicate that the latter may contain disordered stretches (Fig. 5) as has been observed for seed storage globulins from other plant species such as soybean [52].

The second group included those allergens whose spectra clearly showed no fingerprints for tertiary structure (Fig. 1). These were whole caseins from cows' and goats' milk (Bos d 8, WCC) and tropomyosin from brown shrimp (Pen a 1). The spectra for caseins are consistent with other observations of protein mobility

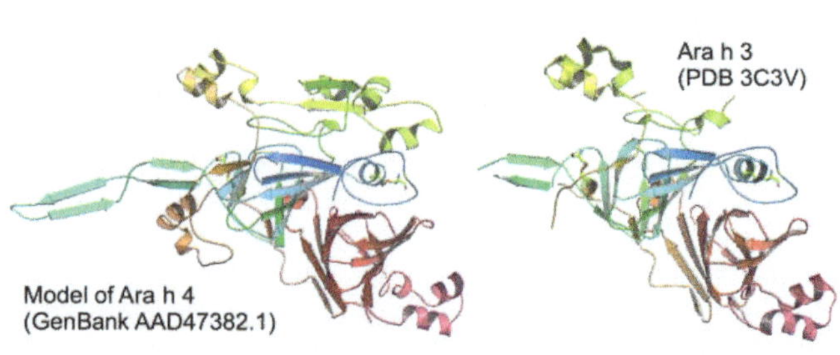

Figure 7. Modelled and experimental structures of Ara h 3/4 isoforms. Experimental structure of Ara h 3/4 (PDB 3c3b) and model of its sequenced isoform (Q9SQH7 GenBank AAD47382.1; 530 residues) based on PDB 3c3v as template. The presence of mobile parts is indicated by the many extended loops of the model, corresponding to similar extended loops or to unresolved regions of the template. Disulphide bonds are rendered as sticks. Modelled residue range: 21–521. Sequence Identity [%]: 75. QMEAN Z-score = −1.933.

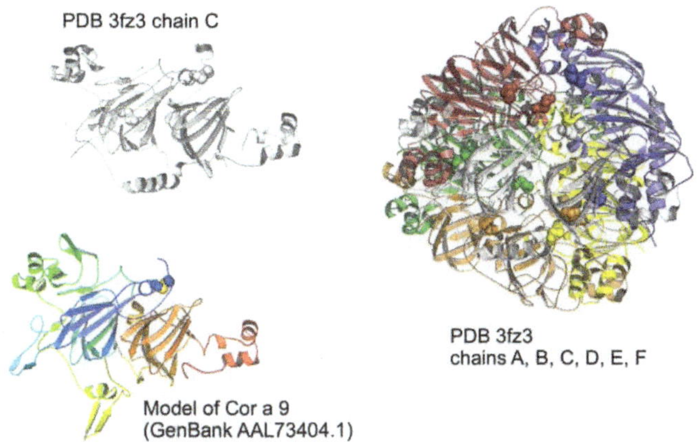

Figure 8. Modelled and experimental structures of 11S globulins from hazelnut and almond. Model of Cor a 9 (11S globulin from hazelnut), based on template PDB 3fz3 (11S globulin from almond) chain C (515 residues). Disulphide bonds are rendered as spheres. Both the monomer and the hexamer of the template are shown. The template's chain C is rendered in light gray, with the same orientation, either as monomer or in the hexamer. The presence of mobile parts is indicated by the many extended loops of the model, corresponding to similar extended loops or to unresolved regions of the template. Modelled residue range: 34 to 496. Sequence Identity [%]: 51. QMEAN Z-score = −3.084.

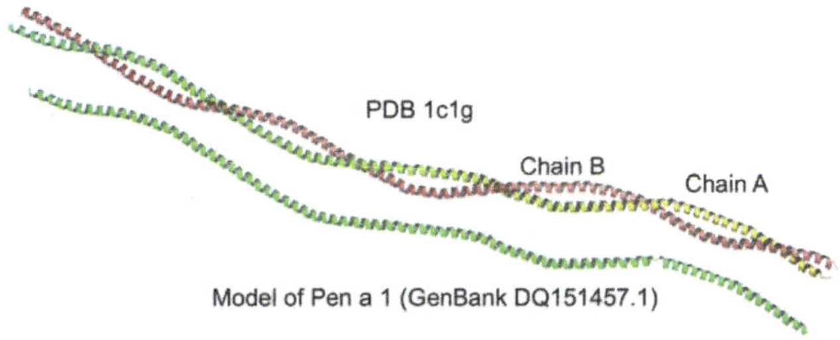

Figure 9. Structures of tropomyosin from brown shrimp (modelled) and pig (experimental). Model of Pen a 1, the tropomyosin from brown shrimp (284 residues) based on tropomyosin (PDB 1c1g chain A) from cardiac muscle of pig (*Sus scrofa*). Tropomyosins can pass from a coiled coil to molten-like structure before complete dissociation of the two chains. Chains are flexible and can be unfolded at physiological temperature. Modelled residue range: 1 to 283. Sequence Identity [%]: 56. QMEAN Z-score = −0.371. QMEAN score 4 = 0.755 (0.732 on tropomyosin from striated-muscle of *R. norvegicus* 2b9c chain A).

which has led to them being termed rheomorphic [19].

The third group included allergens whose spectra revealed an intermediate structure: the 11S globulin Cor a 9 and the 7/8S globulin Ara h 1. Their spectra (Fig. 5) indicated that the protein could be structured with well organized rigid regions with an ordered tertiary structure, interspersed with disordered regions (as indicated by temperature factors in the x-ray structures of certain seed storage globulins and the fact certain regions had not been resolved and appear to be highly mobile even in a crystal lattice [41]. Alternatively these data indicate the sample could be a mixture of folded and unfolded or differently folded proteins. The spectrum of the 11 S globulin Ara h 3/4 (Fig. 5) also indicated the presence of both disordered and ordered parts.

It is worth noting that some of the allergens investigated displayed molecular masses, (e.g. 60 kDa without considering possible aggregations) that can be considered beyond the limitations of the method and the instruments adopted.

Concluding remarks

High quality allergen batches with defined physicochemical features are essential for reliable and sensitive *in vitro* diagnosis for allergy. The 3-dimensional structures of the most important allergen families have important impacts on their IgE binding activity. It has become evident that food processing can affect the structure and thus allergenicity. Therefore, methods to assess the structural integrity of purified allergens are urgently needed. The present study has shown that 1D NMR can be used to generate a fingerprint containing the overall structural and dynamic information of allergenic proteins in a high throughput manner.

Author Contributions

Conceived and designed the experiments: SA KHS. Performed the experiments: SA. Analyzed the data: SA KHS. Contributed reagents/materials/analysis tools: SA AS SV CM JMW PS NR KHS. Wrote the paper: SA KHS.

References

1. Hoffmann-Sommergruber K, Mills EN (2009) Food allergen protein families and their structural characteristics and application in component-resolved diagnosis: new data from the EuroPrevall project. Anal Bioanal Chem 395:25–35.
2. Nicolaou N, Poorafshar M, Murray C, Simpson A, Winell H, et al. (2010) Allergy or tolerance in children sensitized to peanut: prevalence and differentiation using component-resolved diagnostics. J Allergy Clin Immunol 125:191–197.
3. Hansen KS, Ballmer-Weber BK, Sastre J, Lidholm J, Andersson K, et al. (2009) Component-resolved in vitro diagnosis of hazelnut allergy in Europe. J Allergy Clin Immunol 123:1134–1141.
4. Bublin M, Pfister M, Radauer C, Oberhuber C, Bulley S, et al. (2011) Component-resolved diagnosis of kiwifruit allergy with purified natural and recombinant kiwifruit allergens. J Allergy Clin Immunol 125:687–694.
5. Hoffmann-Sommergruber K, Mills EN, Vieths S (2008) Coordinated and standardized production, purification and characterization of natural and recombinant food allergens to establish a food allergen library. Mol Nutr Food Res 52 Suppl 2:S159–165.
6. Sancho AI, Hoffmann-Sommergruber K, Alessandri S, Conti A, Giuffrida MG, et al. (2010) Authentication of food allergen quality by physicochemical and immunological methods. Clin Exp Allergy 40:973–986.
7. Johnson P, Philo M, Watson A, Mills EN (2011) Rapid Fingerprinting of Milk Thermal Processing History by Intact Protein Mass Spectrometry with Nondenaturing Chromatography. J Agric Food Chem 59(23):12420–7.
8. Vissers YM, Iwan M, Adel-Patient K, Stahl Skov P, Rigby NM, et al. (2011) Effect of roasting on the allergenicity of major peanut allergens Ara h 1 and Ara h 2/6: the necessity of degranulation assays. Clin Exp Allergy 41:1631–1642.
9. Rosner HI, Redfield C (2009) The human alpha-lactalbumin molten globule: comparison of structural preferences at pH 2 and pH 7. J Mol Biol 394:351–362.
10. Rehm T, Huber R, Holak TA (2002) Application of NMR in structural proteomics: screening for proteins amenable to structural analysis. Structure 10:1613–1618.
11. Page R, Peti W, Wilson IA, Stevens RC, Wuthrich K (2005) NMR screening and crystal quality of bacterially expressed prokaryotic and eukaryotic proteins in a structural genomics pipeline. Proc Natl Acad Sci U S A 102:1901–1905.
12. Jenkins JA, Griffiths-Jones S, Shewry PR, Breiteneder H, Mills EN (2005) Structural relatedness of plant food allergens with specific reference to cross-reactive allergens: an in silico analysis. J Allergy Clin Immunol 115:163–170.
13. Jenkins JA, Breiteneder H, Mills EN (2007) Evolutionary distance from human homologs reflects allergenicity of animal food proteins. J Allergy Clin Immunol 120:1399–1405.
14. Wijesinha-Bettoni R, Alexeev Y, Johnson P, Marsh J, Sancho AI, et al. (2010) The structural characteristics of nonspecific lipid transfer proteins explain their resistance to gastroduodenal proteolysis. Biochemistry 49:2130–2139.
15. Pasquato N, Berni R, Folli C, Folloni S, Cianci M, et al. (2006) Crystal structure of peach Pru p 3, the prototypic member of the family of plant non-specific lipid transfer protein pan-allergens. J Mol Biol 356:684–694.

16. Shewry PR, Napier JA, Tatham AS (1995) Seed storage proteins: structures and biosynthesis. Plant Cell 7:945–956.
17. Albrecht M, Alessandri S, Conti A, Reuter A, Lauer I, et al. (2008) High level expression, purification and physico- and immunochemical characterisation of recombinant Pen a 1: a major allergen of shrimp. Mol Nutr Food Res 52 Suppl 2:S186–195.
18. Frye J, Klenchin VA, Rayment I (2010) Structure of the tropomyosin overlap complex from chicken smooth muscle: insight into the diversity of N-terminal recognition. Biochemistry 49:4908–4920.
19. Farrell HM Jr, Jimenez-Flores R, Bleck GT, Brown EM, Butler JE, et al. (2004) Nomenclature of the proteins of cows' milk–sixth revision. J Dairy Sci 87:1641–1674.
20. Oberhuber C, Ma Y, Marsh J, Rigby N, Smole U, et al. (2008) Purification and characterisation of relevant natural and recombinant apple allergens. Mol Nutr Food Res 52 Suppl 2:S208–219.
21. Gaier S, Marsh J, Oberhuber C, Rigby NM, Lovegrove A, et al. (2008) Purification and structural stability of the peach allergens Pru p 1 and Pru p 3. Mol Nutr Food Res 52 Suppl 2:S220–229.
22. Rigby NM, Marsh J, Sancho AI, Wellner K, Akkerdaas J, et al. (2008) The purification and characterisation of allergenic hazelnut seed proteins. Mol Nutr Food Res 52 Suppl 2:S251–261.
23. Marsh J, Rigby N, Wellner K, Reese G, Knulst A, et al. (2008) Purification and characterisation of a panel of peanut allergens suitable for use in allergy diagnosis. Mol Nutr Food Res 52 Suppl 2:S272–285.
24. Blanc F, Bernard H, Alessandri S, Bublin M, Paty E, et al. (2008) Update on optimized purification and characterization of natural milk allergens. Mol Nutr Food Res 52 Suppl 2:S166–175.
25. Brereton IM, Field JM, Irving G, Doddrell DM (1989) Water Suppression with Bo Filed Gradient Homospoil Pulse in High-Resolution NMR Spectroscopy. Magnetic Resonance in Medicine 9:18–125.
26. Peitsch M (1995) Protein modelling by E-mail/. Nature Biotechnology (N Y) 13:658–660.
27. Pieper U, Eswar N, Braberg H, Madhusudhan MS, Davis FP, et al. (2004) MODBASE, a database of annotated comparative protein structure models, and associated resources. Nucleic Acids Res 32:D217–222.
28. Arnold K, Bordoli L, Kopp J, Schwede T (2006) The SWISS-MODEL workspace: a web-based environment for protein structure homology modelling. Bioinformatics 22:195–201.
29. Kiefer F, Arnold K, Kunzli M, Bordoli L, Schwede T (2009) The SWISS-MODEL Repository and associated resources. Nucleic Acids Res 37:D387–392.
30. Benkert P, Kuenzli M, Schwede T (2009) QMEAN Server for Protein Model Quality Estimation. Nucleic Acids Research 37:Web server issue: W510–W514.
31. Benkert P, Schwede T, Tosatto SC (2009) QMEANclust: estimation of protein model quality by combining a composite scoring function with structural density information. BMC Struct Biol 9:35.
32. Benkert P, Biasini M, Schwede T (2011) Toward the estimation of the absolute quality of individual protein structure models. Bioinformatics 27:343–350.
33. Scheich C, Leitner D, Sievert V, Leidert M, Schlegel B, et al. (2004) Fast identification of folded human protein domains expressed in *E. coli* suitable for structural analysis. BMC Struct Biol 4:4.
34. Baum J, Dobson CM, Evans PA, Hanley C (1989) Characterization of a partly folded protein by NMR methods: studies in the molten globule state of guinea pig alpha-lactalbumin. Biochemistry 28:7–13.
35. Ohgushi M, Wada A (1983) 'Molten-globule state': a compact form of globular proteins with mobile side-chains. FEBS Lett 164:21–24.
36. Toda M, Reese G, Gadermaier G, Schulten V, Lauer I, et al. (2011) Protein unfolding strongly modulates the allergenicity and immunogenicity of Pru p 3, the major peach allergen. J Allergy Clin Immunol 128:1022–1030 e1027.
37. Perrocheau L, Bakan B, Boivin P, Marion D (2006) Stability of barley and malt lipid transfer protein 1 (LTP1) toward heating and reducing agents: relationships with the brewing process. J Agric Food Chem 54:3108–3113.
38. Burks AW, Cockrell G, Stanley JS, Helm RM, Bannon GA (1995) Recombinant peanut allergen Ara h I expression and IgE binding in patients with peanut hypersensitivity. J Clin Invest 96:1715–1721.
39. Cabanos C, Urabe H, Tandang-Silvas MR, Utsumi S, Mikami B, et al. (2011) Crystal structure of the major peanut allergen Ara h 1. Mol Immunol 49:115–123.
40. Fukuda T, Maruyama N, Salleh MR, Mikami B, Utsumi S (2008) Characterization and crystallography of recombinant 7S globulins of Adzuki bean and structure-function relationships with 7S globulins of various crops. J Agric Food Chem 56:4145–4153.
41. Cabanos C, Urabe H, Masuda T, Tandang-Silvas MR, Utsumi S, et al. (2010) Crystallization and preliminary X-ray analysis of the major peanut allergen Ara h 1 core region. Acta Crystallogr Sect F Struct Biol Cryst Commun 66:1071–1073.
42. Chruszcz M, Maleki SJ, Majorek KA, Demas M, Bublin M, et al. (2011) Structural and Immunologic Characterization of Ara h 1, a Major Peanut Allergen. J Biol Chem 286:39318–39327.
43. Zhang YZ, Jin T, Guo F, Chen YW, Howard A (2009) Crystal structure of Ara h 3, a major allergen in peanut. Molecular Immunology 46:1796–1804.
44. Kleber-Janke T, Crameri R, Appenzeller U, Schlaak M, Becker WM (1999) Selective cloning of peanut allergens, including profilin and 2S albumins, by phage display technology. Int Arch Allergy Immunol 119:265–274.
45. Rouge P, Culerrier R, Sabatier V, Granier C, Rance F, et al. (2009) Mapping and conformational analysis of IgE-binding epitopic regions on the molecular surface of the major Ara h 3 legumin allergen of peanut (*Arachis hypogaea*). Mol Immunol 46:1067–1075.
46. Lauer I, Foetisch K, Kolarich D, Ballmer-Weber BK, Conti A, et al. (2004) Hazelnut (Corylus avellana) vicilin Cor a 11: molecular characterization of a glycoprotein and its allergenic activity. Biochem J 383:327–334.
47. Beyer K, Grishina G, Bardina L, Grishin A, Sampson HA (2002) Identification of an 11S globulin as a major hazelnut food allergen in hazelnut-induced systemic reactions. J Allergy Clin Immunol 110:517–523.
48. Jin T, Albillos SM, Guo F, Howard A, Fu TJ, et al. (2009) Crystal structure of prunin-1, a major component of the almond (*Prunus dulcis*) allergen amandin. J Agric Food Chem 57:8643–8651.
49. Reese G, Schicktanz S, Lauer I, Randow S, Luttkopf D, et al. (2006) Structural, immunological and functional properties of natural recombinant Pen a 1, the major allergen of Brown Shrimp, *Penaeus aztecus*. Clin Exp Allergy 36:517–524.
50. Whitby FG, Phillips GN Jr. (2000) Crystal structure of tropomyosin at 7 Angstroms resolution. Proteins 38:49–59.
51. Greenfield NJ, Huang YJ, Palm T, Swapna GV, Monleon D, et al. (2001) Solution NMR structure and folding dynamics of the N terminus of a rat non-muscle alpha-tropomyosin in an engineered chimeric protein. J Mol Biol 312:833–847.
52. Mills EN, Mackie AR (2008) The impact of processing on allergenicity of food. Curr Opin Allergy Clin Immunol 8:249–253.

9

Targeting a Cross-Reactive Gly m 5 Soy Peptide as Responsible for Hypersensitivity Reactions in a Milk Allergy Mouse Model

Renata Curciarello[1,5], Paola L. Smaldini[1], Angela M. Candreva[1,5], Virginia González[2], Gustavo Parisi[2], Ana Cauerhff[3], Ivana Barrios[4], Luis Bruno Blanch[4], Carlos A. Fossati[1], Silvana Petruccelli[5]☯, Guillermo H. Docena[1,5]☯*

1 Laboratorio de Investigaciones del Sistema Inmune-LISIN, Departamento de Ciencias Biológicas, Facultad de Ciencias Exactas, Universidad Nacional de La Plata, La Plata, Buenos Aires, Argentina, **2** Centro de Estudios e Investigaciones, Departamento de Ciencias y Tecnología Universidad Nacional de Quilmes, Quilmes, Buenos Aires, Argentina, **3** Centro de Investigación y Desarrollo en Fermentaciones Industriales, CINDEFI (UNLP y CONICET) and Instituto de Investigaciones Bioquímicas de Buenos Aires (IIBBA-CONICET), Fundación Instituto Leloir, Buenos Aires, Argentina, **4** Cátedra de Química Medicinal, Departamento de Ciencias Biológicas, Facultad de Ciencias Exactas, Universidad Nacional de La Plata, La Plata, Buenos Aires, Argentina, **5** Centro de Investigaciones y Desarrollo en Criotecnología de Alimentos-CIDCA, Facultad de Ciencias Exactas, Universidad Nacional de La Plata, La Plata, Buenos Aires, Argentina

Abstract

Background: Cross-reactivity between soybean allergens and bovine caseins has been previously reported. In this study we aimed to map epitopes of the major soybean allergen Gly m 5 that are co-recognized by casein specific antibodies, and to identify a peptide responsible for the cross-reactivity.

Methods: Cow's milk protein (CMP)-specific antibodies were used in different immunoassays (immunoblotting, ELISA, ELISA inhibition test) to evaluate the *in vitro* recognition of soybean proteins (SP). Recombinant Gly m 5 (α), a truncated fragment containing the C-terminal domain (α-T) and peptides of α-T were obtained and epitope mapping was performed with an overlapping peptide assay. Bioinformatics tools were used for epitope prediction by sequence alignment, and for modelling the cross-recognized soy proteins and peptides. The binding of SP to a monoclonal antibody was studied by surface Plasmon resonance (SPR). Finally, the *in vivo* cross-recognition of SP was assessed in a mouse model of milk allergy.

Results: Both α and α-T reacted with the different CMP-specific antibodies. α-T contains IgG and IgE epitopes in several peptides, particularly in the peptide named PA. Besides, we found similar values of association and dissociation constants between the α-casein specific mAb and the different milk and soy components. The food allergy mouse model showed that SP and PA contain the cross-reactive B and T epitopes, which triggered hypersensitivity reactions and a Th2-mediated response on CMP-sensitized mice.

Conclusions: Gly m 5 is a cross-reactive soy allergen and the α-T portion of the molecule contains IgG and IgE immunodominant epitopes, confined to PA, a region with enough conformation to be bound by antibodies. These findings contribute to explain the intolerance to SP observed in IgE-mediated CMA patients, primarily not sensitised to SP, as well as it sets the basis to propose a mucosal immunotherapy for milk allergy using this soy peptide.

Editor: Guillermo H. Giambartolomei, National Council of Sciences (CONICET), Argentina

Funding: This work was supported by the Consejo Nacional de Investigaciones Científicas y Técnicas de Argentina (CONICET) (grant PIP 5475), by Agencia Nacional de Promoción Científica y Tecnológica (grants PICT2007-0049 and PICT 2010-2366 to SP, PICT 2008-2202 to GHD) and by Universidad Nacional de La Plata, Argentina (grants X498 to SP and X455 to CAF). The funders had no role in study design, data collection and analysis, decision to publish, or preparation of the manuscript.

Competing Interests: The authors have declared that no competing interests exist.

* E-mail: guidoc@biol.unlp.edu.ar

☯ These authors contributed equally to this work.

Introduction

Food allergy is an increasing health care concern. Cow's milk protein (CMP) is the leading cause of food allergy in children younger than 3 years in many regions, including our country [1,2]. This is reflected by most of the position papers and guidance with statements and recommendations for food allergy that are focused on CMP allergy (CMA) [3].

If symptoms were relevant and CMA were suspected, a diagnostic dietary elimination of CMP should be initiated for a certain period of time (days to 4 weeks) [4,5]. Once a diagnosis of allergy to milk proteins has been confirmed, it is important to avoid CMP and to ensure a healthy balanced diet that promotes an adequate child growth and development. Depending on the age and other food allergies a restriction or milk free diet is indicated as therapy.

Soy-based formulas have been available for almost 100 years and have been widely used as a milk substitute in children intolerant to cow's milk protein-based formula [6]. However, there are some indications and contraindications of soy formulas since gastrointestinal reactions, including hypersensitivity, have been described for more than 50 years [7], and because of the nutritional quality of soy proteins [8]. More recently, it has been reported that a small proportion of children with IgE and non IgE-mediated milk allergy develop a clinical intolerance to soy-protein-based formula during the restriction treatment, which may be explained by cross-reactivity once milk contamination has been discarded [6,9,10]. We focused our work in investigating the cross-recognition between CMP and soy components. We identified bovine caseins, the main allergens of milk [11,12], and the soybean Gly m 6 G4 as cross-reactive allergens [13–15]. The analysis of a soy variety that naturally lacks the Gly G4 led us to detect that a residual cross-reactivity may lie on Gly m 5.0101, the α subunit of the β-conglycinin. Besides, both seed proteins have been characterized as allergens in patients with IgE-mediated atopic dermatitis [16], food allergy [17,18], asthma [19] and anaphylaxis [20,21]. Therefore, we propose that the clinical intolerance observed in a restricted proportion of milk allergic patients, with documented IgE specific to milk proteins, may be due to the presence of these relevant cross-reactive allergens in soy protein-based formulas.

In this study, we immunochemically and biologically characterized the α subunit of β-conglycinin, and a C-terminal fragment called α-T, containing putative cross-reactive epitopes with bovine caseins. Using bioinformatic, immunochemical and biological tools we demonstrated the presence of B epitopes on this molecule, and we identified a polypeptide that contains critical epitopes for cross-recognition. The results presented here may shed some light to understand the concomitant soy allergy that occurs in infants with IgE-mediated CMA, and not primarily sensitised to soy proteins. However, and more challenging for us, the identification of cross-reactive B and T epitopes would set the basis to propose a soy-based immunotherapy for milk and soy allergies, taking advantage of the lower immunogenicity of soy proteins.

Methods

Protein Extracts

Cow's milk protein extract was prepared from skimmed dry milk (Svelty, Nestle). Proteins were extracted with phosphate saline buffer pH 7.4 (10 mg/ml) and filtered. Soy protein (SP) extract was prepared from *Glycine max.* L merr genotype Asgrow seeds as described previously [14]. Briefly, proteins were extracted from crushed seeds with 0.01N $NaHCO_3$ at 90°C. The extract was centrifuged (2,500×g-20 min at room temperature) and lipids were extracted with chloroform (overnight at 4°C). Finally, the extract was dialyzed against distilled water. The total protein content was quantified with the Bicinchoninic acid kit (Pierce BCA Protein Assay), using bovine serum albumin (BSA) as standard.

Production of the α Subunit of β-conglycinin and α-T Fragment in *Escherichia coli*

The cDNA coding sequence for α (GenBank: X17698) was obtained by PCR amplification of cDNA library from developing *Glycine max* L. Merr. seeds [22]. pET-mα and pET α-T [22] were transformed into *Escherichia coli* strain BL21(DE3) for protein expression of α subunit of β-conglycinin (α) and α-T, its truncated polypeptide containing three alpha helix and one cupin domain typical of the cupin superfamily [23]. Production and purification of the recombinant proteins are described elsewhere [14].

PA and PN Peptide Constructs, Expression and Purification

The oligonucleotide primers used for expression of peptides A and N (PA and PN, amino acids 357–418 and amino acids 438–499 of the pre-pro α subunit, respectively) were: F-pepA (CACCCTGTTTAGTAGAGAGGAAG) and R-pepA (TCACT-TGTTGGAGTAGATGGG), F-pepN (CACCATCTTCCTCA-GTATTGTGG) and R-pepN (TCATTCGGCTCTATATT-TCCGC). Amplified PCR products were cloned directionally into pENTR/D TOPO (Life Technology, S.A. Buenos Aires, Argentina), and then transferred to pDEST destination vector for expression [24]. E. coli BL21 Codon Plus competent cells transformed with the construct "pDEST His-PA" and "pDEST His-PN", were induced for protein expression. Recombinant proteins were purified as described previously [14] and protein concentration was determined by BCA protein assay.

Production of Polyclonal and Monoclonal Antibodies

CMP- and SP-specific polyclonal antisera obtained in rabbit using complete or incomplete Freund's Adjuvant, and a specific α-casein monoclonal antibody (1D5 mAb) were all obtained as described in Docena et al [11]. 1D5 mAb was biotinylated for the SPR biosensor assay. Briefly, 1D5 mAb (1 mg/ml in 0.1M borate buffer, pH 8.8) was incubated with 10 mg/ml solution of N-hidroxisuccinimide-biotin in DMSO (250 μg:1 mg of biotin:mAb ratio) for 4 h at room temperature. The biotinylated mAb was desalted by dialysis against PBS and biotinylation was assessed by ELISA using alkaline phosphatase-conjugated streptavidin (Sigma Aldrich, St Louis, MO). For this assay wells were coated with CMP (1 μg/well), and after blocking, dilutions (1:100 to 1:100,000) of the biotinylated-1D5 mAb were added, followed by the alkaline phosphatase-conjugated streptavidin (1:4,000). Color was developed with *p*-nitrophenylphosphate in buffer pH 9.6, and optical density (OD) at 405 nm was measured in an ELISA reader (Sirio S SAECS, Roma, Italy).

Patient Sera Used for *In Vitro* Characterization of the Allergen Content

Sera obtained from 15 atopic children (ages ranging from 3 months to 10 years, mean age: 4.5 years) with documented IgE-mediated CMA by history, and recruited for other studies, were used. Double blind placebo-controlled food challenge was not done since it is not performed in Argentina for diagnosis. Patients showed clinical pictures of immediate reactions associated to the ingestion of milk or milk-derived products (vomiting, diarrhoea, dermatitis, bronchospasm, urticaria and rhinorrhea). Histories showed no evidence of soybean sensitization. CMP-specific IgE antibodies were detected by immunoblotting, ELISA and EAST (Class 2 or higher) as described previously [12]. Skin prick test with commercial extracts (CMP and common environmental allergens) (Alergo Pharma, Buenos Aires, Argentina) was performed. Histamine (10 μg/ml) and PBS (pH 7.4) were used as positive and negative control, respectively.

Besides, sera from 20 subjects (age- and sex-matched) with no history of food allergy, no clinical manifestations after ingestion of CM, with normal level of serum total IgE according to age, and no specific serum IgE antibodies were used as negative controls.

SDS PAGE and Immunoblotting

SDS-PAGE and immunoblotting were performed as described before [14]. Samples prepared in sample buffer were loaded on gels (10–20 μg/lane for CMP or SP, or 7–10 μg/lane for the recombinant proteins) and electrotransferred onto nitrocellulose membranes. Membranes were probed with the 1D5 mAb (1:1,500 in TBS-Tween 20), cow's milk-specific rabbit polyclonal antiserum (1:1,000 in TBS-Tween 20) for 1 h at 37°C, or with patient sera (1:4 in blocking buffer) overnight at 4°C, as primary antibody, followed by the appropriate conjugated secondary antibody which were: biotinylated goat anti-mouse immunoglobulin G (1:3,000, Chemicon Int., Temecula, CA), biotinylated mouse monoclonal antibodies specific to rabbit immunoglobulins (1:3,000, Sigma-Aldrich, St Louis, MO) and horseradish peroxidase-conjugated avidin (1:4,000, Sigma-Aldrich, St Louis, MO), or horseradish peroxidase-conjugated anti-human IgE antibodies (dilution 1:1,000, Sigma Aldrich, St Louis, MO) for 4 h at 37°C. Protein bands were visualized by enhanced chemiluminescence (ECL Plus, GE Healthcare, Bucks, UK) according to manufacturer's instructions. X-ray-sensitive films (Amersham Hypefilm^{TM} MP, GE Healthcare Limited, Pollarsd Wood, UK) were used and images were acquired with a Hewlett Packard scanner.

Indirect ELISA for IgE Reactivity

Polystyrene microtiter plates (NUNC, Maxisorp, Denmark) were coated with 1.25 μg/well of CMP, 0.05 μg/well of SP or with 0.05 μg/well of α or α-T, in 50 mM carbonate buffer (pH 9.6). Plates were blocked with 5% horse serum in PBS (pH 7.4), and the ELISA was carried out using the patient or negative control sera as primary antibody, as previously described [11,14]. Cut-off values were statistically obtained (SEM+2 SD) from the readings of the negative control sera used.

Sequential Competitive ELISA

ELISA plates were coated overnight with 1 μg/well of CMP and blocked with 5% horse serum in PBS (pH 7.4) for 1 hr at 37°C. CMP-specific rabbit antiserum diluted 1:200,000 in 3% horse serum in PBS (pH 7.4), or α-casein specific mAb diluted 1:300,000 in the same buffer, were mixed (1:1) with different concentrations of inhibitors: CMP, α α-T or bovine serum albumin (BSA) (Sigma Aldrich, St Louis, MO) for 2 h at 37°C. Then 100 μl of this pre-mixed dilution was added in triplicates to the antigen-coated wells and incubated for 30 min at 37°C. Biotinylated mouse monoclonal antibodies specific to rabbit immunoglobulins (1:3,000, Sigma-Aldrich, St Louis, MO) or biotinylated goat anti-mouse immunoglobulin G (1:3,000, Chemicon Int., Temecula, CA) were added for 1 h at 37°C. Finally, horseradish peroxidase-conjugated avidin (1:3,000, Sigma-Aldrich, MO, USA) was added (30 min at 37°C) and color was developed with *o*-phenylenediamine and 30% H_2O_2 in 0.1M citrate-phosphate buffer pH 5.0. Optical density was measured at 492 nm in an ELISA reader. Additionally, 96-well plates were coated with α or α-T (0.1 μg/well) and blocked. CMP-specific polyclonal antiserum diluted 1:6,000 was used in the inhibition mix with same inhibitors. Then, 100 μl of the pre-mixed dilution was added to the coated wells and developed as described above.

Cross-reactive Epitope Mapping on α-T

Overlapping 15-mer peptides, frame shifted by five residues, covering the entire aminoacid sequence of α-T were synthesized on a cellulose membrane (PepSpot JPT Peptide Technologies GMBH, Germany). Spots membrane-based immunoassay was carried out by incubation of the blocked membranes with different primary antibodies (pools of sera containing CMP specific IgE, CMP-specific rabbit polyclonal antiserum or 1D5 mAb), followed by the appropriate secondary antibody. Membranes were developed by chemiluminescence as described above.

Binding Kinetics Analysis Using the BIACORE Assay

Affinity sensor analysis experiments were conducted on an IAsys Plus apparatus (Affinity Sensors, Saxon Hill, Cambridge, U.K.). Streptavidin (Sigma Aldrich, USA) (100 μg/ml in acetate buffer, pH 5.0) was covalently coupled to carboxymethyl dextran sensor chips (Affinity Sensors, Saxon Hill, Cambridge, U.K.) (5 ng of protein per cuvette). Then, a solution of 20 μg/ml in saline buffer of the biotinylated 1D5 mAb (the ligand) was added to the cuvette during 10 minutes, the antibody excess was removed by adding 1M NaCl and 10 mM acetate buffer at pH 4.5. Binding reactions with the ligate were carried out in PBS, 0.05% Tween 20 at 25°C, with constant stirring set up at 90%. Data were collected at intervals of 0.3 sec. Ligate binding to the immobilized ligand was monitored at multiple ligate concentrations, ranging 10-fold below to at least 10-fold above preliminary estimates of equilibrium dissociation constants (K_D) for each reaction. Kinetic and Scatchard analysis were performed by using the FAST FIT software (Affinity Sensors, Saxon Hill, Cambridge, U.K.).

Bioinformatics Analysis

Caseins and subunits of soybean β-conglycinin were compared using bioinformatics tools. The sequences of α (gi:9967357: 543 aa), α′ (gi:15425631: 621 aa) and β (gi: 9967359: 416 aa) subunits of β-conglycinin, and αs1- (gi:162792: 214 aa), αs2- (gi:27806963:222 aa), β- (gi:162931:224 aa) and κ- (gi:1228078: 190 aa) caseins were retrieved from the GenBank database. Several epitope prediction methods available in the B Cell Epitope Prediction Tools at the Immune Epitope Database (IEDB) [25] (http://www.immuneepitope.org) were applied. These methods included Chou & Fasman Beta-Turn Prediction [26], Emini Surface Accessibility Prediction [27], Karplus & Schulz Flexibility Prediction [28], Kolaskar & Tongaonkar Antigenicity [29], and Parker Hydrophilicity Prediction [30]. Peptides identified as putative epitopes based on these predictions were collected in a database. A second database was built using overlapping peptides (15 residues long) of the cow milk and soybean proteins mentioned above. Both databases were aligned with the BLASTP program using parameters fixed to short peptides (Expect Value = 20,000, Score Matrix = PAM30, Word Size = 2, SEG Filter = off) [31] and a shorter region of α located on the α-T segment, containing most amino acid coincidences with bovine caseins epitopes, and named "Peptide A (PA)", was selected. We have used MODELLER [32] to build structural models of α protein based on templates found with FFAS03 fold assignment method [33]. Three-D models were assessed using ProsaII [34] and the PyMOL (http://www.pymol.org) was employed to map α-T and PA on the best 3D models obtained. Calculation of the electrostatic potential surface was made with the web-based graphical user interface PBEQ-Solver [35] and the electrostatic map was visualized in PyMOL.

The hit distribution graph was done to represent those similar amino acid positions shared by soybean α, α-T, and bovine casein peptides. The amino acid sequence of 73 peptides of αS1-, αs2-, β- and κ-casein, described as T and/or B epitopes (IEDB, (http://www.immuneepitope.org/), were aligned with α-T sequence by the ClustalW2 server (http://www.ebi.ac.uk/Tools/msa/clustalw2/). The hits represent the accumulation of consensus amino acid in every position of the sequence analyzed. A score of "3" was assigned for conserved aminoacid (identity), "2" for similar, but not identical amino acids (punctuation over 0.5 on

Gonnet or PAM 250 matrixes), and "1" for slightly similar amino acids (punctuation below 0.5 on Gonnet or PAM 250 matrixes).

Secondary Structure Prediction

Bioinformatics studies described above allowed us to find out that the PA fragment has a primary structure alignment with a fragment of bovine α-casein. Different secondary structure prediction servers and softwares were used to analyze both fragments. Prediction programs belong to the Network Protein Sequence Analysis server [36], which contains SOPM, SOPMA, Hierarchical Neural Network, GOR I, GOR III, GOR IV, DPM, DSC, PHD, PREDATOR, SIMPA 96 and Secondary consensus prediction. Other programs such as CFSSP [37], Jpred [38], JUFO 3D [39], NetSurfP and Multivariate Linear Regression Combination were also used. The final secondary structure prediction was the average of all structures obtained with those prediction programs. Besides, the alignments were performed using the BLAST program.

Mice and Experimental Model of IgE-mediated Food Allergy

Sensitization and Antigenic Challenge. Male 6- to 8-week old Balb/c mice were purchased from the School of Animal Sciences, University of La Plata, and kept under pathogen-free conditions with water and commercial diet provided *ad libitum.* Cow's milk sensitization protocol was carried out as previously described [15]. Briefly, mice received 6 weekly intragastric (ig) doses of CMP (20 mg/dose) plus cholera toxin (10 μg/dose) (Sigma Aldrich, St Louis, MO, USA) in a final volume of 200 μl of bicarbonate buffer (sensitization group), or CMP (20 mg/dose) without cholera toxin (control group). Mice were fasted for 2 h before sensitization, and 3% sodium bicarbonate solution was given 30 min before the immunization. Ten days following the last boost mice were ig challenged with different proteins: 20 mg of CMP, 5 mg of SP or 10 mg of OVA (Sigma-Aldrich, St Louis, MO, USA) as an unrelated antigen. Additionally, some animals were sublingual (sl) challenged with 10 μg of purified proteins [β-lactoglobulin (β-lg), α, α-T, PA or OVA]. Symptoms immediately triggered after the oral challenge were scored in a blinded manner by two independent observers.

In vivo evaluation of the allergic state

Assessment of Clinical Signs. Symptoms were observed 30–60 min following the oral challenge, in a blinded fashion by 2 independent researchers, and scored on a scale from 0 to 5. Some animals received sl 10 μg of recombinant soybean proteins, β-lg (positive control), or OVA (unrelated negative control), and elicited symptoms were scored.

Cutaneous Tests. Mice were shaved on both flanks and subcutaneously injected with 200 μg of CMP, 400 μg of SP, 10 μg of α, α-T or PA in 50 μl of sterile saline in one flank, and 10 μg of saline in the other flank, as a negative control. Mice were also intravenous injected in the tail vein with 100 μl of 0.1% Evans blue dye (Anedra, Buenos Aires, Argentina). The presence of blue color in the skin 15 to 30 min following the injection was considered a positive cutaneous test.

In vitro evaluation of the allergic state

Specific IgE Detection. Serum specific IgE antibodies were measured by EAST using the method described by Ceska et al [40]. Briefly, cyanogen bromide -activated cellulose paper discs were coupled with CMP (1.75 mg/ml), SP (0.5 mg/ml), or the recombinant proteins (0.2 mg/ml). Discs were blocked with 0.5 mM ethanolamine, and incubated overnight at 4°C with 50 μl of undiluted serum samples. Then, the assay was developed as described by Smaldini et al [15].

Specific IgG1 and IgG2a Detection. serum CMP- or SP-specific IgG1 and IgG2a were measured by ELISA as described by Smaldini et al [15]. Briefly, microtitre plates were coated with 1 μg/100 μl of either CMP, SP, α, α-T or PA in carbonate-bicarbonate buffer, pH 9.6. The assay was developed as indicated [15].

Cytokine Response of Antigen-stimulated Splenocytes. 24 h following the oral challenge mice were killed, spleens were removed and cells were isolated. Splenocytes (4×10^6 cells/well) were plated in complete medium (RPMI-1640 supplemented with 10% FBS, 100 U/ml penicillin and 100 mg/ml streptomycin), and stimulated for 72 h with CMP (350 μg/ml), SP (200 μg/ml), ConA (5 μg/ml), α (15 μg/100 μl), α-T (15 μg/100 μl) or PA (15 μg/100 μl). Supernatants were collected, and cytokines were quantified by ELISA: IL-5, IFN-γ (Invitrogen, Invitrogen Corporation, USA).

Ethics Statement

All experimental protocols of this study were conducted in strict agreement with international ethical standards for animal experimentation (Helsinki Declaration and its amendments, Amsterdam Protocol of welfare and animal protection and National Institutes of Health, USA NIH, guidelines: Guide for the Care and Use of Laboratory Animals) and were approved by the local Institutional Animal Care and Use Committee at the School of Animal Science (University of La Plata). Anesthetized mice (intraperitoneal injection of 100 mg/kg ketamine and 5 mg/kg xylacine) were killed by cervical dislocation by experienced research personnel, which performed it humanely and effectively. All efforts were made to alleviate suffering during the whole experiment.

For the human sample analysis a written informed consent was obtained from parents of patients and the project was approved by the Ethics Committee of the Argentinean Association of Allergy and Clinical Immunology (February 2012). Sera were obtained from patients assisted at Hospital San Juan de Dios de La Plata.

Statistical Analysis

All statistical analyses were carried out using GraphPad Prism 5 software. The significance of the difference was determined using an independent-sample t-test or ANOVA test. A p-value<0.05 was regarded as statistically significant.

Results

Beta conglycinin Alpha Subunit and the Polypeptide Fragment α-T are Specifically recognized by Different CMP specific Antibodies

We previously showed that although the soybean variety Raiden lacks the cross-reactive G4 glycinin, a residual cross-reactivity, probably due to the 7S seed globulin α-subunit of β-conglycinin (Gly m 5.0101), was detected [14]. In this work, recombinant Gly m 5.0101 (α) and a 235 amino acid residue polypeptide fragment (~27 kDa) containing the three helix and one cupin domain, α-T, were immunochemically evaluated. Different CMP-specific antibodies were used to assess the cross-reactivity of these soy components (Figure 1). The amount of different coated antigens was adjusted in the indirect ELISA to have the same molar relationship. We found that all sera recognized CMP (100%), while most of the milk allergic patient sera presented IgE antibodies that recognized α (86.6%) and α-T (93.3%) (Figure 1A). The pattern reactivity obtained by immunoblotting revealed that human and rabbit polyclonal sera recognized caseins

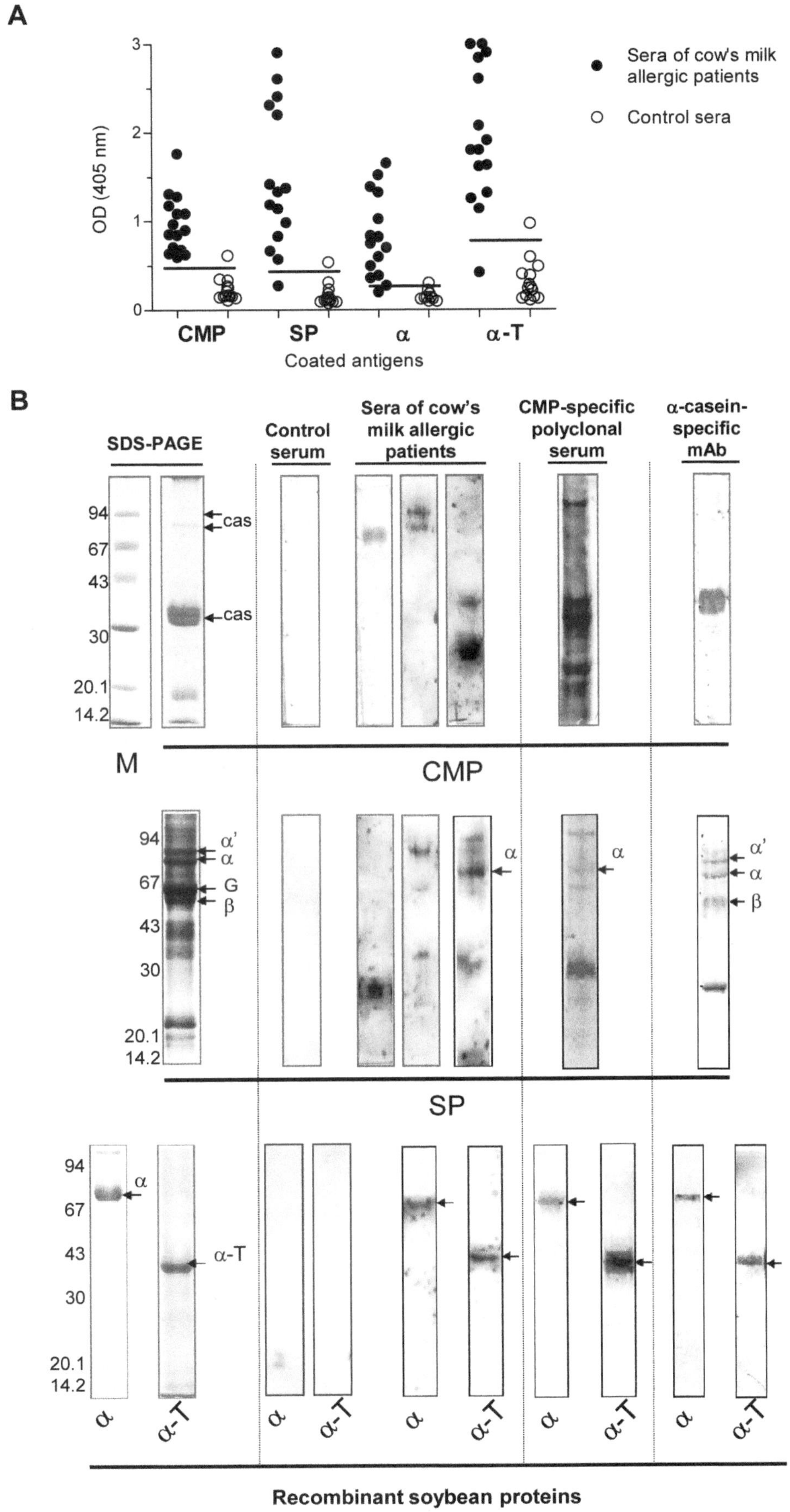
A
OD (405 nm)
3
2
1
0
Sera of cow's milk allergic patients
Control sera
CMP
SP
α
α-T
Coated antigens
B
SDS-PAGE
Control serum
Sera of cow's milk allergic patients
CMP-specific polyclonal serum
α-casein-specific mAb
94
67
43
30
20.1
14.2
cas
cas
M
CMP
α'
α
G
β
SP
α-T
Recombinant soybean proteins

Figure 1. Immunochemical cross-reactivity. A) Detection of specific human serum IgE antibodies by indirect ELISA. Microtiter plates were coated with CMP, SP, recombinant α-subunit of β-conglycinin "α" or α-T, and sequentially incubated with sera of CMA patients and anti-human IgE specific conjugate. 15/15 sera contained IgE antibodies specific for CMP, 13/15 sera contained IgE antibodies specific for α and 14/15 sera contained IgE antibodies for α-T. **B) SDS-PAGE and immunoblotting of CMP and SP.** SDS-PAGE was performed under non reducing conditions for CMP (**upper panel**), SP (**middle panel**), and purified recombinant α and the α-T fraction (**lower panel**). Immunoblottings were developed with patient sera containing milk-specific IgE antibodies or control sera (from non-allergic patients) (1:4), CMP-specific rabbit polyclonal antiserum (1:1,000), and α-casein-specific monoclonal antibody (1D5 mAb 1:1,500). *CMP: Cow's milk protein, cas: caseins, SP: soybean protein, G: 11S glycinin subunits; β-conglycinin subunits are indicated as α, α' and β. M: Molecular masses are given on the left in kilo Daltons (kDa).*

as monomers or aggregates (Figure 1B upper panel), whereas the 1D5 mAb bound α- casein. As it can be seen in the medium panel, these sera recognized soy components of 30 kDa and higher MW, corresponding to α, α′, and β subunit of β-conglycinin. The 30 kDa-band may correspond to the processed polypeptide A5A4B3 of G4 glycinin, previously described as cross-reactive protein [13,14]. The lower panel shows that recombinant α and α-T were recognized by the different milk specific antibodies.

We next investigated the specificity of the antigen-antibody interaction with a sequential competitive ELISA. To enhance the sensitivity and the detection capacity of the assay, the CMP-specific antiserum or the mAb were pre-incubated with different concentrations of soluble inhibitors (reactant proteins). Then, soluble unbound CMP-specific antibodies were allowed to react with the coated antigen. The sigmoid shape of the dose-response curve obtained confirmed the specificity of the Ag-Ab binding (Figure 2). The binding of the CMP-specific polyclonal antiserum to the immobilized CMP was 100% inhibited with 3 mg/ml of soluble CMP, while 50% of inhibition (IC50) was achieved with 0.002 mg/ml CMP and 0.2 mg/ml α (Figure 2A). On the other hand, when any of the recombinant polypeptides was coated to the solid phase, sigmoid curves were obtained with a lower dilution of the polyclonal antiserum (1:6,000), as compared with that used when CMP was coated to the solid phase. This assay rendered an IC50 of 0.1 mg/ml for CMP (Figure 2B). Taken together, and not surprisingly, CMP binding to milk-specific antibodies was more efficiently inhibited with CMP than with soybean components. However, the recombinant soy polypeptides could specifically inhibit the binding of the milk-specific antibodies to the coated homologous antigen. Figure 2C shows the sigmoid curves obtained with the α-casein-specific mAb used in the immunoblottings depicted in figure 1B. More than 95% of inhibition was achieved with a minimum of 0.01 mg/ml CMP as soluble inhibitor, while none of the other proteins could achieve such values at the range of the concentration assessed. The IC50 was 0.0015 mg/ml for CMP, 0.019 mg/ml for α-T and 0.13 mg/ml for α. A non-related control protein (BSA) rendered a constant basal inhibition of less than 10% in all assays (Figures 2A and C).

Kinetic and Equilibrium Constants between α-casein-specific mAb 1D5 and Bovine α-casein and the Recombinant Soybean Proteins

The 1D5 mAb was employed to analyse the kinetic, equilibrium and affinity constants with α-casein and soy components (Table 1). According to the affinity constant (K_A) value of $1.18 \times 10^7\ M^{-1}$ for α-casein we consider that this antibody recognizes with a medium affinity its identity antigen. Interestingly, similar values were found for α and α-T. However, a lower K_A ($4.06 \times 10^6\ M^{-1}$) was measured for PA, which may be due to the smaller size of this fragment, and hence to fewer contacts with the antibody, as compared to α and α-T. Besides, a discrete increase in association constant (k_{ass}) was observed for α as compared with its specific antigen, α-casein. This result may be explained by a different conformation or a different charge on the surface of the epitope in α, which produced more productive contacts with the 1D5 mAb.

Peptides containing Cross-reactive Epitopes were identified in α-T

Once we have detected that α-T contained B epitopes, 24 overlapping 15-mer peptides with 5 amino acid overlaps were synthesized on modified cellulose paper covering the whole sequence of α-T. Spots were probed with different CMP-specific antibodies to identify IgE and IgG cross-recognized zones (Figure 3). We observed similar reactivity patterns with the rabbit polyclonal antiserum and human sera: spots 1, 2 and 9 exhibited strong human IgE binding, while spots 1 and 2 showed a strong reactivity with the rabbit antiserum. We observed a faint reactivity on spots 16 and 22 with the pooled sera, and, on spots 9 and 12 with the rabbit antiserum. Peptides on spots 14 and 23 were only recognized by the rabbit antiserum. On the other hand, the α-casein-specific monoclonal antibody recognized peptides on spots 1, 2, 9, 12, 16 and 22 with high or middle intensity, and, unlike human IgE and rabbit IgG, it also recognized peptides on spots 4, 10 and 14. In summary, 10 peptides along the aminoacidic sequence of α-T were recognized by the different CMP-specific antibodies, indicating that cross-reactivity is not due to a single epitope (spots marked with grey boxes).

Furthermore, we calculated the net charge of the peptides and remarkably we found that reactive peptides are all positive, but peptide 14 (charge −2.2), whereas non reactive peptides are all negatively charged at pH 7.5 (Figure S1 A).

In Silico Analysis showed that Conformational and Linear Epitopes are implicated in Cross-reactivity

In agreement with the epitope mapping of α-T done *in vitro* (Figure 3), sequence alignment analysis in figure 4A and figure S2 showed a high aminoacidic similitude (hits) in those positions where positive spots were obtained in the overlapping assay. High hit values along the α-T sequence where observed around amino acid positions 20 and 40 (region corresponding to positive spots 2 and 4), 77 and 90–100 (spots 9 and 10), 150 (spot 16), and 220 (spots 22 and 23). In figure 4B the sequence of α-T is depicted along with the peptides analyzed in the overlapping assay and the secondary structure predicted with different bioinformatics tools. As it can be observed, the selected PA peptide contains the region with the highest hits (peptides 9, 10 and 12).

The *in silico* predicted secondary structure (Figure 4B) showed that PA contains α-helix and β-sheet conformations. PN peptide was proposed as a control peptide since no secondary structure was predicted in this sequence and it contains low hit regions.

In addition, the amino acid composition was analyzed and we found hydrophilic (serine, asparagine, alanine and lysine) and hydrophobic amino acids (phenylalanine, isoleucine and leucine) as the most frequent amino acids in the different positive peptides in the overlapping assay of α-T. PA contains a compositional bias to hydrophilic amino acids such as glutamic acid (E), serine (S),

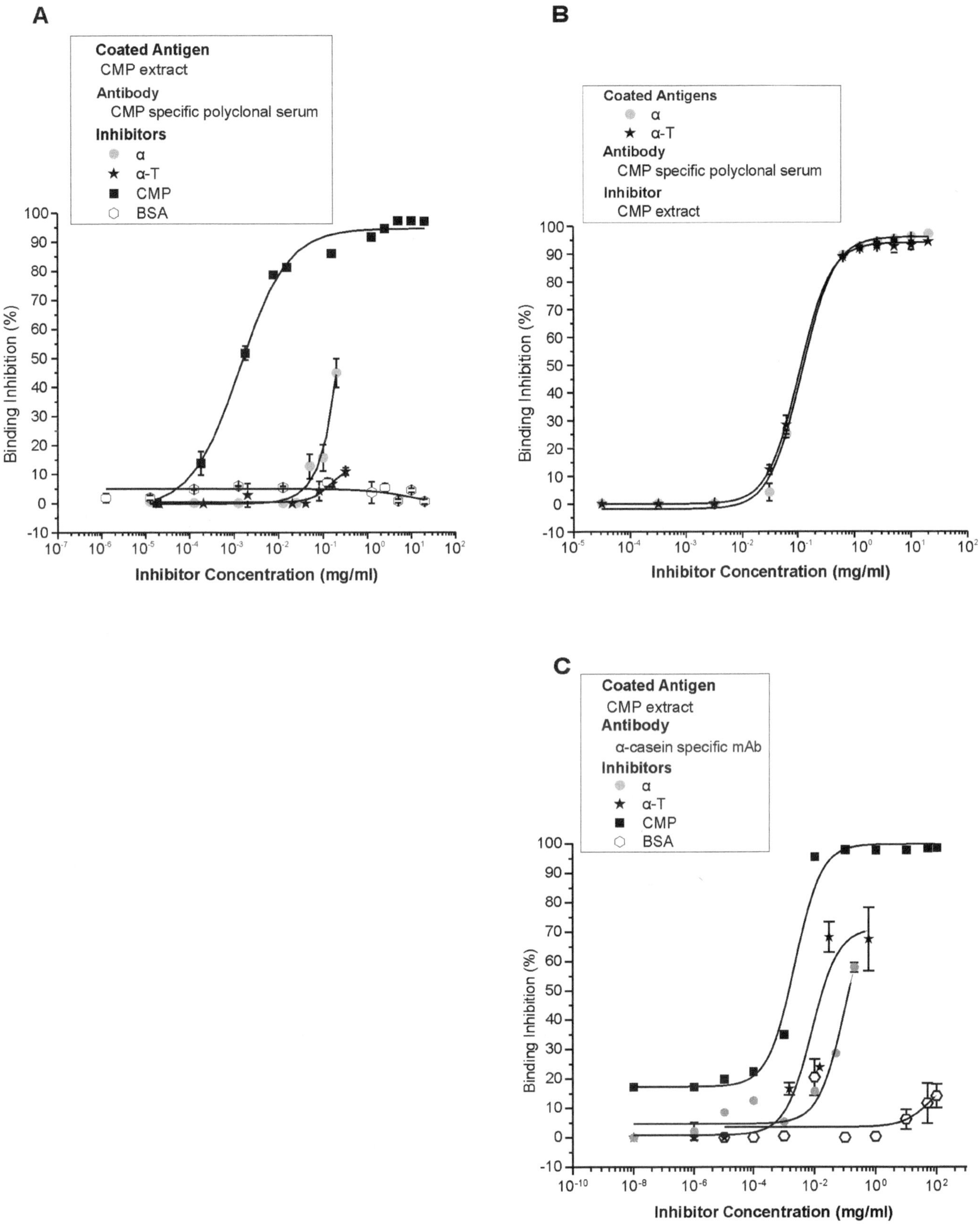

Figure 2. Sequential competitive ELISA with the CMP-specific rabbit polyclonal antiserum and 1D5 mAb. Microtiter plates were coated with CMP (1 μg/well) (**A** and **C**), α (0.1 μg/well) or α-T (0.1 μg/well) (**B**). CMP-specific polyclonal antiserum (**A**: 1:200,000; **B**: 1:6,000) or α-casein-specific mAb (**C**: 1:300,000) were pre-incubated with different inhibitors at several concentrations and then added to Ag-coated wells. Then the appropriate conjugated secondary antibodies were added and the color was developed.

Table 1. Kinetic and equilibrium constants for complexes formed by α-casein, α subunit of β-conglycinin (α), α-T and PA with the 1D5 mAb, specific for α-casein.

	k_{ass} (M^{-1} s^{-1})	k_{diss} (s^{-1})	K_A (M^{-1})	K_D (M^{-1})
Bovine α-casein	$1.05\times10^{4}\pm0.14\times10^{4}$	$8.88\times10^{-4}\pm0.22\times10^{-4}$	$1.18\times10^{7}\pm0.13\times10^{7}$	$8.44\times10^{-8}\pm1.48\times10^{-8}$
α	$1.89\times10^{4}\pm0.18\times10^{4}$	$9.79\times10^{-4}\pm1.47\times10^{-4}$	$1.93\times10^{7}\pm0.22\times10^{7}$	$5.18\times10^{-8}\pm0.60\times10^{-8}$
α-T	$3.14\times10^{4}\pm0.44\times10^{4}$	$2.70\times10^{-3}\pm0.40\times10^{-3}$	$1.16\times10^{7}\pm0.06\times10^{7}$	$8.60\times10^{-8}\pm0.44\times10^{-8}$
PA	$6.92\times10^{3}\pm0,48\times10^{3}$	$1.70\times10^{-3}\pm1.15\times10^{-3}$	$4.06\times10^{6}\pm2.75\times10^{6}$	$2.46\times10^{-7}\pm1.67\times10^{-7}$

k_{ass}: Association constant, k_{diss}: Dissociation constant, K_A: Affinity constant, K_D: Equilibrium Dissociation constant.

lysine (K) and arginine (R) in the α-helix secondary structures (Figure S2).

Since conformational epitopes may be involved in this cross-recognition, homology models of α, α-T and PA were built (Figure 5A). As it can be seen in figure 5A the α-helix and β-sheet conformations are highly critical for the spatial distribution of all components. It became evident that peptides containing the cross-reactive domains are surface exposed and accessible to the solvent (Figure 5B).

The 3D models obtained were built using the structure of the soy α′ subunit of β-conglycinin from soybean (PDB 1UIK), which shows 90% identity with α subunit of β-conglycinin, as derived from fold assignment. The best structural model was evaluated using ProsaII and a Z-score = −7, indicating a high reliability.

According to the peptide reactivity and localization on the surface of the α subunit of β-conglycinin, three putative epitopes can be proposed (Figures 5B I and II). The region 1 would be contained in the PA fragment, while regions 2 and 3 could be structurally close, but on the opposite side of PA in the molecule.

Analyzing the secondary structure of the three immune reactive regions, and taking into account homology modeling results (Modeller) and the superficial residues visualized by PyMol, we found that α-helices, β-strands and connecting loops are relevant for the region 1-containing PA, which includes the positive spots 9, 10 and 12 of the overlapping assay. Instead, region 2 (contains P16, P22 and P23) and region 3 (contains P1, P2 and P4) would be mainly composed of superficial connecting loops. Furthermore, we studied the electrostatic potential on the surface of the three reactive regions using the PBEQ-Solver interface [35] on the web. The surface charge of the region 1 is positive (Figure S1B I) suggesting the predominance of electrostatic interactions with antibodies. On the other hand, the analysis of the electrostatic potential of the accessible solvent surface of region 2 and 3 (located on the opposite side of the molecule) (Figure S1B II) showed different features which may imply different interactions with antibodies. As judge for the electrostatic potential, surface epitopes contained in region 2 may be recognized by antibodies through hydrophobic or non-ionic interactions, while for the region 3 hydrophobic forces may be mainly involved, with a component of electrostatic bonds.

Immunoassays showed the Presence of Linear and Conformational Epitopes on PA

Immunoblotting with different cow's milk-specific antibodies was assessed to validate the cross-reactivity of recombinant PA and PN. The immunoblotting pattern reactivity observed for PA indicates the presence of IgG- and IgE-binding epitopes, whereas PN showed no reactivity (Figure 5C). Elucidation of conformational epitopes involved in the cross-recognition of PA was assessed by dot-blot under different denaturing conditions (Figure 5D). Peptides heated or treated with urea and SDS showed a lower intensity when membranes were revealed with the CMP-specific antibodies (human sera containing IgE, the rabbit polyclonal antiserum and the mAb specific for α-casein), as compared to untreated PA. However, the reactivity observed with the rabbit polyclonal antiserum with DTT- and urea-treated PA led us to speculate that this antiserum also contains milk-specific antibodies capable of recognizing linear IgG epitopes.

In Vivo and *In Vitro* Cross-reactivity of Soybean Components was confirmed with a CMA Murine Model

To further investigate the clinical relevance of the immunochemical cross-reactivity described, orally sensitized Balb/c mice with CMP were challenged with soy proteins (Figure 6A). Signs and symptoms were observed and scored on a scale from 0 to 5 according to the criteria shown in Table 2. We found that milk sensitized mice developed hypersensitivity symptoms immediately following the oral exposure to soy (SP, α, α-T and PA) or milk components (CMP and β-lg) (Figure 6A and B). No symptoms were observed in sensitized mice exposed to OVA, or in sham mice exposed to the different antigens. Remarkably, the sl challenge with individual proteins triggered immediate clinical signs (Figure 6B), thus reflecting the compromise of the mouth mucosa in animals that were intragastrically sensitized. These findings correlated with the high serum specific IgE levels (Figure 6C) and positive skin tests (Figure 6D) found in milk allergic mice injected with α, α-T and PA. Positive skin tests were also obtained with CMP and SP (pictures not shown). In addition, control mice rendered negative skin tests when injected with CMP, SP or soy recombinant components (pictures not showed). Every mice were injected with saline as control in the contra-lateral side and in all cases the reaction was negative (one is showed in Figure 6D). Moreover, Th2-associated IgG1 antibodies that were induced during the sensitization phase with cholera toxin, also recognized the different soy components. Specific IgG2a remained undetectable during the experiment (data not showed), indicating no Th1 induction during the sensitization phase.

Finally, we found an increased secretion of IL-5 by spleen cells stimulated with CMP, SP, α and α-T (Figure 6E). PA showed a slight increase in the production of this Th2-associated cytokine, while IFN-γ remained low, as expected. These findings clearly indicate that CMP-specific T cells elicited during the sensitization phase can be *in vitro* stimulated with soy components.

Discussion

The characterization of the cross-reactivity between milk and soy allergens may shed light on the structural and immunologic

Spot #	Sequence
1	**LITLAIPVNKPGRFE**
2	**IPVNKPGRFE**SFFLS
3	SFFLSSTEAQQSYLQ
4	QSYLQ**GFSRN**ILEAS
5	ILEASYDTKFEEINK
6	EEINKVLFSREEGQQ
7	EEGQQQGEQRLQESV
8	LQESVIVEISKEQIR
9	KEQIR**ALSKRAKSSS**
10	**AKSSSRKTIS**SEDKP
11	SEDKPFNLRSRDPI
12	SRDPI**YSNKL**GKFFE
13	GKFFEITPEKNPQLRD
14	NPQLRD**LDIFL**SIVD
15	LSIVDMNEGALLLPH
16	LLLPH**FNSKA**IVILV
17	IVILVINEGDANIEL
18	ANIELVGLKEQQQEQ
19	QQQEQQQEEQPLEVR
20	PLEVRKYRAELSEQD
21	LSEQDIFVIPAGYPV
22	AGYPV**VVNATSNLNF**
23	**SNLNFFAIGI**NAENN
24	NAENNQRNFL

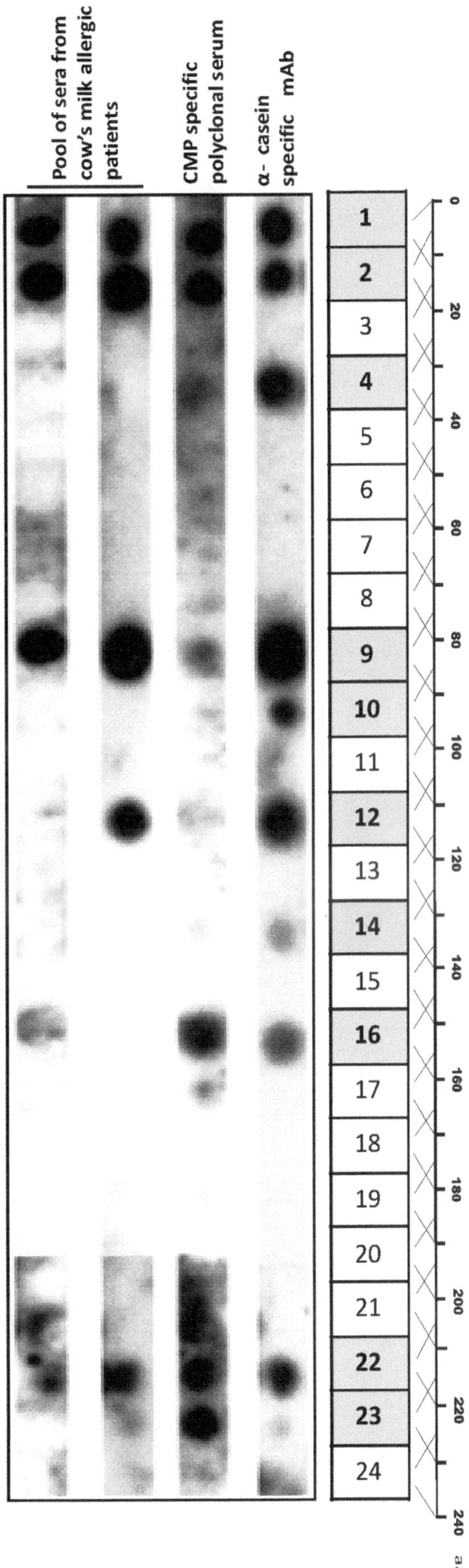

Figure 3. Epitope mapping of α-T. SPOTs array depicting the overlapping 15-aminoacid peptides covering the complete sequence of α-T, and probed with two different pools of serum from cow's milk allergic patients, a rabbit CMP-specific polyclonal serum and the 1D5 α-casein-specific mAb, followed with the appropriate conjugated secondary antibodies. Positive spots are shaded in grey boxes and recognized amino acids are bolded in the sequence depicted for spotted peptides.

relationships between phylogenetically unrelated allergens. Our recent studies show that members of the 11S (Gly m 6) and 7S (Gly m 5) globulin storage soy proteins are cross-reactive allergens with bovine caseins [13–15]. The immunochemical cross-reactivity described has been biologically confirmed using an IgE-mediated mouse model of food allergy with mice exclusively sensitized to CMP [15]. This finding highlights the potential clinical relevance of this phenomenon in allergic patients, although limitations are obvious with conclusions extrapolated from animal models. However, we consider they provide a useful biological tool when ethics is concerning, and in situations in which co-sensitization in patients is almost impossible to disprove. There are some studies reporting the occurrence of clinical intolerance to soy-based formula in milk allergic patients without previous sensitization to soy allergens [9,10]. Although they show that it occurs in a small proportion of patients (<15%), this intolerance is a clinical common concern in our population. Milk allergic patients may develop hypersensitivity reactions following accidental exposure to soy after the ingestion of soy-containing foods, or during the restrictive treatment with soy-based formula.

In this study, we have focused on investigating shared B and T epitopes of Gly m 5 with bovine caseins, which are relevant allergens of soy and milk respectively [11,20]. Of note, the soy recombinant components were recognized as soluble antigens by a rabbit CMP-specific polyclonal antiserum and the α-casein specific monoclonal antibody in a competitive ELISA. These findings discard the possibility of neo epitopes created during the coating of antigens to the solid phase as responsible for this cross-reactivity

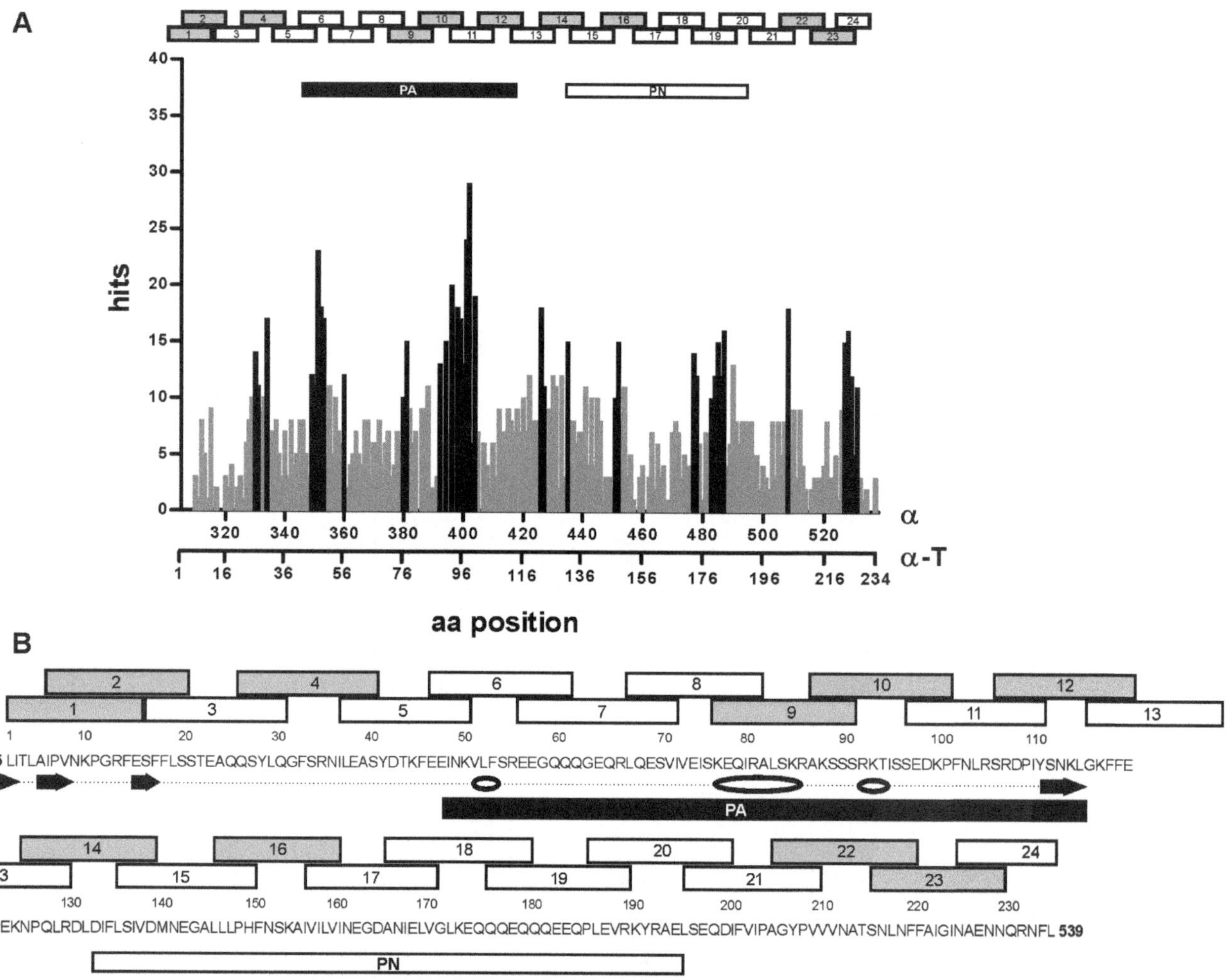

Figure 4. Schematic localization of the identified spots along the α-T sequence and sequence alignment analysis. A) Analysis of the sequence alignment of α-T with IgE epitopes in bovine caseins (IEDB) shown as hit distribution of amino acid similitude per position along the sequence of α-T. Positions of α-T with high hit values (black columns) correlate with positive spots of the overlapping assay (spots 9, 10 and12); **B**) The sequence of α-T (1–234 aa) is depicted along with overlapped peptides, PA and PN (305–539 aa correspond to α). *In silico* predicted alpha-helix (white ovals) and beta-sheet (black arrows) zones are indicated. PA contains the amino acid positions with the highest hits and the α-helix and β strand secondary structures.

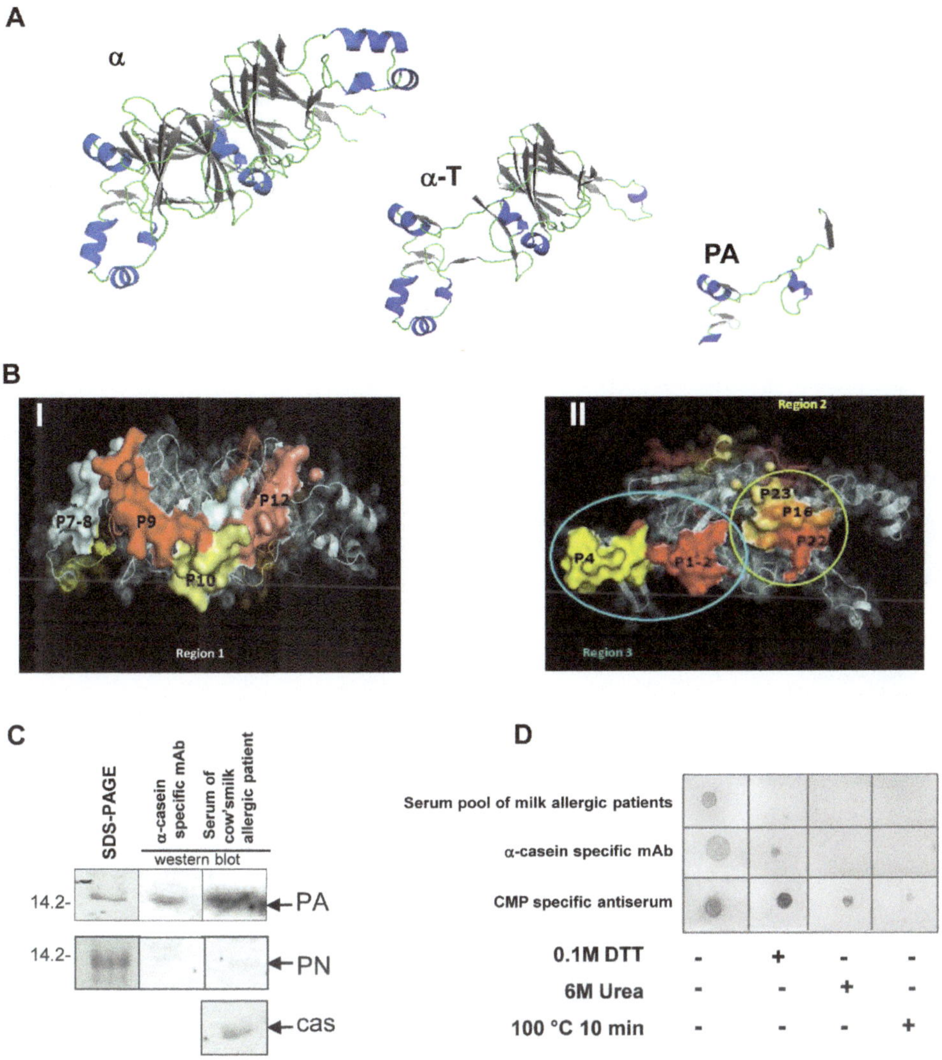

Figure 5. ***In silico* and *in vitro* analysis of α, α-T and PA. A**) Homology model obtained using the Modeller and visualized by PyMOL of α-subunit of β-conglycinin, α-T and PA, based on NCBI Conserved Domain Search results with α′ subunit as template (α-helices are shown in blue and β-sheets as dark grey arrows on the structure). **B**) Surface representation of positive overlapped peptides marked in different colors according to the intensity of the reaction (from pale yellow to red); I and II correspond to opposite sides of the α molecule. Positive peptides localized on the surface of the molecule seem to converge in three regions or putative epitopes. The remaining part of the molecule is represented in transparent spheres showing the secondary structure. **C**) SDS-PAGE of recombinant PA and PN and immunoblotting developed with 1D5 α-casein-specific mAb and a representative serum of CMA patients. Alpha-s1 casein was used as positive control (Molecular masses are shown on the left as kDa). **D**) Dot-blot of recombinant treated and untreated PA revealed with a pool of CMA patient sera, α-casein-specific mAb and CMP-specific polyclonal rabbit antiserum. Denaturing conditions consisted on: 0.1M DTT solution, 6M urea or 100°C for 10 minutes. *Cas: Alpha-s1 casein.*

and confirm that α and α-T contain cross-reactive B epitopes. This assay rendered a higher IC50 for α than that for CMP with the polyclonal and monoclonal antibodies (150 and 86 times respectively), which is reasonable since these antibodies are primary specific for milk components. These results and the shape of the dose-response curves indicate that the antigen-antibody interaction is specific, that the α protein and its fraction α-T bear cross-reactive epitopes with bovine α-casein, and that a restricted population of CMP-specific antibodies specifically recognized B epitopes in α and α-T polypeptides. These findings were further characterized with the biosensor binding assay, which showed that α-casein, α and α-T present similar affinity constant to the α-casein-specific mAb. The higher k_{ass} value found for α-T as compared with that for α and α-casein can be due to stronger favourable contacts in the interface formed between mAb 1D5 and α-T. However, the k_{diss} value means that this complex is more unstable than those formed with α and α-casein. Likewise, the smaller k_{ass} value found for PA as compared to the other components analyzed can be explained by lower contacts with 1D5, which may be due to its smaller size and conformational changes. As expected, we found medium affinities for this monoclonal antibody with different cross-reactive antigens, which may reflect an overall approach to understand the cross-reactivity implicated in a hypersensitivity reaction. Recently, and using synthetic allergens, it has been shown that IgE antibodies do not necessarily need to have a high affinity with its specific antigen to trigger mast cell degranulation [41]. In this study we have shown that even a 64 amino acid residue peptide of moderate affinity triggers a specific allergic response in milk allergic mice, thus indicating that it can activate sensitized cells.

To gain more insight into the molecular feature of this cross-reactivity we next characterized B epitopes (IgG and IgE) on

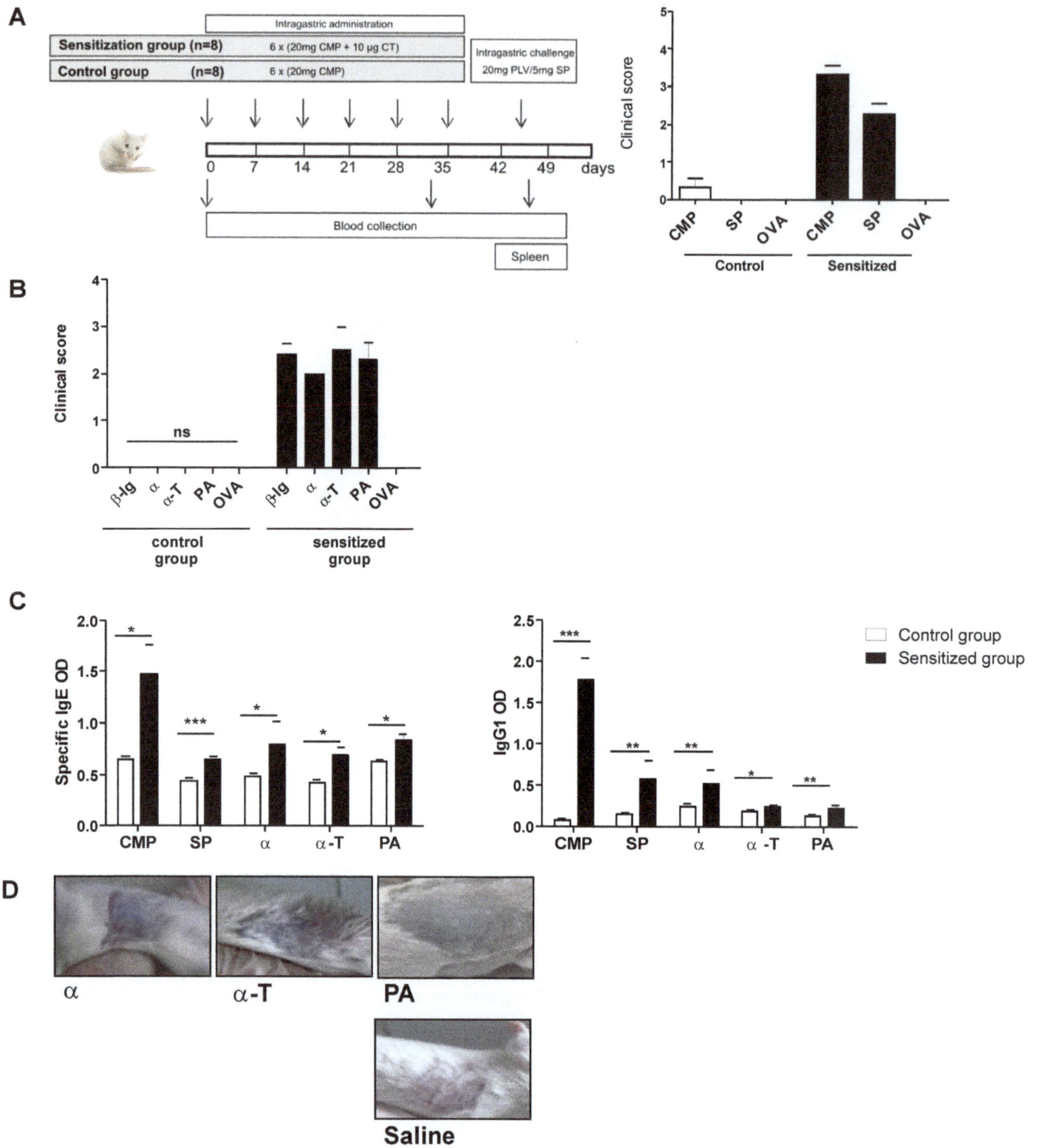
A
Intragastric administration
Sensitization group (n=8)
6 x (20mg CMP + 10 µg CT)
Control group (n=8)
6 x (20mg CMP)
Intragastric challenge
20mg PLV/5mg SP
0 7 14 21 28 35 42 49 days
Blood collection
Spleen
Clinical score
CMP SP OVA CMP SP OVA
Control
Sensitized
B
Clinical score
ns
β-lg α α-T PA OVA β-lg α α-T PA OVA
control group
sensitized group
C
Specific IgE OD
IgG1 OD
CMP SP α α-T PA
Control group
Sensitized group
D
α
α-T
PA
Saline
E
IL-5 pg ml -1
p=0.058
IFN γ pg ml -1
CMP SP α α-T PA
Control group
Sensitized group

Figure 6. *In vivo* cross-reactivity assessed in a food allergy mouse model. A) Schematic representation of the experimental protocol: BALB/c mice were subjected to weekly intragastric sensitization with cholera toxin and CMP from day 0 through day 35. Challenge was performed at day 45 by ig administration of proteins (CMP, SP or OVA). Control mice only received CMP and then they were challenged with the different antigens. Symptoms were observed 30 min following the oral challenge and scored according to Table 2. **B**) Clinical scores assigned to symptoms observed 30 min following the sublingual challenge with 10 μg of β-lg, α, α-T, PA or OVA. **C**) Specific IgE and IgG1 in serum of milk-sensitized and control mice were assessed by EAST or indirect ELISA at day 45, respectively (mean values ± SEM). **D**) Cutaneous test performed in sensitized mice subcutaneously injected with 10 μg of antigens (α, α-T or PA) in the right flank and with saline in the left flank. The presence of blue color in the skin within minutes was considered a positive cutaneous test. **E**) Levels of IL-5 and IFN-γ assayed on stimulated splenocyte supernatants by ELISA (mean values ± SEM). Results correspond to a single experiment with five mice per condition, representative of three separate experiments that gave similar results. Statistically significant differences are denoted as starred values (*) ***$p<0.005$, **$p<0.01$, *$p<0.05$.

different peptides of α (α-T and PA) using overlapping synthetic peptides, recombinant allergenic fragments and unfolded fragments. Besides, the overlapped peptide scanning revealed that cross-reactivity is not due to a unique shared epitope. The overlapping peptide assay showed that the epitope-bearing 15-mer peptides contain 33.8% of hydrophobic (A: alanine, F: phenylalanine and L: leucine), 29% of neutral hydrophilic (S: serine and N: asparagine) and 9.6% of charged hydrophilic aminoacids (K: lysine, E: glutamic acid) with a positive net charge, suggesting that different ways of antibody-antigen recognition may be possible in this type of cross-reactivity (Figure S1). Since the combining site of an antibody may present different zones with different charges, and furthermore, different conformers of the paratope can be found in unbound antibodies exhibiting different surfaces of interaction with antigens in this regard, a single antibody can interact with different epitopes even on the same antigen. In the particular case of the PA, which is mainly positively charged, the interactions with antibodies are expected to be electrostatic with a net negatively charged paratope. Regarding epitopes present in the region 2, the type of interactions are mainly hydrophobic, but analyzing epitopes in the region 3 those interaction could be a combination of hydrophobic and electrostatic ones. Thus, the studied cross-reactivity implies a more complex interpretation than just considering the presence of a unique and shared epitope.

The *in silico* analysis for prediction of cross-reactive epitopes, secondary structure and modeling of Gly m 5 indicated that PA contains cross-recognized conformational and linear epitopes that are exposed on the surface of the allergen to interact with antibodies. Then, IgG and IgE cross-reactive epitopes were confirmed in PA using different milk-specific antibodies and immunoassays. It has been described that the feature of the epitope in caseins is critical for the history of milk allergy in allergic patients [42–44], and the recognition of conformational epitopes is a predictive factor for a later acquisition of tolerance to CMP. Therefore, monitoring the reactivity of serum antibodies against PA might constitute an additional prognostic tool for achievement of immune tolerance in patients. Although the disruption of dominant epitopes in PA using chaotropic agents provided preliminary data, further investigations with structural biology techniques such as X-ray crystallography and nuclear magnetic resonance are necessary to visualize these conformational cross-reactive epitopes. In this sense, the combination of different mapping techniques with the visualization of the 3D models is needed to assess the structural integrity of allergens. Food antigens, which have mainly linear epitopes following food processing or digestion, also contain conformational epitopes that can be affected by food processing, thus interfering with the conformation, IgE binding activity and hence the allergenicity.

The use of different sequence databases of caseins allergenic epitopes provided no information of shared sequences with the soy component studied here. However, the sequence database obtained by us, using the describe techniques above, provided of several peptides of α-subunit of β-conglycinin that presented homology with milk caseins and their cross-reactivity was *in vitro* confirmed. Therefore, based on *in silico* and experimental data we have selected a peptide from the sequence of α-T (PA) that matched the identified IgE-binding epitopes in caseins [42,45,46]. Fu et al [47] identified IgG sequential and solvent-exposed epitopes (185–231) in the N-terminus domain of the α-subunit of the β-conglycinin, which is not coincident with the epitope here described in the C-terminus domain. Therefore this peptide of Gly m 5 represents a new IgE-binding epitope that occurs in a conformational region of the protein exposed to the solvent.

In this study, the combination of bioinformatics tools for prediction of epitopes, secondary structure, surface electrostatic charge, sequence alignment, molecular modeling and visualization of immunodominant regions in 3D modeled molecules, with immunochemical techniques (immunoblotting, indirect ELISA and competitive ELISA), SPR biosensor and *in vivo* experiments, allowed us to strongly demonstrate the existence of cross-reactivity between Gly m 5 and caseins. Besides, we have selected a candidate peptide that contains linear and conformational B, and T epitopes, which could be easily rendered hypoallergenic for a potential and safe therapeutic treatment.

The clinical symptoms elicited after the sublingual challenge with α, α-T and PA, and the positive skin prick tests confirmed the presence of at least two IgE-binding epitopes on the Gly m 5.0101 soy fractions. Of note, the presence of linear T epitopes could be evidenced when

Table 2. Clinical scores assigned to symptoms triggered following the oral or sublingual challenge.

Score	Symptoms
0	No symptoms
1	Scratching and rubbing around the snout and head
2	Puffiness around the eyes and mouth, pilar-erecti, diarrhea, reduced activity and/or decreased activity with increased respiratory rate
3	Respiratory distress, cyanosis around snout and tail
4	No activity upon stimuli, convulsion
5	Death

spleen cells were stimulated with these fractions, with the secretion of IL-5. The ability of α, α-T and mainly PA for T cell activation encourage us to propose them in a potential mucosal therapy for tolerance induction in patients with milk and/or soy allergy.

As a conclusion, using *in vitro*, *in vivo* and *in silico* approaches we have identified a peptide of Gly m 5 that contains B and T cross-reactive epitopes with bovine casein. This information sheds light on the characterization of this relevant soybean allergen, and may provide a molecular explanation for the complex IgE cross-reactivity between the phylogenetically unrelated milk and soy allergens. This phenomenon may explain the secondary soy allergy elicited during the treatment of some cow's milk allergic patients. Finally, this knowledge may be exploited to develop a mucosal tolerizing immunotherapy using PA for intervention in soy and milk allergy.

Supporting Information

Figure S1 Electrostatic and charge analysis of α-T. **A**) pI and charge at pH = 7.5 for peptides of the overlapping assay estimated with the Protein Calculator v3.3 (http://www.scripps.edu/~cdputnam/protcalc.html). **B**) Electrostatic potential surface on the α subunit of β-conglycinin showing **I**) region 1, which contains the PA fragment, and **II**) regions 2 and 3. Note that the region 1 is mostly positively charged, region 2 is mostly hydrophobic and region 3 is hydrophobic and slightly positively charged.
(TIF)

Figure S2 Multiple sequence alignment between sequences of α-T and epitopes on bovine casein peptides. A total of 73 peptides of α-S1 (1–55), α-S2 (56–63), β (64–67) and κ (68–73) bovine caseins, described as T and/or B epitopes (IEDB, (http://www.immuneepitope.org/) were aligned with α-T sequence using the ClustalW2 server (http://www.ebi.ac.uk/Tools/msa/clustalw2/). Common amino acids are shaded in red on casein peptide sequences, or in grey in the α-T sequence. Blue rectangles delimit the highest frequencies of similitude observed (which correspond to the high hit values in Figure 4 A). Green and yellow boxes underneath the α-T sequence correspond to PA and PN respectively.
(TIF)

Acknowledgments

GP, AC, CAF, SP and GHD are scientists' members of the CONICET; AMC is a post-doctoral fellow of CONICET.

Author Contributions

Conceived and designed the experiments: AC LBB GP AMC RC PLS SP GHD. Performed the experiments: RC AMC PLS AC IB VG. Analyzed the data: RC AMC PLS VG GP AC SP GHD. Contributed reagents/materials/analysis tools: CAF LBB AC GP SP GHD. Wrote the paper: RC SP AC GHD. Performed bioinfomatic analysis: VG GP AC SP AMC RC.

References

1. Rona RJ, Keil T, Summers C, Gislason D, Zuidmeer L, et al. (2007) The prevalence of food allergy: a meta-analysis. J Allergy Clin Immunol 120: 638–646. doi:10.1016/j.jaci.2007.05.026.
2. Sicherer SH (2011) Food allergy. Mt Sinai J Med New York 78: 683–696. doi:10.1002/msj.20292.
3. Fiocchi A, Brozek J, Schünemann H, Bahna SL, von Berg A, et al. (2010) World Allergy Organization (WAO) Diagnosis and Rationale for Action against Cow's Milk Allergy (DRACMA) Guidelines. World Allergy Organ J 3: 57–161. doi:10.1097/WOX.0b013e3181defeb9.
4. Koletzko S, Niggemann B, Arato A, Dias JA, Heuschkel R, et al. (2012) Diagnostic approach and management of cow's-milk protein allergy in infants and children: ESPGHAN GI Committee practical guidelines. J Pediatr Gastroenterol Nutr 55: 221–229. doi:10.1097/MPG.0b013e31825c9482.
5. Dupont C (2011) Food allergy: recent advances in pathophysiology and diagnosis. Ann Nutr Metab 59 Suppl 1: 8–18. doi:10.1159/000334145.
6. Bhatia J, Greer F (2008) Use of soy protein-based formulas in infant feeding. Pediatrics 121: 1062–1068. doi:10.1542/peds.2008-0564.
7. COOK CD (1960) Probable gastrointestinal reaction to soybean. N Engl J Med 263: 1076–1077. doi:10.1056/NEJM196011242632109.
8. Agostoni C, Axelsson I, Goulet O, Koletzko B, Michaelsen KF, et al. (2006) Soy protein infant formulae and follow-on formulae: a commentary by the ESPGHAN Committee on Nutrition. J Pediatr Gastroenterol Nutr 42: 352–361. doi:10.1097/01.mpg.0000189358.38427.cd.
9. Zeiger RS, Sampson HA, Bock SA, Burks AW Jr, Harden K, et al. (1999) Soy allergy in infants and children with IgE-associated cow's milk allergy. J Pediatr 134: 614–622.
10. Klemola T, Vanto T, Juntunen-Backman K, Kalimo K, Korpela R, et al. (2002) Allergy to soy formula and to extensively hydrolyzed whey formula in infants with cow's milk allergy: a prospective, randomized study with a follow-up to the age of 2 years. J Pediatr 140: 219–224. doi:10.1067/mpd.2002.121935.
11. Docena GH, Fernandez R, Chirdo FG, Fossati CA (1996) Identification of casein as the major allergenic and antigenic protein of cow's milk. Allergy 51: 412–416.
12. Docena G, Rozenfeld P, Fernández R, Fossati CA (2002) Evaluation of the residual antigenicity and allergenicity of cow's milk substitutes by in vitro tests. Allergy 57: 83–91.
13. Rozenfeld P, Docena GH, Añón MC, Fossati CA (2002) Detection and identification of a soy protein component that cross-reacts with caseins from cow's milk. Clin Exp Immunol 130: 49–58.
14. Curciarello R, Lareu JF, Fossati CA, Docena GH, Petruccelli S (2008) Immunochemical characterization of Glycine max L. Merr. var Raiden, as a possible hypoallergenic substitute for cow's milk-allergic patients. Clin Exp Allergy J Br Soc Allergy Clin Immunol 38: 1559–1565. doi:10.1111/j.1365-2222.2008.03062.x.
15. Smaldini P, Curciarello R, Candreva A, Rey MA, Fossati CA, et al. (2012) In vivo evidence of cross-reactivity between cow's milk and soybean proteins in a mouse model of food allergy. Int Arch Allergy Immunol 158: 335–346. doi:10.1159/000333562.
16. Ogawa T, Bando N, Tsuji H, Nishikawa K, Kitamura K (1995) Alpha-subunit of beta-conglycinin, an allergenic protein recognized by IgE antibodies of soybean-sensitive patients with atopic dermatitis. Biosci Biotechnol Biochem 59: 831–833.
17. Ballmer-Weber BK, Holzhauser T, Scibilia J, Mittag D, Zisa G, et al. (2007) Clinical characteristics of soybean allergy in Europe: a double-blind, placebo-controlled food challenge study. J Allergy Clin Immunol 119: 1489–1496. doi:10.1016/j.jaci.2007.01.049.
18. Krishnan HB, Kim W-S, Jang S, Kerley MS (2009) All three subunits of soybean beta-conglycinin are potential food allergens. J Agric Food Chem 57: 938–943. doi:10.1021/jf802451g.
19. Codina R, Ardusso L, Lockey RF, Crisci CD, Jaén C, et al. (2002) Identification of the soybean hull allergens involved in sensitization to soybean dust in a rural population from Argentina and N-terminal sequence of a major 50 KD allergen. Clin Exp Allergy J Br Soc Allergy Clin Immunol 32: 1059–1063.
20. Holzhauser T, Wackermann O, Ballmer-Weber BK, Bindslev-Jensen C, Scibilia J, et al. (2009) Soybean (Glycine max) allergy in Europe: Gly m 5 (beta-conglycinin) and Gly m 6 (glycinin) are potential diagnostic markers for severe allergic reactions to soy. J Allergy Clin Immunol 123: 452–458. doi:10.1016/j.jaci.2008.09.034.
21. Ogawa A, Samoto M, Takahashi K (2000) Soybean allergens and hypoallergenic soybean products. J Nutr Sci Vitaminol (Tokyo) 46: 271–279.
22. Petruccelli S, Chirdo FG, Añón MC (n.d.) Immunochemical reactivity of soybean b-conglycinin subunits. Food Agric Immunol 16: 17–28.
23. Mills EN, Jenkins J, Marigheto N, Belton PS, Gunning AP, et al. (2002) Allergens of the cupin superfamily. Biochem Soc Trans 30: 925–929. doi:10.1042/.
24. Nallamsetty S, Austin BP, Penrose KJ, Waugh DS (2005) Gateway vectors for the production of combinatorially-tagged His6-MBP fusion proteins in the cytoplasm and periplasm of Escherichia coli. Protein Sci Publ Protein Soc 14: 2964–2971. doi:10.1110/ps.051718605.
25. Peters B, Sidney J, Bourne P, Bui H-H, Buus S, et al. (2005) The immune epitope database and analysis resource: from vision to blueprint. PLoS Biol 3: e91. doi:10.1371/journal.pbio.0030091.
26. Chou PY, Fasman GD (1978) Prediction of the secondary structure of proteins from their amino acid sequence. Adv Enzymol Relat Areas Mol Biol 47: 45–148.
27. Emini EA, Hughes JV, Perlow DS, Boger J (1985) Induction of hepatitis A virus-neutralizing antibody by a virus-specific synthetic peptide. J Virol 55: 836–839.
28. Karplus PA, Schulz GE (1985) Prediction of chain flexibility in proteins. Naturwissenschaften 72: 212–213.
29. Kolaskar AS, Tongaonkar PC (1990) A semi-empirical method for prediction of antigenic determinants on protein antigens. FEBS Lett 276: 172–174.
30. Parker JM, Guo D, Hodges RS (1986) New hydrophilicity scale derived from high-performance liquid chromatography peptide retention data: correlation of

predicted surface residues with antigenicity and X-ray-derived accessible sites. Biochemistry (Mosc) 25: 5425–5432.
31. Altschul SF, Madden TL, Schäffer AA, Zhang J, Zhang Z, et al. (1997) Gapped BLAST and PSI-BLAST: a new generation of protein database search programs. Nucleic Acids Res 25: 3389–3402.
32. Marti-Renom MA, Madhusudhan MS, Fiser A, Rost B, Sali A (2002) Reliability of assessment of protein structure prediction methods. Struct Lond Engl 1993 10: 435–440.
33. Jaroszewski L, Rychlewski L, Li Z, Li W, Godzik A (2005) FFAS03: a server for profile–profile sequence alignments. Nucleic Acids Res 33: W284–288. doi:10.1093/nar/gki418.
34. Wiederstein M, Sippl MJ (2007) ProSA-web: interactive web service for the recognition of errors in three-dimensional structures of proteins. Nucleic Acids Res 35: W407–410. doi:10.1093/nar/gkm290.
35. Jo S, Vargyas M, Vasko-Szedlar J, Roux B, Im W (2008) PBEQ-Solver for online visualization of electrostatic potential of biomolecules. Nucleic Acids Res 36: W270–275. doi:10.1093/nar/gkn314.
36. Combet C, Blanchet C, Geourjon C, Deléage G (2000) NPS@: network protein sequence analysis. Trends Biochem Sci 25: 147–150.
37. Chou PY, Fasman GD (1974) Prediction of protein conformation. Biochemistry (Mosc) 13: 222–245.
38. Cole C, Barber JD, Barton GJ (2008) The Jpred 3 secondary structure prediction server. Nucleic Acids Res 36: W197–201. doi:10.1093/nar/gkn238.
39. Jones DT (1999) Protein secondary structure prediction based on position-specific scoring matrices. J Mol Biol 292: 195–202. doi:10.1006/jmbi.1999.3091.
40. Ceska M (1981) Radioimmunoassay of IgE using paper disks. Methods Enzymol 73: 646–656.
41. Handlogten MW, Kiziltepe T, Alves NJ, Bilgicer B (2012) Synthetic allergen design reveals the significance of moderate affinity epitopes in mast cell degranulation. ACS Chem Biol 7: 1796–1801. doi:10.1021/cb300193f.
42. Chatchatee P, Järvinen KM, Bardina L, Vila L, Beyer K, et al. (2001) Identification of IgE and IgG binding epitopes on beta- and kappa-casein in cow's milk allergic patients. Clin Exp Allergy J Br Soc Allergy Clin Immunol 31: 1256–1262.
43. Chatchatee P, Järvinen KM, Bardina L, Beyer K, Sampson HA (2001) Identification of IgE- and IgG-binding epitopes on alpha(s1)-casein: differences in patients with persistent and transient cow's milk allergy. J Allergy Clin Immunol 107: 379–383. doi:10.1067/mai.2001.112372.
44. Vila L, Beyer K, Järvinen KM, Chatchatee P, Bardina L, et al. (2001) Role of conformational and linear epitopes in the achievement of tolerance in cow's milk allergy. Clin Exp Allergy J Br Soc Allergy Clin Immunol 31: 1599–1606.
45. Cerecedo I, Zamora J, Shreffler WG, Lin J, Bardina L, et al. (2008) Mapping of the IgE and IgG4 sequential epitopes of milk allergens with a peptide microarray-based immunoassay. J Allergy Clin Immunol 122: 589–594. doi:10.1016/j.jaci.2008.06.040.
46. Cocco RR, Järvinen K-M, Sampson HA, Beyer K (2003) Mutational analysis of major, sequential IgE-binding epitopes in alpha s1-casein, a major cow's milk allergen. J Allergy Clin Immunol 112: 433–437.
47. Fu CJ, Jez JM, Kerley MS, Allee GL, Krishnan HB (2007) Identification, characterization, epitope mapping, and three-dimensional modeling of the alpha-subunit of beta-conglycinin of soybean, a potential allergen for young pigs. J Agric Food Chem 55: 4014–4020. doi:10.1021/jf070211o.

10

Purification and Immunobiochemical Characterization of a 31 kDa Cross-Reactive Allergen from *Phaseolus vulgaris* (Kidney Bean)

Ramkrashan Kasera[1,2], Anand Bahadur Singh[1], Shakuntala Lavasa[3], Komarla Nagendra[4], Naveen Arora[1,2]*

1 Allergy and Immunology Section, CSIR-Institute of Genomics and Integrative Biology, Delhi, India, **2** University of Pune, Ganeshkhind, Pune, India, **3** USLavasa Medical and Research Center, Chandigarh, India, **4** Bengaluru Allergy Centre, Bangalore, India

Abstract

Background: Legumes are a rich source of proteins but are also potential elicitors of IgE-mediated food allergy. This study aimed to isolate and characterize a major allergen of *Phaseolus vulgaris* (kidney bean) and determine its allergenicity.

Methodology: Kidney bean allergen was purified using Q Sepharose column (anion exchanger) and eluates with high intensity were pooled to purify protein using Superdex 75 (gel filtration) and C_{18} column (RP-HPLC). Patients with history of kidney bean allergy were skin prick tested (SPT) with crude kidney bean extract and the purified protein. Specific IgE was estimated in sera by enzyme-linked immunosorbent assay (ELISA). Characterization of purified protein and its cross-reactivity was investigated by immunobiochemical methods. Identification of purified protein was carried out by tandem mass spectrometry.

Principal Findings: Purified protein appeared as a single band at 31 kDa on SDS-PAGE and showed IgE binding to 88% patients' sera by ELISA and immunoblotting. SPT with purified protein identified 78% hypersensitive patients of kidney bean. Significant release of histamine from sensitized basophils was observed after challenge with purified protein. PAS staining suggested it to be a glycoprotein, but no change in IgE binding was observed after periodate oxidation. The 31 kDa protein remained stable for 60 min on incubation with pepsin. The purified protein had high allergenic potential since it required only 102 ng of self protein for 50% IgE inhibition. Mass spectrometric analysis identified it as Phytohemagglutinin. It also showed hemagglutination with human RBCs. Cross-reactivity was observed with peanut and black gram with IC_{50} of 185 and 228 ng respectively.

Conclusion/Significance: A 31 kDa major allergen of kidney bean was purified and identified as phytohemagglutinin with cross-reactivity to peanut and black gram.

Editor: William R. Abrams, New York University, United States of America

Funding: No current external funding sources for this study. Thus, the funders had no role in study design, data collection and analysis, decision to publish, or preparation of the manuscript.

Competing Interests: The authors have declared that no competing interests exist.

* E-mail: naveen@igib.res.in

Introduction

Legumes are rich source of proteins but are also potential elicitor of IgE-mediated food allergy. It has been well documented that legumes such as kidney bean, peanut, chick pea, black gram pigeon pea, lentil are an important source of IgE mediated hypersensitivity [1–5]. The clinical manifestations of the allergy to legumes range from oral allergy syndrome, urticaria, angioedema, rhinitis to asthma [6]. Recently, kidney bean has been identified as an emerging cause of food allergy among Indian population [2]. Kidney bean is consumed in Latin America, Africa, Middle East, Mediterranean area and India [1–7]. It contains high amounts of protein, abundant fibre and essential minerals like iron, zinc, calcium, and phosphorus [8]. Rouge and coworkers have also reported anaphylaxis to kidney bean [9]. Kidney bean has been identified as the major sensitizer among the atopic Indian population. Sensitization of about 22% (SPT positive) has been reported in suspected patients of food allergy [2].

So far, specific immunotherapy is the only approved curative treatment available, but it harbors drawbacks, such as side effects [10–11] and the use of crude allergen extracts [12]. Immunotherapy with crude extracts may result in additional sensitization to irrelevant components and can hamper in reaching the optimal maintenance dose during treatment. Moreover, not all the components present in extracts are allergenically relevant for diagnosis and therapy. To overcome this, use of purified and well-defined allergen preparations has been recommended [13]. Great efforts have been made to identify, characterize and purify food allergens from various sources. Three major allergens, Ara h 1, Ara h 2 and Ara h 3 [14–16], and four minor allergens, Ara h 4, Ara h 5, Ara h 6 and Ara h 7 [17], were identified from peanut.

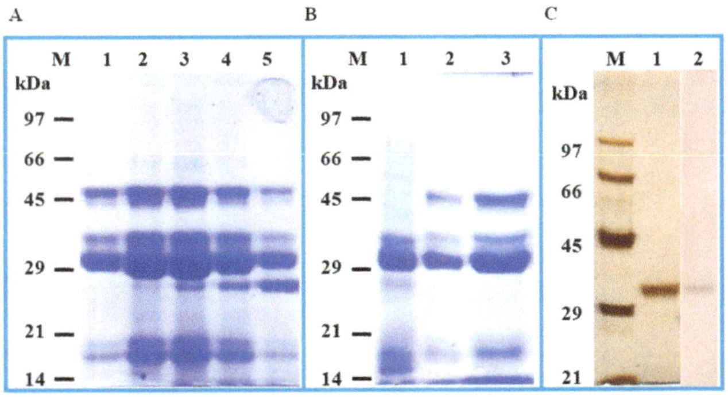

Figure 1. Protein profile of eluted fractions containing 31 kDa as a major eluted kidney bean protein. Kidney bean extract was subjected to anion exchange chromatography (A). Lane 1–5: fractions (10 to 14). Protein profile of gel filtration eluted fractions containing 31 kDa as a major eluted protein (B). Lane 1–3: fractions (17 to 19). Elution profile of purified 31 kDa protein after HPLC (C). Lane 1: purified protein after silver staining on SDS-PAGE, lane 2: immunoblot of purified protein using kidney bean hypersensitive pooled patients' sera.

With the exception of profilin Ara h 5, these allergens are seed storage proteins. Ara h 8 is a homologue of Bet v 1 and was identified as a major allergen in birch-pollen-allergic patients with concomitant peanut allergy [18]. Oleosin, a family of proteins involved in the formation of oil bodies, was also identified as important peanut allergen. This protein also has cross-reactivity with soybean [19]. Ara h 9, a lipid transfer protein was identified as a major allergen in peanut among allergic patients from the Mediterranean area [20]. Lentil has been ranked as the fourth most important allergen in Spain, where the frequency of its allergy is high in pediatric population. Three important allergens from lentil (Len c 1, Len c 2 and Len c 3), two from soybean (β-conglycinin and n-conglycinin), Pha v 3 from green bean and Vig r 1 from *Vigna radiata* were identified, isolated and characterized [21–26].

The availability of purified proteins paves the way for component resolved diagnosis which increases the sensitivity of the test and allows the design of patient-tailored risk profile. Development and progress made in the field of purified allergens have allowed for the development of a new concept in allergy diagnosis, molecular diagnosis, which makes it possible to identify potential disease-eliciting molecules. Therefore, there is a need for well-defined purified food allergens for component resolved diagnosis which may decrease the need for provocation testing and also improve the specificity of allergen-specific immunotherapy [24]. Moreover, purified proteins can also be used to develop antibodies which could provide a valuable tool for sensitive detection of respective allergenic products in food [27]. However, further efforts should be taken to assess the range of cross-reactivity and to identify marker allergen for the most important food allergen sources. This data will affect the management of dietary requirement or recommendation of individual patient with food allergy.

Our earlier study had identified kidney bean as an important legume allergen with 15 IgE binding components. Kidney bean's cross-reactivity has also been observed with other legumes. However, no allergen has been purified and characterized from kidney bean [2,9]. Thus, kidney bean being the major sensitizer among atopic Indian population the present investigation was undertaken to isolate and characterize a major allergenic protein of kidney bean using column chromatographic techniques and standard immunobiochemical methods.

Materials and Methods

Ethics Statement

The present study protocol was approved by the human ethics committee of CSIR-Institute of Genomics and Integrative Biology, Delhi. Informed written consents were obtained from patients and non-allergic volunteers for participation in the study.

Study Subjects

Allergic rhinitis and asthma patients with confirmed history of kidney bean allergy were included in the study from the two centres; Bangalore Allergy Centre, Bangalore and USLavasa Medical and Research Centre, Chandigarh, India. The diagnosis of asthma and rhinitis was ascertained following American Thoracic Society guidelines, 1991 and Allergic Rhinitis and its Impact on Asthma guidelines, 2001 [28–29]. Skin prick tests (SPT) were performed with kidney bean extract (1:10 w/v) in 50% glycerinated solution. Histamine diphosphate (5 mg/ml) and PBS

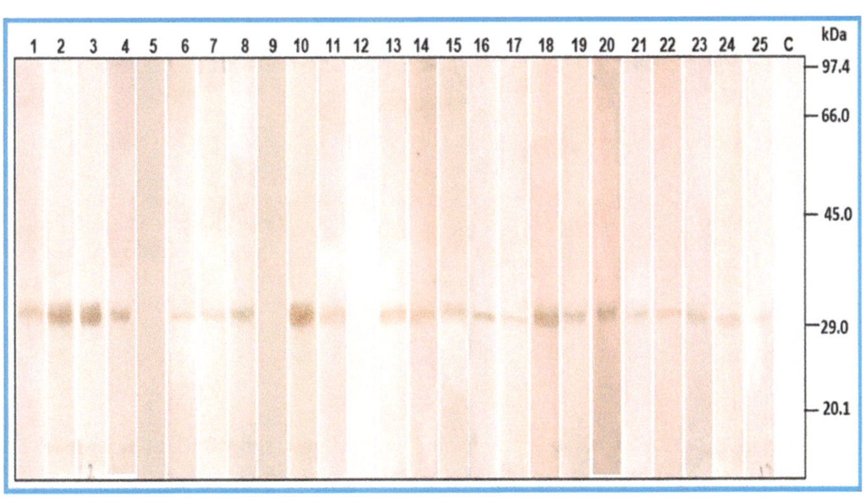

Figure 2. IgE binding of purified 31 kDa protein by immunoblotting. Lane 1–25: with individual patients' sera and lane C: purified protein probed with normal human sera (control).

Table 1. SPT and specific IgE among the patients (1−25) and controls (C1−C5) against raw kidney bean extract and 31 kDa protein.

Patient No.	Age/Sex	Wheal area (mm^2)			Specific IgE (O.D.) to kidney bean[a]	Specific IgE (O.D.) to 31 kDa[b]
		Histamine	Kidney bean extract	31 kDa protein		
1*	51/F	7×7	6×3	4×4	1.822	1.066
2*	34/F	5×5	6×5	n.d.	2.621	0.562
3	32/M	7×5	5×4	4×3	0.808	0.491
4*	35/M	5×6	6×5	n.d.	2.318	1.034
5	56/F	7×4	4×3	2×2	0.426	0.071
6	34/M	7×4	5×5	5×4	1.262	0.909
7	40/F	7×6	5×5	4×3	1.316	0.559
8*	52/M	6×6	6×4	3×3	2.230	0.482
9	49/M	7×5	4×3	n.d.	0.434	0.119
10	25/F	7×5	5×4	n.d.	0.839	0.577
11	60/M	7×5	5×5	n.d.	1.121	0.706
12	63/F	5×5	5×4	2×3	0.789	0.102
13	28/M	5×6	5×5	4×4	1.593	1.041
14	24/M	7×6	5×5	5×5	1.342	0.892
15	32/M	6×5	5×5	n.d.	0.919	0.622
16	48/M	6×5	4×4	n.d.	0.471	0.493
17	23/F	7×5	5×4	2×2	0.704	0.390
18	57/F	7×6	4×4	5×4	0.547	0.508
19	22/F	6×5	5×4	4×4	0.700	0.417
20	28/F	7×5	4×5	n.d.	0.565	0.533
21*	32/M	6×6	5×6	n.d.	1.631	1.046
22*	40/F	6×5	7×6	n.d.	3.161	1.137
23	48/M	5×5	3×3	3×3	0.407	0.431
24	62/F	8×4	5×4	n.d.	0.636	0.416
25	59/M	7×5	5×5	5×5	0.932	0.587
C1	28/M	5×4	1×1	1×1	0.047	0.038
C2	32/M	4×5	1×2	1×1	0.105	0.059
C3	26/F	5×4	1×1	1×1	0.087	0.052
C4	22/F	4×3	2×1	2×1	0.029	0.027
C5	38/M	3×3	1×1	1×1	0.047	0.035

[a]specific IgE cut off 0.189 OD.
[b]specific IgE cut off 0.126 OD.
*used for making patient's pooled sera.
n.d. = SPT not done.

in 50% glycerine were used as positive and negative controls respectively. SPT was also performed with purified protein (1 mg/ml) in kidney bean sensitive patients i.e. patients skin test positive to crude kidney bean extract (n = 14). SPT reactions were observed after 20 min and wheal diameters were recorded. Patients showing SPT positivity to kidney bean with symptoms such as anaphylaxis, redness of mouth, urticaria, nausea, vomiting, diarrhea, abdominal cramps, running nose or breathlessness after ingestion of kidney bean were recruited for the study. Blood was collected from patients who showed the reversal of their respective symptoms after elimination of kidney bean from their diet (n = 25). Blood was also collected from healthy non-allergic individuals (controls, n = 5).

Preparation of Extracts

The extraction of whole kidney bean antigen was carried out following the protocol as described earlier [30]. Briefly, healthy seeds of kidney bean were dried, crushed and defatted in diethyl ether at 4°C. The antigens were extracted in 1:20 (w/v) ammonium bicarbonate buffer (50 mM, pH 8.0) with 5 mM ethylene diamine tetra acetate and 1 mM phenyl methyl sulfonyl fluoride by continuous stirring for 8 h at 4°C. The suspension was centrifuged at 12,000 rpm for 30 min at 4°C. The supernatant was dialyzed overnight with several changes of distilled water. The extracts were again centrifuged at 12,000 rpm for 30 min at 4°C and then passed through a 0.22 μm pore size nitro cellulose membrane filter, aliquotted in small vials and lyophilized. Protein was estimated in the extract using modified lowry's method [31]. Similarly, the extracts for other legumes namely peanut, black

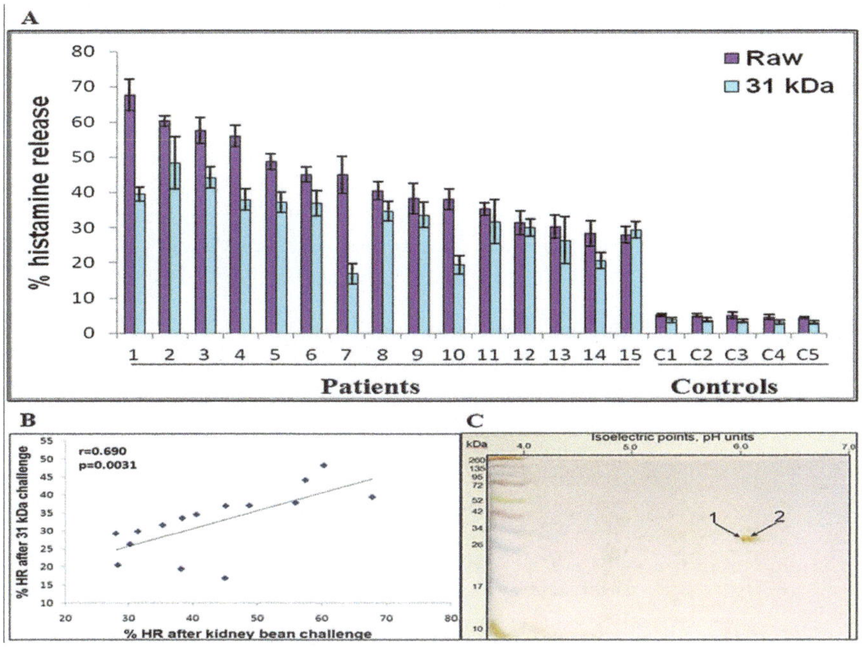

Figure 3. Histamine released from stripped basophils re-sensitized with individual patients' sera (n = 15) on challenge with kidney bean extract and 31 kDa purified protein, separately. Lane C1–C5: controls (A). Scatter plot of the correlation analysis between % histamine released by patients (n = 15) and controls on challenge with crude kidney bean extract and purified protein (B). 2-DE of purified 31 kDa protein showing two close spots (1 & 2) at the same molecular weight. Both the spots were identified as PHA-E after mass spectrometric analysis (C).

gram and pigeon pea were also prepared for cross-reactivity studies.

Purification of Kidney Bean Allergen

Three chromatographic steps were used to obtain purified 31 kDa protein.

Ion Exchange Chromatography

Kidney bean extract was subjected to anion exchange chromatography using fast protein liquid chromatography. The extract (75 mg) was reconstituted in 20 mM Tris buffer (pH 7.9) and loaded onto Q Sepharose column equilibrated with the same buffer. After washing away the unbound protein, the bound proteins were eluted with a linear NaCl gradient (0–1000 mM). Fractions of each resolved peak were pooled, dialyzed, lyophilized and run on SDS-PAGE.

Gel Filtration Chromatography

Pooled fractions containing allergenic protein (identified by immunoblot) were further loaded on Superdex^{TM} 75 column prior equilibrated with 20 mM phosphate buffer, pH 7.0. Fifty fractions (0.5 mL) were collected and protein content was determined, concentrated, analyzed by immunoblot with hypersensitive pooled kidney bean patients' sera. Allergenic protein fractions were pooled for further purification.

Reverse-phase Chromatography

Pooled fractions (after gel filtration chromatography) were loaded on C-18 column and further purified using high pressure liquid chromatography (HPLC). Unbound proteins were washed out with distilled water till the absorbance at 280 nm became zero. The bound proteins were eluted with 50% acetonitrile in water containing 0.1% trifluoroacetic acid. The eluted fraction was analyzed by SDS-PAGE and immunoblotting using pooled sera of kidney bean hypersensitive patients.

Estimation of Specific IgE

Levels of specific IgE in SPT positive patients' sera was determined by enzyme linked immunosorbent assay (ELISA) by following the protocol described earlier [30]. Briefly, crude kidney bean extract or the purified protein was coated in carbonate buffer (1 μg/100 μl/well), overnight at 4°C in a microtitre plate (Nunc, USA). After washing with PBS-Tween 20 (0.05%), the nonspecific sites were blocked with 1% bovine serum albumin (BSA) for 2 h at 37°C. The plate was washed and incubated with diluted sera (1:10 v/v) of kidney bean positive patients, overnight at 4°C. Pool of normal human sera was used as control. After washing antihuman IgE-horse radish peroxidase (1:1000 v/v; Sigma Chemical Co., St Louis, MO, USA) was added for 4 h at 37°C. Colour was developed with orthophenylene diamine. The reaction was stopped by adding 2.5 M H_2SO_4 and the absorbance was read at 492 nm. Specific IgE value ≥3 times of control was considered as positive.

ELISA Inhibition Assay

The allergenic potency of crude kidney bean extract and purified protein was determined by ELISA inhibition (competitive ELISA) using hypersensitive pooled patients' sera as described earlier [2]. Briefly, the extract (1 μg/100 μl per well) or purified protein was coated in carbonate buffer overnight at 4°C in a microtitre plate. The kidney bean patients' pooled serum (1:10 v/v) for respective antigen was preincubated with 10, 50, 100, 1000 and 10000 ng of self protein at 4°C overnight and the mixture was then added to the microtitre plate coated with same extract. Normal human sera was used as control. The protein required for 50% inhibition of IgE binding was calculated using the formula given below.

Table 2. Peptide mass fingerprint database search of selected spots from 2-DE of purified 31 kDa kidney bean proteins.

Spot No.	Accession	Identification	Matches of peptides	Sequence Coverage (%)	MASCOT score	Mass/pI	Proposed function
1	P05088	Full = Erythroagglutinating phytohemagglutinin; AltName: Full = PHA-E	39(21)	32	593	29.7/5.15	defensive protein
2	P05088	Full = Erythroagglutinating phytohemagglutinin; AltName: Full = PHA-E	39(19)	28	494	29.7/5.15	defensive protein

$$1-\frac{\text{OD of sample with inhibitor}}{\text{OD of sample without inhibitor}}\times 100$$

Competitive ELISA was also performed to determine cross-reactivity of purified protein with other legumes. Here, pooled patients' sera was inhibited with different legume extracts (peanut, black gram and pigeon pea) and ELISA was performed with preinhibited sera and purified protein on solid phase.

SDS-PAGE and Immunoblotting

The 31 kDa protein (2.5 μg) was resolved on 12% reducing gel and silver stained or commassie brilliant blue (CBB) stained for visualization.

For immunoblot, the resolved proteins were transferred on to nitrocellulose membrane as described earlier [2]. The unbound sites were blocked with 3% BSA for 3 h at 37°C. The nitrocellulose membrane strips were washed and incubated with kidney bean-hypersensitive patients' sera (1:10 v/v, preinhibited with bromelain) at 4°C. Normal human serum pool was taken as control. The strips were washed with PBS-Tween 20 and incubated with antihuman IgE-peroxidase (1:1000 v/v) (Sigma Chemical Co., St Louis, MO, USA). The IgE binding was detected by diaminobenzidine with hydrogen peroxide in sodium acetate buffer (pH 5.0).

Stripped Basophil Histamine Release Assay

Histamine release assay was performed in 15 kidney bean sensitive individuals having significantly high specific IgE values following the protocol by Kasera *et al.* [2]. In brief, peripheral blood was drawn from nonallergic donors and basophils were separated. Bound IgE was stripped off using lactic acid buffer. Subsequently, the cells were resensitized with serum IgE of individual patients ($n = 15$) and non allergic individuals serum as controls ($n = 5$). The histamine release assay was standardized using a graded amount of protein (1 ng–1 mg) and the protein concentration inducing optimal histamine release (10 ng for crude extract and 5 ng for purified protein) was determined. After passive sensitization, cells were stimulated with either kidney bean (10 ng) or with purified protein (5 ng) for 1 h. The histamine released was determined by the fluorometric method, using o-phthalaldehyde (Sigma Chemical Co., St Louis, MO, USA). Spontaneous histamine release was measured in the supernatant of unstimulated cells. The total histamine content was determined by lysis of cells with 3% perchloric acid. The allergen-induced histamine release was calculated as a percent of the total histamine content after correcting for spontaneous release. A histamine release of more than 10% was considered as positive.

Two Dimensional Gel Electrophoresis (2-DE)

It was performed to confirm the purity of 31 kDa protein following the protocol as described earlier [32]. Purified 31 kDa protein was precipitated using 2-DE clean up kit (GE Healthcare Biosciences Corporation, Piscataway, NJ), as per instructions from the supplier. The clean protein was solubilized in rehydration buffer and applied to 7 cm nonlinear (pH 4−7) IPG strip (BioRad, CA, USA) and left overnight for rehydration. Following incubation, the strip was transferred to the focusing tray. After adding mineral oil over the strip, the separation of proteins in the first dimension was performed in an IEF cell (BioRad, CA, USA) as per manufacturer's instructions. After focusing, a two step equilibration (reduction and alkylation) was performed. After equilibration

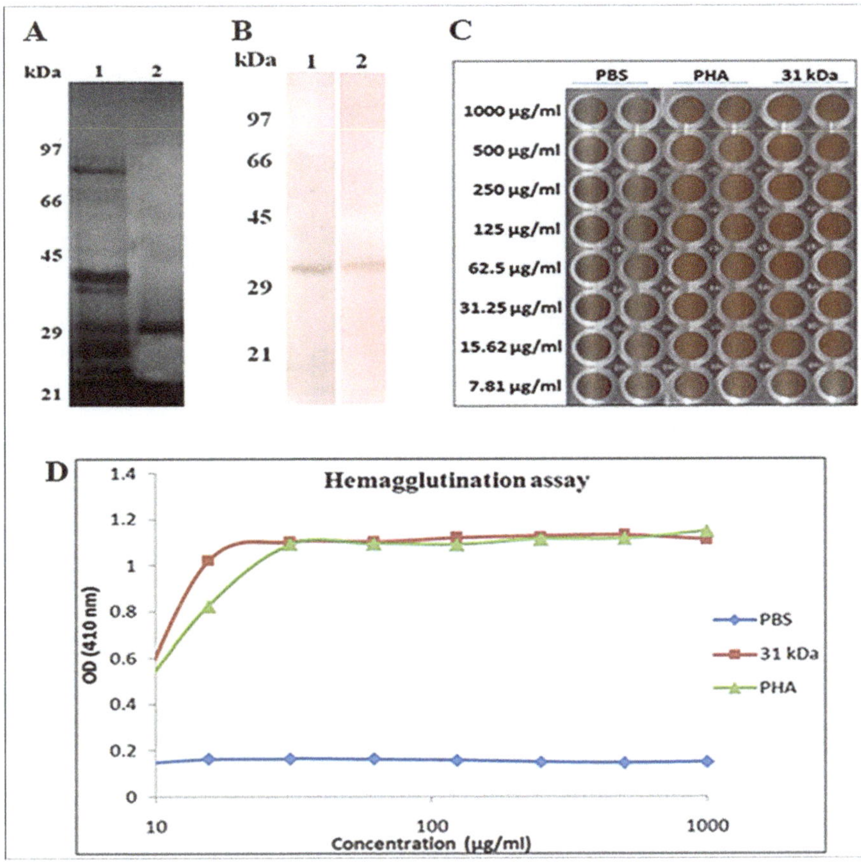

Figure 4. Glycoprotein detection by Periodic Acid Schiff's (PAS) staining. Lane 1: kidney bean extract, lane 2: purified 31 kDa protein (A). Immunoblot of purified protein after periodate treatment. The 31 kDa protein was electro-transfered onto nitrocellulose membrane and then periodate oxidation was done. The strip was washed, blocked with 3% defatted milk and immunoblotted with pooled patients' sera. Lane 1: 31 kDa protein (untreated), lane 2: 31 kDa protein after periodate treatment (B). Hemagglutination assay of 31 kDa protein, PHA (positive control) and PBS (negative control). Both 31 kDa and PHA formed uniform reddish color across the well with a minimum concentration of 15.62 µg/ml (C). Agglutination of human erythrocytes using purified protein and PHA (Sigma) (D).

the strip was placed over 1 mm thick 12.5% vertical acrylamide gel and held in position with molten 0.4% agarose containing bromophenol dye. The second dimension separation was performed in mini Protean III assembly (BioRad, CA, USA). After electrophoresis, the gel was subjected to silver staining.

Silver Staining

It was performed following the method described by Blum *et al.* [33]. Briefly, the gel was incubated in fixative solution containing 50% methanol and 12% acetic acid on shaker for 1.5 h at room temperature. The fixative was removed and saved for use in later step of the experiment. The gel was washed alternatively with 50% and 30% ethanol for 30 min each. Subsequent to washing with ethanol, the gel was treated with sodium thiosulphate solution (0.002%) for 60 sec and washed thrice with distilled water for 20 sec each. The gel was placed in staining solution (12 mM $AgNO_3$ and 0.028% formaldehyde) for 20 min. After incubation, the gel was washed with distilled water thrice to remove traces of silver stain and then developed. The developing solution was consisted of sodium carbonate (6%), formaldehyde (0.0185%) and sodium thiosulphate (4%). The gel was then placed in fixative solution for 10 min to stop the reaction. After that the gel was washed with double distilled water for 10 min and stored in 5% acetic acid solution. The stained gel was scanned at a resolution of 300 dpi using a scanner to acquire the image.

Mass Spectrometric Analysis

Spots were excised from silver stained gels and digested with trypsin. The solution was injected into Agilent nanoLC-1100 (Agilent, Palo Alto, CA, USA) for analysis as described earlier [2].

Periodic Acid Schiffs (PAS) Staining

This staining was used for detection of carbohydrate moieties in purified protein and kidney bean extract. For PAS staining, approximately 30 µg of purified protein or kidney bean extract was run on SDS-PAGE. The gel was incubated in 1% periodic acid in 3% acetic acid solution for 15 min and stained in Schiff's reagent for 15 min in dark. After staining, the gel was washed with 5% sodium metabisulfite solution for 5 min followed by distilled water to visualize the protein bands [34].

Periodate Oxidation

After electro-transfer of proteins onto nitrocellulose membrane strip, it was incubated in dark with 20 mM sodium metaperiodate, overnight at 4°C. Periodate was inactivated for 5−10 min by adding ethylene glycol. To this, 1 mg/ml of sodium borohydride was added and kept overnight at 4°C. The reaction was stopped

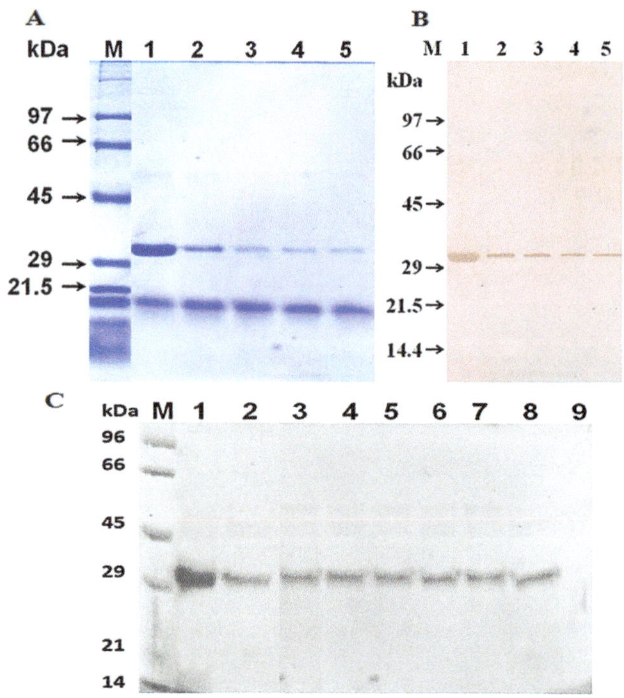

Figure 5. SDS-PAGE profile and immunoblot of 31 kDa kidney bean protein. Lane 1 : untreated, Lane 2–5 : boiled at 100°C for 15, 30, 45 and 60 min, Lane M: molecular weight markers. Protein fractions were stained with Coomassie brilliant blue (A) and immunoblotted (B). SGF digestion of 31 kDa protein Lane M:molecular weight markers, Lane 1: 31 kDa protein (undigested), lanes 2–8: 31 kDa protein incubated in SGF for 0.5, 1, 5, 10, 15, 30 and 60 min, lane 9: pepsin. The digested protein was electrophoresed on SDS-PAGE and visualized by CBB staining (C).

by adding a drop of acetic acid. The strip was washed with water and PBS and protein free sites were blocked with 3% defatted milk in PBS. The remaining steps of western blot were carried out as described earlier [34].

Hemagglutination Assay (HA)

Hemagglutination activity of purified 31 kDa protein was determined by HA assay. Briefly, PBS (50 µl/well) was first added to microtitre plate. To these wells, either 50 µl of purified protein (2 mg/ml) or PHA (Sigma Chemical Co., St Louis, MO, USA) was added. PBS was used as a negative control. Then 50 µl of 0.5% RBC suspension was added to each well and mixed gently. The plate was left undisturbed at room temperature for 1 h at an angle of 45°. In the absence of hemagglutination activity, the RBCs settled and appeared as dots at the corner of plates. Positive reaction resulted in a uniform reddish color across the well. HA titre was recorded as the highest dilution factor that produced a positive reading. OD of the supernatant was taken at 410 nm without disturbing the pellet.

Heat Stability

Purified protein was boiled for 15, 30, 45 and 60 min at 100°C and analyzed by SDS-PAGE and immunoblot.

Simulated Gastric Fluid (SGF) Digestion

The digestibility of purified kidney bean protein was examined in the SGF, as described earlier [34]. Briefly, purified protein (6.8 µg) was treated with 200 µL of prewarmed SGF (US Pharmacopoeia) containing 0.0032% (w/v) of pepsin A (Sigma Chemical Co., St Louis, MO, USA). Digestion was proceeded at 37°C with continuous shaking, and an aliquot (20 µL) of this digest was periodically withdrawn at 0.5, 1, 5, 15, 30, 45, and 60 min for analysis on SDS-PAGE.

Immunoblot Inhibition

Immunoblot inhibition was performed to establish cross-reactivity of 31 kDa kidney bean allergen with other kidney bean proteins. Kidney bean positive sera from 7 patients' (>1.0 O.D.) were pooled and preincubated with 100 µg of 31 kDa kidney bean protein. Whole kidney bean proteins were transferred on to nitrocellulose membrane, strips were cut, blocked and incubated with the preinhibited pooled sera. The rest of the procedure was similar to immunoblotting as described earlier in the methodology section.

Statistical Analysis

Values are represented as mean±SD. Correlation analysis was carried out using MS EXCEL, Prism V software (Graph Pad Prism, San Diego, California, USA). Statistical significance was calculated using one way analysis of variance using software Epi Info 3.3.2. and SISA. The significance level was considered to be $p<0.05$.

Results

Purification of 31 kDa Kidney Bean Protein

The adsorbed proteins of kidney bean on Q Sepharose column were eluted using NaCl gradient and fractions were run on SDS-PAGE. Fraction nos. 10 to 14 showing high intensity band at 31 kDa were pooled (Fig. 1A) and IgE binding was confirmed with immunoblotting using kidney bean hypersensitive pooled patients' sera. The protein was further purified using gel filtration and the fraction nos. 17 to 19 with 31 kDa fractions (Fig. 1B) were pooled and purified using C_{18} columns. The major peak of interest, 31 kDa was eluted at a retention time of 4.57 min which appeared as a single band on SDS-PAGE after silver staining and was recognized by kidney bean hypersensitive pooled patients' sera on immunoblotting (Fig. 1C).

Allergenicity Assessment of Purified 31 kDa Protein

Specific IgE binding of purified protein (31 kDa) and crude kidney bean extract was determined by ELISA using 25 kidney bean sensitive patients' sera (SPT positive). Specific IgE binding of 31 kDa protein, and kidney bean extract showed elevated IgE levels (OD 0.479 to 3.161) against kidney bean extract whereas 22/25 sera showed positive IgE values (OD 0.390 to 1.137) against purified protein (Table 1). There was a significant correlation of specific IgE reactivity of purified protein and kidney bean extract ($r=0.6757$, $p<0.01$).

IgE binding of 31 kDa protein was further assessed by immunoblotting with individual patients' sera ($n=25$) having elevated specific IgE levels to kidney bean. Of these, 22 (88%) sera showed IgE binding with purified protein demonstrating it to be a major allergen (Fig. 2). Sera of three patients' (patient nos. 5, 9 and 12) did not show IgE binding to 31 kDa protein. These patients might be sensitized to other proteins present in kidney bean.

Biopotency of Purified Protein

Out of 25 kidney bean positive patients, 31 kDa protein was skin prick tested on 14 subjects and 11 showed marked positive skin reaction. There was a significant correlation between skin reactivity of purified protein and kidney bean extract ($r=0.615$,

A

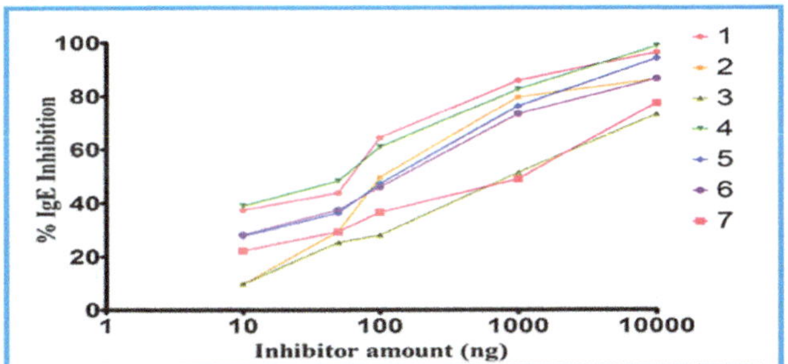

Line No.	Solid phase	Inhibitor	50% inhibition (ng)
1	31 kDa	31 kDa	102
2	Kidney bean	Kidney bean	67.3
3	Kidney bean	31 kDa	976
4	31 kDa	Kidney bean	56
5	31 kDa	Peanut	185
6	31 kDa	Black gram	228
7	31 kDa	Pigeon pea	1300

B

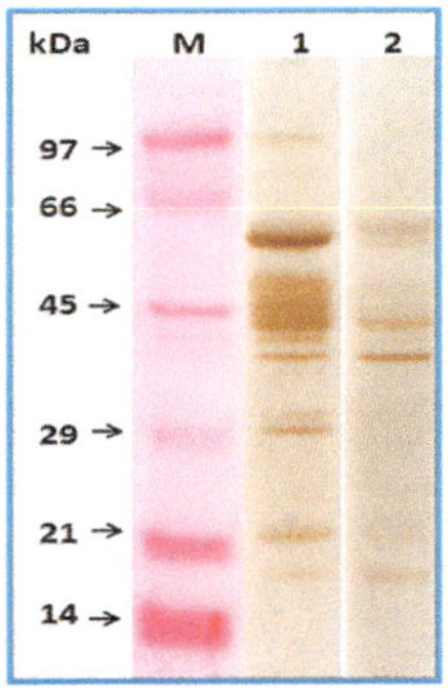

Figure 6. IgE ELISA inhibition of kidney bean extract and 31 kDa protein. Kidney bean protein and extracts of different legumes were used as inhibitor (A). Kidney bean positive patients' pooled sera (1:10 v/v) was preincubated with 5, 10, 50, 100, 1000, 10000 ng of inhibitor. ELISA was carried out on solid phase coated kidney bean extract (2 μg/100 μl/well) or 31 kDa protein (500 ng/100 μl/well) and preincubated sera. Immunoblot inhibition of kidney bean extract with 31 kDa protein (B). Kidney bean positive pooled patients' sera was preincubated with 100 μg of 31 kDa protein (lane 2). Immunoblot using kidney bean positive pooled patients' sera without inhibitor was used as a control (lane 1).

$p = 0.05$). Specific IgE levels were significantly elevated in sera of all 11 SPT positive patients against both kidney bean and purified protein in ELISA (Table 1). Healthy subjects did not demonstrate positive skin reaction with any of the allergen extract.

Histamine Release

Basophils sensitized with kidney bean sensitive individual patients' sera exhibited elevated histamine release after challenge with kidney bean extract and the purified 31 kDa protein in the range of 28–67% and 17–48% respectively (Fig. 3A). Basophils sensitized with sera from healthy individuals released less than 5% histamine. Statistically significant correlation ($r = 0.6903$, $p < 0.01$) was observed between histamine released by kidney bean extract and 31 kDa protein (Fig. 3B).

Mass Spectrometric Analysis

The 31 kDa protein resolved as two discrete spots by 2-DE (Fig. 3C). Both the spots on mass spectrometric analysis were identified as erythroagglutinating Phytohemagglutinin (PHA-E). Sequence coverage of both the isoforms was more than 28%. A total of 39 peptides were matched to the database and 21 and 19 peptides showed extensive homology ($p < 0.05$) in the respective isoforms. Phytohemagglutinin is a defensin protein which functions as host defense protein (Table 2).

PAS Staining and Periodate Treatment

The 31 kDa protein was identified as a glycoprotein after PAS staining (Figure 4A). No change in the IgE binding was observed after periodate treatment on immunoblot with patients' sera (Figure 4B). This ruled out the possibility of any carbohydrate specific IgE binding (non specific) to 31 kDa protein.

Hemagglutination Assay

Both 31 kDa protein and PHA (Sigma Chemical Co., St Louis, MO, USA) showed positive HA assay as compared to the negative control. Human erythrocytes remained suspended in the wells giving uniform reddish color across the well due to agglutinating activity in 31 kDa protein as well purified PHA. However, in case of PBS, erythrocytes were settled down at the corner of the plate showing absence of agglutination (Fig. 4C). The HA titre of 31 kDa was found to be 15.62 μg/ml (Fig. 4D).

Heat Stability

Purified protein remained stable on boiling for up to 60 min at 100°C. However the intensity of protein band decreased as the time of boiling was increased (Fig. 5A). On immunoblot purified protein showed IgE binding even after 60 min of boiling (Fig. 5B).

SGF Digestion

Enzymatic stability of purified 31 kDa kidney bean protein was assessed by SGF digestion. The 31 kDa protein remained undigested (stable) even after 1 h treatment in SGF (Fig. 5C). The negative control, BSA was digested completely by SGF within 1 min and positive control, lactoglobulin remained stable to digestion even after 1 h of treatment.

Allergenic Potency of 31 kDa Protein and its Cross-reactivity

The 31 kDa protein showed a dose dependent inhibition of IgE binding with self protein in competitive ELISA. A maximum inhibition of 98% was achieved with 1 μg of 31 kDa protein as inhibitor whereas 50% inhibition of IgE binding was obtained with 102 ng of self protein (31 kDa) as inhibitor.

However, a maximum inhibition of 61% was observed in IgE binding to crude kidney bean extract (solid phase) when when 1 μg of 31 kDa protein was used as an inhibitor. Whereas, for 50% IgE inhibition to crude kidney bean extract 976 ng of purified protein was required as inhibitor. For 50% IgE inhibition to solid phase crude kidney bean extract only 67.3 ng of self protein extract was required (Fig. 6A).

Cross-reactivity of 31 kDa protein was assessed with black gram, peanut and pigeon pea by ELISA inhibition using serum pools from patients SPT positive only to kidney bean extract and negative to the tested cross-reactive antigen. Here, purified 31 kDa protein from kidney bean was coated on solid phase and different legume extracts (kidney bean, black gram, peanut and pigeon pea) were used as inhibitors. Fifty six ng of kidney bean protein (inhibitor) was required for 50% inhibition of IgE binding to solid phase 31 kDa in ELISA, whereas peanut, black gram and pigeon pea caused same inhibition with 185, 228 and 1300 ng of protein(s), respectively (Fig. 6A).

Electrophoretically transferred kidney bean proteins were incubated with preinhibited serum pool. Preabsorption of pooled patients' sera with 100 μg of 31 kDa protein reduced its IgE reactivity (Fig. 6B, lane 2). IgE binding of proteins corresponding to 120, 95, 70, 34, 31 kDa proteins was inhibited in kidney bean indicating presence of cross reactive components. However, IgE binding of proteins separated at 55 and 50 kDa, were not completely inhibited and 45 and 42 kDa proteins remained uninhibited by purified protein. Therefore, it can be inferred that these proteins are specific allergens of kidney bean.

Discussion

Legumes are consumed worldwide, India being at the top. In India studies on food allergens are very limited and restricted to only few foods such as egg, milk, cereals and few legumes [35–37]. Legumes such as peas, peanut, lentils, black gram, soy bean and chickpeas have been associated with severe allergic reactions [1,18,25,26]. Presently, crude protein extracts are used in the allergic diagnosis. But their use has several pitfalls like batch to batch variation, low expression or concentration of many important allergens in whole extracts. Apart from this many endogenous enzymes may degrade allergens during extraction procedures. However, these problems can be overcome by using purified protein for component resolved diagnosis and patient-tailored therapy [38].

Over the years, many allergens have been purified from diverse sources such as pollen, fungi, insects, mites, and foods including legumes. These have also proved promising in selective diagnosis/therapy of allergy. For example, the major allergen Bet v 1 from birch pollen was purified from natural sources by employing ammonium sulfate precipitation, hydrophobic interaction chromatography and size exclusion chromatography [39]. Marsh *et al.* [40] purified native peanut allergens Ara h 1, 2, 3, 4 and 6 for diagnosis of peanut allergy. Ara h 1, a 63 kDa protein was purified on a ConA Sepharose-4B affinity column after ammonium sulfate precipitation. Ara h 2 and 6 were purified after ammonium sulfate precipitation and gel filtration followed by anion exchange and reverse phase HPLC. Ara h 3/4 were purified following anion exchange and gel filtration chromatography. A major allergen from soy (Gly m Bd), was purified by immunoaffinity column using mAb as a ligand [41]. Anion-exchange chromatography and reverse-phase HPLC were also used to purify Len c 1.01- a major allergen from lentil [42]. A seed storage 24 kDa protein was purified from the seeds of *Lathyrus sativus* by ammonium sulfate fractionation and ion-exchange chromatography [43]. Another 25 kDa legume protein from *Vigna unguiculata* extract was fractionated using ammonium salt precipitation followed by gel chromatographic separation which led to separation of this protein in pure form [44]. Moreover, for component resolved diagnosis with kiwifruit allergy, 4 specific marker allergens were identified out of the panel of 11 kiwifruit allergens and showed the potential of component resolved diagnosis in increasing sensitivity and specificity of *in vitro* tests [45].

In the present study, we have used combination of anion exchange and gel filtration chromatography on FPLC followed by reverse phase HPLC on C_{18} column to get purified 31 kDa kidney bean allergen. Moreover, IgE binding of the purified 31 kDa protein was assessed by *in vivo* (SPT), *in vitro* (ELISA and immunoblotting) and *ex vivo* (histamine release assay) methods. The allergenic relevance of purified 31 kDa protein was showed by IgE binding with more than 88% of kidney bean sensitive patient's sera. Later, when a subset of 14 sensitive patients out of 25 were skin tested, 11/14 (78%) kidney bean sensitive patients showed SPT positive reaction to 31 kDa protein. Thus, being a major allergen it can be used as a marker in the diagnosis of kidney bean allergy. Purified protein inhibited up to 73% IgE binding in competitive ELISA when 10 μg of purified protein was used as inhibitor and crude kidney bean extract on solid phase. Earlier, in a case report by Schiavino et al. [46], anaphylaxis has been reported after SPT with phytohaemoagglutinin.

In the present study, 31 kDa protein demonstrated significant histamine release from kidney bean positive patients' samples (n = 15) as compared to controls, indicating that purified protein is a potent allergen having clinical relevance in diagnosis. Specific IgE values and histamine release with purified 31 kDa protein and kidney bean extract correlated significantly ($p<0.01$). This suggested the importance of purified allergen and its use for diagnosis and therapy of kidney bean allergy. In an earlier study by Kumari *et al.* [34], 7/9 black gram sensitive patients were found SPT positive to its 28 kDa purified protein whereas, 77% black gram patients showed significant IgE binding. López-Torrejón *et al.* [42] in their study on lentil and its purified protein, showed IgE binding of Len c 1.01 to ≥80% of the patient's sera.

In the present study, 102 ng of 31 kDa protein was required for 50% inhibition of self protein whereas, 976 ng of 31 kDa protein was required for kidney bean extract showing it to be a potent allergen. Cross-reactivity has been reported previously among legume allergens [1,2,47]. In the present study, 56 ng of kidney bean extract was required to obtain 50.0% inhibition of IgE binding on solid phase 31 kDa, whereas 185 and 228 ng of peanut and black gram were required respectively for the same. In another study inhibition of 65% IgE binding was observed with 2 μg of purified lentil protein as inhibitor and whole lentil extract on solid phase in immunoblot inhibition [42]. IgE binding protein components of kidney bean corresponding to 120, 95, 70, 34 kDa were completely inhibited when pooled patients' sera was preabsorbed with 100 μg of self protein in immunoblot inhibition. Inhibition of these proteins suggests presence of shared epitopes.

Resistance to proteolytic enzymes and heat is a property associated with food allergens. Many food allergens or stable allergen fragments have been shown to resist conditions of the gastrointestinal tract, and thus have the potential to sensitize the immune system. In the present study, pepsin digestion of 31 kDa protein showed no cleavage products in the SDS-PAGE. This suggested that the protein is available to be taken up by the immune cells and have role in sensitizing system. However, Kumari *et al.* [34] showed the formation of stable protein fragments of 14–16 kDa after digestion with pepsin. The 31 kDa protein was also found stable to heat as the protein is visible on SDS-PAGE even after 1 h of boiling and also showed IgE binding on immunoblot. This further provides evidence that heat stable proteins are much more likely to be allergenic. Rouge *et al.* [9] identified phaseolin and PHA as putative allergens in kidney bean. Both phaseolin (>150 kDa) and PHA (120 kDa) were resistant to heat denaturation and digestive proteolysis, exhibiting an extended surface susceptible to display IgE-binding epitopes that probably account for their allergenic propensity.

The purified 31 kDa protein was identified as PHA-E after mass spectrometric analysis which is a defensive protein. PAS staining identified it as a glycoprotein. Periodate oxidation did not reduce the IgE binding of 31 kDa protein as observed on immunoblot. Thus, ruling out the possibility of any non-specific binding due to the presence of carbohydrate moieties. The 31 kDa protein in the present study showed agglutination activity similar to commercial PHA obtained from Sigma.

In conclusion, a 31 kDa kidney bean protein was purified and identified as phytohemagglutinin. This may be implicated in possible strategies for component resolved diagnosis and therapy of kidney bean allergy. However, further *in vivo* studies are warranted with purified 31 kDa protein to confirm its contribution to various symptoms of food allergy.

Acknowledgments

RK is a Senior Research fellow of Indian Council of Medical Research, New Delhi.

Author Contributions

Conceived and designed the experiments: RK ABS NA. Performed the experiments: RK SL KN. Analyzed the data: RK NA. Contributed reagents/materials/analysis tools: RK. Wrote the paper: RK ABS NA.

References

1. Kumari D, Kumar R, Sridhara S, Arora N, Gaur SN, et al. (2006) Sensitization to black gram in patients with bronchial asthma and rhinitis: clinical evaluation and characterization of allergens. Allergy 61: 104–110.
2. Kasera R, Singh BP, Lavasa S, Prasad KN, Sahoo RC, et al. (2011) Kidney bean: a major sensitizer among legumes in asthma and rhinitis patients from India. PLoS One, 6: e27193.
3. Verma AK, Kumar S, Tripathi A, Chaudhari BP, Das M, et al. (2012) Chickpea (*Cicer arietinum*) proteins induce allergic responses in nasobronchial allergic patients and BALB/c mice. Toxicol Lett 210: 24–33.
4. Misra A, Prasad R, Das M, Dwivedi PD (2009) Probing novel allergenic proteins of commonly consumed legumes. Immunopharmacol Immunotoxicol 31: 186–194.
5. Misra A, Kumar R, Mishra V, Chaudhari BP, Tripathi A, et al. (2010) Partial characterization of red gram (*Cajanus cajan* L. Millsp) polypeptides recognized by patients exhibiting rhinitis and bronchial asthma. Food Chem Toxicol 48: 2725–2736.
6. Pereira MJ, Belver MT, Pascual CY, Martín Esteban M (2002) The allergenic significance of legumes. Allergol Immunopathol (Madr) 30: 346–353.
7. Food and Agriculture Organization [FAO] (1993) Production yearbook, 1992. Vol. 26. Rome, Food and Agriculture Organization of the United Nations.
8. Carvalho LM, Corrêa MM, Pereira EJ, Nutti MR, Carvalho JL, et al. (2012) Iron and zinc retention in common beans (*Phaseolus vulgaris* L.) after home cooking. Food Nutr Res 56. doi, 10.3402/fnr.v56i0.15618.
9. Rougé P, Culerrier R, Thibau F, Didier A, Barre A (2011) A case of severe anaphylaxis to kidney bean, phaseolin (vicilin) and PHA (lectin) identified as putative allergens. Allergy 66: 301–302.
10. Valenta R (2002) The future of antigen-specific immunotherapy of allergy. Nat Rev Immunol 2: 446–453.
11. Larche M, Akdis CA, Valenta R (2006) Immunological mechanisms of allergen-specific immunotherapy. Nat Rev Immunol 6: 761–771.
12. Moverare R, Elfman L, Vesterinen E, Metso T, Haahtela T (2002) Development of new IgE specificities to allergenic components in birch pollen extract during specific immunotherapy studied with immunoblotting and Pharmacia CAP System. Allergy 57: 423–430.
13. Hamilton RG, Franklin Adkinson N Jr (2004) *In vitro* assays for the diagnosis of IgE-mediated disorders. J Allergy Clin Immunol 114: 213–225.
14. Burks AW, Williams LW, Helm RM, Connaughton C, Cockrell G, et al. (1991) Identification of a major peanut allergen, Ara h 1, in patients with atopic dermatitis and positive peanut challenges. J Allergy Clin Immunol 88: 172–179.
15. Burks AW, Williams LW, Connaughton C, Cockrell G, O'Brien TJ, et al. (1992) Identification and characterization of a second major peanut allergen, Ara h II, with use of the sera of patients with atopic dermatitis and positive peanut challenge. J Allergy Clin Immunol 90: 962–969.
16. Rabjohn P, Helm EM, Stanley JS, West CM, Sampson HA, et al. (1999) Molecular cloning and epitope analysis of the peanut allergen Ara h 3. J Clin Invest 103: 535–542.
17. Kleber-Janke T, Crameri R, Appenzeller U, Schlaak M, Becker WM (1999) Selective cloning of peanut allergens, including profilin and 2S albumins, by phage display technology. Int Arch Allergy Immunol 119: 265–274.
18. Mittag D, Akkerdaas J, Ballmer-Weber BK, Vogel L, Wensing M, et al. (2004) Ara h 8, a Bet v 1-homologous allergen from peanut, is a major allergen in patients with combined birch pollen and peanut allergy. J Allergy Clin Immunol 114: 1410–1417.
19. Pons L, Chery C, Romano A, Namour F, Artesani MC, et al. (2002) The 18 kDa peanut oleosin is a candidate allergen for IgE-mediated reactions to peanuts. Allergy 57: 88–93.
20. Lauer I, Dueringer N, Pokoj S, Rehm S, Zoccatelli G, et al. (2009) The non-specific lipid transfer protein, Ara h 9, is an important allergen in peanut. Clin Exp Allergy 39: 1427–1437.
21. Mittag D, Vieths S, Vogel L, Wagner-Loew D, Starke A, et al. (2005) Birch pollen-related food allergy to legumes, identification and characterization of the Bet v 1 homologue in mung bean (*Vigna radiata*), Vig r 1. Clin Exp Allergy 35: 1049–1055.
22. Blanc F, Bernard H, Alessandri S, Bublin M, Paty E, et al. (2008) Update on optimized purification and characterization of natural milk allergens. Mol Nutr Food Res 52: S166–S175.
23. Rigby NM, Marsh J, Sancho AI, Wellner K, Akkerdaas J, et al. (2008) The purification and characterisation of allergenic hazelnut seed proteins. Mol Nutr Food Res 52: S251–S261.
24. Treudler R, Simon JC (2012) Overview of Component Resolved Diagnostics. Curr Allergy Asthma Rep [PMID: 23076421].
25. Zoccatelli G, Pokoj S, Foetisch K, Bartra J, Valero A, et al. (2010) Identification and characterization of the major allergen of green bean (*Phaseolus vulgaris*) as a non-specific lipid transfer protein (Pha v 3). Mol Immunol 47: 1561–1568.
26. Akkerdaas J, Finkina EI, Balandin SV, Santos Magadán S, Knulst A, et al. (2012) Lentil (*Lens culinaris*) lipid transfer protein Len c 3, a novel legume allergen. Int Arch Allergy Immunol 157: 51–57.
27. Liu B, Teng D, Wang X, Yang Y, Wang J (2012) Expression of the soybean allergenic protein P34 in Escherichia coli and its indirect ELISA detection method. Appl Microbiol Biotechnol 94: 1337–1345.
28. Bousquet J, Cauwenberge PV, Khaltaev N (2001) Allergic Rhinitis and its Impact on Asthma. J Allergy Clin Immunol 108: 147–334.
29. American Thoracic Society. (1991) Lung Function Testing: Selection of Reference Values and Interpretative Strategies. Am Rev Respir Dis 144: 1202–1218.
30. Kasera R, Singh AB, Kumar R, Lavasa S, Prasad KN, et al. (2012) Effect of thermal processing and γ-irradiation on allergenicity of legume proteins. Food Chem Toxicol 50: 3456–3461.
31. Singh BP, Sridhara S, Arora N, Gangal SV (1992) Evaluation of protein assay methods for pollen and fungal spore extracts. Biochem Int 27: 477–484.
32. Singh S, Gupta S, Singh B, Sharma SK, Gupta VK, et al. (2012) Proteomic Characterization of *Aspergillus fumigatus* Treated with an Antifungal Coumarin for Identification of Novel Target Molecules of Key Pathways. J Proteome Res [Epub ahead of print, PMID: 22533410].
33. Blum H, Beier H, Gross HJ (1987) Improved silver staining of plant proteins, RNA and DNA in polyacrylamide gels. Electrophoresis 8: 93–99.
34. Kumari D, Arora N, Kasera R, Sridhara S, Kumar R, et al. (2012) Isolation and characterization of a 28 kDa major allergen from blackgram (*Phaseolus mungo*). Immunobiology 217: 895–904.
35. Parihar H, Kumar L, Puri R, Kumar V (1984) The incidence of allergic diseases and feeding patterns in children upto 2 years of age. Indian J Pediatr 51: 7–12.
36. Kumar R, Srivastava P, Kumari D, Fakhr H, Sridhara S, et al. (2007) Rice (*Oryza sativa*) allergy in asthma and rhinitis patients: a clinico-immunological study. Immunobiology 212: 141–147.
37. Sharman J, Kumar L, Singh S (2000) Allergenicity of common foods restricted in respiratory allergy. Indian J Paediatr 67: 713–720.
38. Hoffmann-Sommergruber K, Mills EN, Vieths S (2008) Coordinated and standardized production, purification and characterization of natural and recombinant food allergens to establish a food allergen library. Mol Nutr Food Res 52: S159–S165.
39. Bollen MA, Garcia A, Cordewener JH, Wichers HJ, Helsper JP, et al. (2007) Purification and characterization of natural Bet v 1 from birch pollen and related allergens from carrot and celery. Mol Nutr Food Res 51: 1527–1536.
40. Marsh J, Rigby N, Wellner K, Reese G, Knulst A, et al. (2008) Purification and characterisation of a panel of peanut allergens suitable for use in allergy diagnosis. Mol Nutr Food Res 52: S272–S285.
41. Tsuji H, Bando N, Hiemori M, Yamanishi R, Kimoto M, et al. (1997) Purification of characterization of soybean allergen Gly m Bd 28K. Biosci Biotechnol Biochem 61: 942–947.
42. López-Torrejón G, Salcedo G, Martín-Esteban M, Díaz-Perales A, Pascual CY, et al. (2003) Len c 1, a major allergen and vicilin from lentil seeds, protein isolation and cDNA cloning. J Allergy Clin Immunol 112: 1208–1215.
43. Qureshi IA, Sethi DK, Salunke DM (2006) Purification, identification and preliminary crystallographic studies of an allergenic protein from *Lathyrus sativus*. Acta Crystallogr Sect F Struct Biol Cryst Commun 62: 869–872.
44. Chanana V, Kaur KJ, Salunke DM (2004) Purification, identification and preliminary crystallographic characterization of a novel seed protein from *Vigna unguiculata*. Acta Crystallogr D Biol Crystallogr 60: 2100–2103.
45. Bublin M, Pfister M, Radauer C, Oberhuber C, Bulley S, et al. (2010) Component-resolved diagnosis of kiwifruit allergy with purified natural and recombinant kiwifruit allergens. J Allergy Clin Immunol 125: 687–694.
46. Schiavino D, Nucera E, Murzilli F, Schinco G, Papa G, et al. (1992) Anaphylactic shock after skin test with phytohaemoagglutinin. Allergy 47: 121–122.
47. Ibáñez MD, Martínez M, Sánchez JJ (2003) Fernández-Caldas E. Legume cross-reactivity. Allergol Immunopathol 31: 1511–61.

11

Effects of Different Up-Dosing Regimens for Hymenoptera Venom Immunotherapy on Serum CTLA-4 and IL-10

Anna Maria Riccio[1], Daniele Saverino[2], Giampaola Pesce[3], Anthi Rogkakou[1], Maurizio Severino[4], Patrizia Bonadonna[5], Erminia Ridolo[6], Marina Mauro[7], Giorgio Walter Canonica[1], Marcello Bagnasco[3], Giovanni Passalacqua[1]*

1 Allergy and Respiratory Diseases, Department of Internal Medicine, University of Genoa, Genoa, Italy, **2** Section of Human Anatomy, Department of Experimental Medicine, University of Genoa, Genoa, Italy, **3** Medical and Radiomethabolic Therapy, Department of Internal Medicine, University of Genoa, Genoa, Italy, **4** Allergy Unit, Ospedale San Giovanni di Dio, Florence, Italy, **5** Allergy Service, Verona General Hospital, Verona, Italy, **6** Experimental and Internal Medicine, University of Parma, Parma, Italy, **7** Allergy Unit, Sant'Anna Hospital, Como, Italy

Abstract

Background: Cytotoxic T lymphocyte associated antigen-4 (CTLA-4) is involved in the activation pathways of T lymphocytes. It has been shown that the circulating form of CTLA-4 is elevated in patients with hymenoptera allergy and can be down regulated by immunotherapy.

Objective: to assess the effects on CTLA-4 of venom immunotherapy, given with different induction protocols: conventional (6 weeks), rush (3 days) or ultra rush (1 day).

Methods: Sera from patients with hymenoptera allergy were collected at baseline and at the end of the induction phase. CTLA-4 and IL-10 were assayed in the same samples. A subset of patients were assayed also after 12 months of VIT maintenance.

Results: Ninety-four patients were studied. Of them, 50 underwent the conventional induction, 20 the rush and 24 the ultra-rush. Soluble CTLA-4 was detectable in all patients at baseline, and significantly decreased at the end of the induction, irrespective of its duration. Of note, a significant decrease of sCTLA-4 could be seen already at 24 hours. In parallel, IL-10 significantly increased at the end of the induction. At 12 months, sCTLA-4 remained low, whereas IL-10 returned to the baseline values.

Conclusions: Serum CTLA4 is an early marker of the immunological effects of venom immunotherapy, and its changes persist after one year of maintenance treatment.

Editor: Jianqing Xu, Fudan University, China

Funding: These authors have no support or funding to report.

Competing Interests: The authors have declared that no competing interests exist.

* E-mail: passalacqua@unige.it

Introduction

Allergy is the clinical manifestation of the "atopic status" that is characterized by an abnormal IgE response to ubiquitous substances, including pollens, foods, drugs and venoms of stinging insects. When the contact with the offending allergen is occasional and isolated (e.g. hymenoptera venom allergy, HVA, or food allergy) a "pure" IgE-mediated reaction takes place. This is essentially characterized by the sudden release of mast cell derived mediators (mainly histamine), triggered by IgE. The pure IgE-mediated diseases represent a very "clean" model to study the allergic reaction and its modulation by specific immunotherapy (SIT). T lymphocytes are responsible for the "deviation" towards the atopic status, and this deviation seems to be driven by T regulatory (Treg) cells [1,2], so that impairment in the function of Treg cells may lead to either autoimmunity or allergy.

Many different signalling molecules intervene in the immune response, and an increasing interest is currently devoted to the activation pathways of T lymphocytes. An effective T-cell activation requires a primary signal delivered by the antigenic peptide presented by major histocompatibility complex molecules and a non-specific signal (co-stimulation) mediated by the interaction of CD28 with B7 family members (CD80, CD86) expressed on antigen-presenting cells [3]. Cytotoxic T lymphocyte-associated antigen 4 (CTLA-4), a member of the Ig superfamily, is able to bind B7 antigens, as its homologue CD28 [3]. There is evidence that CTLA-4, as distinct from CD28, is a negative regulator of T-cell activation [4]. A native soluble form of CTLA-4 (sCTLA-4), which may have immunoregulatory functions [5,6] has also been described. High serum

Table 1. Characteristics of patients.

	Conventional	Rush	Ultra-rush
N	50	20	24
Male/Female	38/12	11/9	20/4
Mean age (range)	48 (16–74)	45,5 (16–69)	35 (9–66)
Grade of reaction			
I	3	0	2
II	2	5	4
III	26	13	6
IV	19	2	12
VIT *Apis mellifera*	6	9	8
VIT *Polistes spp*	9	2	4
VIT *Vespula spp*	34	8	15
VIT *Vespa Crabro*	1	1	1

concentrations of sCTLA-4 have been detected in patients with various disorders, including autoimmune thyroid diseases, celiac disease and allergic asthma [6–8]. In addition, we have recently shown that sCTLA-4 is elevated in the serum of hymenoptera allergic patients, and decreases after venom immunotherapy (VIT) [9]. In this sense, sCTLA-4 can be regarded as a hallmark of the immunological effect of VIT.

VIT can be given according to different regimens, which essentially differ in the duration of the induction phase. In the classical protocols (often defined conventional or modified rush), the build-up lasts 6 weeks or more, whereas in rush regimens the maintenance dose is achieved in 3 days or less. All those protocols are similarly effective, but there is no evidence on the timing of the immunological changes according to the induction. Based on this background, we assessed and compared the changes in sCTLA-4 induced by different regimens of VIT. Serum IL-10 was also studied in parallel.

Methods

Patients diagnosed as having HVA, and undergoing different VIT protocols, were studied. Blood samples were collected as per routine procedures, and sCTLA-4 and IL-10 were measured at baseline and immediately after the termination of the induction phase of VIT. In a subgroup of patients, the assays were repeated after 12 months of VIT maintenance. The study is observational, and all the procedures are part of the standard clinical practice in HVA. Therefore the study was simply notified to the Ethical Committees of the participating centres, each using its approved induction protocol, according to the Italian law. The Ethical Committee approved the study. All patients (and parents in the case of minors) signed a written informed consent for the treatment of their personal data, for the diagnostic procedure and for the vaccination, according to our routine practice.

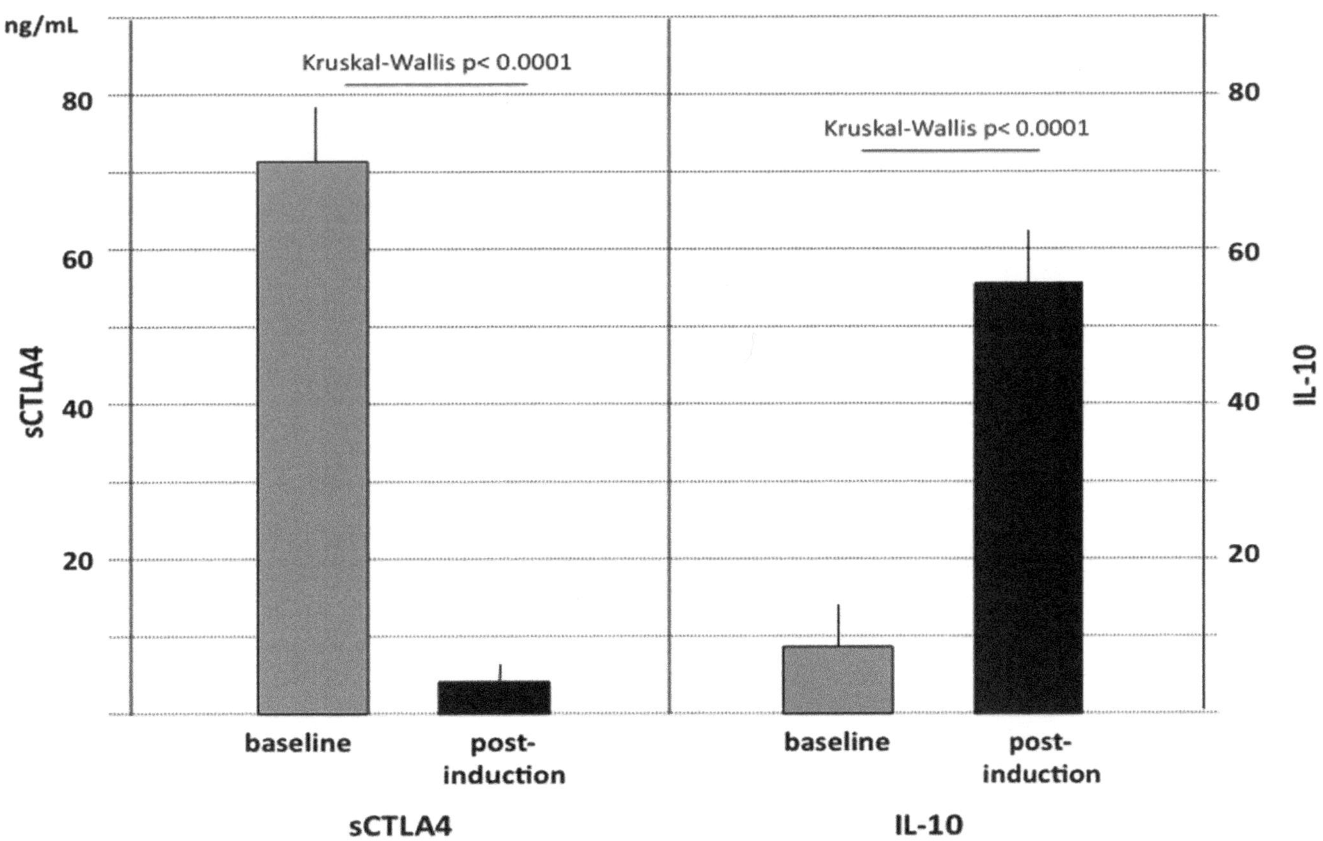

Figure 1. Serum CTLA4 (left) and IL-10 (right) at baseline and at the end of VIT induction phase in the whole population. Values are expressed as mean and SD. Kruskal-Wallis comparisons are also shown.

Patients and Diagnosis

Ninety-four patients with HVA were included in this study. The diagnosis of HVA was made according to current guidelines [10], and all centres used the same diagnostic procedures. Prick tests were performed at increasing concentrations from 0.01 to 100 µg/mL, and intradermal tests involved the injection of 0.02 mL extract at 0.001 to 1 µg/mL concentrations. The tests were carried out with *Apis mellifera, Vespula species* (Stallergènes, Milan, Italy), *Polistes dominulus* and *Vespa crabro* (Anallergo, Florence, Italy). The Cap-RAST assay was performed with the same venoms.

VIT Protocols

The patients were prescribed with VIT for the responsible venom, but with different induction protocols as follows: a) conventional, b) rush, c) ultra-rush. The conventional induction lasted 6 weeks. On Day 1, increasing doses of 0.01, 0.1, 1 and 3 µg were administered. The subsequent doses of 10, 20, 40, 75 and 100 µg were given weekly subdivided in two injections. In the rush protocol the doses were given as follows: 0.01, 0.1, 1 and 3 µg on day 1, 5, 10 and 20 µg on day 2, 30, 35, 35 µg on day 3. Injections were given at 30-minute intervals. The ultra-rush induction lasted 210 minutes. A cumulative dose of 111.1 µg was divided into 6 injections, with an initial dose of 0.1 µg followed by 1, 10 and 20 µg at 30-minute intervals. Then 30 and 40 µg injections were given every 60 minutes. For all protocols the maintenance dose was 100 µg, given at 4–6 week intervals, and the planned duration was 3–5 years as per guidelines.

sCTLA-4 and IL10 Assay

A blood sample was collected at the time of diagnosis (baseline), and immediately after completing the induction phase of immunotherapy. In a subset of patients, blood samples were obtained also after 12 months of maintenance VIT, and in 4 patients receiving the conventional VIT induction, sCTLA4 was measured every week from baseline to week 6. sCTLA-4 was measured by an ELISA kit (Bender Med System, Milano, Italy), according to the manufacturer's instructions. Each sample was diluted 1:10 and tested in triplicate. Deviation within triplicates was <10% for any reported value. The sensitivity threshold was 0.1 ng/mL. The analytical response was linear approximately between 0.162 and 1.200 of absorbance values, corresponding to 0.1–50 ng/mL (data not shown). Serum IL-10 was measured by an ELISA method (Diaclone Research, Besançon, France). The lower sensitivity threshold of the method was 5 pg/mL. Specific IgG4 were assayed by ImmunoCAP Phadia.

Statistical Analysis

The Kruskall-Wallis nonparametric test was used to compare the paired samples, since a normal distribution could not be assumed. A p value <0.05 was considered significant. Nonpara-

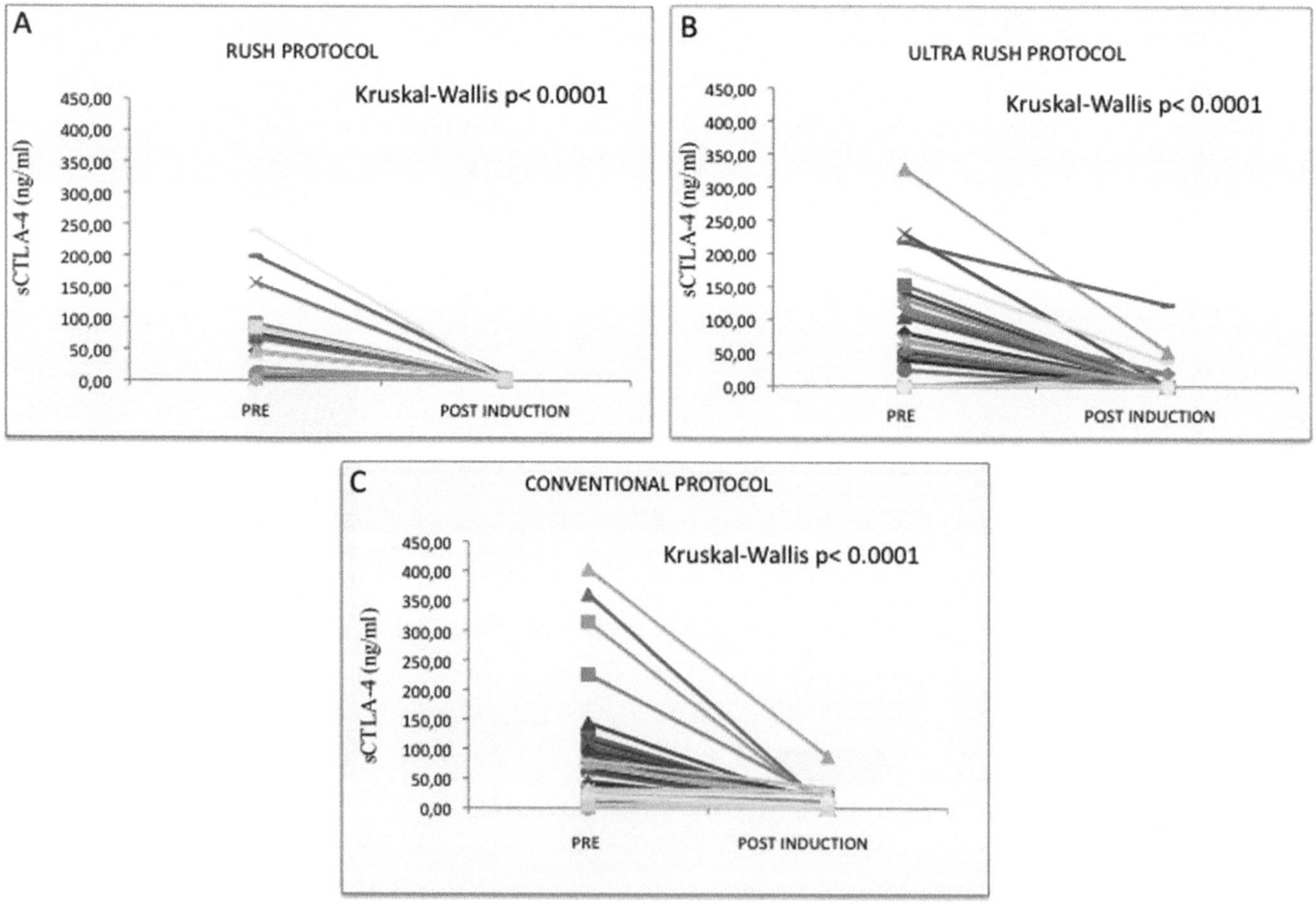

Figure 2. Serum CTLA4 at baseline and at the end of the induction. Three different protocols: rush (Panel A), ultra-rush (panel B) and conventional (panel C).

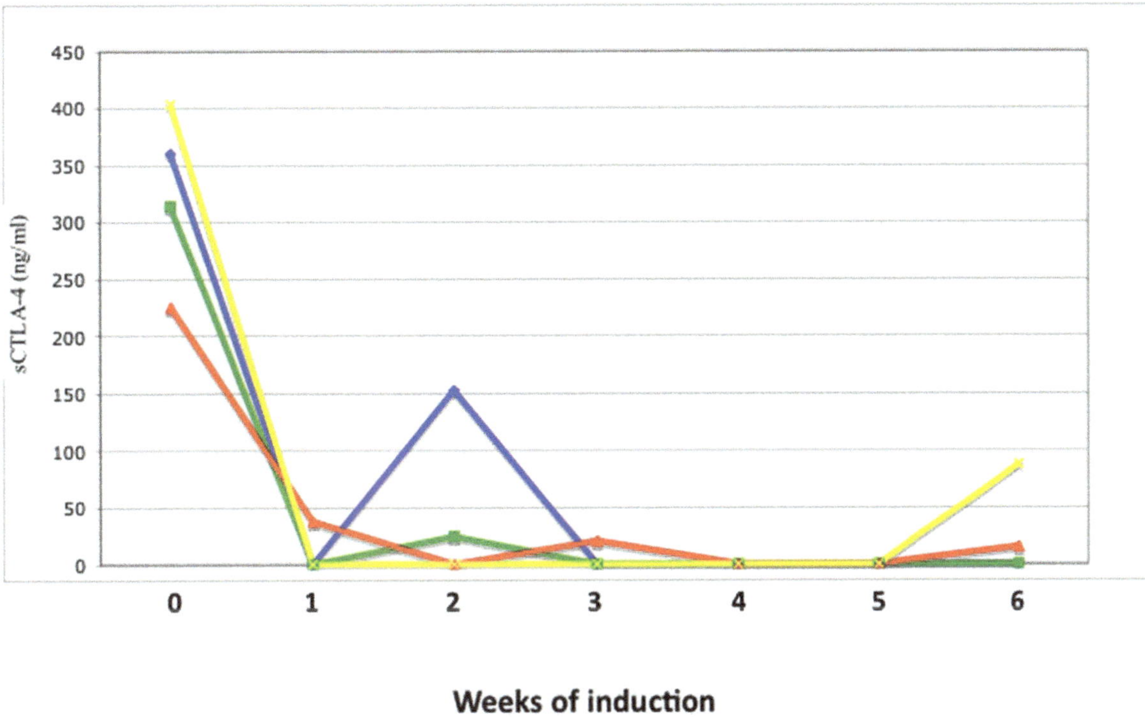

Figure 3. Serum CTLA4 week by week in four patients receiving the conventional 6-week induction.

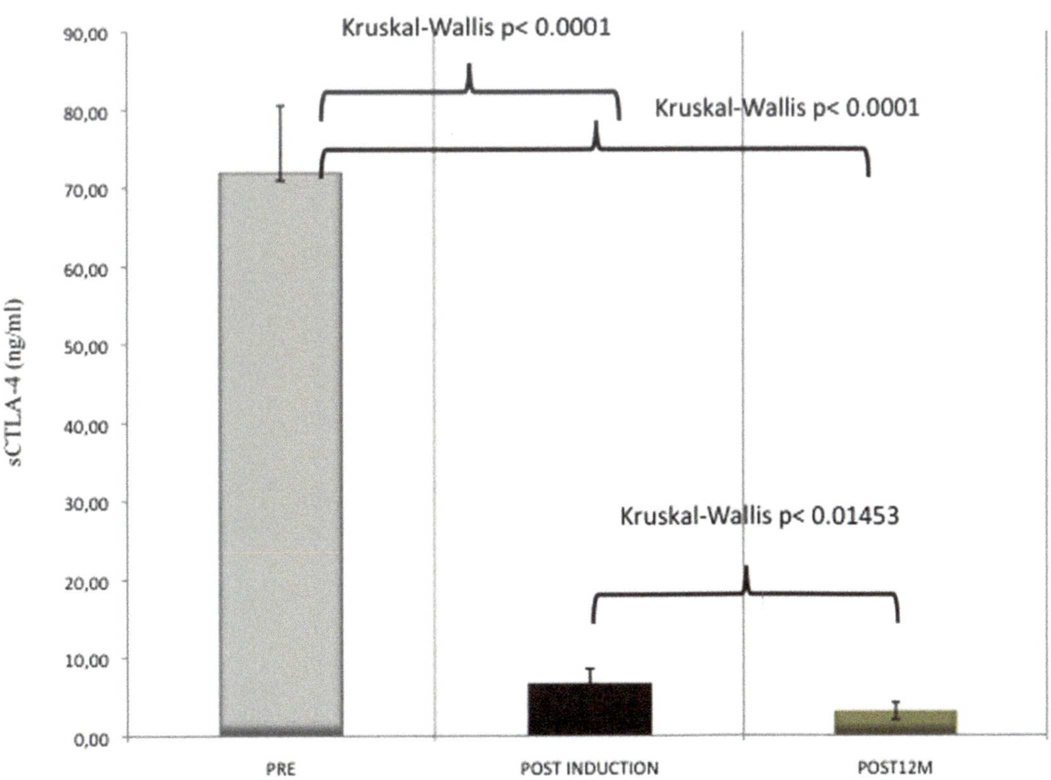

Figure 4. Serum CTLA4 at baseline, at the end of induction phase and after 1 year of VIT (mean, SD, and Kruskal-Wallis comparisons).

metric ANOVA was used to test the differences in % change before versus after induction among groups.

Results

Ninety-four patients (69 male and 25 female, mean age 45, age range 9–74 years) were studied. None of them had a previous history of anaphylaxis due to food or drugs. Fifty subjects received the conventional induction (6 weeks), 20 the rush (3 days), and 24 the ultra-rush (24 hours) regimen. VIT was prescribed for the following venoms: 15 *Polistes*, 61 *Vespula* species, 23 *Apis Mellifera*, 3 *Vespa Crabro*. The main characteristics of the patients in the three groups are summarized in **table 1**. Out of 94 patients, 53 had one or more field re-sting, none during the induction phase. None of those 53 subjects had systemic reactions of grade II or higher, 12 had a grade I reaction and the remaining had only local reactions.

The overall results of sCTLA4 assays before and after the induction phase of VIT are reported in **Figure 1**. According to our previous observations, all patients showed detectable levels of sCTLA4 at baseline, although distributed over a wide range of values. There was no appreciable correlation between baseline sCTLA4 and severity of the reaction. At the end of VIT induction sCTLA4 concentrations sharply decreased, irrespective of the induction protocol used, that is, independently of the duration of the induction phase (**Figure 2**). In fact, sCTLA-4 was significantly reduced as early as 24 hours also in the ultra-rush induction group (Kruskal-Wallis $p<0.001$). The percentage change in sCTLA4 did not differ among the three groups (one way ANOVA: R square 0.0003, $p=0.987$). At the end of the induction phase the serum levels of IL-10 were significantly increased with respect to the baseline values (mean 10,39±2,82 pg/mL VS 57,58±6,10 pg/mL; $p<0.0001$) (**Figure 1**). Also in this case, the increase was apparent at the end of the induction phase whatever the induction protocol (not shown). The percentage change in IL-10 did not differ among the three groups (one way ANOVA: R square 0.025, $p=0.3427$). In the four patients who had sCTLA4 measured week by week, a sharp decrease of sCTLA-4 could be observed starting from the first week (**Figure 3**).

Both sCTLA-4 and IL-10 were measured after 12 months of maintenance VIT in 69 patients. The concentration of sCTLA-4 remained lower than at baseline at post-induction, with a further significant decrease at 12 months of maintenance (Kruskal-Wallis $p=0.015$) (**Figure 4**). On the contrary, the concentration of IL-10 at 12 months returned to baseline levels (mean 10,46±1,74 VS 10,39±2,82 p = ns) (**Figure 5**).

Discussion

CTLA-4 is recognized as a negative regulator of T-cell activation. In fact, the binding of CTLA-4 to the T-cell surface initiates a cascade of biochemical events that attenuates the ongoing immune response [6]. The most convincing data supporting such a role for CTLA-4 come from experiments in knockout mice where the *CTLA-4* gene is inactivated [11]. These mice display severe polyclonal lymphoproliferative disorders that infiltrate most organs, and die in a few weeks. CTLA-4 may play a role also in atopy, where the activation of T cells is crucial for the regulation of the immune response [12,13]. Since CTLA-4 can be present as a native soluble form in the serum, and sCTLA-4 is able to bind its ligands and displays functional activities [5,6], we previously assessed its behaviour in a pure IgE mediated disease such as HVA [9]. We showed that sCTLA-4 was increased in all patients with HVA, but not in respiratory allergy or in healthy subjects. Of note, the role of sCTLA-4 is not well ascertained in respiratory allergy, as demonstrated by controversial results [14–16]. On the other hand, CTLA-4 appears to be consistently elevated in HVA and sharply decreased after the induction phase of VIT. This reduction parallels the increase in IL-10 [9]. As such,

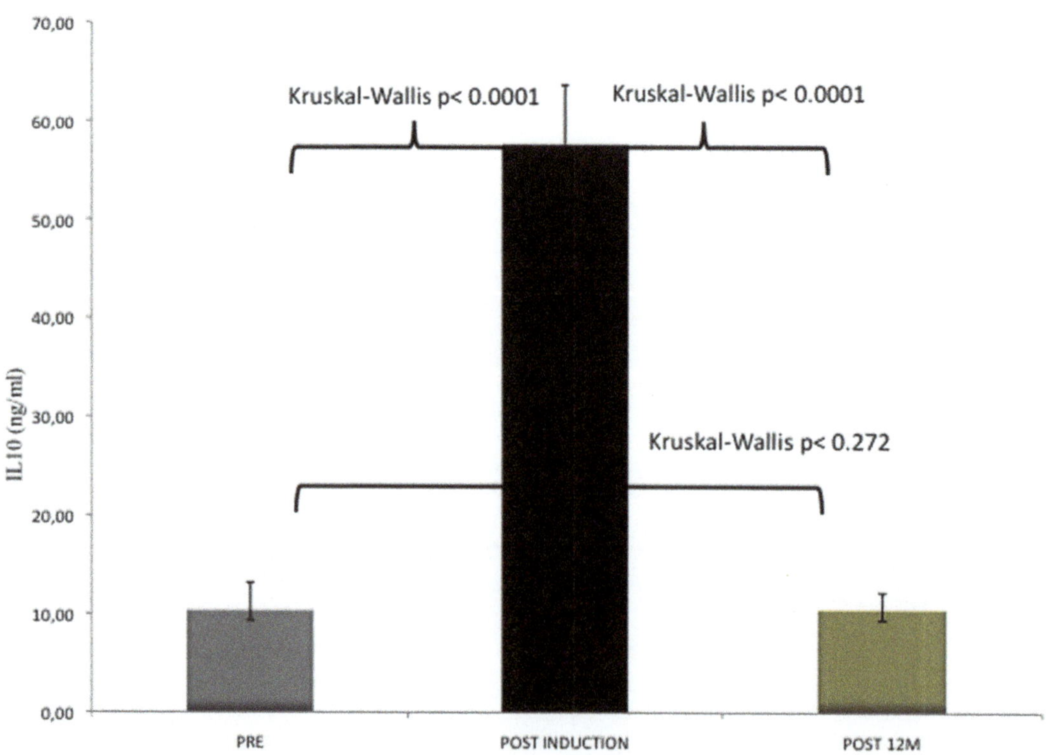

Figure 5. Serum IL-10 at baseline, at the end of induction phase and after 1 year of VIT (mean, SD, Kruskal-Wallis comparison).

serum sCTLA-4 seems to discriminate patients with HVA with respect to healthy subjects and patients with allergic respiratory diseases. In the present study we aimed at assessing if the duration of the VIT induction phase influences the behavior of circulating sCTLA-4, and if there are modifications on the long-term. We observed that the decrease in CTLA-4 is a very early phenomenon that occurs immediately after induction whatever the induction protocol: the faster was the induction, the earlier sCTLA4 decrease. The magnitude of decrease seems to be merely related to the amount of allergen administered, without any relationship with induction timing. Long-term follow-up demonstrated that sCTLA4 concentrations remained low as long as 12 months after starting VIT. Of note, the changes in IL-10 are very early, within 24 hours. On the other hand IL-10 returned to baseline level after one year, thus suggesting that this cytokine intervenes only in the early phases of specific immunotherapy [17], whereas sCTLA4 testifies for the persistence of the immunologic effects of vaccination.

Thus, although the two phenomena (sCTLA4 decrease and IL10 rise) occur abruptly and nearly simultaneously, they are not strictly dependent between each other, in other words, sustained IL10 secretion is not required to maintain low sCTLA4 levels in serum. This is perhaps not surprising, since it is well conceivable that other cytokines/regulatory signals play some role. It is worth noting, in addition, that IL10 secretion following VIT is likely due to different cell types (T-cells and monocytes) with different timing and kinetics [18,19]. In any case, we hypothesize that sCTLA4 reduction may reflect subsiding of sustained T-cell activation in patients under VIT maintenance. It is conceivable that production of sCTLA4 primarily depends upon T- cell activation (irrespective to their specificity or cytokine secretion capability), and that sCTLA4, which proved to be a functional molecule, plays a role in perpetuating the activation state of T-cells by interfering with negative signalling through membrane CTLA4 [6]. Thus, VIT, that is expected to redirect the immune response to the allergen(s), results in stable reduction of sustained activation state of T-cells. Of note, it is possible that sCTLA4 also derives from cell types other than T-lymphocytes; in addition and more importantly, as previously discussed [6] the interaction of sCTLA4 with resting T-cells may act in an inhibitory way, by interfering with stimulatory signalling through membrane CD28 expressed by resting T-cells.

In conclusion, serum sCTLA4 reduction following VIT induction, whatever the protocol used, is a very early marker of VIT effectiveness, and it is possible to envisage that the persistence of low sCTLA4 levels indicates sustained protection against clinical reactions to field-resting.

Author Contributions

Conceived and designed the experiments: AMR DS GP MB GP GWC. Performed the experiments: AMR DS GP MB AR MS PB ER MM. Analyzed the data: AMR DS GP MB GP GWC AR MS PB ER MM. Contributed reagents/materials/analysis tools: AR MS PB ER MM. Wrote the paper: AMR DS GP MB GP GWC AR MS PB ER MM.

References

1. Romagnani S (2006) Regulation of the T cell response. Clin Exp Allergy 36: 1357–1366.
2. Palomares O, Yaman G, Azkur AK, Akkoc T, Akdis M, et al. (2010) Role of Treg in immune regulation of allergic diseases. Eur J Immunol. 40: 1232–40.
3. Linsley PS, Brady W, Urnes M, Grosmaire LS, Damle K, et al. (1991) CTLA-4 is a second receptor for the B cell activation antigen B7. J Exp Med 174: 561–569.
4. Thompson B, Allison JP (1997) The emerging role of CTLA-4 as an immune attenuator. Immunity 7: 445–450.
5. Burr JS, Kimzey SL, Randolph DR, Green JM (2001) CD28 and CTLA-4 coordinately regulate airway inflammatory cell recruitment and T-helper cell differentiation after inhaled allergen. Am J Respir Cell Mol Biol 24:563–568.
6. Oaks MK, Hallett KM (2000) A soluble form of CTLA-4 in patients with autoimmune thyroid disease, J Immunol 164: 5015–5018.
7. Saverino D, Brizzolara R, Simone R, Chiappori A, Milintenda Floriani F, et al. (2007) Soluble CTLA-4 in autoimmune thyroid diseases: Relationship with clinical status and possible role in the immune response dysregulation. Clin Immunol 123: 190–198.
8. Wong CK, Lun SWM, Ko FWS, Ip WK, Hui DS (2005) Increased expression of plasma and cell surface co-stimulatory molecules CTLA-4, CD28 and CD86 in adult patients with allergic asthma. Clin Exp Immunol 141: 122–129.
9. Saverino D, Riccio AM, Rogkakou A, Bagnasco M, Bonadonna P, et al. (2009) Serum cytotoxic T lymphocyte-associated antigen 4 in Hymenoptera venom allergy and its modulation by specific immunotherapy J Allergy Clin Immunol. 123: 258–60.
10. Bilò MB, Rueff F, Mosbech H, Bonifazi F, Oude-Elberinck A (2005) The EAACI interest group on insect venom hypersensitivity. Diagnosis of Hymenoptera venom allergy. Allergy 60:1339–49.
11. Waterhouse P, Penninger JM, Timms E (1995) Lymphoproliferative disorders with early lethality in mice deficient in CTLA-4. Science 270: 985–988.
12. Perez VL, Van Parijs L, Biuckians A (1997) Induction of peripheral T cell tolerance in vivo requires CTLA-4 engagement. Immunity 6:411–417.
13. Keane-Myers A, Gause WC, Linsley PS (1997) B7-CD28/CTLA-4 costimulatory pathways are required for the development of T helper cell 2-mediated allergic airway responses to inhaled antigens. J Immunol 158:2042–2049.
14. Jasek M, Łuszczek W, Obojski A, Winiarska B, Hałubek K, et al. (2006) Distribution of CTLA-4 polymorphisms in allergic asthma. Int Arch Allergy Immunol.141: 223–9.
15. Ip WK, Wong CK, Leung TF, Lam CW (2006) Plasma concentrations of soluble CTLA-4, CD28, CD80 and CD86 costimulatory molecules reflect disease severity of acute asthma in children. Pediatr Pulmonol. 41: 674–82.
16. Kawayama T, Kinoshita T, Imaoka H, Gauvreau GM, O'Byrne PM, et al. (2008) Effects of inhaled fluticasone propionate on CTLA-4-positive CD4+CD25+ cells in induced sputum in mild asthmatics. Respirology. 13: 1000–1007.
17. Akdis CA, Akdis M (2011) Mechanisms of allergen specific immunotherapy J Allergy Clin Immunol. 127: 18–27;
18. Dreschler K, Bratke K, Petermann S, Bier A, Thamm P, et al. (2011) Impact of immunotherapy on blood dendritic cells in patients with Hymenoptera venom allergy ImmunotherapyJ Allergy Clin Immunol. 127 (2):487–494.
19. Bussmann C, Xia J, Allam JP, Maintz L, Bieber T, et al. (2010) Early markers for protective mechanisms during rush venom immunotherapy Allergy. 65(12):1558–65.

12

Sensitization to Food and Inhalant Allergens in Relation to Atopic Diseases in Early Childhood: A Birth Cohort Study

Chih-Yung Chiu[1,2,3], Yu-Lin Huang[2,4], Ming-Han Tsai[1,2], Yu-Ling Tu[2,4], Man-Chin Hua[1,2], Tsung-Chieh Yao[2,4], Kuo-Wei Yeh[2,4*], Jing-Long Huang[2,4*]

1 Department of Pediatrics, Chang Gung Memorial Hospital, Keelung, Taiwan, **2** Community Medicine Research Centre, Chang Gung Memorial Hospital, Keelung, Taiwan, **3** Division of Pediatric Pulmonology, Chang Gung Memorial Hospital, College of Medicine, Chang Gung University, Taoyuan, Taiwan, **4** Division of Allergy, Asthma, and Rheumatology, Department of Pediatrics, Chang Gung Memorial Hospital, and Chang Gung University College of Medicine, Taoyuan, Taiwan

Abstract

Objectives: A correct interpretation of sensitization to common allergens is critical in determining susceptibility to allergic diseases. The aim of this study was to investigate the patterns of sensitization to food and inhalant allergens, and their relation to the development of atopic diseases in early childhood.

Methods: Children aged 0 through 4 years from a birth cohort in the Prediction of Allergies in Taiwanese Children (PATCH) study were enrolled. Specific IgE antibody against food and inhalant allergens were measured and their association between total serum IgE levels and atopic diseases were assessed.

Results: A total of 182 children were regular followed up at clinics for a four-year follow-up period. The prevalence of food allergen sensitization increased markedly after 6 months of age, reaching up to 47% at 1.5 years of age and then declined significantly to 10% in parallel with a considerable increase in the prevalence of sensitization to inhalant allergens up to 25% at age 4. Food allergen sensitization appeared to be mainly associated with the elevation of serum total IgE levels before age 2. A combined sensitization to food and inhalant allergens had an additive effect on serum IgE levels after age 2, and was significantly associated with the risk of developing atopic diseases at age 4.

Conclusions: Sensitization to food occurs early in life, in parallel with the rising prevalence of sensitization to inhalant allergens at older age. A combined sensitization to food and inhalant allergens not only has an additive increase in serum IgE antibody production but also increases the risk of developing allergic respiratory diseases in early childhood.

Editor: Nades Palaniyar, The Hospital for Sick Children and The University of Toronto, Canada

Funding: This work was supported by CMRPG2B0050-52 from the Chang Gung Medical foundation, Chang Gung University, Taiwan. The funders had no role in study design, data collection and analysis, decision to publish, or preparation of the manuscript.

Competing Interests: The authors have declared that no competing interests exist.

* Email: kwyeh@adm.cgmh.org.tw (KWY); long@adm.cgmh.org.tw (JLH)

These authors contributed equally to this work.

Introduction

The prevalence of atopic diseases in childhood has significantly been increasing in the past few decades [1–3]. As the prevalence of atopic diseases in the population increases, early identification of atopic children is desirable. Potential predictors for atopic diseases in childhood or later in life have been studied widely [4,5]. Early sensitization to allergens has consistently been identified as a risk factor for developing allergic respiratory diseases [6]. Assessment of allergen sensitization therefore is considered to be important in diagnosing and managing atopic diseases throughout childhood [7]. However, the interpretation of allergen sensitization and its clinical application in children sensitized to various allergens is challenging.

Allergic sensitization in infancy generally occurs first to food allergens. As children grow older, the majority of sensitization is directed against inhalant allergens [8]. Long-lasting sensitization to food allergens during the first two years of life has been regarded as a major risk factor for the development of allergic airway diseases [6]. In early childhood, the relationship between specific sensitization to food and inhalant allergens and their relevance to the occurrence of atopic diseases however has not been well determined.

Immunoglobulin E (IgE) is a critical component of allergic diseases. Although several studies have shown an association between the prevalence of atopic diseases and total serum immunoglobulin E (IgE) levels, total serum IgE levels are most useful in screening for atopic predisposition, rather than in the diagnosis or management of atopic diseases [9–11]. However, a moderate amount of specific IgE to a particular allergen may have much greater significance for a relatively lower total IgE levels [12]. Allergen-specific IgE antibodies also provide useful serological information in the differential diagnosis on IgE-mediated atopic diseases in young children with allergy-like symptoms [13]. Some persons with significant allergy problems can have normal, moderately or strongly elevated IgE levels. Although an elevated IgE level is associated with an increased risk of atopic diseases, the impact of sensitization to different allergens on the total serum IgE levels and the development of allergic diseases is still not well-defined.

The aim of this study was to determine sensitization to most common food and inhalant allergens in children aged 0 through 4 years from a birth cohort in the Prediction of Allergies in Taiwanese Children (PATCH) study. The patterns of sensitization to different allergens were assessed, and their relationship between total serum IgE levels and the development of atopic diseases were also examined.

Materials and Methods

Study Population

The Prediction of Allergies in Taiwanese Children (PATCH) study is a population-based birth cohort study initiated in 2007 to investigate the epidemiology and predictive factors of asthma and allergies in Taiwanese children. New born babies delivered at Chang Gung Memorial Hospital (CGMH), Keelung from October 1, 2007 to September 30, 2010 were recruited voluntarily and followed-up until the age of 4 years. Neonates born at more than 34 weeks of gestation with birth weight ≥2500 g were enrolled. Infants with any perinatal insult, significant neonatal respiratory difficulties, or congenital anomalies were excluded. Subjects who dropped out during the follow-up period were likewise excluded. This study was approved by the Ethic Committee of Chang Gung Memory Hospital (No. 100-0201B). Informed written consent was obtained from the parents of all study subjects.

Data Collection

The parents of enrolled subjects were invited and underwent a standardized interview conducted by well-trained investigators for answering a questionnaire at birth and at 1, 2, 3 and 4 years of follow-up. The questionnaire was derived from the well-validated International Study of Asthma and Allergies in Childhood (ISAAC) questionnaire [14]. The details of information regarding demographic data, family atopy history and the health care of children including medical conditions were collected. Detailed questionnaire in regard to clinical symptoms and diagnosis of allergic diseases were also collected.

Evaluation and Diagnosis of Atopic Diseases

The atopic diseases of childhood consist of atopic dermatitis, allergic rhinitis, and asthma. Information of current and past allergic symptoms for the diagnosis of atopic diseases was obtained from the validated ISAAC questionnaire [14]. Specific questions related to the development of allergic/atopic diseases and symptoms were also inquired and evaluated by a pediatric pulmonologist at outpatient clinics. Eczema was diagnosed as a pruritic rash over the face and/or extensors with a chronic relapsing course as described by Hanifin and Rajka [15]. Rhinitis was diagnosed as ever having the symptoms representing rhinitis such as sneezing, nasal congestion, itching, rhinorrhea or current use of medication for these symptoms [16]. Asthma was diagnosed as ever having asthma with the occurrence of wheeze or current use of asthma medication.

Total and Allergen-Specific Serum Immunoglobulin E

Serum samples were collected and measured at 6 months, and 1, 1.5, 2, 3 and 4 years of age. The serum level of total IgE was measured by ImmunoCAP (Phadia, Uppsala, Sweden). Specific IgE was determined by a commercial assay for IgE (ImmunoCAP Phadiatop Infant; Phadia) against food and inhalant allergens. Egg and milk allergy are the most prevalent food allergies in infant and young Asian children [17]. In addition to egg and cow's milk, wheat based supplementary food is most commonly supplied for young children in Taiwan. In contrast, *D. pteronyssinus* and *D. farina* are the two most common inhalant allergens causing sensitization in more than 95% of children in Taiwan [18]. In addition, molds are ubiquitously present in homes because of the warm and humid subtropical climate in Taiwan and *C. herbarum* is the most prevalent species [19]. Specific IgE antibody testing therefore included a mix of three most common food allergens (egg white, milk and wheat) and three most common inhalant allergens (*D. pteronyssinus*, *D. farina* and *C. herbarum*). The cut-off values for each ImmunoCAP Phadiatop Infant class 0, 1, 2, 3 and >3 are 0, 0.35, 0.7, 3.5 and ≥17.5 kU/L, respectively. Values of ImmunoCAP Phadiatop Infant of ≥0.35 kU/L (≥ class 1) were considered indicative of allergic sensitisation [10,20].

Statistical Analysis

Demographic data of population characteristics obtained by questionnaire and the prevalence of physician-diagnosed atopic diseases were collected and analysed. The Student t test was used to compare continuous variables, and the χ^2 or Fisher exact test was used to compare the nominal data. Differences between continuous variables with non-normal distribution were estimated with the Mann-Whitney test. The association of atopic diseases measured as a binary outcome with sensitization to food or inhalant allergens was calculated by the odds ratio (OR), using standard methods of logistic regression analysis. Statistical analysis was performed by using the Statistical Program for Social Sciences (IBM SPSS Statistics for Windows, Version 20.0. Armonk, NY: IBM) and graphs were drawn using GraphPad Prism Version 5.01 software (GraphPad Software Inc, California, USA). All statistical hypothesis tests were two tailed and a P value of less than 0.05 was considered to be significant.

Results

Population Characteristics

A total of 258 children who fulfilled the inclusion criteria were voluntarily enrolled; 226 (87.6%), 210 (81.4%), 198 (76.7%) and 182 (70.5%) children were regular followed up at clinics for a one, two, three and four year follow-up respectively. The major reasons for dropout were the fear of blood drawing and parents' unwillingness of regular outpatient follow-up. Blood test for allergies was performed in 138 children at age 1, 109 children at age 2, 102 children at age 3 and 91 children at age 4. Atopic diseases including eczema, rhinitis and asthma were diagnosed in 20, 58 and 26 children, respectively, at 4 years of age (Fig. 1).

Prevalence of Sensitization to Food and Inhalant Allergens

Allergen-specific serum IgE for food and inhalant allergens was measured at 6 months, and 1, 1.5, 2, 3 and 4 years of age during follow-up. In food sensitization, the sensitization patterns of milk and egg white were similar. The prevalence of sensitization to milk

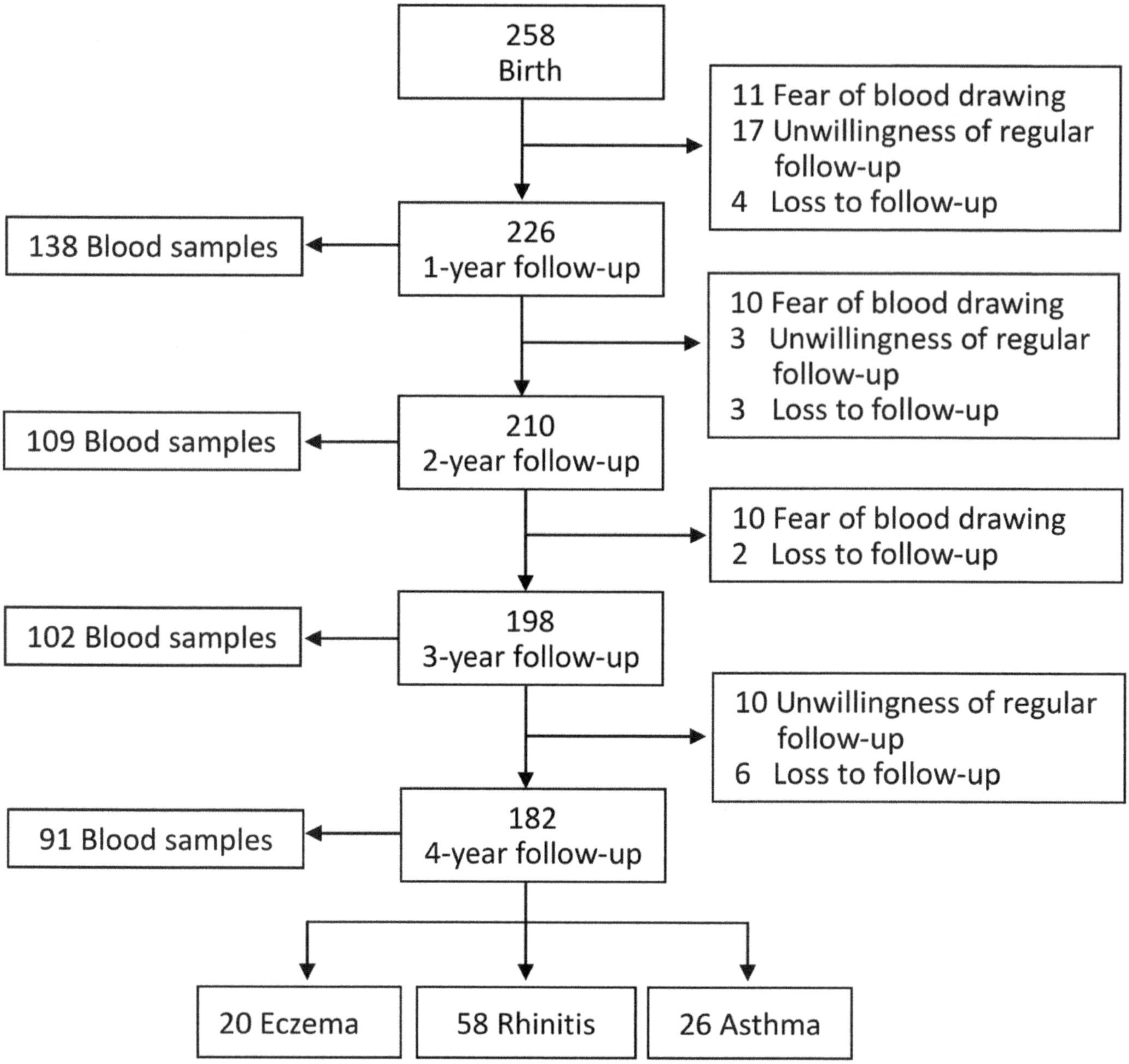

Figure 1. Schematic presentation of the recruitment process of the study subjects.

and egg white allergens increased with increasing age until 1.5 years of age. By contrast, the prevalence of sensitization to wheat allergen was persistent low with approximately only 5%. Sensitization patterns to food and inhalant allergens are shown in Fig. 2. The prevalence of all food allergen sensitization increased markedly after 6 months of age and reached up to 47% at 1.5 years of age. In contrast, the prevalence of sensitization to inhalant allergens was only 5% at age 2, but increased markedly after 2 years of age. At 4 years of age, the prevalence of sensitization to food allergens declined significantly to 10% but there was a considerable increase in the prevalence of sensitization to inhalant allergens up to 25%. Furthermore, the prevalence of a combined sensitization to food and inhalant allergens showed to be increased gradually with increasing age, from 3% at 6-month-old to 26% at 4-year-old. Moreover, approximately fifty percent of the food-sensitized children at different ages had become sensitized to aeroallergens simultaneously at 4 years of age.

Association between Food, Inhalant Allergen Sensitization and Serum IgE Levels

Fig. 3 shows the changes of total serum IgE levels in children with sensitization to food and inhalant allergens at different years of age. In children with food allergen sensitization, the total serum IgE levels appeared to be decreased with increasing age after age 1. In contrast, serum IgE levels showed to be increased gradually in children with inhalant allergen sensitization after age 2. In comparison to children with inhalant allergen sensitization, a significantly higher serum IgE level was found in children with food allergen sensitization at age 1 and 1.5. However, a statistically significant increase in serum IgE level was found in children with a

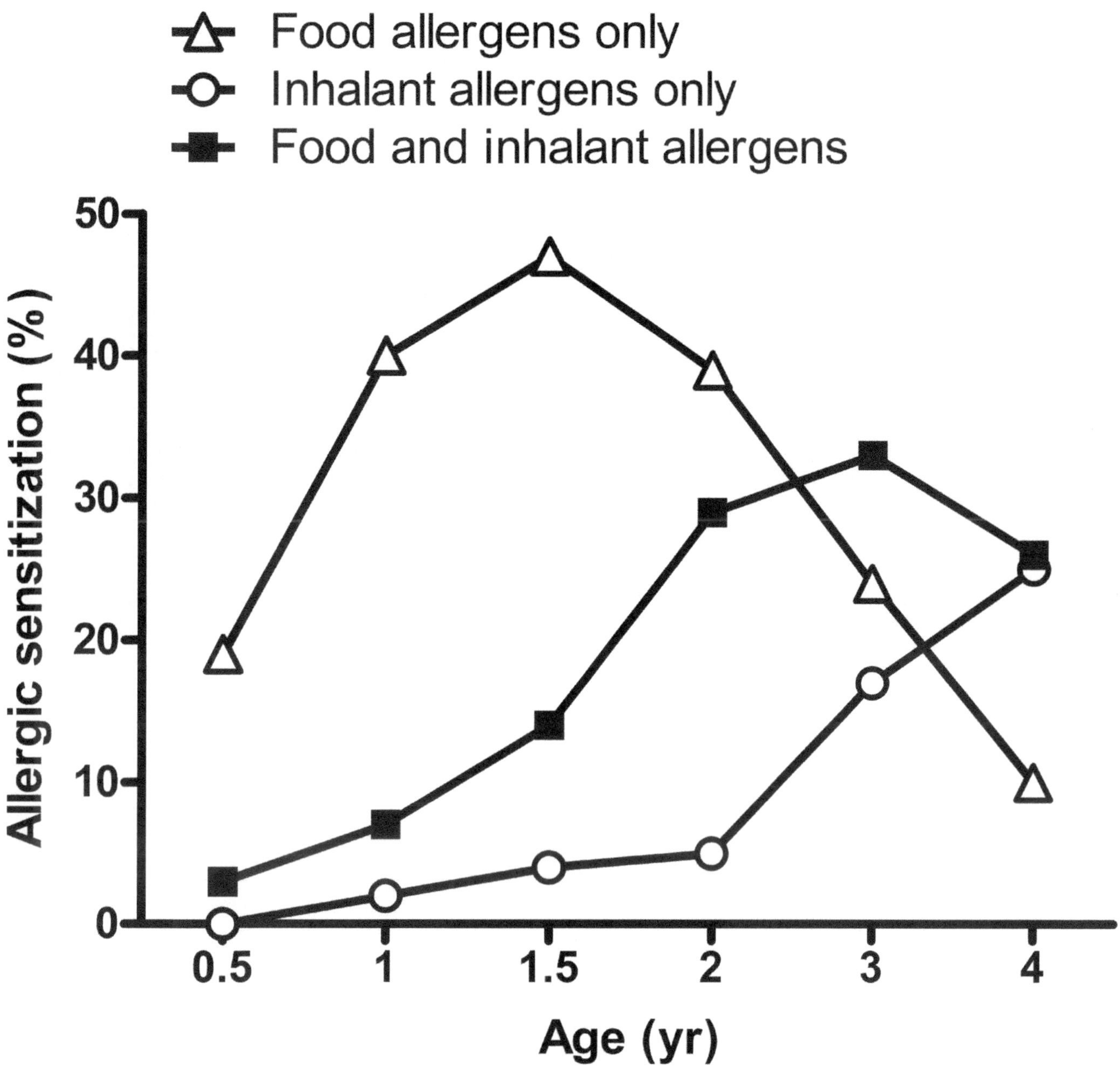

Figure 2. Sensitization patterns to food and inhalant allergens from age 0 to age 4.

combined sensitization to food and inhalant allergens with an addition effect after age 2.

Association between Food, Inhalant Allergen Sensitization and Atopic Diseases

Table 1 presents the relationships between food, inhalant allergen sensitization and risk of atopic diseases by the age of 4 years. At 6 months of age, sensitization to food allergens, only egg white but not milk or wheat, showed a statistically significant risk in association with atopic diseases including eczema, rhinitis and asthma at age 4. In contrast, there was a significant increased risk for developing asthma and rhinitis but not eczema in children with sensitization to inhalant allergens after age 1 and age 2, respectively. A combined sensitization to food and inhalant allergens showed a significant risk in relation to all three atopic diseases before age 2 but it appeared to be more specific to rhinitis and asthma after age 2.

Discussion

Atopic diseases are among the most common chronic disorders of childhood. In young children, the diagnosis of atopic diseases is mainly based on clinical evaluation. Although assessment of allergen-specific IgE antibodies provides helpful information to the clinician, a correct interpretation of sensitization to common allergens is critical in determining susceptibility to allergic diseases. In this study, the prevalence of sensitization to food allergens appeared to occur and increase in early infancy as in previous publication [6]. However, it declined significantly after age 2 and there was concomitantly a compensatory increase in the preva-

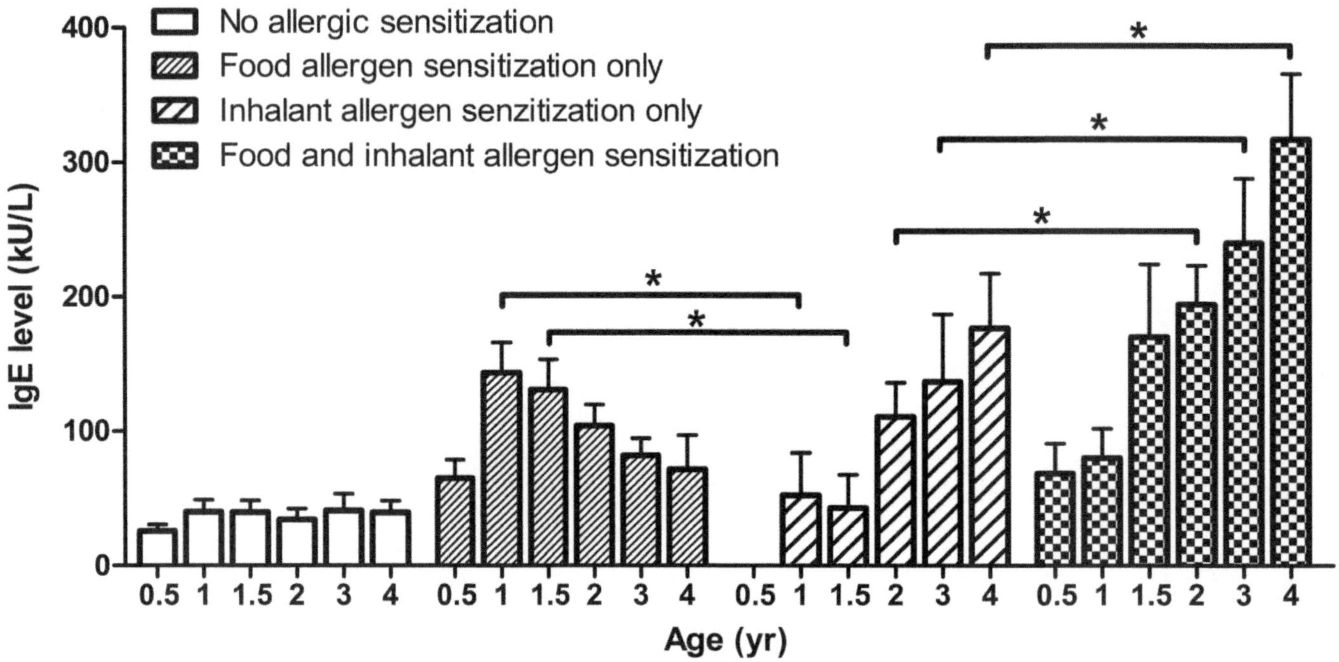

Figure 3. Changes of total serum IgE levels in children with sensitization to food and inhalant allergens at different years of age. Data shown are mean ± SEM. *P* values refer to the comparisons indicated by the marker. $^{*}P<0.05$.

lence of sensitization to inhalant allergens [21]. Most importantly, the prevalence of a combined sensitization to food and inhalant allergens showed to be increased with increasing age. These findings indicate that changes in sensitization to food and inhalant allergens varies with age in early childhood, which may play an important role in allergic response and the development of atopic disorders.

An allergic reaction occurs when the immune system overreacts to the allergen by producing IgE antibodies. IgE is a type of antibody that is present in minute amounts in the body but plays a major role in allergic diseases [22]. In this study, the changes of serum IgE levels were consistent with the sensitization patterns to food and inhalant allergens in relation to age. A high prevalence of sensitization to food allergens and a significantly elevated IgE levels in children with food allergen sensitization at age 1 and 1.5 indicates that food allergen sensitization may mainly be associated with the elevation of serum IgE levels before the age of 2. With the decline in the IgE levels induced by food allergen sensitization, the prevalence of sensitization to inhalant allergens increased after age 2 and an additive increase in serum IgE levels was in parallel with an increase in the prevalence of a combined sensitization to food and inhalant allergens, indicating that sensitization to inhalant allergens may play an important role in allergic responses after age 2. Clinically, total serum IgE levels have shown to be associated with the severity of allergies among young children [23]. In this study, the total serum IgE values was strongly associated with the striking cosensitization between food and inhalant allergens, suggesting that increased IgE levels induced by multiple allergen sensitizations may contribute to a severe allergic response and increase a risk for developing atopic diseases [24].

Sensitization to allergens has been recognized as the most important risk factor for atopic diseases. Many studies have suggested that the occurrence and severity of symptoms in later childhood are directly related to allergen sensitization in infancy [6,25]. Sensitization to food allergens is more common in early life and has been thought to be a significant factor for infantile eczema as in this study [6,26]. However, approximately half of young infants with food allergen sensitization were more likely to be allergic to inhalant allergens, and were at increased risk for developing respiratory allergic diseases by the age of 4 years. Furthermore, egg sensitization in infancy was associated the most strongly with the development of atopic diseases. These findings support the previous report that the presence of egg-specific IgE antibodies constitutes the earliest marker of atopy [21]. Filaggrin gene defects are strongly associated with atopic eczema [27]. Furthermore, the increased skin permeability may increase the risk of sensitization to food and other allergens, and the risk of developing atopic diseases [28]. An infant with a genetic predisposition has been reported to develop antibodies to foods at a very early age, mostly to egg white and milk [29]. Although it has been proposed that exposure to egg proteins occurs via mother's milk due to the lack of egg white in the young infant's diet [30], a genetic susceptibility to allergy may also potentially play an important role in such instances.

The environmental factor has been studied most extensively as a potential risk for allergic sensitization and manifestation of atopy. In sensitized children, early exposure to inhalant allergens not only determines the risk of asthma, but also the time of the onset of the disease [31]. In this study, sensitization to inhalant allergens mainly occurred after age 2 and appeared to be more specific to the development of asthma. This finding may explain why the majority of school-aged asthmatic children have their onset of asthma during the first 2 to 3 years of life [32,33]. Furthermore, food allergen sensitization in infancy not only increased the risk of sensitization to inhalant allergens but also the risk for developing atopic diseases at older age. It must be emphasized that a well recognition and interpretation of the changes in sensitization to food and inhalant allergens in early life may help clinician to predict the occurrence of atopic diseases and determine possible prevention strategies in clinical practice.

Limitations of this study include a relatively small sample size of only 182 case subjects and a limited power to detect a statistically

Table 1. Relationships between food allergen sensitization, inhalant allergen sensitization and risk of atopic diseases by the age of 4 years.

Age (yr)	Allergic sensitization	Eczema		Rhinitis		Asthma	
		OR	95% CI	OR	95% CI	OR	95% CI
0.5	Food allergens only	8.22	(1.72–39.51)*	5.29	(1.41–19.85)*	7.59	(1.75–33.00)*
	Inhalant allergens only	5.33	(0.45–63.22)	1.60	(0.14–18.29)	1.91	(0.11–32.01)
	Food and inhalant allergens	8.22	(0.67–101.03)	2.11	(0.18–24.37)	2.85	(0.17–48.86)
1	Food allergens only	3.00	(0.77–11.65)	1.16	(0.47–2.84)	3.00	(0.86–10.43)
	Inhalant allergens only	3.33	(0.59–18.72)	2.39	(0.58–9.93)	3.56	(0.71–17.79)
	Food and inhalant allergens	6.00	(0.88–40.87)	1.82	(0.39–8.51)	4.80	(0.74–31.08)
1.5	Food allergens only	1.00	(0.25–4.03)	1.82	(0.69–4.81)	9.00	(1.04–78.17)*
	Inhalant allergens only	7.60	(0.57–101.79)	5.18	(0.48–56.09)	38.0	(1.66–870.45)*
	Food and inhalant allergens	7.60	(1.07–54.09)*	8.64	(1.59–46.81)*	57.0	(4.36–744.71)*
2	Food allergens only	1.07	(0.23–5.05)	2.40	(0.81–7.14)	7.47	(0.82–68.10)
	Inhalant allergens only	4.00	(0.20–78.79)	8.00	(0.76–83.88)	48.0	(2.31–997.18)*
	Food and inhalant allergens	5.60	(1.15–27.37)*	8.40	(2.31–30.60)*	38.4	(3.95–373.09)*
3	Food allergens only	1.00	(0.15–6.85)	3.14	(0.85–11.67)	3.00	(0.40–22.30)
	Inhalant allergens only	3.50	(0.59–20.68)	4.50	(1.02–19.90)*	10.5	(1.50–73.67)*
	Food and inhalant allergens	3.50	(0.76–16.12)	6.29	(1.81–21.80)*	10.0	(1.71–58.63)*
4	Food allergens only	2.86	(0.63–12.92)	13.8	(1.18–161.71)*	34.5	(2.35–505.75)*
	Inhalant allergens only	4.38	(0.79–24.45)	4.22	(1.15–15.51)*	9.86	(1.61–60.24)*
	Food and inhalant allergens	6.13	(1.03–36.45)*	13.8	(3.40–55.96)**	13.8	(2.13–89.52)*

yr, year; OR, odds ratio; CI, confidence interval.
*$P<0.05$;
**$P<0.001$.

significant association for subanalyses. A 4-year follow-up in this birth cohort study may not predict whether children with allergic sensitization will develop atopic diseases in later years. The strength of the present study lies in its longitudinal design, allowing sequential and concurrent measurements of serum total IgE, allergen-specific IgE for allergic sensitization and the accurate diagnostic evaluations for atopic diseases at outpatient clinics. Although a larger and longer study may be needed to confirm the findings presented in this study, this birth cohort study has demonstrated the importance of allergic sensitization patterns in developing atopic diseases in early childhood.

In conclusion, sensitization to food is mostly common in early life, in parallel with the rising prevalence of sensitization to inhalant allergens at older age. Serum total IgE levels appear to be associated with the response to different types of allergens. Sensitization to food, especially egg white is highly related to eczema, whereas sensitization to inhalant allergens appears to be more specific to the development of rhinitis and asthma. A combined sensitization to food and inhalant allergens not only has an additive effect on serum IgE antibody production but also increases the risk of developing atopic diseases. A fully understanding of the prevalence of allergen sensitization in different age would help early diagnosis and intervention of atopic diseases in early childhood.

Acknowledgments

We are extremely grateful to all the families who took part in this study, all pediatricians for their help in recruiting them and the whole PATCH team, which includes interviewers, nurses, computer and laboratory technicians and research assistants.

Author Contributions

Conceived and designed the experiments: CYC KWY JLH. Performed the experiments: MHT YLT MCH TCY. Analyzed the data: CYC YLH. Contributed reagents/materials/analysis tools: YLH. Contributed to the writing of the manuscript: CYC KWY JLH.

References

1. Bousquet J (2002) Allergy as a global problem: 'think globally, act globally'. Allergy 57: 661–662.
2. Downs SH, Marks GB, Sporik R, Belosouva EG, Car NG, et al. (2001) Continued increase in the prevalence of asthma and atopy. Arch Dis Child 84: 20–23.
3. Law M, Morris JK, Wald N, Luczynska C, Burney P (2005) Changes in atopy over a quarter of a century, based on cross sectional data at three time periods. BMJ 330: 1187–1188.
4. Moore MM, Rifas-Shiman SL, Rich-Edwards JW, Kleinman KP, Camargo CA Jr, et al. (2004) Perinatal predictors of atopic dermatitis occurring in the first six months of life. Pediatrics 113: 468–474.
5. Szefler SJ, Wenzel S, Brown R, Erzurum SC, Fahy JV, et al. (2012) Asthma outcomes: biomarkers. J Allergy Clin Immunol 129: S9–23.
6. Kulig M, Bergmann R, Tacke U, Wahn U, Guggenmoos-Holzmann I (1998) Long-lasting sensitization to food during the first two years precedes allergic airway disease. The MAS Study Group, Germany. Pediatr Allergy Immunol 9: 61–67.
7. Host A, Andrae S, Charkin S, Diaz-Vazquez C, Dreborg S, et al. (2003) Allergy testing in children: why, who, when and how? Allergy 58: 559–569.
8. Hattevig G, Kjellman B, Bjorksten B (1993) Appearance of IgE antibodies to ingested and inhaled allergens during the first 12 years of life in atopic and non-atopic children. Pediatr Allergy Immunol 4: 182–186.
9. Satwani H, Rehman A, Ashraf S, Hassan A (2009) Is serum total IgE levels a good predictor of allergies in children? J Pak Med Assoc 59: 698–702.
10. Sunyer J, Anto JM, Castellsague J, Soriano JB, Roca J (1996) Total serum IgE is associated with asthma independently of specific IgE levels. The Spanish Group of the European Study of Asthma. Eur Respir J 9: 1880–1884.
11. Burrows B, Martinez FD, Halonen M, Barbee RA, Cline MG (1989) Association of asthma with serum IgE levels and skin-test reactivity to allergens. N Engl J Med 320: 271–277.
12. Busse W, Kraft M (2005) Cysteinyl leukotrienes in allergic inflammation: strategic target for therapy. Chest 127: 1312–1326.
13. Halvorsen R, Jenner A, Hagelin EM, Borres MP (2009) Phadiatop infant in the diagnosis of atopy in children with allergy-like symptoms. Int J Pediatr 2009: 460737.
14. Asher MI, Keil U, Anderson HR, Beasley R, Crane J, et al. (1995) International Study of Asthma and Allergies in Childhood (ISAAC): rationale and methods. Eur Respir J 8: 483–491.
15. Seymour JL, Keswick BH, Hanifin JM, Jordan WP, Milligan MC (1987) Clinical effects of diaper types on the skin of normal infants and infants with atopic dermatitis. J Am Acad Dermatol 17: 988–997.
16. Togias AG (2000) Systemic immunologic and inflammatory aspects of allergic rhinitis. J Allergy Clin Immunol 106: S247–250.
17. Lee AJ, Thalayasingam M, Lee BW (2013) Food allergy in Asia: how does it compare? Asia Pac Allergy 3: 3–14.
18. Yong SB, Wu CC, Tzeng YC, Hung WC, Yang KD (2013) Different profiles of allergen sensitization in different ages and geographic areas in Changhua, Taiwan. J Microbiol Immunol Infect 46: 295–301.
19. Leung R, Ho P, Lam CW, Lai CK (1997) Sensitization to inhaled allergens as a risk factor for asthma and allergic diseases in Chinese population. J Allergy Clin Immunol 99: 594–599.
20. Ballardini N, Nilsson C, Nilsson M, Lilja G (2006) ImmunoCAP Phadiatop Infant–a new blood test for detecting IgE sensitisation in children at 2 years of age. Allergy 61: 337–343.
21. Kulig M, Bergmann R, Klettke U, Wahn V, Tacke U, et al. (1999) Natural course of sensitization to food and inhalant allergens during the first 6 years of life. J Allergy Clin Immunol 103: 1173–1179.
22. Galli SJ, Tsai M (2012) IgE and mast cells in allergic disease. Nat Med 18: 693–704.
23. Borish L, Chipps B, Deniz Y, Gujrathi S, Zheng B, et al. (2005) Total serum IgE levels in a large cohort of patients with severe or difficult-to-treat asthma. Ann Allergy Asthma Immunol 95: 247–253.
24. de Jong AB, Dikkeschei LD, Brand PL (2011) Sensitization patterns to food and inhalant allergens in childhood: a comparison of non-sensitized, monosensitized, and polysensitized children. Pediatr Allergy Immunol 22: 166–171.
25. Sun BQ, Zheng PY, Zhang XW, Huang HM, Chen DH, et al. (2014) Prevalence of allergen sensitization among patients with allergic diseases in Guangzhou, Southern China: a four-year observational study. Multidiscip Respir Med 9: 2.
26. Hill DJ, Hosking CS, de Benedictis FM, Oranje AP, Diepgen TL, et al. (2008) Confirmation of the association between high levels of immunoglobulin E food sensitization and eczema in infancy: an international study. Clin Exp Allergy 38: 161–168.
27. Worth A, Sheikh A (2010) Food allergy and atopic eczema. Curr Opin Allergy Clin Immunol 10: 226–230.
28. van den Oord RA, Sheikh A (2009) Filaggrin gene defects and risk of developing allergic sensitisation and allergic disorders: systematic review and meta-analysis. BMJ 339: b2433.
29. Martorell Aragones A, Bone Calvo J, Garcia Ara MC, Nevot Falco S, Plaza Martin AM (2001) Allergy to egg proteins. Food Allergy Committee of the Spanish Society of Pediatric Clinical Immunology and Allergy. Allergol Immunopathol (Madr) 29: 72–95.
30. Vance GH, Lewis SA, Grimshaw KE, Wood PJ, Briggs RA, et al. (2005) Exposure of the fetus and infant to hens' egg ovalbumin via the placenta and breast milk in relation to maternal intake of dietary egg. Clin Exp Allergy 35: 1318–1326.
31. Lau S, Illi S, Sommerfeld C, Niggemann B, Bergmann R, et al. (2000) Early exposure to house-dust mite and cat allergens and development of childhood asthma: a cohort study. Multicentre Allergy Study Group. Lancet 356: 1392–1397.
32. Yunginger JW, Reed CE, O'Connell EJ, Melton LJ 3rd, O'Fallon WM, et al. (1992) A community-based study of the epidemiology of asthma. Incidence rates, 1964–1983. Am Rev Respir Dis 146: 888–894.
33. Martinez FD (2002) Development of wheezing disorders and asthma in preschool children. Pediatrics 109: 362–367.

Anaphylaxis to Iodinated Contrast Media: Clinical Characteristics Related with Development of Anaphylactic Shock

Min-Hye Kim[1,2,3,4], Suh-Young Lee[1,2], Seung-Eun Lee[1,2], Min-Suk Yang[1,2,5], Jae-Woo Jung[2,6], Chang Min Park[7], Whal Lee[7], Sang-Heon Cho[1,2,3], Hye-Ryun Kang[1,2,3]*

1 Department of Internal Medicine, Division of Allergy and Clinical Immunology, Seoul National University Hospital, Seoul, Republic of Korea, **2** Institute of Allergy and Clinical Immunology, Seoul National University Medical Research Center, Seoul, Republic of Korea, **3** Seoul National University Hospital Regional Pharmacovigilance Center, Seoul, Republic of Korea, **4** Department of Internal Medicine, Ewha Womans University School of Medicine, Seoul, Republic of Korea, **5** Department of Internal Medicine, SMG-SNU Boramae Medical Center, Seoul, Republic of Korea, **6** Department of Internal Medicine, Chung-Ang University College of Medicine, Seoul, Republic of Korea, **7** Department of Radiology and Institute of Radiation Medicine, Seoul National University College of Medicine, Seoul, Republic of Korea

Abstract

Objective: Anaphylaxis is the most severe form of radiocontrast media (RCM) induced hypersensitivity and can be life-threatening if profound hypotension is combined. With increased use of iodine based RCM, related hypersensitivity is rapidly growing. However, the clinical characteristics and risk factors of RCM induced anaphylaxis accompanied by hypotension (anaphylactic shock) are not clearly defined. This study was performed to investigate the risk factors of RCM induced anaphylactic shock and the clinical value of RCM skin testing to identify causative agents in affected patients.

Methods: We analyzed the data of RCM induced anaphylaxis monitored by an inhospital pharmacovigilance center at a tertiary teaching hospital from January 2005 to December 2012 and compared the clinical features and skin test results according to the accompanying hypotension.

Results: Among total of 104 cases of RCM induced anaphylaxis, 34.6% of patients, developed anaphylaxis on their first exposure to RCM. Anaphylactic patients presenting with shock were older (57.4 vs. 50.1 years, $p = 0.026$) and had a history of more frequently exposure to RCM (5.1 ± 7.8 vs. 1.9 ± 3.3, $p = 0.004$) compared to those without hypotension. Among RCMs, hypotension was more frequent in anaphylaxis related to iopromide compared to other agents (85.0% vs. 61.4%, $p = 0.011$). Skin tests were performed in 51 patients after development of RCM induced anaphylaxis. Overall skin test positivity to RCM was 64.7% and 81.8% in patients with anaphylactic shock.

Conclusion: RCM induced anaphylactic shock is related to multiple exposures to RCM and most patients showed skin test positivity to RCM.

Editor: Jacques Zimmer, Centre de Recherche Public de la Santé (CRP-Santé), Luxembourg

Funding: This research was supported by a grant from Ministry of Food and Drug Safety to operation of the regional pharmacovigilance center in 2014. The funders had no role in study design, data collection and analysis, decision to publish, or preparation of the manuscript.

Competing Interests: The authors have declared that no competing interests exist.

* E-mail: helenmed@snu.ac.kr

Introduction

Anaphylaxis is a rapid-onset severe hypersensitivity reaction that can be fatal. Although death from anaphylaxis is not common and most episodes of anaphylaxis can be reversed by a single dose of epinephrine, severe anaphylaxis accompanied with cardiovascular collapse can be resistant to treatment and result in death.

As the use of computed tomography (CT) is rapidly growing, iodine based radiocontrast media (RCM) is administered about 75,000,000 times per year worldwide [1]. As low osmolality non-ionic contrast agents replaced high-osmolality ionic ones, the incidence of immediate RCM hypersensitivity diminished remarkably from 3.8–12.7% to 0.7–3.1% [2–4]. Similarly, the incidence of severe immediate RCM hypersensitivity also decreased from 0.1–0.4% to 0.01–0.04%. However, anaphylactic deaths still occur in 1–3 per 100,000–1,000,000 administrations regardless of ionicity [5,6]. Presently, the clinical characteristics and risk factors for the development of anaphylactic shock are not clearly defined.

The principle of post-anaphylaxis management is to avoid the causative agents. Although other imaging can be used as an alternative test in RCM hypersensitivity patients, CT imaging has its own advantage and unavoidable in some clinical situations. Although antihistamines and systemic steroids can be used as preventive measures, they cannot ensure complete prevention of RCM induced anaphylaxis [7,8]. Currently, there are no established guidelines on premedication for RCM induced anaphylaxis [9]. Therefore, information on a causal agent and safer substitutes will be very useful for patients who need contrast enhanced CT scan despite previous history of RCM induced anaphylaxis. Until recently, diagnostic value of RCM skin test has been underestimated and there are only a limited number of studies which evaluated the sensitivity of RCM skin testing to various RCM [10–12].

This study was performed to investigate the risk factors for the development of hypotension and the clinical value of RCM skin testing to identify causative agents in RCM induced anaphylaxis.

Methods

1. Study Subjects

This study protocol was approved by the institutional review board (IRB) of Seoul National University Hospital. Informed consents of patients were exempted from IRB because this study only used retrospective chart review data and all personal data was eliminated and coded as arbitrary number which were not personally-identifiable. Research data was accessed only by researchers using password.

We extracted all the cases of RCM induced hypersensitivity based on ATC code of causative agents (V08A: X-ray contrast media, iodinated, V08B: X-ray contrast media, non-iodinated)' and WHOART (ARRN: 0712 allergic reaction, 0713 anaphylactic shock, 0714 anaphylactoid reaction, 2237 anaphylactic reaction, 2268 documented hypersensitivity to administered drug) from our inhospital pharmacovigilance database collected from January 2005 to December 2012 at Seoul National University Hospital, in Seoul, Korea. Demographic and clinical data of affected patients such as age, sex, number of contrast exposures, laboratory test results, and underlying diseases based on ICD-10 were collected from electronic medical records. This study dealt only with CT procedures, not with other procedures such as cardiac catheterization or coronary angiography.

All the medical records were thoroughly re-evaluated by two allergy specialists to assess clinical features of anaphylaxis and the presence of previous contrast hypersensitivity reactions. Anaphylaxis was diagnosed if cases satisfied the criteria of anaphylaxis suggested by the National Institute of Allergy and Infectious Disease and Food Allergy and the Anaphylaxis Network [13]. Hypotension was considered as a systolic blood pressure less than 90 mmHg or greater than 30% decrease from an individual's baseline. [13] Hypotension unrelated with underlying diseases or other drugs was considered a manifestation of anaphylaxis.

After completing review, patients with anaphylaxis were classified into two groups depending on combined hypotension. We analyzed the data to identify risk factors for the development of anaphylactic shock by comparing anaphylactic patients combined with and without hypotension.

2. Skin Tests with Iodinated Contrast Agents

Skin tests were carried out after experiencing RCM induced anaphylaxis for those patients who agreed to undergo skin testing. Skin prick and intradermal tests were performed on the volar part of the forearm with 6 different RCM used in our hospital - iopromide (Ultravist®, Bayer Healthcare, Brussels, Belgium), iopamidol (Pamiray®, Dongkook Pharm. Co., Ltd, Korea), iomeprol (Iomeron®, Bracco, Milan, Italy), iohexol (Omnipaque®, Armersham Health, Princeton, NJ), iodixanol (Visipaque®, Armersham Health, Princeton, NJ), and iobitridol (Xenetics®, Guerbet, Gorinchem, Netherlands). Undiluted solution and 1:10 diluted solution were used for the skin prick test and intradermal

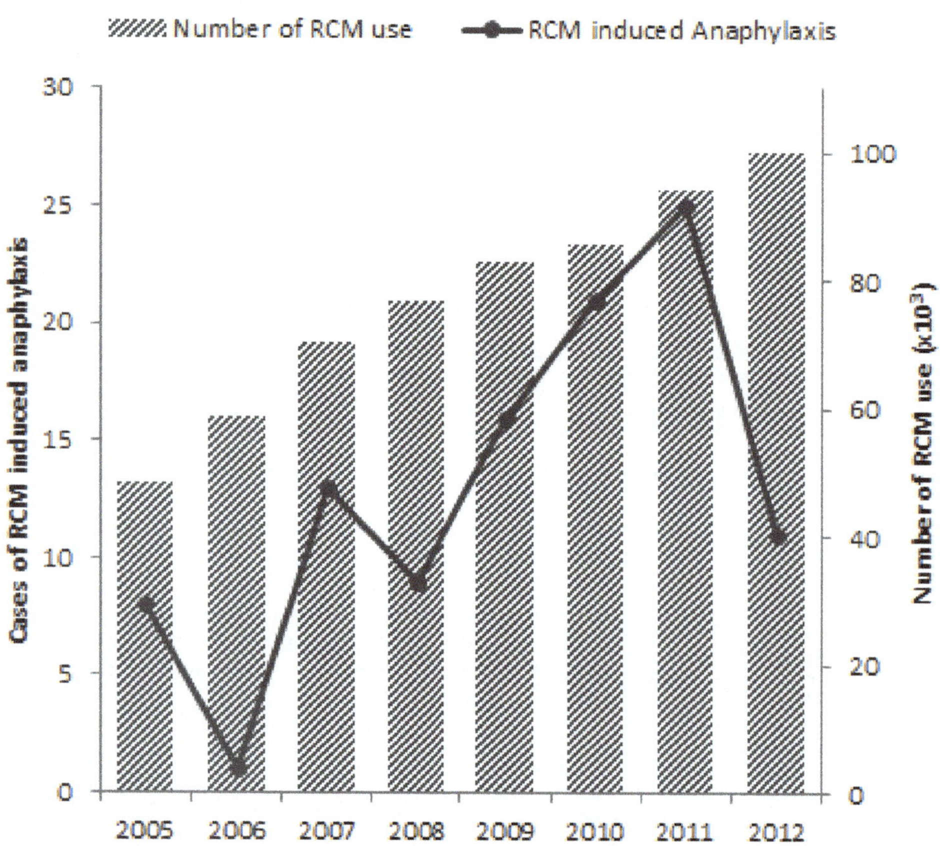

Figure 1. Anaphylactic reactions and total number of RCM use in every year of the study period.

Table 1. Clinical characteristics according to the development of hypotension.

	Total (N, %)	Anaphylactic shock (N, %)	Normotensive anaphylaxis (N, %)	P-value
Number	104	78	26	
Age (years)*	55.6±13.4	57.4±13.2	50.1±13.0	0.024
Male gender, %	43 (41.3)	35 (44.9)	8 (30.8)	0.254
Number of previous exposure to RCM*	4.3±7.1	5.1±7.8	1.9±3.3	0.004
None	36 (34.6)	24 (30.8)	12 (46.2)	0.369
1	17 (16.3)	13 (16.7)	4 (15.4)	
≥2	51 (49.0)	41 (52.6)	10 (38.5)	
Previous RCM reactions	21/68 (30.9)	18/54 (33.3)	3/14 (21.4)	0.362
WBC count (/μL)	5,844.7±1,883.8	5,886±1,921	5,617±1,720	0.668
Eosinophil count (/μL)	62.0±84.4	64.2±86.9	50.0±71.4	0.574
Hypersensitivity Symptoms				
Skin symptoms	69 (66.3)	49 (62.8)	20 (76.9)	0.235
Urticaria/erythema	53 (51.0)	36 (46.2)	17 (65.4)	0.114
Angioedema	34 (32.7)	21 (26.9)	13 (50.0)	0.052
Respiratory symptoms*	50 (48.1)	32 (41.0)	18 (69.2)	0.022
Dyspnea†	42 (40.4)	24 (30.8)	18 (69.2)	0.001
Cardiovascular symptoms†	88 (84.6)	78 (100.0)	10 (38.5)	<0.001
Gastrointestinal symptoms	20 (19.2)	16 (20.5)	4 (15.4)	0.775
Underlying allergic diseases	12 (11.5)	8 (10.3)	4 (15.4)	0.464
Radiocontrast media‡				
Iopromide*	60 (57.7)	51 (65.4)	9 (34.6)	0.011
Iopamidol	12 (11.6)	8 (10.3)	4 (15.4)	0.726
Iomeprol	11 (10.6)	8 (10.3)	3 (11.5)	1.000
Iohexol	7 (6.7)	3 (3.8)	4 (15.4)	0.064
Iobitridol	3 (2.9)	3 (3.8)	0 (0.0)	0.571
Iodixanol	4 (3.8)	3 (3.8)	1 (3.8)	1.000
Unidentified agents*	7 (6.7)	2 (2.6)	5 (19.2)	0.010
Positive skin test†	33/51 (64.7)	27/33 (81.8)	6/18 (33.3)	0.001
Skin prick test	1/51 (2.0)	1/33 (3.0)	0/18 (0.0)	1.000
Intradermal test†	33/51 (64.7)	27/33 (81.8)	6/18 (33.3)	0.001

Continuous variables are expressed as mean ± standard deviation.
*$P<0.05$, †$P<0.01$. ‡Among the total 104 subjects, radiocontrast media involved in anaphylaxis could not be identified in seven patients who had experienced anaphylaxis prior to the introduction of electronic medical recording system.

test, respectively, as used in previous studies [10,12,14,15]. Histamine and normal saline were used as positive and negative control, respectively. The results were interpreted 15 minutes after the prick or the intradermal injection. Skin prick test was determined to be positive when wheal diameter was greater than 3 mm, and intradermal test was determined to be positive when wheal diameter increased 3 mm or more than the initial bleb [12]. The rate and factors contributing to the positivity of RCM skin test were analyzed.

3. Statistical Analysis

SPSS (version 19.0) was used to analyze the data. To compare the clinical features of two groups, Student t-test or Mann-Whitney test was used for continuous variables, and Chi-square test or Fisher's exact test was used for categorical variables. To identify the risk factors related with anaphylactic shock and a positive skin test, multiple logistic regression was used. We included adjustment factors that had a P-value less than 0.1 in the univariate analysis, and other clinically important factors such as age and sex. A P-value less than 0.05 was considered statistically significant.

Results

1. Clinical Characteristics of the Study Subjects and Accompanied Anaphylaxis

A total number of contrast-enhanced CT scans during the study period was 632,513. A total of 104 cases of RCM related anaphylaxis were monitored during the study period. The incidence of contrast-induced anaphylaxis was 0.016%. As the total number of RCM use increased over the study period, the RCM related anaphylaxis also showed increasing tendency in number (Figure 1). The mean age was 55.6±13.1 years and 41.3% (43/104) of them were male (Table 1).

The median number of previous RCM exposures was 1.0 (interquartile range (IQR), 0.0–5.0) before the development of the

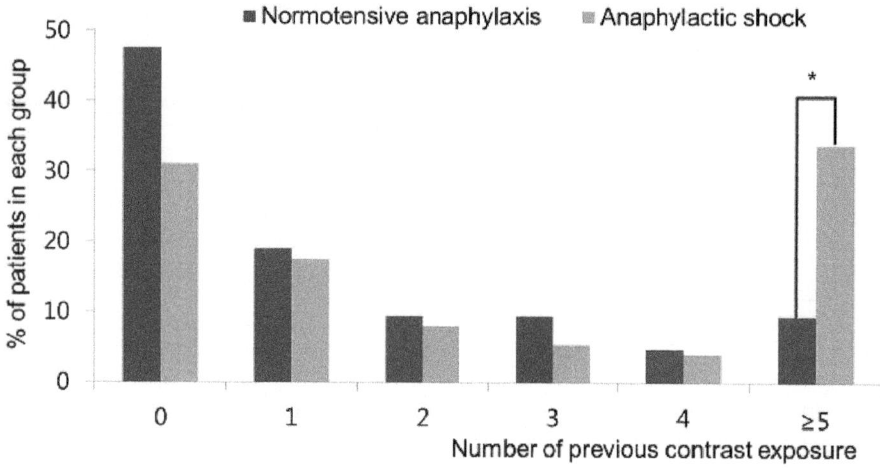

Figure 2. Comparison of the number of contrast exposures according to the presence of hypotension. *$p<0.05$.

first anaphylaxis. While anaphylaxis developed at the first exposure to RCM in 34.6% (36/104) of patients, 65.4% (68/104) of patients experienced anaphylaxis on repeated exposure to RCM and 21 of 68 (30.9%) had a milder form of hypersensitivity reactions in previous exposure to RCM.

Among hypersensitivity symptoms present in patients with anaphylaxis, cardiovascular symptoms were the most common (88/104, 84.6%), followed by skin symptoms (69/104, 66.3%) and respiratory symptoms (50/104, 48.1%) (Table 1). Most symptoms occurred within several minutes after the RCM injection. Seventy-eight patients experienced anaphylaxis with hypotension (anaphylactic shock) and 26 patients had anaphylaxis without hypotension.

2. Comparison of Clinical Characteristics According to the Development of Hypotension

Compared to anaphylactic patients without hypotension, patients who presented with anaphylactic shock were older (57.4 vs. 50.1 years, $p=0.026$) and had significantly higher number of previous RCM exposures (5.1±7.8 vs. 1.9±3.3, $p=0.004$). Of note, the number of patients who underwent previous CT more than two times was 52.6% and 38.5%, respectively in anaphylactic patients with and without hypotension. Especially, the proportion of previous exposure to RCM more than 5 times showed significant difference between anaphylactic patients with and without hypotension (35.4% vs. 9.1%, $p=0.018$, Figure 2).

In terms of the causative contrast agent, hypotension was more frequent among anaphylaxis related to iopromide compared to other agents (85.0% vs. 61.4%, $p=0.011$). Iopromide use was more frequently observed in patients with hypotension than in patients without it among patients with anaphylaxis (65.4% vs 34.6%, $p=0.011$). With multiple logistic regression analysis after adjustment of age, sex, diabetes, and number of previous contrast exposure, iopromide use was still a risk factor for an anaphylactic shock (OR 3.088, 95% confidential interval (CI) = 1.078–8.843, $p=0.036$).

3. Comparison of Clinical Characteristics According to Skin Test Positivity

Fifty-one patients with anaphylaxis followed the recommendation of allergists and underwent RCM skin test and the other 53 patients refused to perform skin test because they did not have a scheduled follow-up CT in the near future.

The mean interval between the time of anaphylaxis and skin test was 14.8 months (IQR 3.4–38.9). Skin test was performed in 41% of patients within one year since they experienced anaphylaxis. The remaining patients underwent skin test at the time when more than one year passed since anaphylaxis occurred (IQR 21.8–64.1).

Among those 51 patients with RCM skin test results, 33 (64.7%) had a positive response to at least one RCM while 18 patients (35.3%) did not show positivity to any RCM tested. In anaphylactic patients accompanied by hypotension, skin test showed 81.8% positivity. Among 33 patients with positive RCM skin test results, mean 1.1 contrast media (1.1±1.1) were positive per person.

Precise information on the culprit RCM was available in 29 patients. Twenty-two (75.9%) patients showed positivity to RCM including their culprit RCM; 14 patients showed single positivity to the culprit RCM; 8 patients showed positivity to other RCMs in addition to the culprit one. Another 7 patients responded to RCM agents other than the culprit one.

The positivity rate of skin test for each contrast agent is varied from 0.0% to 100.0% (Table 2). Iobitridol showed the highest sensitivity (100%) followed by iopromide (59.3%) and iodixanol (50.0%). However, all 5 patients who experienced iohexol induced anaphylaxis were negative in skin test with iohexol.

In patients with a positive RCM skin test, hypotension (79.4% vs. 35.3%, $p=0.004$) and gastrointestinal symptoms (28.1% vs. 0.0%, $p=0.047$) were more frequent compared to patients who had a negative RCM skin test. With multiple logistic regression analysis after adjustment by age, sex and diabetes, the presence of hypotension was a characteristic associated with a RCM skin test positivity (OR 10.0, 95% CI 2.105–47.098, $p=0.004$). However, skin test positive rate was not different according to the history of previous RCM hypersensitivity reactions, accumulated number of exposures to the RCM, and underlying allergic disease.

Discussion

Incidence of anaphylaxis is increasing rapidly and known to be 4–50/100,000 person-years [16]. In adults, drugs are the most common cause of anaphylaxis [16,17] and radiocontrast media was the most commonly involved drug in a study of Korean tertiary care hospital [18]. Although the incidence of RCM hypersensitivity decreased as high-osmolality ionic contrasts were

Table 2. Sensitivity and false negative rate on skin test.

Causative RCM	Sensitivity		False negative rate	
	To any RCM N (%)	To culprit RCM N (%)	To any RCM N (%)	To culprit RCM N (%)
Iopromide	20/27 (74.1)	16/27 (59.3)	7/27 (25.9)	11/27 (40.7)
Iopamidol	2/5 (40.0)	1/5 (20.0)	3/5 (60.0)	4/5 (80.0)
Iomeprol	4/5 (80.0)	2/5 (40.0)	1/5 (20.0)	3/5 (60.0)
Iohexol	1/5 (20.0)	0/5 (0.0)	4/5 (80.0)	5/5 (100.0)
Iobitridol	2/2 (100.0)	2/2 (100.0)	0/2 (0.0)	0/2 (0.0)
Iodixanol	1/2 (50.0)	1/2 (50.0)	1/2 (50.0)	1/2 (50.0)
Total	30/46 (65.2)*	22/46 (47.8)	16/46 (32.6)	24/46 (52.1)

*Five patients in whom causal contrast media could not be identified were excluded from this analysis among 51 patients with skin test results.
Iopromide, iopamidol, iomeprol, iohexol, and iobitridol are low-osmolar contrast media. Iodixanol is an iso-osmolar contrast media.

replaced by low-osmolality non-ionic ones, anaphylactic death still occurred regardless of ionicity [5,6].

Traditionally, immediate hypersensitivity reactions to RCM were considered representative of non-IgE mediated 'anaphylactoid reaction' since it can occur on the first exposure and does not always recur on the repeated exposure [1,10,11,19]. However, a previous report showed that only 30% of immediate RCM hypersensitivity developed at the first exposure to RCM [20] and our study also revealed that only 35% of RCM induced anaphylaxis occurred at the first exposures to RCM. We found that milder hypersensitivity symptoms heralded anaphylaxis in 1/3 of the patients on preceding exposure to RCM. Multiple exposures and a previous hypersensitivity reaction prior to RCM induced anaphylaxis suggest that an immunologic mechanism may have some role in the development of some RCM induced anaphylaxis.

Anaphylaxis is a severe, life-threatening systemic hypersensitivity reaction involving at least two or more organs at the same time. However, diagnosis of anaphylaxis can be made if sudden hypotension develops after exposure to a known allergen. Based upon symptoms, anaphylaxis can be classified into mild, moderate, and severe grade. [21] When hypotension occurs as a manifestation of anaphylaxis either as a sole feature or with other symptoms, physicians should pay attention to the development of potential cardiovascular collapse which is the main cause of mortality in anaphylaxis [22]. There are several known risk factors for a severe RCM hypersensitivity such as previous history of RCM hypersensitivity, asthma, allergies requiring medical treatment, use of beta-adrenergic blockers, female gender, Indian and Mediterranean ethnicity, and malignant tumor [23]. However, there was no data on the risk factors for the development of hypotension in anaphylaxis. In this study, we reported risk factors for anaphylactic shock such as older age, previous multiple exposures to RCM, iopromide use. However, we do not have a clear picture of what the overall anaphylaxis rate is using iopromide or the other study contrast agents, since patients without anaphylaxis are not included in the study. Secondly, the number of administrations of other contrast agents was too small to provide statistically significant results. In other words, we cannot conclude from this study that iopromide is more likely to cause anaphylaxis than any of the other contrast agents, but among the anaphylactic patients, iopromide was associated with more severe forms of anaphylaxis (anaphylaxis with hypotension). In addition, anaphylaxis with hypotension showed stronger association with RCM skin test positivity than anaphylaxis without hypotension. Although skin test positivity might be the result of direct mast cell activation by RCM, it is more likely that IgE mediated hypersensitivity may have a role in the development of RCM induced anaphylaxis when presented with hypotension.

Skin test is widely used to identify the causative agents in IgE mediated hypersensitivity [12,15,16]. Previously, sensitivity of the intradermal test was reported as high as 73% when performed with undiluted solutions [20]. However, this result may have been overestimated by irritation with undiluted RCM and a 1:10 solution has been preferred for intradermal test with RCM in general. The positive rate of the intradermal skin test was variable and reported as low as 4.2% among patients with RCM hypersensitivity [10]. On the other hand, data from the European Network of Drug Allergy multicentre study demonstrated a 50% positive rate of RCM skin test in immediate reactors [14]. Recently, Kim et al. reported that a significantly higher sensitivity positive rate of RCM skin test in severe immediate reactions (57.1%) compared with mild (12.9%) and moderate reactions (25.0%) and suggested their modest utility in evaluating severe adverse reactions retrospectively [24]. In this study, we observed much higher positive rate of RCM skin test in patient with RCM induced anaphylaxis (64.7%). Positive rate went up as high as 81.8% among patients with anaphylactic shock and it is the highest value ever reported in RCM hypersensitivity. Three quarter of patients who showed skin test positivity responded to the very same RCM used at the time of anaphylaxis and cross reactivity rate to other RCMs was low. These findings suggest that a substantial proportion of patients with RCM induced anaphylaxis, especially anaphylactic shock, may have specificity to causative agents and skin tests can provide information on the safe substitutes. However, considering negativity in one third of patients, skin test is not helpful to choose safe alternative RCMs in some populations and clinical reasoning is needed on interpreting the results.

Although we could not perform skin test in negative controls, skin test positivity in the negative control is known to be negligible. There are several studies which elucidated very low positivity of skin test in the negative controls. Brockow et al. reported that positivity of skin test was 0.0% (0/11)–4.2% (3/71) in the negative controls [14]. Kim et al. performed RCM skin testing on 1,048 Korean subjects before contrast-enhanced CT and found only 1 case of positive immediate skin test (0.09%) [24].

There are several limitations in this study. The main limitation is its retrospective design and underreporting of adverse reaction to spontaneous reporting systems. Another limitation is the lack of information on the number of individual RCM used in contrast-enhanced CT during the study period. Thus, large scale prospective studies including sufficient number of patients reacting to each RCM are needed in order to define the exact incidence and risk factors of RCM induced anaphylaxis.

Conclusion

RCM induced anaphylactic shock is related with multiple exposure to RCM and skin test positivity to RCM.

Author Contributions

Conceived and designed the experiments: H-RK S-HC. Performed the experiments: M-HK S-YL S-EL M-SY J-WJ. Analyzed the data: C-MP WL. Contributed reagents/materials/analysis tools: M-HK S-YL S-EL M-SY J-WJ C-MP WL S-HC H-RK. Wrote the paper: M-HK H-RK.

References

1. Brockow K, Ring J (2011) Anaphylaxis to radiographic contrast media. Curr Opin Allergy Clin Immunol 11: 326–331.
2. Kim MH, Park CH, Kim DI, Kim KM, Kim HK, et al. (2012) Surveillance of contrast-media-induced hypersensitivity reactions using signals from an electronic medical recording system. Ann Allergy Asthma Immunol 108: 167–171.
3. Katayama H (1990) Adverse reactions to contrast media. What are the risk factors? Invest Radiol 25 Suppl 1: S16–17.
4. Thomsen HS, Bush WH Jr (1998) Adverse effects of contrast media: incidence, prevention and management. Drug Saf 19: 313–324.
5. Cashman JD, McCredie J, Henry DA (1991) Intravenous contrast media: use and associated mortality. Med J Aust 155: 618–623.
6. Wysowski DK, Nourjah P (2006) Deaths attributed to X-ray contrast media on U.S. death certificates. AJR Am J Roentgenol 186: 613–615.
7. Williams AN, Kelso JM (2007) Radiocontrast-induced anaphylaxis despite pretreatment and use of iso-osmolar contrast. Ann Allergy Asthma Immunol 99: 467–468.
8. Davenport MS, Cohan RH, Caoili EM, Ellis JH (2009) Repeat contrast medium reactions in premedicated patients: frequency and severity. Radiology 253: 372–379.
9. Morcos SK, Thomsen HS, Webb JA (2001) Prevention of generalized reactions to contrast media: a consensus report and guidelines. Eur Radiol 11: 1720–1728.
10. Trcka J, Schmidt C, Seitz CS, Brocker EB, Gross GE, et al. (2008) Anaphylaxis to iodinated contrast material: nonallergic hypersensitivity or IgE-mediated allergy? AJR Am J Roentgenol 190: 666–670.
11. Brockow K, Ring J (2010) Classification and pathophysiology of radiocontrast media hypersensitivity. Chem Immunol Allergy 95: 157–169.
12. Caimmi S, Benyahia B, Suau D, Bousquet-Rouanet L, Caimmi D, et al. (2010) Clinical value of negative skin tests to iodinated contrast media. Clin Exp Allergy 40: 805–810.
13. Sampson HA, Munoz-Furlong A, Campbell RL, Adkinson NF Jr, Bock SA, et al. (2006) Second symposium on the definition and management of anaphylaxis: summary report–Second National Institute of Allergy and Infectious Disease/Food Allergy and Anaphylaxis Network symposium. J Allergy Clin Immunol 117: 391–397.
14. Brockow K, Romano A, Aberer W, Bircher AJ, Barbaud A, et al. (2009) Skin testing in patients with hypersensitivity reactions to iodinated contrast media - a European multicenter study. Allergy 64: 234–241.
15. Goksel O, Aydin O, Atasoy C, Akyar S, Demirel YS, et al. (2011) Hypersensitivity reactions to contrast media: prevalence, risk factors and the role of skin tests in diagnosis–a cross-sectional survey. Int Arch Allergy Immunol 155: 297–305.
16. Lee JK, Vadas P (2011) Anaphylaxis: mechanisms and management. Clin Exp Allergy 41: 923–938.
17. Greenberger PA, Rotskoff BD, Lifschultz B (2007) Fatal anaphylaxis: postmortem findings and associated comorbid diseases. Ann Allergy Asthma Immunol 98: 252–257.
18. Yang MS, Lee SH, Kim TW, Kwon JW, Lee SM, et al. (2008) Epidemiologic and clinical features of anaphylaxis in Korea. Ann Allergy Asthma Immunol 100: 31–36.
19. Maddox TG (2002) Adverse reactions to contrast material: recognition, prevention, and treatment. Am Fam Physician 66: 1229–1234.
20. Dewachter P, Laroche D, Mouton-Faivre C, Bloch-Morot E, Cercueil JP, et al. (2011) Immediate reactions following iodinated contrast media injection: a study of 38 cases. Eur J Radiol 77: 495–501.
21. Muraro A, Roberts G, Clark A, Eigenmann PA, Halken S, et al. (2007) The management of anaphylaxis in childhood: position paper of the European academy of allergology and clinical immunology. Allergy 62: 857–871.
22. Khan BQ, Kemp SF (2011) Pathophysiology of anaphylaxis. Curr Opin Allergy Clin Immunol 11: 319–325.
23. Morcos SK (2005) Review article: Acute serious and fatal reactions to contrast media: our current understanding. Br J Radiol 78: 686–693.
24. Kim SH, Jo EJ, Kim MY, Lee SE, Kim MH, et al. (2013) Clinical value of radiocontrast media skin tests as a prescreening and diagnostic tool in hypersensitivity reactions. Ann Allergy Asthma Immunol 110: 258–262.

Determinants of Allergic Rhinitis in Young Children with Asthma

Lise Moussu[1], Philippe Saint-Pierre[2], Virginie Panayotopoulos[1], Rémy Couderc[3], Flore Amat[1], Jocelyne Just[1]*

1 Allergology department, Centre de l'Asthme et des Allergies, Hôpital d'Enfants Armand-Trousseau (Assistance Publique Hôpitaux de Paris) - Université Pierre et Marie Curie, Paris, France, **2** Laboratoire de Statistiques Théoriques et Appliquées, Université Pierre et Marie Curie, Paris, France, **3** Service de Biochimie et Biologie Moléculaire, Hôpital d'Enfants Armand-Trousseau (Assistance Publique Hôpitaux de Paris), Paris, France

Abstract

Background: In the preschool period, allergic rhinitis (AR) is infrequent and thus under-diagnosed. However, recent works have highlighted the occurrence of AR in toddlers although the causes of AR in this young population remain unknown. The objective of this study was to identify determinants of AR in young children with asthma.

Methods: We carried out a case-control study of 227 children with active asthma and enrolled in the Trousseau Asthma Program. AR and other allergic diseases (asthma, food allergy and eczema) were diagnosed by medical doctors using standardized questionnaires. Parental history of AR and asthma, biological markers of atopy (total IgE, blood eosinophilia, allergic sensitization towards food and aeroallergens) and environmental parameters were also collected.

Results: Forty one of the children (18.1%) had AR. By univariate logistic regression analysis, AR was mainly associated with peanut sensitization (OR = 6.75; p = 0.002); food allergy (OR = 4.31; p = 0.026); mold exposure (OR = 3.81 $p<0.01$) and parental history of AR (OR = 1.42; p = 0.046). Due to the strong link between food allergy and peanut sensitization three models of multivariate logistic regression were performed and confirmed that AR is associated with peanut sensitization but also food allergy and mold exposure. A random forest analysis was also performed to explain AR. The results reinforced the logistic analysis that peanut sensitization and mold exposure were the principal determinants of AR.

Conclusions & Clinical Relevance: These results stress the importance of investigating AR in young children with asthma to potentially diagnose a particularly severe allergic asthmatic phenotype. Moreover, these data evoke the hypothesis that peanut could be an aeroallergen.

Editor: Luo Zhang, Beijing Instiitute of Otolaryngology, China

Funding: The authors have no support or funding to report.

Competing Interests: The authors have declared that no competing interests exist.

* E-mail: jocelyne.just@trs.aphp.fr

Introduction

Allergic rhinitis (AR) is an atopic manifestation frequently associated with asthma. The prevalence of AR in children has been rising in many countries and is associated with a western lifestyle [1]. The Score for AR (SFAR) [2], which has been validated in the pediatric population after adding the idea of nasal itching [3], is a valuable diagnostic tool. The AR and its Impact on Asthma (ARIA)[4] classification further helps assess the severity of this pathology, as it takes into account the chronology of the symptoms and the discomfort they cause. In addition to causing other ear, nose and throat disorders [5] and harmful effects on quality of life [6], AR has been identified as a risk factor for asthma onset [7,8], severity and poor control [9]. The occurrence of AR in pre-school children is now widely accepted [10–12], but diagnosis has long been overlooked or questioned in early infancy. This is mainly explained by its similarity with infectious symptoms which are frequent in toddlers.

The « Pollution and Asthma Risk: an Infant Study » (PARIS) birth cohort, gave an estimated general prevalence of AR of around 9.1% in 18-month-old infants [13], but other studies give estimates ranging from 3 to 29%, depending on how stringent the applied criteria were [14,15]. AR and asthma are two components of the chronic allergic respiratory syndrome, as they involve the same allergic immunological processes, fostering the concept of unity of the respiratory tract [16]. Nevertheless, because allergen sensitization of asthmatic infants seldom occurs, except for infants having an allergic phenotype [17], the mode of its association with AR is still unknown at this age of life.

Our study set out to identify determinants associated with AR in a case-control study performed in a cohort of young children with asthma.

Materials and Methods

Ethics

Data were collected by standardized questionnaires and the medical examination was conducted by a physician after the parents gave their written informed consent. The Ile de France V ethics committee approved the protocol and this consent procedure.

Population

This case-control study gathered data from January to November 2011 and enrolled children who were part of the TAP (Trousseau Asthma Program). All the children had been referred to the center for recurrent wheezing by a primary care physician and joined the study consecutively.

Inclusion criteria for the study were: age younger than 30 months; persistent asthma (defined as a history of recurrent wheeze, more than three episodes of reversible bronchial obstruction documented within the previous 6 months) [18]; absence of other chronic obstructive pulmonary diseases (congenital or acquired), or exacerbation or acute respiratory illness within the 6 weeks preceding the explorations.

Health outcomes

General data were collected on the children's gender and age.

AR was diagnosed by a medical doctor supported by the SFAR criteria as defined by a score of 7 or more [3]. Based on these data, infants were allocated into two groups – one comprising children diagnosed with AR (the AR group) and the other comprising those without (the control group) – in a randomized manner and adjusted for age and gender.

Personal history of atopy (eczema) was mostly assessed by questions from the International Study of Asthma and Allergies in Childhood (ISAAC) [19]. Food allergy was defined by clinical symptoms of allergy after consumption of a food allergen and a positivity of specific IgE for the same allergen.

Moderate to severe asthma was determined according to the National Asthma Education and Prevention Program [20].

Finally, information about parental history (paternal and/or maternal) of AR and asthma were also gathered.

Environmental factors

Environmental factors were assessed by the questions applied in the PARIS birth cohort. We collected data about exclusive maternal breast-feeding beyond 3 months, exposure to passive smoking (defined by smokers at home smoking more than five cigarettes a day) and overcrowding (less than 9 m^2 for each person living at home). Potential sources of biologic allergens were also evaluated: mold exposure (visible mold and moldy smell) and presence of visible cockroaches at home.

Biological markers

Biological markers of atopy were measured in peripheral blood. These included the multiple allergenic screening test Phadiatop infant and blood levels of specific IgE toward inhaled and food allergens (cow milk, egg, peanut, house dust mite, grass pollen, birch pollen, cat, dog and alternaria) for children testing positive. Children with two or more sensitizations to food and/or aeroallergens were considered to have polysensitization. Aeroallergen sensitization was defined as at least one sensitization to an inhaled allergen. Other inflammatory biological markers, such as total eosinophilia count and serum level of total IgE, were measured too. Thresholds were used to define increased levels: increased blood eosinophilia was defined as a concentration ≥470 eosinophils/mm^3, (cell count by automated Sysmex; France), increased total IgE as a concentration ≥45 kU/L [21] and positive specific IgE ≥0.35 kU/L (ImmunoCAP; Uppsala, Sweden).

Statistical analysis

The chi-square test and Fisher's exact test were used to compare the distribution of each variable (clinical, environmental and environmental) between the control and the AR group. A logistic regression analysis [22] was used to examine the relationships between the binary outcome of interest (presence of AR) and multiple risk factors. Univariate and multivariate models, with and without interaction terms, were constructed to better understand the presence of AR. Spearman's correlation coefficient was computed to examine the association between variables. Risk factors associated with AR in the univariate analysis ($p<0.2$) were included in the multivariate analysis. The multivariate models were selected using the backward stepwise procedure.

A random forest analysis [23] was then applied to classify AR. This ensemble method uses a number of classification trees [24] to improve the classification compared to a single tree. In addition to the good predictive performance, random forests estimate the relevance (discriminating power) of each variable using importance measure (permutation-based mean decrease in accuracy). This non-linear approach provides an alternative to the logistic regression by providing another variables selection. Statistical analysis was performed with R version 2.12.0 (http://www.r-project.org). The R package 'glm', 'Rpart' and 'randomForest' were used to perform the analysis.

Results

Forty-one of the 227 children seen in the TAP between January and November 2011 (18.1%) had AR. Among the remaining 186 asthmatic children without AR, 88 were randomized and enrolled in the control group. The two groups were similar regarding age (17 [6-30] versus 16 [6–29] months in the AR and control group respectively) and gender (54% boys in the AR group vs. 53% in the control group).

Risk factors for AR: descriptive analysis (Table 1, Table 2)

The AR group appeared to have –more features of allergy: food allergy ($p = 0.042$), allergic polysensitization ($p = 0.030$), especially due to peanut sensitization ($p = 0.002$) and greater exposure to mold ($p = 0.030$). Manifestations of food allergy were cutaneous (rash or facial edema) for seven of them and digestive (nausea or vomiting) for three. One child had both types of symptoms.

Risk factors for AR: univariate logistic regression analysis (Table 3)

In univariate logistic regression analysis, AR was found to be mainly associated with food allergy (OR = 4.31; $p = 0.026$); peanut (OR = 6.75; $p = 0.002$) and then with one environmental factor: mold exposure (OR = 3.81; $p<0.01$). Other risk factors were found to be: biological biomarkers identified by Phadiatop infant (OR = 2.27; $p = 0.046$), more precisely polysensitization (OR = 3.22; $p = 0.019$); and egg sensitization (OR = 2.56; $p = 0.048$); and finally a parental history of AR (OR = 1.42; $p = 0.046$).

Table 1. Characteristic features of the entire population, the control group and the AR group.

	Entire population (n = 129)	AR group (n = 41)	Control group (n = 88)	p-value*
Eczema	43 (33.0)	18 (43.9)	25 (28.4)	0.124
Food allergy	11 (8.5)	7 (17.1)	4 (4.5)	0.042
Moderate to severe Asthma	66 (51.2)	26 (63.4)	40 (45.4)	0.080
Parental history of Asthma	3 (2.3)	0 (0)	3 (3.4)	0.770
Parental history of AR	12 (9.3)	6 (14.6%)	6 (6.8)	0.119
Eosinophilia (≥470/mm³)	30 (23.3)	10 (24.4)	20 (22.7)	0.896
Elevated total IgE (≥45 kU/L)	38 (29.5)	12 (29.3)	26 (29.5)	0.885
Phadiatop infant	36 (27.9)	20 (22.7)	16 (39.0)	0.071
Polysensitization	20 (15.5)	11 (26.8)	9 (10.2)	0.030
Sensitizations to food and aeroallergens (≥0.35 kU/L)				
Cow Milk	24 (18,6)	11 (26.8)	13 (14.8)	0.163
Egg	22 (17.1)	11 (26.8)	11 (12.5)	0.078
Peanut	14 (10.9)	10 (24.4)	4 (4.5)	0.002
House dust mite	10 (7.8)	4 (9.8)	6 (6.8)	0.820
Cat	6 (4.7)	3 (7.3)	3 (3.4)	0.381
Dog	1 (0.8)	1 (2.4)	1 (1.1)	0.999
Grass pollen	2 (1.6)	1 (2.4)	1 (1.1)	0.536
Birch pollen	1 (0.8)	1 (2.4)	0 (0)	0.318
Alternaria	2 (1.6)	2 (4.9)	0 (0)	0.099
Any aeroallergen	1 (8.5)	5 (12.2)	6 (6.8)	0.497

All the values are expressed in absolute numbers and percentage in brackets. *Chi-square test when conditions were respected or Fisher's exact tests otherwise. Boldface values indicate statistical significance. Food allergy was defined by clinical symptoms of allergy after consumption of a food allergen and a positivity of specific IgE for the same allergen. Severity of asthma was determined according to the National Asthma Education and Prevention Program [20]. Polysensitization is defined as two or more specific allergen sensitizations.Any aeroallergen is defined as at least one aeroallergen sensitization.

Risk factors for AR: multivariate logistic regression analysis (Table 4)

In the multivariate analysis, model selection using an automatic stepwise procedure led to a model without interaction for the following variables: food allergy ($OR_a = 3.96$; $p = 0.081$), peanut sensitization ($OR_a = 3.40$; $p = 0.075$), mold exposure ($OR_a = 3.20$; $p = 0.013$), familial history of AR ($OR_a = 1.45$; $p = 0.052$) and moderate to severe asthma ($OR_a = 1.24$; $p = 0.124$) (model 1). A correlation study highlighted the association between food allergy and peanut sensitization ($\chi^2 = 11.23$; $p<0.001$). Such a correlation should be avoided as the two variables share common information. We thus constructed a model without peanut sensitization (Model 2) and a model without food allergy (Model 3) (Table 4). The OR associated with peanut sensitization or food allergy were found to be higher in these models. After adjustment, peanut sensitization, food allergy, parental history of AR and the presence of mold were found to increase the risk of AR.

Risk factors for AR: random forest analysis

The importance measure (permutation measure) obtained from the random forest analysis (Fig. 1) can be interpreted as a measure of discriminating power. These measures reinforced the previous results of peanut sensitization, mold exposure, moderate to severe asthma, parental history of AR, polysensitization and food allergy being determinants of AR. The mold exposure and peanut sensitization were associated with the highest values and seems to be the most important variables to explain AR.

Table 2. Environmental characteristics of the entire population, the control group and the AR group.

	Entire population (n= 129)	AR group (n = 41)	Control group (n = 88)	p-value*
Breastfeeding	69 (53.5)	23 (56.1)	46 (52.3)	0.829
Overcrowding	12 (9.3)	2 (4.9)	10 (11.4)	0.336
Mold exposure	33 (25.6)	18 (43.0)	15 (17.0)	0.002
Cockroaches	9 (7.0)	3 (7.3)	6 (6.8)	0.999
Passive smoking	35 (27.1)	13 (31.7)	22 (25)	0.558

All the values are expressed in absolute numbers and percentage in brackets *Chi-square test when conditions were respected or Fisher's exact test otherwise. Boldface values indicate statistical significance. Maternal breast-feeding beyond 3 months, Passive smoking (defined by smokers at home smoking more than 5 cigarettes a day). Overcrowding (less than 9 m² for each person living at home). Mold exposure (visible mold and moldy smell) and cockroaches (visible cockroaches at home).

Table 3. Univariate logistic regression in the entire population (n = 129).

	Odds ratio	95% CI	p-value*
Eczema	1.97	0.91–4.27	0.084
Food allergy	4.32	1.19–15.73	0.026
Moderate to severe Asthma	1.40	0.94–2.10	0.098
Parental history of AR	1.42	1.01–2.02	0.046
Mold exposure	3.81	1.66–8.74	0.002
Phadiatop infant	2.27	1.01–5.07	0.046
Polysensitization	3.22	1.21–8.54	0.019
Cow milk sensitization	2.11	0.85–5.24	0.105
Egg sensitization	2.56	1.01–6.55	0.048
Peanut sensitization	6.77	1.98–23.19	0.002

*Wald test. Only p-value<0.2 are reported. Boldface values indicate statistical significance.
Food allergy was defined by clinical symptoms of allergy after consumption of a food allergen and a positivity of specific IgE for the same allergen. Moderate to severe asthma was determined according to the National Asthma Education and Prevention Program [20]. Mold exposure: visible mold and moldy smell. Allergen sensitization: specific IgE ≥0.35 kU/L. Polysensitization: defined as two or more specific allergen sensitizations.

Discussion

The main result of our study is that independent variables for AR in young asthmatic children are mainly peanut sensitization (linked to food allergy) and a moldy environment. Taking together all the results, in a less constant manner, an association was found between AR and moderate to severe asthma but also a parental history of AR and polysensitization.

Sensitization to peanut results in a fivefold increase in the risk of AR

In school age children, co-morbidities of allergic diseases such as AR and asthma occur more frequently in sensitized children (especially related to aeroallergen) [25,26]. The fact that biological evidence of atopy should lead to a suspicion of AR in infants has already been shown by Herr *et al.* [13] but without identifying a specific allergic sensitization.

In our study, peanut sensitization appeared to be an important determinant of AR in preschool children. Similarly, Kulig *et al.* highlighted the fact that sensitization to a food allergen is a risk factor for further sensitization to an aeroallergen even without clinical food allergy [27]. Moreover, a particular link between peanut sensitization and the severity of allergic disease (such as eczema) has recently been described in the LEAP (Learning Early About Peanut Allergy) study [28]. Finally, it has also recently been described that a certain amount of peanut present in home air could stimulate basophils under IgE immune response [29]. These results, along with ours, point up the possibility that inhaled peanut could be a specific trigger of AR.

Moreover, we showed a significant link between food allergy and AR within the same toddler period. The relatively low importance of food allergy in random forest analysis was explained by the correlation with peanut sensitization [30]. This association between food allergy and allergic respiratory disease could simply reflect a particular severe allergic phenotype in young children with asthma, previously described by our team [17].

Mold exposure an environmental determinants of AR

Our findings identified indoor dampness and the resulting molds as important risk factors for AR in young children with asthma. This risk has also been pointed out by the ISAAC study in the 6 to 7 year-old age group [31]. A Finish cohort of children followed from age 1 to 7 years also linked mold to the *de novo* development of AR (OR = 1.96; CI 95%: 1.29–2.99) and showed the increased risk to be dose-dependent [32]. There are certainly multiple mechanisms involved. Molds enhance direct sensitization

Table 4. Multivariate logistic regression in the entire population (n = 129).

	Model 1 OR (95% CI) [p-value*]	Model 2 OR (95% CI) [p-value*]	Model 3 OR (95% CI) [p-value*]
Food allergy	3.96 (0.84-18.57) [0.081]	5.96 (1.43–24.84) [0.014]	
Peanut sensitization	3.40 (0.86–13.07) [0.075]		5.02 (1.38–18.25) [0.014]
Mold exposure	3.20 (1.28–7.97) [0.013]	3.84 (1.59–9.28) [0.003]	2.86 (1.18–6.94) [0.020]
Parental history of AR	1.45 (0.99–2.12) [0.052]	1.46 (1.01–2.13) [0.043]	1.41 (0.97–2.05) [0.073]
Moderate to severe asthma	1.40 (0.91–2.17) [0.124]	1.41 (0.92–2.16) [0.117]	1.39 (0.90–2.14) [0.136]

*Wald test. Risk factors associated with AR in the univariate analysis (p<0.2) are included in the multivariate analysis. Automatic backward stepwise procedure was used for model selection (Model 1). Due to the correlation between food allergy and peanut sensitization, one of these variables is removed from the selected model (Model 2 and Model 3). Boldface values indicate statistical significance.
Food allergy was defined by clinical symptoms of allergy after consumption of a food allergen and a positivity of specific IgE for the same allergen. Moderate to severe asthma was determined according to the National Asthma Education and Prevention Program [20]. Allergen sensitization: specific IgE ≥0.35 kU/L. Mold exposure: visible mold and moldy smell. Cockroaches: visible cockroaches at home.

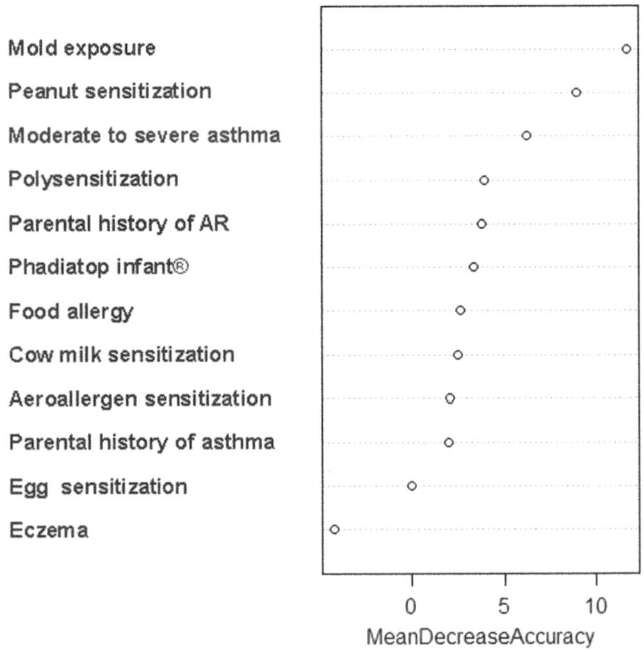

Figure 1. Importance measure (permutation-based mean decrease in accuracy) provided by the random forest analysis. Highest values of the importance measure are associated with a higher discriminating power.

with specific IgE production. However, we believe that the detrimental exposure is more due to irritation than to allergic sensitization towards mold, especially in young children. In fact, it is well known that mold exposure promotes bacterial growth and the release of volatile organic compounds which enhance non-specific inflammation especially in severe asthmatic children [33,34]. The increase of epithelial permeability could thus lead to sensitization to other aeroallergens [35].

Influence of a parental history of AR

Our study shows a link between the development of AR in early childhood and a parental history of AR. This result is in line with previous findings. The follow-up of the PARIS birth cohort estimated that a double parental history is associated with a twofold increased risk of the infant developing AR. In a study of children in Singapore, the risk of AR was 4.5 times higher (CI 95%: 3.3–6.1) when both parents had AR [36]. This transmission of a precise phenotype has also been observed for atopic dermatitis and asthma. In the English ALSPAC cohort, a history of atopic dermatitis in both parents was associated with an OR of 2.72 (CI 95%: 2.09–3.53) in children with atopic dermatitis [37]. Furthermore, the PARIS birth cohort showed that infants having an atopic asthma phenotype were more likely to have asthmatic parents [38]. The awareness of this phenotypic link could sensitize health professionals to the diagnosis of AR in asthmatic infants and improve their treatment and follow-up. In the same way, we recently found an association between mold exposure and AR present in a particularly severe allergic phenotype in young children with asthma [17].

Severe asthma and its link with AR

A link between AR and moderate to severe asthma as independent variables was found by random forest analysis with a borderline association in the three multivariate logistic regression models. It has been well reported in the literature that AR worsens the asthma prognosis [38], while intranasal treatment improves asthma outcomes [39]. Moreover, bronchial hyper-responsiveness is frequent in children with rhinitis especially in those with AR [40]. Finally, AR is also more likely to persist during childhood than non AR [41].

Polysensitization, another risk factor of AR

Simpson *et al.* [42] showed that atopic sensitization is not a dichotomous trait in relation to allergic respiratory disease (especially asthma). They demonstrated that a particular phenotype associated with multiple early allergic sensitizations predicts not only the presence, but also the persistence and severity of childhood asthma.

On a clinical level, Schröder *et al.* [43] confirm this point of view, with a significant association between food allergy and risk of asthma in children from a family-based food allergy cohort. Moreover, in accordance with our study, they demonstrated that the association was stronger in children with multiple food allergies.

Strengths and limitations of the study

The main strength of this study lies in the use of precisely defined clinical parameters and biological markers. AR was assessed by medical doctors, supported by the SFAR criteria, which were more stringent than those used in previous studies [13]. Moreover, we had access (1) to a relatively large group of asthmatic toddlers with AR; (2) who shared close characteristics to toddlers with AR described in general population by Herr *et al.* [13]. Nevertheless, a limitation of our study is that we did not perform food challenges for diagnosing food allergies. Another limitation is that our questionnaire could have been more precise regarding environmental factors by using objective measurements. This fact may explain why our results did not show any link between AR and passive smoking, contrary to other authors [7,44].

Conclusions

Our study reveals that in young children with asthma, AR could be a signal symptom of a severe allergic phenotype with a particular association with peanut sensitization. This data stresses the importance of thoroughly investigating AR so as not to miss potentially diagnosing a particular severe asthmatic phenotype. Finally our results raise the hypothesis that peanut could be considered as an inhaled allergen.

Author Contributions

Conceived and designed the experiments: JJ. Performed the experiments: LM PSP VP RC. Analyzed the data: LM PSP JJ. Contributed reagents/materials/analysis tools: LM PSP VP JJ FA. Wrote the paper: LM JJ VP PSP.

References

1. Strachan D, Sibbald B, Weiland S, Aït-Khaled N, Anabwani G, et al. (1997) Worldwide variations in prevalence of symptoms of allergic rhinoconjunctivitis in children: the International Study of Asthma and Allergies in Childhood (ISAAC). Pediatr Allergy Immunol 8: 161–176.

2. Annesi-Maesano I, Didier A, Klossek M, Chanal I, Moreau D, et al. (2002) The score for allergic rhinitis (SFAR): a simple and valid assessment method in population studies. Allergy 57: 107–114.
3. Braun-Fahrländer C, Wüthrich B, Gassner M, Grize L, Sennhauser FH, et al. (1997) Validation of a rhinitis symptom questionnaire (ISAAC core questions) in a population of Swiss school children visiting the school health services. SCARPOL-team. Swiss Study on Childhood Allergy and Respiratory Symptom with respect to Air Pollution and Cl. Pediatr Allergy Immunol 8: 75–82.
4. Bousquet J, Van Cauwenberge P, Khaltaev N (2001) Allergic rhinitis and its impact on asthma. J Allergy Clin Immunol 108: S147–334.
5. Hellings PW, Fokkens WJ (2006) Allergic rhinitis and its impact on otorhinolaryngology. Allergy 61: 656–664.
6. Silva CHM da, Silva TE da, Morales NMO, Fernandes KP, Pinto RMC (n.d.) Quality of life in children and adolescents with allergic rhinitis. Braz J Otorhinolaryngol 75: 642–649.
7. Wright AL, Holberg CJ, Martinez FD, Halonen M, Morgan W, et al. (1994) Epidemiology of physician-diagnosed allergic rhinitis in childhood. Pediatrics 94: 895–901.
8. Rochat MK, Illi S, Ege MJ, Lau S, Keil T, et al. (2010) Allergic rhinitis as a predictor for wheezing onset in school-aged children. J Allergy Clin Immunol 126: 1170–5.e2.
9. De Groot EP, Nijkamp A, Duiverman EJ, Brand PLP (2012) Allergic rhinitis is associated with poor asthma control in children with asthma. Thorax 67: 582–587.
10. Peroni DG, Piacentini GL, Alfonsi L, Zerman L, Di Blasi P, et al. (2003) Rhinitis in pre-school children: prevalence, association with allergic diseases and risk factors. Clin Exp Allergy 33: 1349–1354.
11. Wang WC, Lue KH, Sheu JN (n.d.) Allergic diseases in preschool children in Taichung City. Zhonghua Min Guo Xiao Er Ke Yi Xue Hui Za Zhi 39: 314–318.
12. Kulig M, Klettke U, Wahn V, Forster J, Bauer CP, et al. (2000) Development of seasonal allergic rhinitis during the first 7 years of life. J Allergy Clin Immunol 106: 832–839.
13. Herr M, Clarisse B, Nikasinovic L, Foucault C, Le Marec A-M, et al. (2011) Does allergic rhinitis exist in infancy? Findings from the PARIS birth cohort. Allergy 66: 214–221.
14. Ballardini N, Nilsson C, Nilsson M, Lilja G (2006) ImmunoCAP Phadiatop Infant—a new blood test for detecting IgE sensitisation in children at 2 years of age. Allergy 61: 337–343.
15. Martinez FD, Wright AL, Taussig LM, Holberg CJ, Halonen M, et al. (1995) Asthma and wheezing in the first six years of life. The Group Health Medical Associates. N Engl J Med 332: 133–138.
16. Togias A (2003) Rhinitis and asthma: evidence for respiratory system integration. J Allergy Clin Immunol 111: 1171–83.
17. Just J, Gouvis-Echraghi R, Couderc R, Guillemot-Lambert N, Saint-Pierre P (2012) Novel severe wheezy young children phenotypes: boys atopic multiple-trigger and girls nonatopic uncontrolled wheeze. J Allergy Clin Immunol 130: 103–10.
18. Tabachnik E, Levison H (1981) Postgraduate course presentation. Infantile bronchial asthma. J Allergy Clin Immunol 67: 339–347.
19. Asher MI, Keil U, Anderson HR, Beasley R, Crane J, et al. (1995) International Study of Asthma and Allergies in Childhood (ISAAC): rationale and methods. Eur Respir J 8: 483–491.
20. NAEPP 2007 Guidelines. Available: http://www.nhlbi.nih.gov/guidelines/asthma/asthsumm.pdf. Accessed 27 April 2014.
21. Just J, Nicoloyanis N, Chauvin M, Pribil C, Grimfeld A, et al. (2008) Lack of eosinophilia can predict remission in wheezy infants? Clin Exp Allergy 38: 767–773.
22. Hosmer D, Lemeshow S (2004) Applied Logistic Regression. Wiley.
23. Breiman L (2001) Random forests. Mach Learn 45:5-32.
24. Breiman L, Olshen RA, Stone CJ (1984) Classification and regression trees. Wadsworth & Brooks/Cole., editor Advanced Books and Software.
25. Arshad SH, Tariq SM, Matthews S, Hakim E (2001) Sensitization to common allergens and its association with allergic disorders at age 4 years: a whole population birth cohort study. Pediatrics 108: E33.
26. Kjaer HF, Eller E, Høst A, Andersen KE, Bindslev-Jensen C (2008) The prevalence of allergic diseases in an unselected group of 6-year-old children. The DARC birth cohort study. Pediatr Allergy Immunol 19: 737–745.
27. Kulig M, Bergmann R, Tacke U, Wahn U, Guggenmoos-Holzmann I (1998) Long-lasting sensitization to food during the first two years precedes allergic airway disease. The MAS Study Group, Germany. Pediatr Allergy Immunol 9: 61–67.
28. Du Toit G, Roberts G, Sayre PH, Plaut M, Bahnson HT, et al. (2013) Identifying infants at high risk of peanut allergy: the Learning Early About Peanut Allergy (LEAP) screening study. J Allergy Clin Immunol 131: 135–43.
29. Brough HA, Santos AF, Makinson K, Penagos M, Stephens AC, et al. (2013) Peanut protein in household dust is related to household peanut consumption and is biologically active. J Allergy Clin Immunol 132: 630–638.
30. Tolosi L, Lengauer T (2011) Classification with correlated features: unreliability of feature ranking and solutions. Bioinformatics 27: 1986–1994.
31. Zacharasiewicz A, Zidek T, Haidinger G, Waldhör T, Vutuc C, et al. (2000) Symptoms suggestive of atopic rhinitis in children aged 6-9 years and the indoor environment. Allergy 55: 945–950.
32. Jaakkola JJK, Hwang B-F, Jaakkola MS (2010) Home dampness and molds as determinants of allergic rhinitis in childhood: a 6-year, population-based cohort study. Am J Epidemiol 172: 451–459.
33. Mudarri D, Fisk WJ (2007) Public health and economic impact of dampness and mold. Indoor Air 17: 226–235.
34. O'Sullivan MM, Brandfield J, Hoskote SS, Segal SN, Chug L, et al. (2012) Environmental improvements brought by the legal interventions in the homes of poorly controlled inner-city adult asthmatic patients: a proof-of-concept study. J Asthma 49: 911–917.
35. Husman T (1996) Health effects of indoor-air microorganisms. Scand J Work Environ Health 22: 5–13.
36. Lee JT, Lam ZCM, Lee WT, Kuo LCT, Jayant V, et al. (2004) Familial risk of allergic rhinitis and atopic dermatitis among Chinese families in Singapore. Ann Acad Med Singapore 33: 71–74.
37. Wadonda-Kabondo N, Sterne JAC, Golding J, Kennedy CTC, Archer CB, et al. (2004) Association of parental eczema, hayfever, and asthma with atopic dermatitis in infancy: birth cohort study. Arch Dis Child 89: 917–921.
38. Clarisse B, Demattei C, Nikasinovic L, Just J, Daures J-P, et al. (2009) Bronchial obstructive phenotypes in the first year of life among Paris birth cohort infants. Pediatr Allergy Immunol 20: 126–133.
39. Lohia S, Schlosser RJ, Soler ZM (2013) Impact of intranasal corticosteroids on asthma outcomes in allergic rhinitis: a meta-analysis. Allergy 68: 569–579.
40. Kim S-W, Han DH, Lee S-J, Lee CH, Rhee C-S (n.d.) Bronchial hyperresponsiveness in pediatric rhinitis patients: the difference between allergic and nonallergic rhinitis. Am J Rhinol Allergy 27: e63–8.
41. Westman M, Stjärne P, Asarnoj A, Kull I, van Hage M, et al. (2012) Natural course and comorbidities of allergic and nonallergic rhinitis in children. J Allergy Clin Immunol 129: 403–408.
42. Simpson A, Tan VYF, Winn J, Svensén M, Bishop CM, et al. (2010) Beyond atopy: multiple patterns of sensitization in relation to asthma in a birth cohort study. Am J Respir Crit Care Med 181: 1200–1206.
43. Schroeder A, Kumar R, Pongracic JA, Sullivan CL, Caruso DM, et al. (2009) Food allergy is associated with an increased risk of asthma. Clin Exp Allergy 39: 261–270.
44. Biagini JM, LeMasters GK, Ryan PH, Levin L, Reponen T, et al. (2006) Environmental risk factors of rhinitis in early infancy. Pediatr Allergy Immunol 17: 278–284.

Severe Eczema in Infancy Can Predict Asthma Development. A Prospective Study to the Age of 10 Years

Marie Ekbäck[1], Michaela Tedner[2], Irene Devenney[1]*, Göran Oldaeus[3], Gunilla Norrman[4], Leif Strömberg[5], Karin Fälth-Magnusson[1]

1 Division of Pediatrics, Department of Clinical and Experimental Medicine, Faculty of Health Sciences, Linköping University and Department of Pediatrics, County Council of Östergötland, Linköping, Sweden, 2 Pediatric Clinic, Täby, Stockholm, Sweden, 3 Pediatric Clinic, County Hospital Ryhov, Jönköping, Sweden, 4 Pediatric Clinic, Hudiksvall, Sweden, 5 Department of Pediatrics in Norrköping, County Council of Östergötland, Norrköping, Sweden

Abstract

Background: Children with atopic eczema in infancy often develop allergic rhinoconjunctivitis and asthma, but the term "atopic march" has been questioned as the relations between atopic disorders seem more complicated than one condition progressing into another.

Objective: In this prospective multicenter study we followed children with eczema from infancy to the age of 10 years focusing on sensitization to allergens, severity of eczema and development of allergic airway symptoms at 4.5 and 10 years of age.

Methods: On inclusion, 123 children were examined. Hanifin-Rajka criteria and SCORAD index were used to describe the eczema. Episodes of wheezing were registered, skin prick tests and IgE tests were conducted and questionnaires were filled out. Procedures were repeated at 4.5 and 10 years of age with additional examinations for ARC and asthma.

Results: 94 out of 123 completed the entire study. High SCORAD points on inclusion were correlated with the risk of developing ARC, ($B = 9.86$, $P = 0.01$) and asthma, ($B = 10.17$, $P = 0.01$). For infants with eczema and wheezing at the first visit, the OR for developing asthma was 4.05($P = 0.01$). ARC at 4.5 years of age resulted in an OR of 11.28($P = 0.00$) for asthma development at 10 years.

Conclusion: This study indicates that infant eczema with high SCORAD points is associated with an increased risk of asthma at 10 years of age. Children with eczema and wheezing episodes during infancy are more likely to develop asthma than are infants with eczema alone. Eczema in infancy combined with early onset of ARC seems to indicate a more severe allergic disease, which often leads to asthma development. The progression from eczema in infancy to ARC at an early age and asthma later in childhood shown in this study supports the relevance of the term "atopic march", at least in more severe allergic disease.

Editor: Jacques Zimmer, Centre de Recherche Public de la Santé (CRP-Santé), Luxembourg

Funding: Financial support was given by the Health Research Council in the South-East of Sweden (FORSS), the Swedish Asthma and Allergy Association's Research Foundation, and grants were received from Lion's Club in the South-East of Sweden, GlaxoSmithKline and Konsul Th C Bergh's Foundation for Scientific Research. The funders had no role in study design, data collection and analysis, decision to publish, or preparation of the manuscript.

Competing Interests: GlaxoSmithKline supported the study with a minor grant in 2004 given as a scholarship to one of the junior researchers in the group. This does not alter the authors' adherence to PLOS ONE policies on sharing data and materials. There are no competing interests, and the funder has no role in the study design, data collection and analysis, decision to publish, or preparation of the manuscript. No products in development or marketed products from GlaxoSmithKline were part of the study.

* E-mail: irene.devenney@lio.se

Introduction

Background

Children with an atopic constitution are at risk of developing allergic symptoms, such as atopic eczema, food allergy, allergic rhinoconjunctivitis (ARC) and asthma [1–3], with multiple factors influencing these immune responses. Especially in countries with a western life style the prevalence of allergy in childhood has increased remarkably in recent decades [2,4,5]. The "atopic march" is a term that has been used to describe the progression from atopic eczema and food allergy during infancy to ARC and subsequently to asthma later in childhood [6–9]. Previous studies have shown that children with atopic eczema or those sensitized to allergens in early childhood more often develop ARC and asthma [8,10–13]. However, the concept of "atopic march" has been questioned. The relations between the allergic disorders seem to be much more complicated than that of one condition progressing into another [7,8].

Wheezing during infancy is common, but is not necessarily caused by asthma. Epidemiological studies have described different phenotypes of asthma [3,8,14,15], many of which are transient conditions with low risk of asthma and allergy later in life. However, 30–50% of the children involved have been reported to develop persistent asthma, especially if they are sensitized [2,3,16].

Several environmental factors have been associated with asthma in epidemiological studies, for example sensitization to aeroallergens early in life, exposure to pets, maternal diet during pregnancy and lactation, breastfeeding, exposure to tobacco smoke during pregnancy and early in life, viral infections, a disturbed balance of microbes, and psychosocial factors [3,17]. Differences in opinion make it controversial to give advice concerning pets and maternal diet. Breastfeeding has been reported to decrease wheezing associated with respiratory infections in early childhood, but there is not enough evidence as to whether it prevents asthma [3,18].

A better understanding of the process of developing allergic airway symptoms, including early warning signs, would be of great value. This could help to identify children at high risk of developing asthma and thereby enable early intervention and treatment and perhaps even aid prevention.

Aim

The aim of the present study was to follow infants with eczema and suspected food allergy over time, focusing on sensitization to allergens, severity of eczema and the development of allergic airway symptoms at 4.5 and 10 years of age. Furthermore, we wanted to identify any early signs that could be associated with a higher risk of developing allergic airway symptoms.

Methods

Ethics statement

The study was approved by the Human Research Ethics Committees at the Faculty of Health Sciences Linköping University and at the Medical Faculty at Uppsala University. Written informed consent was obtained from the children's parents at all ages and from the children at 10 years of age.

Methods

The study population was 123 children (71 boys and 52 girls) with eczema and suspected food allergy recruited to the study from June 1999 to September 2001. They were all under two years of age (median 6 months, range 1–23) and had been referred from their primary care physician to the pediatric clinics in Linköping, Jönköping, Norrköping and Hudiksvall [19].

Factors studied on inclusion and at follow-up examinations are presented in Table 1. At the first visit, the patients were examined by a pediatrician. Questionnaires regarding other atopic manifestations, family history, environmental factors and nutrition were completed by the parents. The diagnostic criteria proposed by Hanifin and Rajka were used to diagnose atopic dermatitis [20]. The severity of eczema was evaluated by a standardized method, "The Severity Scoring of Atopic Dermatitis" (SCORAD). SCORAD was used to classify eczema as mild (≤25 points), moderate (26–50 points) or severe (>50 points) [21]. Standardized skin prick tests (SPT) were performed in a standardized way [22]; a mean wheal diameter of three mm was used as the lower limit for positivity as recommended in the EAACI position paper [22,23]. The SPTs and the SCORAD were assessed by experienced allergy nurses. All children were recommended treatment with emollients and/or topical steroids. Children with a positive SPT were recommended a temporary elimination diet. For food allergic children, milk and eggs were reintroduced in either open standardized or double-blind placebo-controlled oral food challenges when SPT was ≤10 mm and SCORAD ≤25points [19]. Six weeks after inclusion, the patients were reexamined by the same nurse using SCORAD and SPT. Venous blood samples were obtained on inclusion, at the six-week follow-up, at 4.5 and 10 years of age. IgE was analyzed with UniCAP, as previously described [24].

The patients were reexamined by a pediatrician at 4.5 years and 10 years of age. Persisting eczema was assessed using Hanifin-Rajka criteria, severity was graded according to SCORAD at both visits, and venous blood samples were obtained. SPTs were performed for foods and aeroallergens (Table 1). Questionnaires enquiring about other allergic manifestations and tolerance to food were completed. At 10 years of age, lung function tests were performed. A standardized spirometric test combined with a standardized exercise test was performed. It included a period of 6 minutes intense running to increase the pulse rate to 160 beats per minute. Heart rate and oxygen saturation were documented. Spirometric values were measured before and immediately after running, after 10 minutes rest, and 15 minutes after inhalation of 1 mg terbutalin, inhaled from a multi-dose powder inhaler. Exhaled nitric oxide was measured with NIOX MINO (Aerocrine, Solna, Sweden) before and directly after the exercise period.

After the final examination at 10 years of age, the patients were divided into three groups. The first group was patients with no persisting allergic airway problems with or without eczema, the second group was patients suffering from ARC, and the third group was patients suffering from asthma. Patients with both ARC and asthma at 10 years were included in the asthma group.

The diagnostic criterion used for asthma in infants and preschool children in this study was any episode of obstructive airway symptoms in combination with IgE-mediated eczema, as recommended by the Swedish National Pediatric Allergy Group [25].

At the final visit for the 10 year-olds, an increase in FEV1 ≥ 10% after inhaling salbutamol or a reduction in FEV1 ≥10% of baseline levels after effort was considered diagnostic for asthma, as were patients previously diagnosed as fulfilling the criteria for asthma [26,27]. ARC was defined as symptoms of rhinitis or conjunctivitis after exposure to allergens, correlating to a positive SPT or a positive test for specific IgE. Sensitization was defined as either a positive SPT or specific IgE values ≥0.35kUA/l [24].

Statistics

Binary logistic regression with ARC and asthma as covariates was used to calculate odds ratios (ORs) with 95% confidence intervals (CIs). Linear regression was used to study the relationship between different dependent scalar variables, ARC and asthma as independent variables. Significance tests of the regression coefficients, here referred to as B, together with estimates and accompanying CIs are presented. T test was used to analyze differences in SCORAD at the first visit between drop-outs and the study population. Differences combined with p values of < 0.05 were considered statistically significant. Descriptive statistics were used to calculate means and confidence intervals for the groups with no airway symptoms, ARC and asthma seen in the Figures 1–4. All calculations were made with SPSS version 20 for Windows.

Results

Participation and summary of symptoms

At the follow-up at 4.5 years of age, 115 out of 123 children participated and several of them displayed more than one

Table 1. An overview of examinations and tests performed on the children with eczema on inclusion, at 4.5 years and at 10 years.

	Inclusion	4,5 years	10 years
Physical examination	X	X	X
SCORAD	X	X	X
Hanifin-Rajka	X	X	X
SPT	X	X	X
IgE	X	X	X
Questionnaries	X	X	X
Wheezing episodes	X		
ARC		X	X
Asthma		X	X
Spirometry			X
Exhaled NO			X

symptom. Of the 115, 60 still suffered from eczema, 26 had ARC, 37 had asthma and 35 had no symptoms of atopic disease at all. Ninety-four out of 123 completed the entire study until 10 years of age, of whom 60 continued to have eczema, 44 had ARC, 27 had asthma and 13 had no symptoms of allergy at all.

Characteristics on inclusion and later risk of disease

At the first visit, the duration of breastfeeding in months, sensitization to cow's milk and egg, having furred pets at home, SCORAD points, eczema fulfilling Hanifin-Rajka criteria, episodes of wheezing and exposure to tobacco smoke were studied.

Higher SCORAD points on inclusion increased the risk of having ARC, B = 9.86 (95%CI 2.18–17.53; P = 0.01) and asthma, B = 10.17 (95%CI 2.82–17.52; P = 0.01) at 10 years of age.

For infants with eczema and wheezing at the first visit, the OR for being diagnosed with asthma at 10 years was 4.05 (95%CI 1.42–11.56; P = 0.01). Sensitization to egg correlated to the risk of an asthma diagnosis at 10 years of age, OR 2.59 (95%CI 1.00–6.67; P = 0.05). On inclusion, no statistically significant differences were found for fulfilled Hanifin-Rajka criteria, sensitization to milk, breastfeeding, having furred pets, or exposure to tobacco smoke.

Characteristics at 4.5 years and later risk of disease

At 4.5 years of age, exposure to tobacco smoke, having furred pets at home, sensitization to milk, egg and aeroallergens, SCORAD points, eczema fulfilling Hanifin- Rajka criteria, ARC and asthma were studied.

For children with remaining sensitization to egg at 4.5 years of age, the OR for ARC at 10 years of age was 10.30 (95%CI 3.28–32.38; P = 0.00). For an asthma diagnosis at 10 years of age, the OR was 3.63 (95%CI 1.25–10.60; P = 0.02). Sensitization to aeroallergens at 4.5 years of age meant an OR of 4.70 (95%CI 1.50–14.75; P = 0.01) for ARC at 10 years of age and an OR of 6.21 (95%CI 1.83–21.06; P = 0.00) for asthma at 10 years of age. ARC at 4.5 years of age gave an OR of 11.28 (95%CI 3.61–35.28; P = 0.00) for asthma development but an OR of 3.05 (95%CI 0.88–10.60; P = 0.08) for only ARC at 10 years of age. For children diagnosed with asthma at 4.5 years of age, the OR for asthma at 10 years of age was 14.44 (95%CI 4.77–43.72; P = 0.00), whereas the OR for only ARC at 10 years of age was 1.08 (95% CI 0.34–3.47; P = 0.89).

No statistically significant differences were found for SCORAD points, having furred pets, remaining sensitization to milk, and fulfilled Hanifin-Rajka criteria at 4.5 years of age.

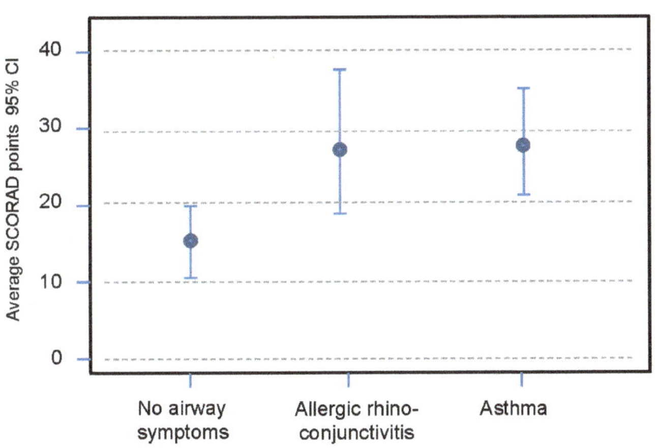

Figure 1. Average SCORAD points on inclusion for children with no airway symptoms, allergic rhinoconjunctivitis or asthma at 10 years.

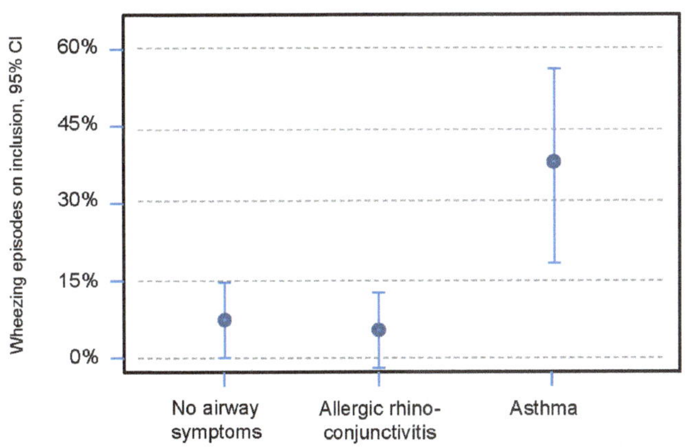

Figure 2. Percentage of children who had had at least one episode of wheezing before inclusion in the groups who had no airway symptoms, allergic rhinoconjunctivitis and asthma at 10 years.

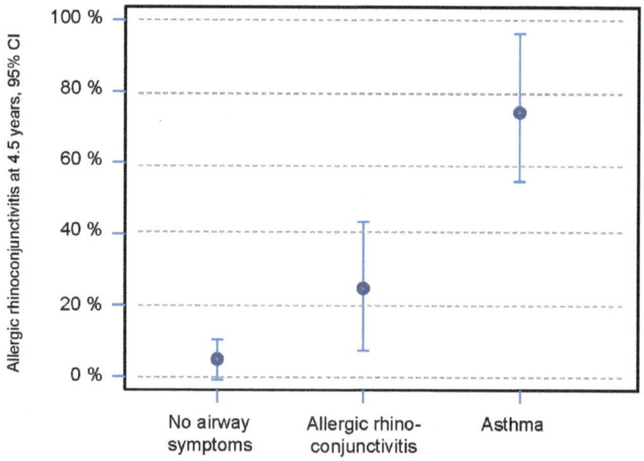

Figure 3. Percentage of children who had allergic rhinoconjunctivitis at 4.5 years among the groups with no airway symptoms, allergic rhinoconjunctivitis and asthma at 10 years.

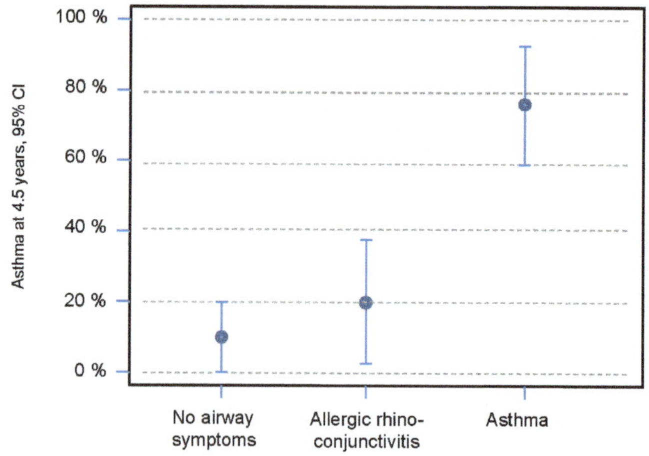

Figure 4. Percentage of children who were diagnosed with asthma at 4.5 years in the groups with no airway symptoms, allergic rhinoconjunctivitis and asthma at 10 years.

Results at 10 years of age

Heredity, gender, exposure to tobacco smoke during the first 10 years, pets at home, sensitization to foods and aeroallergens, SCORAD, eczema fulfilling Hanifin-Rajka criteria, and values of exhaled NO before and after effort were studied at 10 years of age.

For children with eczema sensitized to aeroallergens at 10 years of age, the OR for ARC was 30.25 (CI 3.69-248.25; P = 0.00) and the OR for asthma was 5.84 (CI 1.65–20.71; P0.01). Higher levels of NO before effort resulted in B = 7.16 (CI 0.26–14.06; P = 0.04) for ARC and B = 13.25 (CI 6.61–19.89; P = 0.00) for asthma. For higher NO values after effort, the B for ARC was 7.76 (CI 0.85–14.66; P = 0.03) and for asthma, 13.26 (CI 6.35–20.16; P = 0.00).

The relation between eczema severity on inclusion and SCORAD points at 10 years of age was also studied. There was no significant difference in SCORAD points at 10 years of age between children with mild, moderate and severe eczema as infants.

Comparing the groups with no airway symptoms, ARC and asthma at ten years displayed no significant difference in positive family history of atopy (defined as at least one first-degree family member suffering from allergic symptoms), gender and fulfilled Hanifin-Rajka criteria.

To compare the representativity of the compliant cases with that of the original cohort, we also studied differences in SCORAD points on inclusion between the patients who had dropped out and those who remained in the study at 10 years of age. The drop-outs had a mean SCORAD point of 22.11, whereas those who remained had a mean SCORAD point of 21.47 on inclusion. The difference was not significant, P = 0.84.

Discussion

In this prospective multicenter study we followed 123 children with eczema from infancy to 10 years of age to study factors that might influence and predict the risk of developing allergic airway symptoms.

Of the 123 patients, 94 completed the entire study. At the age of 10 years, 64% of the children still had problems with eczema, 47% had ARC, 29% had asthma, and only 14% had no symptoms of allergy. Therefore eczema in infancy must be considered a serious warning sign for lasting allergic problems rather than a transient condition, although eczema usually gets less severe with time [28]. Atopic disease during childhood often persists into adulthood [9]. The reported risk for children with atopic eczema of developing asthma varies between different studies. Our results are in line with several other studies [29–32]. Compared with the results from the Swedish birth cohort, BAMSE, which followed 810 children with infantile eczema to 12 years of age, the children in our study more often had persisting symptoms [33,34]. This difference might be explained by the fact that the children in the present study who were diagnosed with eczema and referred to a pediatric clinic are likely to have had more severe symptoms than the children in BAMSE, whose were diagnosed with eczema based on questionnaire data.

We found that the risk of developing ARC and asthma before 10 years of age correlated with high SCORAD points during infancy. The SCORAD system has previously shown adequate validity and reliability to measure the severity of eczema [35,36]. Our findings indicate that high SCORAD points in infancy could also be used to predict the risk of developing asthma and that severe eczema is more associated with allergic airway symptoms is than mild eczema. In contrast, high SCORAD points at the ages of 4.5 and 10 years were not associated with a higher risk of asthma or ARC when the patients were 10 years old. It has previously been shown that the severity of atopic dermatitis predicts the prognosis of eczema and the risk of developing other atopic manifestations [32,37]. This study refutes the notion that severe eczema in infancy, classified according to SCORAD, is a predictor of a poorer prognosis of eczema later in childhood, as we did not find any correlation between high SCORAD points in infancy and high SCORAD points at 10 years of age. Nor did we find any correlation between high SCORAD points in infancy and remaining eczema at 10 years of age that fulfilled the Hanifin-Rajka criteria.

Wheezing in infancy is often transient, and infants tend to outgrow their breathing problems [16]. For our patients with eczema, however, wheezing meant a 4 times greater risk of having an asthma diagnosis at the age of 10 compared with infants affected by eczema only. This is not surprising as other atopic manifestations among wheezing infants are known risk factors for remaining asthma [38]. Children who fulfilled the criteria for asthma at 4.5 years had a 14 times higher risk of suffering from asthma at 10 years of age than had children with only eczema and no wheezing.

The children in our study who had symptoms of ARC at 4.5 years of age had a high risk of developing asthma. At 10 years of age, 67% of them were diagnosed with asthma, and the risk of developing asthma was 11 times higher than for 4.5 year olds without ARC. A strong association between ARC and asthma development was expected as Peroni et al found a strong correlation among 3–5 year olds [39]. Among adults, rhinitis is seen as an independent risk factor for developing asthma [40,41]. Our study confirms the correlation between ARC and asthma for children with eczema. It is likely that eczema in infancy combined with early onset of ARC indicates a more severe allergic disease, which tends to lead to asthma development rather than ARC only.

Concerning food allergy, sensitization to hen's egg in infancy was correlated with a risk of developing asthma. Remaining sensitization to egg at 4.5 years of age was associated with both ARC and asthma development, confirming several other studies [37,42]. In early childhood, sensitization to hen's egg has been associated with sensitization to airborne allergens [43]. At the age of 10 we found no correlation for egg sensitization, ARC and asthma. For our patients, sensitization to aeroallergens at 4.5 and 10 years of age was a strong predictor of allergic airway symptoms, as shown in earlier studies [44,45].

Family history is a well-known risk factor for atopic diseases [46,47]. Almost all patients in our study had a positive family history of atopy, with at least one first-degree family member suffering from allergic symptoms, which probably explains why heredity did not have any impact on the results. Parental smoking, before or immediately after birth, may not increase the risk of allergic sensitization in children, but it is a significant risk factor for recurrent wheezing in the first 1.5 years of life [48,49]. In our study, only six children were exposed to tobacco smoke and almost no parents reported indoor smoking. This might explain why we were unable to find any correlation between tobacco smoke and airway problems in this study population.

To our knowledge, this is the only prospective study that has followed infants with eczema to the age of 10 with standardized methods such as SCORAD index and Hanifin-Rajka criteria to objectively describe the eczema, and with spirometric and NO tests for a reliable asthma diagnosis [50]. One concern was that following children for a long time could increase the number of drop-outs. It is plausible to assume that children who did not have any allergic symptoms would be less enthusiastic to continue the study and more likely to be found among our drop-outs, which could affect the result. This, however, has not been the case in other studies [33,51,52]. To minimize the risk of misinterpreting the results, we compared SCORAD points on inclusion for drop-outs with the rest of the study population and found no significant difference between the groups.

Conclusions

This study indicates that high SCORAD points in infants with eczema are associated with a greater risk of asthma at 10 years of age. Children with eczema and wheezing episodes during infancy are more likely to get asthma later in life compared with infants with eczema only. Eczema in infancy combined with early onset of ARC appears to indicate a more severe allergic disease, which often leads to asthma development. The study shows that the progression from eczema in infancy to ARC at an early age and asthma later in childhood could support the relevance of the term "atopic march", at least for children with a more severe allergic disease.

Acknowledgments

We would like to thank all the children and their parents who participated. We would also like to express our gratitude to the participating nurses. Thanks to Karl Wahlin for invaluable statistical advice. Thanks also to Dr. Lennart Nilsson for valuable advice. The advice on language from Maurice Devenney is gratefully acknowledged.

Author Contributions

Conceived and designed the experiments: MT ID GO GN LS KFM. Performed the experiments: ME MT ID GO GN LS KFM. Analyzed the data: ME ID. Wrote the paper: ME ID KFM.

References

1. Van Bever HP (2009) Determinants in early life for asthma development. Allergy Asthma Clin Immunol 9;5(1):6.
2. Host A, Halken S (2000) The role of allergy in childhood asthma. Allergy 55(7):600–608.
3. Pedersen SE, Hurd SS, Lemanske RF Jr, Becker A, Zar HJ, et al. (2011) Global strategy for the diagnosis and management of asthma in children 5 years and younger. Pediatr Pulmonol 46(1):1–17.
4. Burgess JA, Lowe AJ, Matheson MC, Varigos G, Abramson MJ, et al. (2009) Does eczema lead to asthma? J Asthma 46(5):429–436.
5. Leung DY, Bieber T (2003) Atopic dermatitis. Lancet 11;361(9352):151–160.
6. Ker J, Hartert TV (2009) The atopic march: what's the evidence? Ann Allergy Asthma Immunol 103(4):282–289.
7. Scadding GK (2007) Further marches: allergic and non-allergic. Clin Exp Allergy 37(4):485–487.
8. van der Hulst AE, Klip H, Brand PL (2007) Risk of developing asthma in young children with atopic eczema: a systematic review. J Allergy Clin Immunol 120(3):565–569.
9. Nissen SP, Kjaer HF, Host A, Nielsen J, Halken S (2013) The natural course of sensitization and allergic diseases from childhood to adulthood. Pediatr Allergy Immunol 24(6):549–555.
10. Carlsten C, Dimich-Ward H, Ferguson A, Watson W, Rousseau R, et al. (2013) Atopic dermatitis in a high-risk cohort: natural history, associated allergic outcomes, and risk factors. Ann Allergy Asthma Immunol 110(1):24–28.
11. Dharmage SC, Lowe AJ, Matheson MC, Burgess JA, Allen KJ, et al. (2013) Atopic dermatitis and the atopic march revisited. Allergy 14.
12. Saunes M, Oien T, Dotterud CK, Romundstad PR, Storro O, et al. (2012) Early eczema and the risk of childhood asthma: a prospective, population-based study. BMC Pediatr 24;12:168-2431-12-168.
13. von Kobyletzki LB, Bornehag CG, Hasselgren M, Larsson M, Lindstrom CB, et al. (2012) Eczema in early childhood is strongly associated with the development of asthma and rhinitis in a prospective cohort. BMC Dermatol 27;12:11-5945-12-11.
14. Fitzpatrick AM, Teague WG, Meyers DA, Peters SP, Li X, et al. (2011) Heterogeneity of severe asthma in childhood: confirmation by cluster analysis of children in the National Institutes of Health/National Heart, Lung, and Blood Institute Severe Asthma Research Program. J Allergy Clin Immunol 127(2):382–389.e1–13.
15. Just J, Saint-Pierre P, Gouvis-Echraghi R, Boutin B, Panayotopoulos V, et al. (2013) Wheeze phenotypes in young children have different courses during the preschool period. Ann Allergy Asthma Immunol 111(4):256–261.e1.
16. Martinez FD, Wright AL, Taussig LM, Holberg CJ, Halonen M, et al. (1995) Asthma and wheezing in the first six years of life. The Group Health Medical Associates. N Engl J Med 19;332(3):133–138.
17. Agache I, Ciobanu C (2010) Risk factors and asthma phenotypes in children and adults with seasonal allergic rhinitis. Phys Sportsmed 38(4):81–86.
18. Duncan JM, Sears MR (2008) Breastfeeding and allergies: time for a change in paradigm? Curr Opin Allergy Clin Immunol 8(5):398–405.
19. Devenney I, Norrman G, Oldaeus G, Stromberg L, Falth-Magnusson K (2006) A new model for low-dose food challenge in children with allergy to milk or egg. Acta Paediatr 95(9):1133–1139.
20. Hanifin JM Rajka G (1980) Diagnostic features of atopic dermatitis. Acta Derm Venereol 92:44–47.
21. European Task Force on Atopic Dermatitis (1993) Severity scoring of atopic dermatitis: the SCORAD index. Consensus Report of the European Task Force on Atopic Dermatitis. Dermatology 186(1):23–31.
22. Devenney I, Falth-Magnusson K (2001) Skin prick test in duplicate: is it necessary? Ann Allergy Asthma Immunol 87(5):386–389.
23. The European Academy of Allergology and Clinical Immunology (1993) Position paper: Allergen standardization and skin tests. Allergy 48(14 Suppl):48–82.

24. Tomicic S, Norrman G, Falth-Magnusson K, Jenmalm MC, Devenney I, et al. (2009) High levels of IgG4 antibodies to foods during infancy are associated with tolerance to corresponding foods later in life. Pediatr Allergy Immunol 20(1):35–41.
25. Swedish National Pediatric Allergy Group (nd) 1st Asthma in Toddlers - terminology and diagnoses. Available: http://www.barnallergisektionen.se/stenciler_nya06/b1_astmadefinitioner.html. Accessed 2005.
26. Dalen G, Kjellman B (1979) Assessment of lung function on healthy children using an electronic spirometer and an air-flowmeter before and after inhalation of an adrenergic receptor stimulant. Acta Paediatr Scand 68(1):103–108.
27. Silverman M AS (1972) Standardization of exercise test in asthmatic children. Arch Dis Child 47:882–889.
28. Illi S, von Mutius E, Lau S, Nickel R, Gruber C, et al. (2004) The natural course of atopic dermatitis from birth to age 7 years and the association with asthma. J Allergy Clin Immunol 113(5):925–931.
29. van der Hulst AE, Klip H, Brand PL (2007) Risk of developing asthma in young children with atopic eczema: a systematic review. J Allergy Clin Immunol 120(3):565–569.
30. Spergel JM, Paller AS (2003) Atopic dermatitis and the atopic march. J Allergy Clin Immunol 112(6 Suppl):S118–27.
31. Bergmann RL, Edenharter G, Bergmann KE, Forster J, Bauer CP, et al. (1998) Atopic dermatitis in early infancy predicts allergic airway disease at 5 years. Clin Exp Allergy 28(8):965–970.
32. Gustafsson D, Sjoberg O, Foucard T (2000) Development of allergies and asthma in infants and young children with atopic dermatitis—a prospective follow-up to 7 years of age. Allergy 55(3):240–245.
33. Ballardini N, Kull I, Lind T, Hallner E, Almqvist C, et al. (2012) Development and comorbidity of eczema, asthma and rhinitis to age 12: data from the BAMSE birth cohort. Allergy 67(4):537–544.
34. Ballardini N, Bergström A, Böhme M, van Hage M, Hallner E, et al. Infantile Eczema - prognosis and risk of asthma an rhinitis in pre-adolescence. J.Allergy Clin.Immunol. In press.
35. Schmitt J, Langan S, Williams HC (2007) European Dermato-Epidemiology Network. What are the best outcome measurements for atopic eczema? A systematic review. J Allergy Clin Immunol 120(6):1389–1398.
36. Schram ME, Spuls PI, Leeflang MM, Lindeboom R, Bos JD, et al. (2012) EASI, (objective) SCORAD and POEM for atopic eczema: responsiveness and minimal clinically important difference. Allergy 67(1):99–106.
37. Ricci G, Patrizi A, Baldi E, Menna G, Tabanelli M, et al. (2006) Long-term follow-up of atopic dermatitis: retrospective analysis of related risk factors and association with concomitant allergic diseases. J Am Acad Dermatol 55(5):765–771.
38. Frank PI, Morris JA, Hazell ML, Linehan MF, Frank TL (2008) Long term prognosis in preschool children with wheeze: longitudinal postal questionnaire study 1993–2004. BMJ 21;336(7658):1423–1426.
39. Peroni DG, Piacentini GL, Alfonsi L, Zerman L, Di Blasi P, et al. (2003) Rhinitis in pre-school children: prevalence, association with allergic diseases and risk factors. Clin Exp Allergy 33(10):1349–1354.
40. Shaaban R, Zureik M, Soussan D, Neukirch C, Heinrich J, et al. (2008) Rhinitis and onset of asthma: a longitudinal population-based study. Lancet 20;372(9643):1049–1057.
41. Guerra S, Sherrill DL, Martinez FD, Barbee RA (2002) Rhinitis as an independent risk factor for adult-onset asthma. J Allergy Clin Immunol 109(3):419–425.
42. Gaffin JM, Sheehan WJ, Morrill J, Cinar M, Borras Coughlin IM, et al. (2011) Tree nut allergy, egg allergy, and asthma in children. Clin Pediatr (Phila) 50(2):133–139.
43. Gustafsson D, Sjoberg O, Foucard T (2003) Sensitization to food and airborne allergens in children with atopic dermatitis followed up to 7 years of age. Pediatr Allergy Immunol 14(6):448–452.
44. Govaere E, Van Gysel D, Verhamme KM, Doli E, De Baets F (2009) The association of allergic symptoms with sensitization to inhalant allergens in childhood. Pediatr Allergy Immunol 20(5):448–457.
45. Arshad SH, Tariq SM, Matthews S, Hakim E (2001) Sensitization to common allergens and its association with allergic disorders at age 4 years: a whole population birth cohort study. Pediatrics 108(2):E33.
46. Burke W, Fesinmeyer M, Reed K, Hampson L, Carlsten C (2003) Family history as a predictor of asthma risk. Am J Prev Med 24:160.
47. Litonjua AA, Carey VJ, Burge HA, Weiss ST, Gold DR (1998) Parental history and the risk for childhood asthma. Does mother confer more risk than father? Am J Respir Crit Care Med 158(1):176–181.
48. Strachan DP, Cook DG (1998) Health effects of passive smoking .5. Parental smoking and allergic sensitisation in children. Thorax 53(2):117–123.
49. Halken S (2004) Prevention of allergic disease in childhood: clinical and epidemiological aspects of primary and secondary allergy prevention. Pediatr Allergy Immunol 15 Suppl 16:4–5, 9–32.
50. Jenkins C, Seccombe L, Tomlins R (2012) Investigating asthma symptoms in primary care. BMJ 344:e2734.
51. Savenije OE, Granell R, Caudri D, Koppelman GH, Smit HA, et al. (2011) Comparison of childhood wheezing phenotypes in 2 birth cohorts: ALSPAC and PIAMA. J Allergy Clin Immunol 127(6):1505–12.e14.
52. Ostblom E, Lilja G, Pershagen G, van Hage M, Wickman M (2008) Phenotypes of food hypersensitivity and development of allergic diseases during the first 8 years of life. Clin Exp Allergy 38(8):1325–1332.

16

Identification of Critical Amino Acids in the IgE Epitopes of Ric c 1 and Ric c 3 and the Application of Glutamic Acid as an IgE Blocker

Natalia Deus-de-Oliveira[1], Shayany P. Felix[1], Camila Carrielo-Gama[1], Keysson V. Fernandes[1], Renato Augusto DaMatta[2], Olga L. T. Machado[1]*

1 Laboratório de Química e Função de Proteínas e Peptídeos/Centro de Biociências e Biotecnologia, Universidade Estadual do Norte Fluminense - Darcy Ribeiro, Campos dos Goytacazes, Rio de Janeiro, Brazil, **2** Laboratório de Biologia Celular e Tecidual/Centro de Biociências e Biotecnologia, Universidade Estadual do Norte Fluminense - Darcy Ribeiro, Campos dos Goytacazes, Rio de Janeiro, Brazil

Abstract

Background: The allergenicity of *Ricinus communis* L. (castor bean, Euphorbiaceae) is associated with components of its seeds and pollen. Castor bean allergy has been described not only in laboratory workers, but also in personnel working in oil processing mills, fertilizer retail, the upholstery industry and other industrial fields. In the present study, we describe the critical amino acids in the IgE-binding epitopes in Ric c 1 and Ric c 3, two major allergens of *R. communis*. In addition, we also investigate the cross-reactivity between castor bean and some air and food allergen extracts commonly used in allergy diagnosis.

Methodology/Principal Findings: The IgE reactivity of human sera from atopic patients was screened by immune-dot blot against castor bean allergens. Allergenic activity was evaluated *in vitro* using a rat mast cell activation assay and by ELISA. Cross-reactivity was observed between castor bean allergens and extracts from shrimp, fish, gluten, wheat, soybean, peanut, corn, house dust, tobacco and airborne fungal allergens. We observed that treatment of rat and human sera (from atopic patients) with glutamic acid reduced the IgE-epitope interaction.

Conclusions/Significance: The identification of glutamic acid residues with critical roles in IgE-binding to Ric c 3 and Ric c 1 support the potential use of free amino acids in allergy treatment.

Editor: Jean Kanellopoulos, University Paris Sud, France

Funding: This work was supported by grants CNPq, CAPES (graduate fellowships), and FAPERJ. The funders had no role in study design, data collection and analysis, decision to publish, or preparation of the manuscript.

Competing Interests: The authors have declared that no competing interests exist.

* E-mail: olgauenf@yahoo.com.br

Introduction

Castor bean (*Ricinus communis* L.) contains approximately 50% oil, which has special characteristics such as a high viscosity, a high stability under heat and pressure, a low freezing point, and the ability to form waxy substances upon chemical treatment. As 0energy demands increase and fossil fuels are limited, the development of alternative renewable fuels becomes imperative. Interest in biodiesel has been increasing owing to its environmental benefits and renewability [1–3]. As castor beans are a good biofuel source [3], castor bean cultivation is likely to increase, posing a risk of exposure to pollen allergens [4–6]. In previous studies, major castor bean allergens were identified [7–11]. We have recently reported the identification of IgE-binding epitopes of castor bean seed allergens, defining four continuous epitopes in Ric c 3 and two in Ric c 1 [12].

In the present study we identify critical amino acids for IgE binding and investigate cross-reactivity with allergens typically used for allergy diagnosis. Initially, we utilized the glutamic acid-specific Woodward's Reagent K, WRK, (*N*-ethyl-5-phenylisoxazolium-3′-sulfonate) [13] to demonstrate the importance of the glutamic acid carboxylic group in the Ric c 1 and Ric c 3 epitopes in IgE binding. In addition, pre-incubation of atopic patient serum with free amino acids (glutamic acid) blocked IgE epitope interaction sites. We also have observed cross-reactivity between castor bean and airborne and food allergens, which was also reduced by incubation with dicarboxylic amino acids.

Methods

Plant material and 2S albumin purification

Castor bean (*R. communis L.*, cultivar IAC-226) seeds were obtained from the Instituto Agronômico de Campinas, São Paulo/Brazil. The 2S albumin fractions were isolated and characterized by SDS-PAGE and immunoblotting experiments as described previously [9]. The 2S albumin isoforms, Ric c 1 and Ric c 3 as well as their polypeptide chains were isolated as described by [12].

Animals and antiserum

Isogenic female R/A Tor rats, generally high producers of IgE, were obtained from the animal facility of the Universidade Federal

Fluminense, Niteroi, RJ – Brazil, and all experimental procedures were approved by the animal research ethics committee of this University (Proc. CEUA-UENF/112). Immunizations with the 2S albumin pool (Ric c 1 plus Ric c 3) and serum separation were conducted as previously described [12].

Extraction of IgG by affinity chromatography

IgG and IgE from human and rat sera were separated by affinity chromatography using protein G-Sepharose beads in batch mode with 1.5 mL polypropylene tubes (Sigma protocols). Thirty micro litres of total serum of immunized R/A Tor rat was mixed with the 100 µL of resin and with 50 µL of equilibration buffer. This mixture was incubated for 16 hours under stirring at 4°C. The mixture was centrifuged and the supernatant denoted FE (fraction likely enriched in IgE) was removed and stored at 4°C. After removal of the supernatant, the resin was washed ten times with 100 µL of equilibration buffer to remove the remaining uncoupled material. The immunoglobulin coupled to protein G-Sepharose was eluted using 100 µL of a 0.5 M acetic acid. The acidic solution was immediately neutralized by the addition of 1 M Tris-HCl pH 9.0. After washing and centrifugation, the eluted fraction, denoted FG (fraction likely enriched in IgG), was isolated. The presence of IgG was investigated in both FE and FG by dot blotting. Mast cell degranulation assays in the presence of FG or FE were also performed to identify the immunoglobulin involved in mast cell activation.

Affinity Dot Blotting

Human serum analysis: sera from five patients who had total IgE values of 106 to 1527 KU/L were evaluated for their ability to recognize 2S albumin from *R. communis* by dot blotting. After the first evaluation, patient serum with high intensity recognition of castor bean allergens was used in subsequent assays.

For dot blot assays, 2S albumin or synthetic peptide (10 µg in 10 µL/dot) was spotted onto a nitrocellulose membrane and allowed to dry. The nitrocellulose membrane was incubated with total serum (1:50) or affinity supernatant or eluted fractions, FE and FG, from human or rat serum. Secondary anti-rat IgG or anti-human biotin IgE (0.5 mg/mL) (both diluted 1:2000) was then added to the membrane for 1 hour. Two hours later, IgG was detected using a rabbit anti-rat IgG- HRP conjugate (1:2500). For IgE detection, the membrane was subsequently incubated with streptavidin-biotinylated HRP complex for 1 h. The colour of all probes was developed with a substrate mixture: 5 mg of DAB in 4.9 mL of water, 300 µL of 0.1 M imidazole, 100 µL of Tris-HCl 2 M buffer (pH 7.5) and 5 µL of 30% H_2O_2.

Rat peritoneal mast cells

Wistar rats were obtained from the animal facility of the Universidade Estadual do Norte Fluminense Darcy Ribeiro (UENF). All experimental procedures were approved by the animal research ethics board of the UENF (Proc. CEUA-UENF/112). Rats (weighing ~250 g) were euthanized with CO_2 and a peritoneal wash was performed by injection of 20 mL of DMEM (Dulbecco's Modified Eagle Medium) containing 12 U/mL of heparin. The abdomen was gently massaged for approximately 90 s. The peritoneal cavity was carefully opened and the fluid containing peritoneal cells was aspirated with a Pasteur pipette. Thereafter, the cells were transferred to Petri plates and incubated for 30 min at 37°C. Two-thirds of the supernatant was aspirated and discarded. The mast cell-rich supernatant (1.8×10^5 mast cells/mL) was separated into 100 µL aliquots and kept at room temperature.

Mast cell degranulation assays and cross-reactivity

Rat peritoneal mast cells (100 µL) were incubated with pre-immune serum (control) and activated for 60 min at 37°C using 2S albumin polyclonal anti-rat IgE (2S alb AR IgE). After sensitization with 2S alb AR IgE, cells were washed twice with DMEM. Each experiment was carried out in the presence or absence of the synthetic peptides and a 2S albumin pool (100 ng). After incubation with antibodies and potential allergens (synthetic peptides, 2S albumin), histamine contents were determined (see below) and the cells (in 10 µL) were stained for 15 min with 10 µL of a solution containing 0.1% toluidine blue, 10% formaldehyde and 1% acetic acid, pH 2.8, allowing the visualization of degranulated mast cells. Granulated and degranulated mast cells were counted under a light microscope using the 40 X objective in a Neubauer chamber.

In order to investigate cross-reactivity between 2S albumin from *R. communis* and allergens used for allergy diagnosis, mast cells previously sensitized by 2S alb AR IgE were incubated with airborne and food allergens from FDA Allergenic (FDA-PRICKIT-Lot 04AK00001 and FDA-FOODKIT lot 04AK00004).

The airborne allergens that were tested were from dust, airborne fungi, wool, dust mites, grass, flowers, tobacco, cat epithelium, dog epithelium, horse epithelium, bovine epithelium, epithelia mix, feathers, cotton, horsehair, grass, chamomile, cockroaches, pyrethrum, silk, and cattails. The food allergens were from poultry, shrimp, beef, pork, egg, egg yolk, milk, fish, rice, gluten, corn, wheat, soybean, pepper, pineapple, cocoa, cashew, peanuts, orange, lemon, tomato and strawberry. Protein content measurements of the allergen solutions from FDA allergenic were performed using the Bradford method using egg albumin as a standard. Stock solutions containing 10 µg/mL were prepared and each test used 10 µL of these allergen solutions. Mast cell activation was evaluated by taking the percentage of granulated and degranulated cells as described previously and by the quantification of histamine released.

Histamine quantification

After incubation with antibodies and allergens, the cell suspensions (100 µL) were centrifuged at 170 xg for 10 min. An aliquot of the supernatant (20 µL) was removed for histamine detection. The released histamine was submitted to ion exchange chromatography and quantified using a previously described protocol [12].

Identification of amino acids involved in IgE binding.

The peptides previously identified as IgE-binding epitopes in Ric c 1 or Ric c 3 allergens by Felix et al. [12] were synthesized utilizing the solid phase method. The synthetic peptide sequences are displayed in Table 1. All six peptides (P0 to P5) contained two or more dicarboxylic amino acid residues. In order to investigate which amino acid was able to bind to sensitized mast cells, two strategies were employed: chemical modification of synthetic peptides using Woodward's Reagent K (WRK) and treatment of IgE-mast cells with free amino acids as a potential IgE blocker.

Modification with Woodward's Reagent K (WRK)

WRK is a specific reagent for modifying dicarboxylic amino acids [3]. Samples (500 µg of peptides or 1000 µg of the "pool" of 2S albumin) were treated with the WRK solution (250 mM in 0.001 M HCl). Fifty micro litres of samples and 50 µL of WRK solution were kept at 35°C for 3 hours. Peptide re-purification and chemical modification were evaluated by reverse-phase HPLC and mass spectrometry. The allergenicity of treated peptides or 2S

Table 1. Identification of IgE epitopes from Ric c 1 and Ric c 3.

Sample/Amino acid sequences of the peptide	Degranulationin the presence of total serum	Degranulation in the presence of IgE (affinity FE)	Degranulation in the presence of IgG (affinity FG)
Mast cell isolation (negative control)	30 (+1,0)	30 (+1,0)	30 (+1,0)
2S albumin (positive control)	70 (+1,0)	78,0 (+1,6)	38,8 (+1,7)
P0/EGLRQAI**E**QQQSQGQ	74 (+0,9)	75,0 (+0,5)	33,1 (+1,8)
P1/ESKG**E**R**E**GSSSQQCR	64 (+0,4)	69,9 (+1,7)	38,4 (+0,1)
P2/Q**E**VQRKDLSSC**E**RYL	70 (+0,5)	67,9 (+1,1)	39,0 (+0,7)
P3/Q**E**QQNLRQCQ**E**YIK	65 (+0,7)	65,7 (+0,3)	39,7 (+0,3)
P4/D**E**CQC**E**AIKYIA**E**DQ	67 (+0,5)	67,2 (+0,6)	38,4 (+0,9)
P5/LHG**EE**S**E**RVAQRAG**E**	54 (+0,2)	64,4 (+0,6)	36,0 (+0,8)

albumin was analysed by the mast cell degranulation assay as described above.

Evaluation of chemical modifications using reverse-phase high performance liquid chromatography

To verify the modifications on the proteins after chemical treatments, the samples, synthetic peptides and 2S albumin were subjected to reverse-phase liquid chromatography on a C18 column (Sephasil peptide C18 5 µST 4.6/250, flow rate of 0.7 mL min^{-1} using 0.1% trifluoroacetic acid (TFA) as solvent A and 80% of acetonitrile containing 0.1% TFA as solvent B.) using a Shimadzu apparatus. The elution profile was monitored by on-line measurement of the absorbance at 220 nm. Fractions containing the major peaks were dried in a speed Vac system. The UV spectrum was obtained using a photo-diode detector.

Blockage of IgE

Mast cells sensitized with IgE were treated with 100 ng of aspartic acid, glutamic acid or a mixture containing 100 ng of each other amino acids present in the synthetic peptide (Gly, Leu, Arg, Gln, Ala, Ile, Ser for P_0; Ser, Lys, Gly, Arg, Gln, Cys for P_1; Gln, Val, Arg, Lys, Leu, Ser, Cys, Tyr, for P_2; Gln, Asn, Leu, Arg, Cys, Tyr, Ile, Lys for P_3; Cys, Gln, Ala, Ile, Lys, Tyr, for P_4 and Leu, His, Gly, Ser, Arg, Val, Ala, Gln, for P_5). Amino acids were dissolved in DEMEN. After free amino acid treatment, cells were incubated with 100 ng of each synthetic peptide or allergenic fractions (Ric c 1 or Ric c 3). Mast cell degranulation was evaluated as described, and the percentages of degranulation and histamine release were compared with those triggered by synthetic peptides or by allergenic isoforms in the absence of free amino acid treatment.

Quantification of human IgE using ELISA

During the development of this project, there was no contact with atopic patients. Sera were used after performing security tests, and this project was not submitted to the human ethics committee because patients were not identified. Specific IgE levels were tested by ELISA with 20 µg/well of castor bean allergen. Plates were incubated with serum from one atopic patient diluted 1:50. Bound IgE antibodies were detected with biotin-anti-human IgE (1:2000 diluted) followed by streptavidin-peroxidase conjugate (1:1000 diluted) (Pharmingen). The peroxidase reaction was developed and the optical density (OD) was measured at 492 nm. Each value represents the mean of two assays. OD Values <0.1 were considered negative.

ELISA inhibition and mast cell activation assay for analysis of glutamic acid as an IgE blocker

The ability of glutamic acid to inhibit the binding of allergic patients' IgE to Ric c 1 and Ric c 3 was assessed by ELISA inhibition and mast cell activation assays. Briefly, serum from an atopic patient (427 KU/L- 1:5 diluted) and Wistar rats were preincubated for 1 h with glutamic acid (end concentration 10 µg/mL). The ELISA or mast cell degranulation assays were performed as previously described. The percentage of IgE binding inhibition achieved by the pre-incubation treatment was calculated as follows: percentage of IgE binding $= 100-(OD_I/OD_T \times 100)$; OD_I represents the absorbance after incubation of glutamic acid-treated human serum; and OD_T represents the absorbance of untreated human sera. Mast cell granulation or degranulation was counted by optical microscopy and histamine release was quantified as described above.

Results

Fractionation of serum immunoglobulins by affinity chromatography

Initially, the serum immunoglobulins (IgG and IgE) were separated by affinity chromatography. Two fractions denoted FE

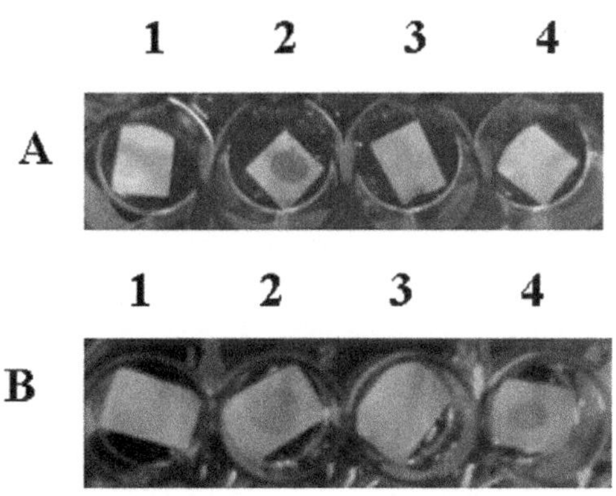

Figure 1. Analysis of rat affinity chromatography fractions FE and FG by dot blotting using a rabbit anti-rat IgG- HRP conjugate. A1 and B1) negative controls: water plus rat serum anti-2S albumin; A2 and B2) positive controls: 2S albumin plus rat serum anti-2S albumin; A3 and B3) affinity buffer plus anti-rat IgG; A4) 2S albumin incubated with FE plus anti-rat IgG; B4) 2S albumin incubated with FG plus anti-rat IgG.

Table 2. Percent of mast cell degranulation induced by Ricinus communis-derived synthetic peptides.

Peptide number	Mast cell degranulation by untreated peptide	Mast cell degranulation by WRK-treated peptide
Control cells	30±3	30±3
P0	74±4	37±1
P1	62±2	37±2
P2v	65±4	30±1
P3	63±2	33±2
P4	65±4	37±1
P5	53±2	39±1

(supernatant fraction) and FG (eluted fraction) were obtained and the presence of IgG was investigated in both fractions by dot blotting. Figure 1 shows the lack of IgG in the supernatant fraction FE (spot A4), while IgG was detected in eluted fraction (spot B4), confirming that this immunoglobulin was removed by affinity chromatography. The supernatant fraction FE was used during mast cell degranulation assays.

The synthetic peptides present in Ric c 1 and Ric c 3 structures, which were recognized by the pool of sera and induced mast cell degranulation as described by Felix et al. [12], were tested in the presence of the FG or FE fractions. Table 1 shows the sequences of these peptides and indicates that mast cell degranulation is mediated only by IgE. The values of mast cell degranulation in the presence of total serum or FE fractions were similar, ranging from 64 to 78%, whereas degranulation mediated by FG was disregarded as it was similar to the negative control (approximately 30%).

Importance of carboxylic groups in IgE binding

We found that the peptides identified as IgE epitopes had at least two glutamic acid residues (Table 1, residues marked in bold). To verify that these residues are essential for IgE binding, we examined mast cells incubated with IgE in the presence of synthetic peptides modified by Woodward's Reagent K. The first step of the reaction with WRK is the formation of an irreversible ketoketenimine that can be identified by a peak of absorbance at 340 nm [14]. The modification of the synthetic peptides by the WRK reagent was confirmed by specific spectra and by the increase of the peptide molecular weights by 254 Dalton or multiples of this value, indicating the inclusion of at least one *N*-ethyl-5-phenylisoxazolium-3′-sulfonate group (data not shown) by each glutamic residue. WRK-modified peptides were employed in mast cell degranulation assays and the results are shown in Table 2. After WRK treatment, peptide-induced mast cell degranulation was severely reduced to levels (30–39%) similar to that observed for the negative controls (30–39%). These data indicate the importance of carboxylic groups on IgE binding and in the mast cell degranulation.

Dicarboxylic amino acids inhibit mast cell degranulation

Mast cells preloaded with IgE from rat serum were pre-incubated with free amino acids and exposed to a 2S albumin pool or IgE epitopes (synthetic peptides). The rationale of our experiment is illustrated in Figure S1.

The process of isolation of mast cells from rat peritoneal cavities induces ~30% degranulation and 2% histamine release; thus, these values were set as a baseline for the negative controls. Castor bean 2S albumin induced 70% mast cell degranulation and more than 40% histamine release when incubated in the presence of IgE (Table 3).

When mast cells were incubated with untreated serum or with serum treated with neutral or basic amino acids, degranulation triggered by allergens could be observed (Table 3, column 4). However, dicarboxylic amino acids protected IgE-bound mast cells from degranulation as described in Table 3 columns 5 to 7, implying that binding of IgE to castor bean 2S albumin was specifically blocked by glutamic or aspartic acid.

Glutamic acid inhibits IgE binding to castor bean allergens.

Initially, the presence of anti-2S albumin IgE specific for castor bean allergen in sera from five atopic patients was evaluated by dot blotting, and the results are presented on Table 4. The serum from patient number 3 (total IgE- 427 KU/L) was the most positive for 2S albumin IgE and was selected for further study. This serum was fractionated by affinity chromatography and the presence of IgE was confirmed by dot blotting analysis to be only in the FE supernatant fraction as presented in Figure 2 (spot 3). We also used ELISA to examine the binding of this atopic patient serum to the 2S albumin pool and their isolated light and heavy chains and synthetic peptides P0 to P5. Higher affinity was observed for the

Table 3. Critical role of dicarboxylic amino acid in mast cell degranulation induced by 2S albumin: percent of mast cell degranulation in the presence of the total serum that had been incubated with or without pooled amino acids.

Sample/Degranulation in the presence of total serum	% of Histamine released	Degranulation in the presence of total serum incubated with pooled amino acids	Degranulation in the presence of total serum incubated with Asp	Degranulation in the presence of total serum incubated with Glu	% of Histamine released after incubation with Glu
30 (+1.0) (negative control)	2	30.0 (±1.0)	30.0 (±1.0)	30.0 (±1.0)	2
70 (+1.0) (Positive control)	64	69.5 (±0.5)	36.8 (±.47)	29.7 (±0.1)	6
P0/74(+0.9)	80	63.0 (±0.7)	40.6 (±0.6)	37.6 (±0.6)	52
P1/64(+0.4)	58	67.1 (±0.7)	39.6 (±1.8)	37.0 (±1.9)	6
P2/70(+0.5)	64	63.5 (±0.4)	40.4 (±0.4)	30.3 (±1.6)	12
P3/65 +0.7)	58	65.2 (±0.7)	40.3 (±0.2)	33.8 (±1.7)	4
P4/67(+0.5)	60	63.8 (±0.8)	39.2 (±0.2)	36.7 (±0.6)	8
P5/54 +0.2)	56	63.4 (±0.9)	41.5 (±0.3)	38.8 (±1.4)	4

Table 4. Detection of IgE anti 2S albumin in Human serum by dot blotting.

Patient	SerumTotal IgE (KU/L)	Dot Blotting
Control cells	1527	-
1	266	+
2	427	+++
3	143	-
4	108	-
5	1527	-

2S albumin pool, P2 and for the Ric c 1 light chain (Figure 3); however, binding was also observed for all tested samples.

The possible blocking effect of glutamic acid was evaluated by ELISA experiments with serum from an allergic patient, and the results are presented in Figure 3. Pre-incubation of serum with glutamic acid inhibited by 78% the IgE binding when 2S albumin pool or Ric c 1 light chain was tested and inhibited by 56% when Ric c 1 heavy chain or both chains from Ric c 3 were used. The IgE binding to P0 and P1 were inhibited by 70% and was completely inhibited to other IgE epitopes, P2, P4 and P5 (Figure 3), confirming the results obtained with sensitized mast cells (Table 3).

Cross-reactivity between castor bean 2S albumin and airborne/food allergens

The results obtained with mast cells previously sensitized with castor bean allergens and triggered by cross-reactivity with commercial allergens are shown in Table 5. Considering positive reactions to be above 50% degranulation, significant IgE reactivity to food extracts from shrimp, fish, gluten, wheat, soybean and peanut were observed. Cross-reactivity was also observed with inhalable allergens as house dust, tobacco and airborne fungus (Table 5). Mast cell degranulation for other foods tested as strawberry, birds, beef, pork, egg white, egg yolk, tomato, milk, rice, pineapple, cocoa, cashew, orange and lemon and for other aeroallergens as mites, wool, grass-plot, flowers, cat dander, dog epithelium, equine epithelium, bovine epithelium, mixed epithelium, feather mix, cotton, mane, grass, silk, flax, cockroach and cattail were below 35% (data not shown).

Glutamic acid protects against cross-reactivity

As observed in Table 5 (columns 4 and 5), pre-absorption of serum with glutamic acid resulted in inhibition of IgE reactivity to both inhalable and food allergens, indicating that the carboxyl

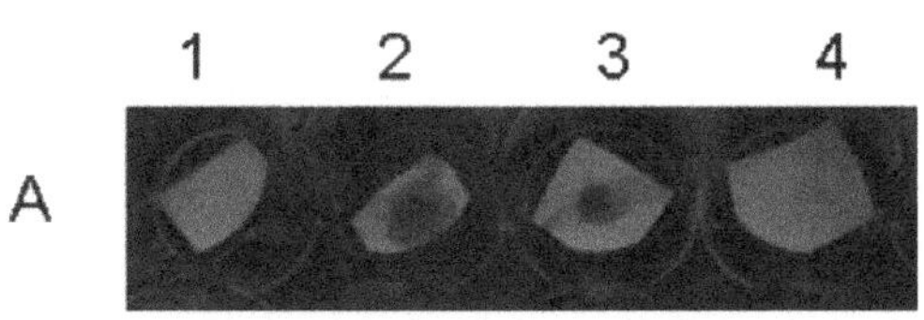

Figure 2. Analysis of human serum and affinity chromatography fractions, FE and FG by dot blotting using anti-human biotin IgE/streptavidin-biotinylated-HRP. A1) negative control: buffer plus human (patient 3) total serum; A2) 2S albumin plus human (patient 3) total serum; A3) 2S albumin incubated with affinity chromatography fraction, FE; A4) 2S albumin incubated with affinity chromatography fraction, FG.

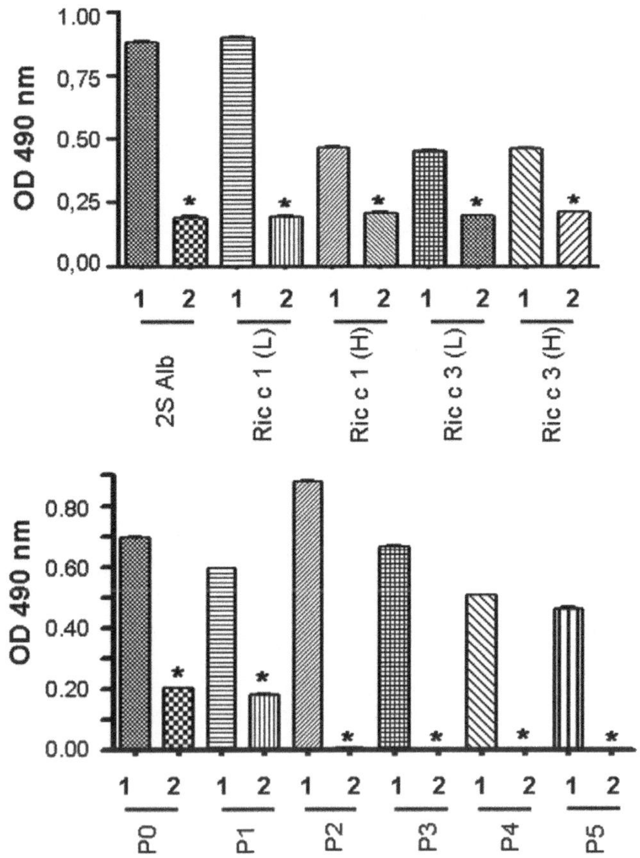

Figure 3. Glutamic acid reduces human IgE binding. ELISA binding assays of 2S albumin pool, 2S albumin light chain (L), heavy chain (H) and synthetic peptides with IgE from human serum without treatment (1) and with human serum treated with glutamic acid (2). Mean values from 5 experiments ± SD are presented. Statistical analysis was performed using one-way ANOVA followed by Turkey's post-test. * $p<0.001$.

group of these amino acids could be important in IgE-epitope interactions.

Discussion

The use of castor bean oil in biodiesel production will result in the increased planting of castor beans. Castor bean allergens are present not only in the seeds but also in the pollen of this plant [5,15]. Thus, identifying the allergenic epitopes and reactive amino acids are critical steps toward the development of strategies to reduce IgE binding, which will undoubtedly help protect rural workers or those in direct contact with the seeds.

To determine which amino acids are involved in IgE binding, the chemical modification of synthetic peptides by WRK was employed. Yost and Anderson [16] suggested the importance of a carboxyl group in the NAD-glycohydrolase activity of a *Bungarus fasciatus venom* protein as this enzyme is rapidly inactivated by WRK treatment. To confirm the importance of carboxylic groups in IgE binding, we have performed blocking assays using free amino acids (glutamic and aspartic acids) (Table 3). The dicarboxylic amino acids protected mast cell activation by IgE from degranulation when these cells were incubated with 2S albumin or an IgE epitope (synthetic peptides). Here we provided the first experimental evidence supporting the fundamental role of amino acids with side chains containing acidic groups (mainly

Table 5. Percentage of degranulation triggered by cross-reaction between 2S albumin from *Ricinus communis* L. and food or aero allergens.

Samples	Degranulation (%) in the absence of total serum (± S.D.)	Degranulation (%) in the presence of total serum (± S.D.)	Degranulation (%) after blockage with Glu (± S.D.)	Degranulation (%) after blockage with Asp (± S.D.)
Negative control	27.6 (±1.2)	30.0 (±1.0)	30.0 (±1.0)	30.0 (±1.0)
2S Albumin	32.6 (±1.3)	70.0 (±1.0)	29.7 (±0.1)	36.8 (±0.4)
Shrimp	34.0 (±0.7)	53.8 (±0.8)	34.0 (±1.0)	41.6 (±1.0)
Fish	38.8 (±1.0)	57.6 (±0.3)	34.9 (±0.2)	40.6 (±0.3)
Gluten	38.6 (±1.0)	56.3 (±0.5)	35.5 (±0.3)	40.6 (±0.3)
Wheat	38.8 (±0.2)	56.0 (±0.9)	36.8 (±0.5)	41.6 (±0.2)
Soybean	27.4 (±0.4)	62.5 (±0.4)	32.7 (±0.3)	39.7 (±0.3)
Peanut	30.2 (±0.3)	51.4 (±0.3)	35.2 (±0.5)	40.6 (±0.4)
Corn	34.4 (±1.0)	54.4 (±1.5)	34.1 (±0.3)	40.6 (±0.5)
House dust	36.7 (±0.2)	51.4 (±0.4)	33.9 (±0.7)	40.0 (±0.2)
Tobacco	34.8 (±0.2)	55.0 (±0.9)	34.6 (±0.1)	43.2 (±0.5)
Air fungus	48.7 (±0.7)	51.9 (±0.9)	32.3 (±0.4)	40.0 (±0.6)

Dicarboxylic amino acids (glutamic or aspartic acid) were used as IgE blocker.

glutamic acid) in the formation of IgE epitopes of castor bean allergens. Worldwide, 10–20 million people suffer from pollen allergies [17,18]. Vieths et al. [19] have indicated that between 50% and 93% of birch pollen allergic individuals develop hypersensitivity reactions towards certain foods (e.g., apples, carrots, hazelnut, celery), which is mediated by cross-reactive IgE antibodies primarily directed against Bet v 1, a major birch pollen allergen [18,19]. This type of hypersensitivity was described as pollen-food syndrome (PFS) [18,20]. The identification of aeroallergens and food allergens that cross-react with castor bean is an important step towards developing strategies for the prevention and treatment of allergies triggered by these components. The cross-reactivity between castor bean 2S albumin and allergens from shrimp, fish, wheat, soybean, peanut and corn causes concern because individuals who live in regions close to castor bean farms could become sensitive to these foods. The involvement of charged amino acids in Blo t 5, the most prevalent Blomia tropicalis allergen, with IgE binding was observed in another study [21]. These authors have demonstrated that four charged residues: Glu76, Asp81, Glu86, and Glu91 (peptide ELKRTDLNILERFNYE), localized to the region connecting the alpha helices 2 and 3, have been found to be involved in IgE binding. The pre-absorption of the serum of atopic individuals with glutamic acid decreased IgE binding to *R. communis* allergens (Table 3). We note that this amino acid also affected mast cell degranulation and histamine release, not only triggered by Ric c 1 and Ric c 3, but also triggered by other allergens that showed cross-reactivity with Ric c 1 and Ric c 3. There is continuing concern with the development of new drugs for the treatment of allergy and allergic rhinitis. A list of the medications used in allergic rhinitis, including their mechanisms of action and side effects, was presented by two other studies [22,23]. The results presented in this manuscript support a new strategy for drug development based on IgE blocking (Machado et al., Brazilian patent 00320/2005) [24].

Supporting Information

Figure S1 (A) Hypersensitivity reactions: a) Allergenic proteins are processed by antigen-presenting cells (APC) by the MHC class II pathway with subsequent increases in IgE production; b) IgE sensitizes mast cells by binding to FcεRI; c) A second exposure to the allergen activates these cells to degranulate and release vasoactive amines. (B) Blockage of IgE: a) Sensitized mast cells are incubated with glutamic or aspartic acid; b) These dicarboxylic amino acids bind to IgE-sensitized mast cells resulting in protection from mast cell degranulation.
(TIF)

Author Contributions

Conceived and designed the experiments: OLTM. Performed the experiments: NDO SPF KVF CCG RAD. Analyzed the data: OLTM NDO SPF KVF CCG RAD. Contributed reagents/materials/analysis tools: OLTM RAD. Wrote the paper: OLTM.

References

1. Conceição MM, Candeia R, Dantas HJ, Soledade LEB, Fernandes VJ, et al. (2005) Rheological behavior of castor oil biodiesel. Energ Fuel 19: 2185–2188.
2. Azam MM, Waris A, Nahar NM (2005) Prospects and potential of fatty acid methyl esters of some non-traditional seed oils for use as biodiesel in India. Biomass Bioenerg:– 29: 293–302.
3. Ogunniyi D (2006) Castor oil: A vital industrial raw material. Bioresour Technol 97: 1086–1091.
4. Garcia-Gonzalez JJ, Bartolome-Zavala B, Trigo-Perez MD, Barcelo-Munoz JM, Fernandez-Melendez S, et al. (1999) Pollinosis to *Ricinus communis* (castor bean): an aerobiological, clinical and immunochemical study. Clin Exp Allerg 29: 1265–1275.
5. Singh A, Panzani RC, Singh AB (1997) Specific IgE to castor bean *(Ricinus communis)* pollen in the sera of clinically sensitive patients to seeds. J Investig Allergol Clin Immunol 7: 169–174.
6. Thorpe D, Kemeny R, Panzani M, Lessof MH (1988) Allergy to castor bean I. Its relationship to sensitization to common inhalant allergens. J Allerg Clin Immunol 82: 62–66.
7. Thorpe SC, Kemeny DM, Panzani RC, Mcgurl B, Lord M (1988) Allergy to castor bean. 2. Identification of the major allergens in castor bean-seeds. J Allerg Clin Immunol 82: 67–72.
8. Sharief FS, Li SSL (1982) Amino acid sequence of light and heavy subunits of seed storage protein from *Ricinus communis*. J Biol Chem 257: 14753–14759.
9. Irwin SD, Keen JN, Findlay JBC, Lord JM (1990) The *Ricinus communis* 2S Albumin precursor: a single preproprotein may be processed into two different heterodimeric storage proteins. Mol Gen Genet 222: 400–408.
10. Machado OLT, da Silva JG (1992) An allergenic 2S storage protein from *Ricinus communis* seeds which is a part of the 2S albumin precursor predicted by c-DNA data. Braz J Med Biol Res 25: 567–582.

11. daSilva JG, Machado OLT, Izumi C, Padovan JC, Chait BT, et al. (1996) Amino acid sequence of a new 2S albumin from *Ricinus communis* which is part of a 29-kDa precursor protein. Arch Biochem Biophys 336: 10–18.
12. Felix SP, Mayerhoffer RO, Damatta RA, Verícimo MA, Nascimento VV, et al. (2008) Mapping IgE-binding epitopes of Ric c 1 and Ric c 3, allergens from *Ricinus communis*, by mast cell degranulation assay. Peptides 29: 497–504.
13. Dunn BM, Anfinsen CB (1974) Kinetics of Woodward's Reagent K Hydrolysis and Reaction with Staphylococcal Nuclease. J Biol Chem 249: 3717–3723.
14. Sinha U, Brewer JM (1985) A spectrophotometric method for quantitation of carboxyl group modification of proteins using Woodward's Reagent K. Anal Biochem 151: 327–333.
15. Bashir MEH, Hubatsch I, Leinenbach HP, Zeppezauer M, Panzani RC, et al. (1998) Ric c 1 and Ric c 3, the allergenic 2S albumin storage proteins of *Ricinus communis*: Complete primary structures and phylogenetic relationships. Intern Arch Allerg Immunol 115: 73–82.
16. Yost DA, Anderson BM (1982) Studies of bungarus-fasciatus venom NAD glycohydrolase - inhibition, modification, and transglycosilation reactions. J Biol Chem 257: 767–772.
17. D'Amato G, Spieksma FT, Liccardi G, Jager S, Russo M, et al. (1998) Pollen-related allergy in Europe. Allergy 53: 567–578.
18. Klinglmayr E, Hauser M, Zimmermann F, Dissertori O, Lackner P, et al. (2009) Identification of B-cell epitopes of Bet v 1 involved in cross-reactivity with food allergens Allergy 64: 647–651.
19. Vieths S, Scheurer S, Ballmer-Weber B (2002) Current understanding of cross-reactivity of food allergens and pollen. Ann N Y Acad Sci 964: 47–68.
20. Egger M, Mutschlechner S, Wopfner N, Gadermaier G, Briza P, et al. (2006) Pollen-food syndromes associated with weed pollinosis: an update from the molecular point of view. Allergy 61: 461–476.
21. Chan SL, Ong TC, Gao YF, Tiong YS, Wang DY, et al. (2008) Nuclear magnetic resonance structure and IgE epitopes of Blo t 5, a major dust mite allergen. J Immunol 18: 2586–2596.
22. Bousquet J, VanCauwenberge P, Khaltaev N (2002) Allergic rhinitis and its impact on asthma (ARIA) – executive summary. Allergy 57: 841–855.
23. - Bousquet J, Khaltaev N, Cruz AA, Denburg J, Fokkens WJ, et al. (2008) Allergic Rhinitis and its Impact on Asthma (ARIA) 2008 Update (in collaboration with the World Health Organization, GA2LEN and AllerGen) Allergy 63(Suppl. 86): 8–160.
24. Machado OLT, Felix SP, Mayerhoffer RO. Antiallergic pharmaceutical composition using free amino acid. 2005 Brazilian Patent - PI0506648-4 A2.

Expression of High-Affinity IgE Receptor on Human Peripheral Blood Dendritic Cells in Children

Monica Vasudev[9], Dorothy S. Cheung[9], Hannah Pincsak, Shun-Hwa Li, Ke Yan, Pippa Simpson, Trivikram Dasu, Mitchell H. Grayson*

Department of Pediatrics, Medical College of Wisconsin, Milwaukee, Wisconsin, United States of America

Abstract

Background: In a mouse model of viral induced atopic disease, expression of FcεRI on dendritic cells is critical. While adult human conventional (cDC) and plasmacytoid (pDC) dendritic cells have been shown to express FcεRI, it is not known if this receptor is expressed in childhood and how its expression is governed by IgE.

Methods: Following informed consent of subjects (n = 27, aged 12–188 months), peripheral blood was stained for surface expression of CD19, ILT7, CD1c, IgE, FcεRI and analyzed by flow cytometry (cDC: $CD19^{-}$ $ILT7^{-}$ $CD1c^{+}$; pDC: $CD19^{-}$ $ILT7^{+}$ $CD1c^{-}$). Total and specific serum IgE levels to food and inhalant allergens were determined by ImmunoCAP, and the relationship between FcεRI expression on dendritic cells and sensitization, free IgE, cell bound IgE, and age was determined.

Results: Independent of sensitization status, FcεRI expression was noted on cDC and pDC as early as 12 months of age. Serum IgE level correlated with expression of FcεRI on cDC, but not pDC. Based on the concentration of IgE, a complex relationship was found between surface bound IgE and expression of FcεRI on cDC. pDC exhibited a linear relationship of FcεRI expression and bound IgE that was consistent through all IgE concentrations.

Conclusions: In children, FcεRI expression on cDC and pDC is modulated differently by serum and cell bound IgE. IgE governance of FcεRI expression on cDC depends upon a complex relationship. Further studies are needed to determine the functional roles of FcεRI on cDC and pDC.

Editor: Marco Idzko, University Hospital Freiburg, Germany

Funding: Funding was provided by Genentech (www.gene.com), National Institutes of Health grant HL087778 (www.nih.gov), and the Children's Research Institute of the Children's Hospital of Wisconsin (www.chw.org/display/PPF/DocID/30477/router.asp). The funders had no role in study design, data collection and analysis, decision to publish, or preparation of the manuscript.

Competing Interests: Mitchell H. Grayson has received research support from Genentech and the National Institutes of Health. The other authors declare no competing financial interests. This does not alter the authors' adherence to all the PLoS ONE policies on sharing data and materials.

* E-mail: wheeze@allergist.com

[9] These authors contributed equally to this work.

Introduction

Severe viral respiratory infections early in life are associated with increased risk of asthma and atopic disease [1,2,3,4]. Using a mouse model we defined potential mechanisms translating anti-viral immune responses into atopic disease. Mice infected with the murine type 1 parainfluenza virus develop an acute inflammatory response and severe weight loss in the first week of infection. By 10 days post-viral inoculation, the animals clear virus and begin to gain weight; however, by day 21 post-inoculation they manifest chronic airway hyper-reactivity and IL-13 dependent mucous cell metaplasia [5]. In addition, exposure to an environmental antigen during the viral infection is sufficient to generate IgE against the environmental antigen leading to worse atopic disease [6]. We have also shown that a similar response can occur in the gastrointestinal tract [7].

One hallmark of our model is that murine cDC and pDC do not express FcεRI except during severe viral infections, when cognate interactions with a specific neutrophil subset drives FcεRI expression [8]. Cross-linking FcεRI bound IgE on cDC leads to recruitment of IL-13 producing Th2 cells driving the atopic response. We have shown in humans that cross-linking IgE on cDC produces CCL28, the same Th2 chemoattractant critical for the mouse model [9]. Although adult human cDC and pDC are known to express FcεRI, very little is known about induction and regulation of this receptor on human cDC and pDC from children. We undertook this study to answer this issue.

Our study documents expression patterns of FcεRI on peripheral blood cDC and pDC in young children. While the receptors are present early in life, we found a marked differential effect of low and high IgE on cDC FcεRI expression. This finding implies that cDC expressed FcεRI has disparate effects on cDC function depending on serum level of IgE. Further, our data suggest that IgE control of FcεRI may be different in children compared to adults.

Methods

Experimental Design

A cross sectional time analysis was employed. Our primary goal was to determine the age at which human cDC and pDC expressed FcεRI. Our secondary goal was to determine if sensitization to any food or inhalant allergen was associated with FcεRI and IgE expression.

Ethics Statement

This study was approved by the Children's Hospital of Wisconsin IRB. Parental written consent and subject verbal assent was obtained before enrollment of subjects into this study.

Subjects

Once consent and assent was obtained, an abbreviated atopic history was collected and venipuncture performed. Eligible patients were children aged 1–15 years. Exclusion criteria were: atopic dermatitis, persistent controlled asthma, uncontrolled asthma, immunodeficiency, or any co-morbid disease; use of any corticosteroids within the last month; current therapy with any prescribed medication; use of any investigational agent in the last 30 days; women of childbearing age not on contraception or women breastfeeding.

Sensitization status and total serum IgE determination

Total IgE and specific IgE levels to foods (casein, alpha-lactalbumin, beta-lactoglobulin, cheese, egg white, cacao, soybean, peanut, codfish, tuna, oat, rice, wheat) and aeroallergens (*D. farinae*, *D. pteronyssinus*, cockroach, cat dander, dog dander, mouse epithelium, rat epithelium, guinea pig epithelium, mouse serum protein, rat serum protein, mouse urine protein, rat urine protein, June grass, *Alternaria tenuis*, *Cladosporium herbarum*, *Aspergillis fumigatus*, common ragweed, oak, birch, *L. destructor*) were determined by ImmunoCAP (Quest Dignostics/IBT Laboratories). Sensitization was defined as elevated serum specific IgE (>0.35 kU/L) to one or more allergens tested.

Flow Cytometry

Immunophenotyping for evaluation of pDC and cDC was performed within 6 hours of specimen collection. 100 µl of heparinized whole blood was stained with antibodies to human CD19 (PerCP labeled clone SJ25C1, BD Biosciences), ILT7 (PE labeled clone 17G10.2, eBioscience), and CD1c (APC labeled clone BDCA-1, Miltenyi Biotec), as well as either antibodies against FcεRIα (FITC labeled clone AER-37, eBioscience) or IgE (FITC labeled, Kirkegaard & Perry Laboratories, Inc.) for 15 min. at room temperature. Erythrocytes were lysed with 2 ml FACSLyse (BD Biosciences) and stained cells were washed with PBS/0.1% NaN_3 and fixed using 1% paraformaldehyde. Flow cytometry (BD FACSCalibur) was performed with 5×10^5 to 1×10^6 total cellular events collected on each stained specimen. cDC (also referred to as mDC-1) were identified as $CD19^-$/$ILT7^-$/$CD1c^+$ and pDC identified as $CD19^-$/$ILT7^+$/$CD1c^-$. This type of phenotyping strategy has been used before, as ILT7 is a specific marker for pDC and $CD19^-CD1c^+$ cells have been shown to be essentially all cDC [9,10,11,12,13,14,15,16]. Using multi-color flow cytometry and Boolean gating strategy, the expression of IgE and FcεRIα were identified on the cDC and pDC subsets and measured as fold mean florescence (fold MFI) over individual isotype control background using CellQuest Pro software (BD Biosciences) as shown in Figure 1A. Appropriate isotype control antibodies were utilized, and calibration of FcεRIα expression (MEPE) was performed in each run using fluorescent beads as described [17].

Statistical Analysis

Data were expressed as frequency and percent for categorical variables and median and interquartile range for continuous variables. Since the data were skewed, continuous variables were compared using a Mann-Whitney test while doing 2 group comparisons, and continuous variables were examined using scatter plots and Pearson correlations. To investigate the inter-related effects of variables on the outcomes of interest, a regression tree analysis was done using Salford Systems' CART software (http://salford-systems.com/). Regression trees are a non-parametric approach where the data are split recursively into two groups based on an optimizing function, until the specified limits for subgroups are reached. A least absolute deviance from the median was used as the optimizing function, with a limit of 10 in any group to be split and 5 minimally needed for any group. Linear regression was used to fit the data with linear or a polynomial trend with normality of the error term checked with a normal probability plot. cDC IgE was fit to serum IgE using a non-linear regression for a sigmoidal type curve of the form $1/(1+M/\text{serum IgE})^m$, where M is the (fitted) median value of cDC IgE and m is the slope of the curve at that value. We fit linear regression using SAS 9.2 and non-linear regression using JMP 9.0. Given the relatively small sample, we did not use a bootstrap approach or a holdout sample to validate the model results. Therefore, these results will need to be validated on another sample.

Results

Twenty-seven patients aged 12 to 188 months were recruited from June through September 2009. All patients denied symptoms of current allergic disease or respiratory tract infection. A summary of subject characteristics is in Table 1. Subjects were classified as sensitized based on ImmunoCap testing, with a single positive test being considered "sensitized". No correlation was noted between sensitization status and age, and other than total serum IgE there was no significant difference in any demographic information between the sensitized ($n = 12$) and non-sensitized subjects ($n = 15$).

In a linear regression, we found that there was a moderate correlation between age and serum IgE ($r = 0.53$), with about 25% of the variation of IgE explained by the linear relationship with age. However, much of this relationship occurred in the non-sensitized group ($r = 0.56$) compared to the sensitized group ($r = 0.29$). This is not surprising, since serum IgE levels can fluctuate, such as with viral infections, and our data were obtained at only a single time point per subject [18].

Comparing the relative frequencies of conventional (cDC) and plasmacytoid dendritic cells (pDC) amongst all of our subjects, we found 1.26 (0.66–2.55) (median (IQR)) fold more cDC than pDC. This ratio was not significantly different between sensitized and non-sensitized subjects, nor did it correlate with age (data not shown). While this ratio of cDC to pDC is lower than what has been reported in older children, it is similar to what has been reported in adult studies using a dendritic cell phenotyping strategy similar to ours [14,15,19].

Conventional dendritic cells (cDC)

We initially hypothesized that similar to the rodent system, peripheral blood cDC would not express FcεRI early in life. However, as shown in Figure 1B, FcεRI expression was detected on cDC at all ages. Given that viral infections have been shown to upregulate expression of FcεRI on dendritic cells, and that older individuals likely had more viral infections, we supposed that expression of the receptor would increase with age [18]. As shown in Figure 1B, the age of the subject had a marginally linear correlation to level of expression of FcεRI on cDC ($r = 0.36$,

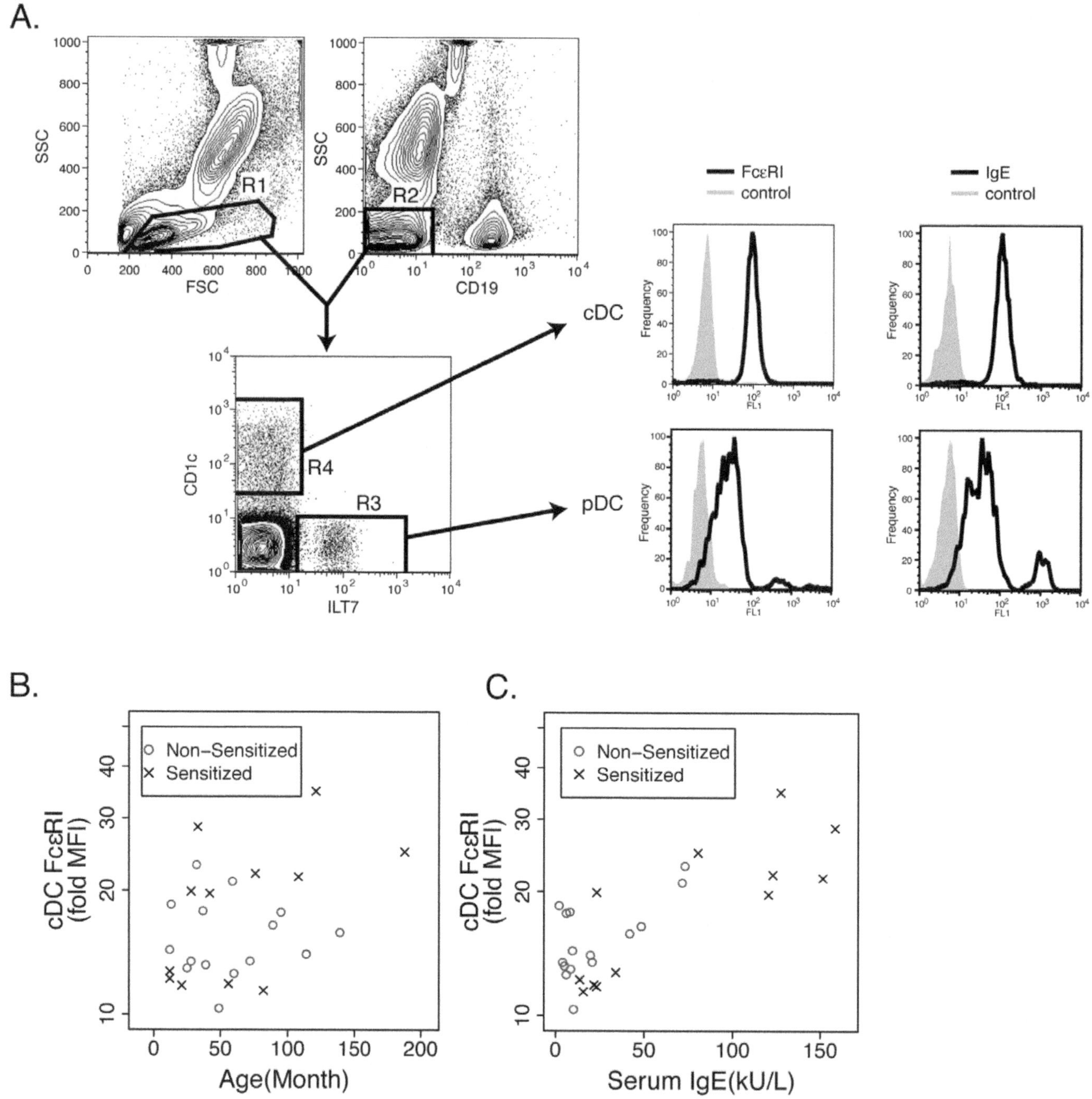

Figure 1. Expression of FcεRI on cDC correlates with serum IgE but not with subject's age. (A) Gating strategy used to identify expression of FcεRI and IgE on cDC and pDC. Cells were gated on scatter (R1) and lack of expression of CD19 (R2, PerCP negative). Those events that satisfied both of these criteria were examined for expression of ILT7 (R3, PE positive) versus CD1c (R4, APC positive). Cells that were $CD19^{-}ILT7^{+}CD1c^{-}$ were considered pDC and $CD19^{-}ILT7^{-}CD1c^{+}$ were considered cDC. The expression of FcεRI (left histograms, FITC positive) or IgE (right histograms, FITC positive) on these cells was then determined and compared to an appropriate isotype control. (B) Expression of FcεRI on peripheral blood cDC was determined by flow cytometry and compared to subject's age or (C) serum IgE level. Data are presented as fold MFI FcεRI versus age in months (B) or serum IgE in kU/L (C), with non-sensitized subjects (n = 15) in circles and sensitized subjects (n = 12) in x's. Sensitization was defined as having at least one positive allergen specific IgE by ImmunoCAP.

$p = 0.07$) and this marginal correlation was found in sensitized ($r = 0.53$, $p = 0.08$) but not non-sensitized ($r = -0.002$, $p = 0.99$) subjects. Further, no association was found between family atopic status and FcεRI expression on cDC ($p = 0.42$, data not shown).

In human mast cells and basophils, IgE modulates FcεRI expression [20]. In fact, in a study with anti-IgE the reduction in IgE directly correlated with subsequent reduction of FcεRI expression on peripheral blood DC of adults [21]. We examined the relationship between serum IgE and cDC expression of FcεRI. As shown in Figure 1C, there was a linear correlation ($r = 0.78$, $p < 0.0001$) between serum IgE levels and cDC expression of FcεRI. This correlation held regardless of sensitization status

Table 1. Subject Characteristics.

Variable	Non-sensitized (n = 15)	Sensitized† (n = 12)
Age (months), median (range)	49 (12–139)	49 (12–188)
Male, n (%)	8 (53%)	5 (42%)
Personal History Atopy*, n(%)	14 (93%)	12 (100%)
Family History Atopy*, n(%)	12 (80%)	7 (58%)
Elevated Food specific IgE, n(%)	0 (0%)	9 (75%)§
Elevated Inhalant allergen specific IgE, n(%)	0 (0%)	9 (75%)

*Atopy history: defined as self reported or MD diagnosed allergic rhinitis/hayfever/environmental allergies, asthma/wheeze, atopic dermatitis, food allergy. Family history of atopy was based on self-reporting only.
†Sensitized: defined as any elevated food or inhalant serum specific IgE.
§Only 4 of these subjects had a clinical history suggestive of an allergy for the foods to which they had IgE against.

($r = 0.83$, $p = 0.0009$ sensitized subjects; $r = 0.64$ non-sensitized subjects, $p = 0.01$).

Sensitization status did not differentiate level of expression of FcεRI on cDC (Table 2). However, a regression tree analysis revealed that when serum IgE was less than 60 kU/L, FcεRI expression was significantly higher on cDC from non-sensitized subjects (median (IQR) = 14.03 (13.2, 16.48) fold MFI) compared to sensitized individuals (median (IQR) = 12.05 (11.77, 12.74) fold MFI), $p = 0.04$.

Since bound IgE modulates expression of FcεRI on human mast cells and basophils, we examined the level of IgE on peripheral blood cDC and correlated this with FcεRI expression. As shown in Figure 2A, the relationship between cDC expression of FcεRI and surface bound IgE was complex. With low level staining of IgE (less than a fold MFI IgE expression of 12) there was no relationship between surface bound IgE and FcεRI. However, at higher levels of surface bound IgE there was a direct correlation between bound IgE and FcεRI expression. Interestingly, fitting curves to the data (the equations are shown in Table 3) showed the relationship between cDC bound IgE and FcεRI expression to be different for sensitized and non-sensitized individuals. In Figure 2A the relationship in sensitized individuals appears to be exponential, while in non-sensitized it was more sigmoidal. However, both curves appear to converge when subjects expressed a fold MFI for IgE of 12 or greater. Analyzing all of the data together (without making a distinction on sensitization status) generated a curve that was sigmoidal and the inflection point remained at a fold MFI IgE expression of 12 (Figure 2A, blue line).

By overlaying serum IgE levels, we found only subjects with a serum IgE above 34–42 kU/L had a cDC fold IgE expression of 12 or greater (Figure 2B). These data suggest serum IgE drives FcεRI expression on peripheral blood cDC only when it crosses this threshold level. Because the two curves converge (Figure 2A), this effect appears to be unrelated to subject's sensitization status.

Plasmacytoid dendritic cells (pDC)

Unlike peripheral blood cDC, pDC expression of FcεRI was minimal (median (IQR) = 15.82 (12.74–21.05) versus 2.47 (1.47–3.25) on cDC and pDC, respectively). In fact, 6 of the 27 subjects appeared to have no expression of FcεRI on their pDC (fold MFI equal to or less than 1.0). As shown in Table 2, analogous to the cDC data, sensitization status did not associate with level of expression of FcεRI on pDC. We also found no linear correlation between age of the subject and pDC expression of FcεRI (Figure 3A; $r = 0.13$, $p = 0.51$ for all subjects; $r = 0.28$, $p = 0.38$ for sensitized subjects; and $r = -0.05$, $p = 0.87$ for non-sensitized subjects). In sum, there was no correlation between a given subject's expression of FcεRI on their cDC or pDC and age.

Unlike with cDC (Figure 1C), serum IgE levels did not correlate with pDC expression of FcεRI (Figure 3B, $r = 0.21$, $p = 0.29$ for all subjects; $r = 0.42$, $p = 0.17$ for sensitized subjects; $r = 0.21$, $p = 0.46$ for non-sensitized subjects). Also, unlike cDC, pDC bound IgE levels correlated linearly with pDC expression of FcεRI in both

Table 2. Comparison of Sensitized and Non-Sensitized Children for Dendritic Cell Expression of IgE and FcεRI.

	Median (IQR)		
Variable	Non-Sensitized (n = 15)	Sensitized (n = 12)	p-value†
Age (month)	49 (28, 89)	49 (24.5, 95)	>0.99
Serum IgE (kU/L)	9.5 (6, 42)	57.25 (22.3, 125)	0.003
pDC bound IgE (fold MFI)	2.42 (1.54, 2.74)	2.13 (1.15, 4.1)	>0.999
pDC FcεRI (fold MFI)	2.65 (1.59, 3.25)	2.02 (1.04, 3.25)	0.39
cDC bound IgE (fold MFI)	4.3 (2.68. 19.2)	17.33 (5.12, 33.5)	0.08
cDC FcεRI (fold MFI)	14.37 (13.2, 17.8)	19.8 (12.1, 23.5)	0.48

†: Mann-Whitney test.
IQR: interquartile range, cDC: conventional dendritic cells, pDC: plasmacytoid dendritic cells.

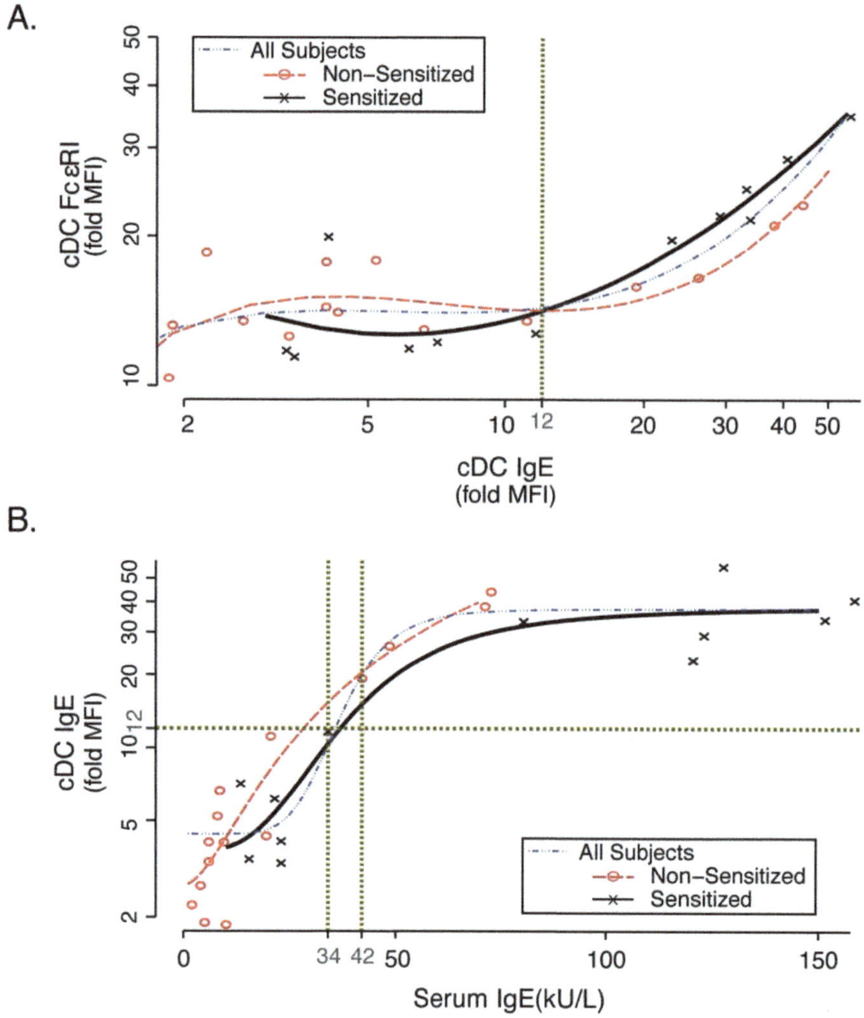

Figure 2. Correlation of cDC expression of FcεRI with IgE. Expression of FcεRI and IgE on the surface of cDC was determined by flow cytometry. (A) Data are presented as fold MFI FcεRI versus fold MFI IgE expression, with non-sensitized subjects (n = 15) in red circles and sensitized subjects (n = 12) in black x's. Note the difference in the slope of the fitted lines (non-sensitized subjects in red dotted line; sensitized subjects in black solid line) above and below a fold MFI IgE of 12, suggesting that there is differential regulation of FcεRI on cDC around this level of cell bound IgE. For all subjects the data was fit with the following cubic equation (blue line): $\text{Ln(cDC FcεRI)} = 2.26+0.72*\ln(\text{cDC IgE})-0.43*\ln(\text{cDC IgE})^2+0.082*\ln(\text{cDC IgE})^3$; r = 0.86; p = 0.045. For equations based on sensitization status, see Table 3. (B) Expression of cell bound IgE on cDC compared with serum (free) IgE levels. Data are presented as in (A) with fold MFI IgE expression versus serum IgE (kU/L). Note that a cell bound IgE fold MFI of 12 correlates with a serum IgE of around 38 (based on statistical fitting of the curve, this value could range between 34 and 42 kU/L).

Table 3. Sensitization status regression models with significant Pearson correlations.

	Regression Equation	Pearson correlation (p-value)
Non-sensitized		
pDC FcεRI Vs. pDC IgE		
	Ln(pDC FcεRI) = 0.26+0.73*ln(pDC IgE)	r = 0.76 (p = 0.001)
cDC FcεRI Vs. cDC IgE		
	Ln(cDC FcεRI) = 2.49+0.13*ln(cDC IgE)	r = 0.65 (p = 0.009)
Sensitized		
pDC FcεRI Vs. pDC IgE		
	Ln(pDC FcεRI) = 0.004+0.8*ln(pDC IgE)	r = 0.98 (p<0.0001)
cDC FcεRI Vs. cDC IgE		
	Ln(cDC FcεRI) = 2.06+0.32*ln(cDC IgE)	r = 0.85 (p = 0.0004)

Ln indicates the natural log transformation.

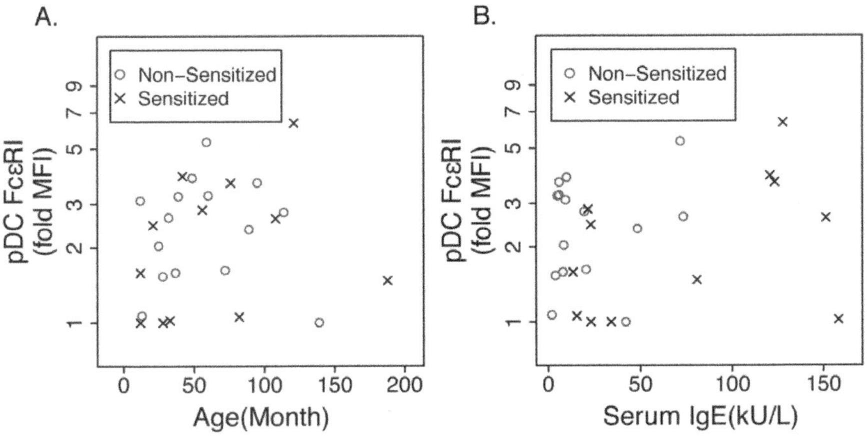

Figure 3. Expression of FcεRI on pDC does not correlate with serum IgE or age of subject. Expression of FcεRI on peripheral blood pDC was determined by flow cytometry and compared to subject's age (panel A) and serum IgE level (panel B). Data are presented as in Figure 1.

sensitized ($r = 0.76$, $p = 0.001$) and non-sensitized subjects ($r = 0.98$, $p < 0.0001$). These data provide further evidence for a direct association between bound IgE and FcεRI expression in pDC but not cDC, suggesting that regulation of FcεRI is dissimilar in cDC and pDC.

Discussion

Other studies have attempted to describe relationships between serum IgE, cell-bound IgE, and FcεRI expression on dendritic cells [17,21]. These prior studies utilized adults, and did not examine expression in children. There is one publication in the literature that looked at children [22]. However, this report examined older children and did not differentiate FcεRI and IgE staining on cDC and pDC, as they used CD11c and MHC-II as markers for dendritic cells—markers that are insufficient to distinguish cDC and pDC cells in humans [23]. Further, our study utilized regression analysis to better understand the role of FcεRI on dendritic cells in children of various ages. We found that as early as 12 months of age, regardless of sensitization status, FcεRI is expressed on peripheral blood cDC and pDC, although pDC expression of some subjects was quite minimal. No association between age and expression of IgE or FcεRI was found, indicating that our initial hypothesis was wrong (i.e., FcεRI expression on dendritic cells would correlate with age). Although we do acknowledge that a longitudinal study would be more appropriate to examine the relationship between age and receptor expression. It does remain possible that early life developmental control of FcεRI expression exists before 12 months of age—especially with pDC. Once induced, FcεRI expression clearly can be modulated by viral infections [18].

Interestingly, we found no association between sensitization status and FcεRI expression. We cannot equate sensitization with atopy because we did not challenge our subjects with the respective allergens. Further, it is quite possible that those subjects we identified as non-sensitized were indeed making specific IgE—just against antigens that were not included in our panels. For these reasons our data may be different from two studies in adults where atopic subjects were noted to have significantly higher FcεRI expression on cDC and pDC [15,21]. Our results do corroborate those of the adult studies in the fact that expression of FcεRI is much higher on cDC than on pDC. What the functional implications are for this difference in expression remains unclear.

The most intriguing finding of our study is the major difference in the role of IgE in receptor expression. Whereas a direct relationship between FcεRI expression and IgE on both cDC and pDC have been reported by others, we found that only pDC FcεRI expression correlated in a linear fashion with bound IgE [21,24]. Our data did not show a relationship between serum IgE and FcεRI expression on pDC. This suggests free IgE may not drive receptor expression, an event that depends singularly upon level of bound IgE. This difference may be due to the low level of expression of FcεRI on pDC, and may explain differences between how IgE drives FcεRI expression on mast cells and basophils when compared to pDC [20,25].

Unlike pDC, expression of FcεRI on cDC correlated directly with serum IgE levels. However, the relationship between bound IgE and FcεRI was more complex. When cell bound IgE was below 12 fold MFI there was little effect of bound IgE on FcεRI expression. Once bound IgE levels crossed the threshold, a direct relationship developed. At low levels of serum IgE (<34–42 kU/L) there is rapid accumulation of bound IgE with little effect on FcεRI expression. At these low levels of IgE, a difference in correlation of bound IgE and FcεRI exists between sensitized and non-sensitized subjects. Both responses are parabolic, however, non-sensitized subjects tend to have an initial increase in FcεRI expression with increasing bound IgE (below 12 fold MFI). Sensitized subjects had the exact opposite effect. Once serum IgE levels reached 34–42 kU/L, corresponding to bound IgE levels of 12 fold MFI, both sensitized and non-sensitized subjects exhibited a direct correlation between IgE and FcεRI.

We have found a threshold effect of bound IgE on cDC FcεRI. The functional implications for this threshold effect are unclear; it is inviting to speculate that FcεRI has disparate functions at low versus high IgE levels. Perhaps at lower levels FcεRI acts as a rheostat, similar to what is seen in rodents, where the receptor functions as a mechanism for cellular recruitment and less for antigen-uptake [5,6]. At higher levels of IgE, the receptor may function more as a means for "antigen-focusing" [26]. It is beyond the scope of this study to elucidate actual mechanisms behind this phenomenon, but the functional implications of IgE regulation of FcεRI expression are tantalizing.

Our study had several limitations. First and foremost, we utilized statistical modeling to evaluate our data, and, as a result, it is important that these findings be validated in a second cohort. Further, our sample size was relatively small and likely limited our ability to detect subtle differences. We did not enroll infants younger than 12 months of age, and we were unable to determine if viral infection relates to induction of FcεRI. Finally, defining sensitization status by selected ImmunoCAP may not be ideal—especially from a clinical perspective. However, given that our results were mostly independent of sensitization status, we believe this is not a major defect. Indeed, most of the limitations of our study would only lessen our ability to define statistically significant differences. Since we were able to document clear relationships between IgE (serum and cell bound) and cDC and pDC expression of FcεRI despite these limitations, their presence only strengthen the importance of our findings.

In summary, our results demonstrate the presence of FcεRI on peripheral blood cDC and pDC in children as young as 1 year old, which is in contrast to what is seen in the rodent system. Our data also provide evidence of differential regulation of FcεRI on cDC and pDC in children. With cDC a complex inter-relationship between serum IgE, cell bound IgE, and expression of FcεRI exists that appears to hinge on an IgE level of 34–42 kU/L. The functional significance of this relationship is unclear, and we do not yet understand the mechanisms responsible for this relationship. Future studies need to be undertaken to examine expression of FcεRI on cDC and how IgE modulates this receptor and cDC function.

Author Contributions

Conceived and designed the experiments: MV DSC MHG. Performed the experiments: MV DSC HP TD. Analyzed the data: MV DSC HP TD SHL KY PS MHG. Contributed reagents/materials/analysis tools: SHL PS MHG. Wrote the paper: MV DSC MHG.

References

1. Sigurs N, Aljassim F, Kjellman B, Robinson PD, Sigurbergsson F, et al. (2010) Asthma and allergy patterns over 18 years after severe RSV bronchiolitis in the first year of life. Thorax 65: 1045–1052.
2. Sigurs N, Gustafsson PM, Bjarnason R, Lundberg F, Schmidt S, et al. (2005) Severe respiratory syncytial virus bronchiolitis in infancy and asthma and allergy at age 13. Am J Respir Crit Care Med 171: 137–141.
3. Escobar GJ, Ragins A, Li SX, Prager L, Masaquel AS, et al. (2010) Recurrent wheezing in the third year of life among children born at 32 weeks' gestation or later: relationship to laboratory-confirmed, medically attended infection with respiratory syncytial virus during the first year of life. Arch Pediatr Adolesc Med 164: 915–922.
4. Johnston SL, Pattemore PK, Sanderson G, Smith S, Campbell MJ, et al. (1996) The relationship between upper respiratory infections and hospital admissions for asthma: a time-trend analysis. Am J Respir Crit Care Med 154: 654–660.
5. Grayson MH, Cheung D, Rohlfing MM, Kitchens R, Spiegel DE, et al. (2007) Induction of high-affinity IgE receptor on lung dendritic cells during viral infection leads to mucous cell metaplasia. J Exp Med 204: 2759–2769.
6. Cheung DS, Ehlenbach SJ, Kitchens T, Riley DA, Grayson MH (2010) Development of atopy by severe paramyxoviral infection in a mouse model. Ann Allergy Asthma Immunol 105: 437–443 e431.
7. Chen X, Leach D, Hunter DA, Sanfelippo D, Buell EJ, et al. (2011) Characterization of intestinal dendritic cells in murine norovirus infection. Open Immunol J 4: 22–30.
8. Cheung DS, Ehlenbach SJ, Kitchens RT, Riley DA, Thomas LL, et al. (2010) Cutting edge: CD49d+ neutrophils induce FcepsilonRI expression on lung dendritic cells in a mouse model of postviral asthma. J Immunol 185: 4983–4987.
9. Khan SH, Grayson MH (2010) Cross-linking IgE augments human conventional dendritic cell production of CC chemokine ligand 28. J Allergy Clin Immunol 125: 265–267.
10. Rissoan MC, Duhen T, Bridon JM, Bendriss-Vermare N, Peronne C, et al. (2002) Subtractive hybridization reveals the expression of immunoglobulin-like transcript 7, Eph-B1, granzyme B, and 3 novel transcripts in human plasmacytoid dendritic cells. Blood 100: 3295–3303.
11. Cao W, Bover L (2010) Signaling and ligand interaction of ILT7: receptor-mediated regulatory mechanisms for plasmacytoid dendritic cells. Immunol Rev 234: 163–176.
12. Cao W, Bover L, Cho M, Wen X, Hanabuchi S, et al. (2009) Regulation of TLR7/9 responses in plasmacytoid dendritic cells by BST2 and ILT7 receptor interaction. J Exp Med 206: 1603–1614.
13. Cao W, Rosen DB, Ito T, Bover L, Bao M, et al. (2006) Plasmacytoid dendritic cell-specific receptor ILT7-Fc epsilonRI gamma inhibits Toll-like receptor-induced interferon production. J Exp Med 203: 1399–1405.
14. Kirsche H, Niederfuhr A, Deutschle T, Fuchs C, Riechelmann H (2010) Ratio of myeloid and plasmacytoid dendritic cells and TH2 skew in CRS with nasal polyps. Allergy 65: 24–31.
15. Lundberg K, Greiff L, Borrebaeck CA, Lindstedt M (2010) FcepsilonRI levels and frequencies of peripheral blood dendritic cell populations in allergic rhinitis. Hum Immunol 71: 931–933.
16. Patterson S, Donaghy H, Amjadi P, Gazzard B, Gotch F, et al. (2005) Human BDCA-1-positive blood dendritic cells differentiate into phenotypically distinct immature and mature populations in the absence of exogenous maturational stimuli: differentiation failure in HIV infection. J Immunol 174: 8200–8209.
17. Foster B, Metcalfe DD, Prussin C (2003) Human dendritic cell 1 and dendritic cell 2 subsets express FcepsilonRI: correlation with serum IgE and allergic asthma. J Allergy Clin Immunol 112: 1132–1138.
18. Subrata LS, Bizzintino J, Mamessier E, Bosco A, McKenna KL, et al. (2009) Interactions between innate antiviral and atopic immunoinflammatory pathways precipitate and sustain asthma exacerbations in children. J Immunol 183: 2793–2800.
19. Silver E, Yin-DeClue H, Schechtman KB, Grayson MH, Bacharier LB, et al. (2009) Lower levels of plasmacytoid dendritic cells in peripheral blood are associated with a diagnosis of asthma 6 yr after severe respiratory syncytial virus bronchiolitis. Pediatr Allergy Immunol 20: 471–476.
20. Saini S, MacGlashan DW, Jr., Adelman D, Jardieu P, Togias A, et al. (1997) Culture with IgE increases IgE density and FcεRI expression on human basophils. J Allergy Clin Immunol 99: S102 (abstr.).
21. Prussin C, Griffith DT, Boesel KM, Lin H, Foster B, et al. (2003) Omalizumab treatment downregulates dendritic cell FcepsilonRI expression. J Allergy Clin Immunol 112: 1147–1154.
22. Dehlink E, Baker AH, Yen E, Nurko S, Fiebiger E (2010) Relationships between levels of serum IgE, cell-bound IgE, and IgE-receptors on peripheral blood cells in a pediatric population. PLoS One 5: e12204.
23. Grayson MH (2006) Lung dendritic cells and the inflammatory response. Ann Allergy Asthma Immunol 96: 643–651; quiz 652–643, 678.
24. Schroeder JT, Bieneman AP, Chichester KL, Hamilton RG, Xiao H, et al. (2010) Decreases in human dendritic cell-dependent T(H)2-like responses after acute in vivo IgE neutralization. J Allergy Clin Immunol 125: 896–901 e896.
25. Thompson HL, Metcalfe DD, Kinet JP (1990) Early expression of high-affinity receptor for immunoglobulin E (Fc epsilon RI) during differentiation of mouse mast cells and human basophils. J Clin Invest 85: 1227–1233.
26. Jurgens M, Wollenberg A, Hanau D, de la Salle H, Bieber T (1995) Activation of human epidermal Langerhans cells by engagement of the high affinity receptor for IgE, Fc epsilon RI. J Immunol 155: 5184–5189.

Evaluation of the Allergenicity Potential of TcPR-10 Protein from *Theobroma cacao*

Sara Pereira Menezes[1⁹], Jane Lima dos Santos[2⁹], Thyago Hermylly Santana Cardoso[1], Carlos Priminho Pirovani[1], Fabienne Micheli[1,3], Fátima Soares Motta Noronha[4], Andréa Catão Alves[4], Ana Maria Caetano Faria[4], Abelmon da Silva Gesteira[5*]

1 UESC, Centro de Biotecnologia e Genética, Ilhéus, Bahia, Brasil, **2** UESC, Centro de Microscopia Eletrônica, Ilhéus, Bahia, Brasil, **3** CIRAD, UMAR AGAP, Montpellier, France, **4** UFMG, Instituto de Ciências Biológicas, Pampulha, Belo Horizonte, Minas Gerais, Brasil, **5** Embrapa Mandioca e Fruticultura, Cruz das Almas, Bahia, Brasil

Abstract

Background: The pathogenesis related protein PR10 (TcPR-10), obtained from the *Theobroma cacao-Moniliophthora perniciosa* interaction library, presents antifungal activity against *M. perniciosa* and acts *in vitro* as a ribonuclease. However, despite its biotechnological potential, the TcPR-10 has the P-loop motif similar to those of some allergenic proteins such as Bet v 1 (*Betula verrucosa*) and Pru av 1 (*Prunus avium*). The insertion of mutations in this motif can produce proteins with reduced allergenic power. The objective of the present work was to evaluate the allergenic potential of the wild type and mutant recombinant TcPR-10 using bioinformatics tools and immunological assays.

Methodology/Principal Findings: Mutant substitutions (T10P, I30V, H45S) were inserted in the *TcPR-10* gene by site-directed mutagenesis, cloned into pET28a and expressed in *Escherichia coli* BL21(DE3) cells. Changes in molecular surface caused by the mutant substitutions was evaluated by comparative protein modeling using the three-dimensional structure of the major cherry allergen, Pru av 1 as a template. The immunological assays were carried out in 8–12 week old female BALB/c mice. The mice were sensitized with the proteins (wild type and mutants) via subcutaneous and challenged intranasal for induction of allergic airway inflammation.

Conclusions/Significance: We showed that the wild TcPR-10 protein has allergenic potential, whereas the insertion of mutations produced proteins with reduced capacity of IgE production and cellular infiltration in the lungs. On the other hand, *in vitro* assays show that the TcPR-10 mutants still present antifungal and ribonuclease activity against *M. perniciosa* RNA. In conclusion, the mutant proteins present less allergenic potential than the wild TcPR-10, without the loss of interesting biotechnological properties.

Editor: Baochuan Lin, Naval Research Laboratory, United States of America

Funding: The work of SPM was supported by the Research Support Foundation of the State of Bahia (FAPESB). This research was supported by FAPESB and Conselho Nacional de Desenvolvimento Científico e Tecnológico (CNPq) - 471849/2004-9, http://www.cnpq.br/. The funders had no role in study design, data collection and analysis, decision to publish, or preparation of the manuscript.

Competing Interests: The authors have declared that no competing interests exist.

* E-mail: Abelmon.Gesteira@embrapa.br

⁹ These authors contributed equally to this work.

Introduction

The development of genetically modified organisms (GMOs) through molecular engineering techniques is an alternative to plant genetic improvement programs for the purpose of promoting resistance against pathogens, herbicides or environmental stresses [1,2]. Among the genes that can be potentially used in the genetic transformation of plants so as to improve resistance against diseases, those coding for pathogenesis-related proteins stand out (PR) [3,4,5,6,7]. According to the structural, enzymatic or biological properties, PR proteins are classified into 17 families, whereas PR 1, 2, 3, 4, 5, 8, 10 and 14 are reported to contain proteins with homology to pollen or food allergens; this fact limits the biotechnological application of these genes [8,9,10,11]. Among the allergenic proteins classified as PR-10, the Bet v 1 isolated from *Betula verrucosa* is the main allergen present in pollen grains [12,13]. Food allergens such as Pru p 1 from pear (*Prunus persica*) [14], Mal d 1 from apple (*Malus domestica*) [15], Pru av 1 from cherry (*P.avium*) [16,17] and Dau c 1 in carrot (*Daucus carota*) [18] are also reported as part of the PR-10 family.

The PR-10 family is characterized by the presence of a highly conserved region called P-loop motif, which is usually associated with ribonuclease activity in some members of this family [19]. Yet, the presence of this domain is also associated with the allergenicity of pollen grains [20,21]. The P-loop motif present in some allergenic proteins such as Mal d 1 (*Malus domestica*) [22], Bet v 1 (*Betula verrucosa*) [12] and Api g 1 (*Apium graveolens*) [23] is also conserved in the *TcPR-10* gene identified in a cDNA library observed in the interaction between *Theobroma cacao* and *Moniliophthora perniciosa*.

The TcPR-10 protein has a promising biotechnological potential to act as a ribonuclease and presents antifungal activity against *M. perniciosa*, the causal agent of witches' broom disease, which is one of the most devastating diseases of cocoa plants [24]. The overexpression of the *TcPR10* gene may open new possibilities for cocoa breeding. However, the development of genetically modified organisms (GMOs) requires the discrimination of allergenic and non-allergenic recombinant proteins and a prediction of the potential cross-linking activity of the proteins of the immune system [25,26]. The assessment of allergenicity potential is a major procedure used to ensure the biosafety of GMOs [27]. Thus, this study has aimed to assess the allergenicity potential of the antifungal protein TcPR-10 using bioinformatic tools and immunological assays, and develop and test a mutant strain with little or no allergenic ability, but that maintains ribonuclease and antifungal activities.

Results

Identification of the Allergenicity Potential of TcPR-10 through Bioinformatics Analysis

The assessment of the allergenicity potential of the TcPR-10 protein by sequence comparison analysis with sequences of allergens from the SDAP (Structural Database of Allergenic Proteins) [28,29] database revealed similarity to 13 different groups of allergens (Table 1). The TcPR-10 sequence shows stretches of 6 continuous and identical amino acids with food allergens like Rub i (red raspberry), Dau c 1.01 (carrot), Act d 8 (kiwi fruit), Api g 1 (celery), Mad 1 (apple), Pru ar 1 (apricot), Cor a 1.04 (hazelnut), Pru p 1 (peach), Pru av 1 (sweet cherry), and also pollen allergens such as Que a 1 (white oak) and Bet v 1 (white birch). Based on the sequence of continuous amino acids, one should note that the *TcPR-10* gene showed similarity to allergenic proteins especially in the region rich in glycine (P-loop motif 47GDGGVGSIK55) (Figure 1). Despite the fact that the P-loop motif of the TcPR-10 protein is not identical to Pru p 1, Pru av 1, Bet v 1, Que a 1 and Cor a 1, these proteins also have a P-loop and there are amino acid sequence variations among glycine residues. At position 48, the Bet v 1, Que a 1 and Cor a 1 sequences contain asparagine residues, whereas the TcPR-10 protein contains aspartic acid residues. At position 51, the Pru p 1, Pru av 1, Bet v 1, Que a 1 and Cor a 1 proteins show a proline residue, whereas TcPR-10 shows a valine residue. In addition to the P-loop domain, theTcPR-10 protein sequence shows the common 129EEEIKAGK136 region with Bet v 1, Cor a 1 and Act d 8, the common 116TSHYHT121 region with Mal d 1, Pru ar 1, Pru p 1.0101 and Pru av 1, the 26DSDNLI31 region only with Que a 1, and 59FPEGSHFKY67, only with Bet v 1 (Figure 1).

Based on the identity parameter greater than 35% in a window of 80 amino acids, the TcPR-10 sequence has an excess of 50% homology with the Mad 1, Pru ar 1, Pru p 1.0101, Bet v 1 Cor a 1.0403 and Cor a 1.0402 sequences. The percentage similarity for these six allergen sequences is consistent with the PD value under 14, thus indicating similarity between the physicochemical properties of such allergens and TcPR-10. It can be noted that the lowest and therefore most significant overall similarity index values (E-value) are also observed for these allergen sequences. *E-value* and *PD* indexes indicate that TcPR-10 and *PD* show similarity to pollen and food allergens (Table 1).

Changes in the Structure of the Hydrophobic Cavity and the Surface of TcPR-10

In order to select sites for insertion of mutations that reduce or eliminate the possible allergenic potential of TcPR-10 shown by bioinformatics analysis using SDAP, molecular modeling has been employed so as to predict changes and determine the implications that they may cause in the tridimensional structure of TcPR-10. The templates were identified by PSI-Blast [30] analyses against protein data banking-PDB [31]. The sequences of wild and mutant-type TcPR-10 showed 51% identity in relation to the templates Pru av 1 (pdb: 1e09_A) and RMSD of 0.345 and 0.351, respectively (Table 2). Identity above 50% and an E-value below $4e^{-43}$ indicate that the crystal structure of Pru av 1 is a good model to be used as a template. The value of RMSD indicates that there was little difference between models and template structures. The models of wild and mutant-type TcPR-10 showed three alpha-helices: α1 (16–26); α2 (89–91); α3 (129–152); six stranded anti-parallel beta-sheets (β1-β6): β1 (3–12); β2 (40–46); β3 (54–58); β4 (80–85); β5 (96–106); β6 (111–121); and 9 loop L1 (13–15); L2 (27–39); L3 (47–53); L4 (59–79); L5 (86–88); L6 (92–95); L7 (107–110); L8 (122–128); L9 (153–158) (Figure 2A).

The stereochemical parameters of the model protein structural wild type and mutant were analyzed using the Procheck (Laskowski et al., 2005) and Anolea softwares (Melo; Feytmans, 1998). The Ramachandran plot showed that 76,1% and 76,6% of residues in most favored regions for wild and mutant-type TcPR-10, respectively. 21,7% and 21,2% of residues in additional allowed regions and only 2,2% and 2,2% residues in disallowed regions for wild and mutant-type TcPR-10, respectively. Analysis of the stereochemical properties with Procheck 3.4 confirms good stereochemical quality of the structure ensemble as mirrored by the fact that more than 97% of the amino acid residues are located in the most favoured regions of the Ramachandran plot.

Cloning and Expression of TcPR-10

The recombinant plasmid pET28a containing the TcPR-10 insert with the T10P, I30V and H45S substitutions was cloned and expressed in *E. coli* BL21 (DE3) under the control of the T7 promoter. The three points of substitutions T10P, I30V and H45S-10 inserted into TcPR-10 were marked underlined in the alignment (Figure 1). The heterologous expression of the protein was confirmed in 15% SDS-PAGE gel stained with Coomassie Brilliant Blue and the expression of peptides of an approximate molecular mass of 19KDa fused to the histidine residues, was observed (His-Tag). The purification of the wild and mutant-type TcPR-10 was confirmed by visualization of single bands on SDS-PAGE gel (Figure 3).

Ribonuclease and Antifungal Activity of the mutanttcpr-10

The verification of possible changes in the catalytic function of the TcPR-10 protein due to the insertion of nucleotide substitutions was performed in vitro, using RNA from *M. perniciosa.* Incubation of the mutant TcPR-10 protein with RNA from *M. perniciosa* at 25°C at different times shows that, although there has been a slight decrease in the degradation rate, the insertions have not altered the activity of the ribonuclease protein. After 10 minutes of incubation with the *TcPR-10* mutant gene, the RNA was not completely degraded, as observed for the wild-type TcPR-10 (Figure 4, line 4). After one hour, the RNA bands incubated with the mutant TcPR-10 were still present, but after 3 hours, the RNA from *M. perniciosa* was observed to be totally degraded both in the wild-type and the mutant protein (Figure 4, row 6).

The *in vitro* effect of the TcPR-10 mutant protein in the survival of *M. perniciosa* shows that changes do not inhibit the antifungal activity of the protein. The survival of the fungus decreases as the concentration of mutant TcPR-10 increases, showing the same profile observed for the wild protein (Figure 5). At a concentration

Table 1. Identification of potential allergenic of TcPR-10 protein in the SDAP[1] allergenic proteins database.

N°	Allergen	Species	Description	Sequence in SDAP[1]	Sequence Length	Matching region of contiguous amino acids	E-value	PD[2]	Start-End of the alignment with TcPr-10	Identity[3]
1	Que a 1.0101	*Quercus Alba*	Major oak pollen allergen	P85126	50	25DSDNLI30	$1.5e^{-07}$	6.13	2–51	17.72
2	Rub i 1.0101	*Rubus idaeus*	Putative allergen	Q0Z8U9	137	38GDGGVG43	$3.8e^{-25}$	13.70	10–146	43.04
3	Dau c 1.0201	*Daucus carota*	Food allergen	AAL76932	154	47GDGGVG52	$8.1e^{-18}$	13.66	1–154	35.44
4	Pet c PR10	*Petroselinum crispum*	Pathogenesis-related protein 1	CAA67246	155	47GDGGVG52	$9.7e^{-21}$	13.94	1–155	39.87
5	Act d 8.0101	*Actinidia deliciosa*	Food allergen and Bet v 1 related allergen	CAM31909	157	47GDGGVG52 131EEEIKAGK139	$4.3e^{-24}$	12.13	1–157	48.73
6	Tar o RAP	*Taraxacum officinale*	Root allergen-and pathogenesis-related protein	AAB92255	157	47GDGGVG52	$9.3e^{-18}$	16.21	1–157	35.44
7	Api g 1.0201	*Apium graveolens*	Food allergen	P92918	159	47GDGGVG52	$3.9e^{-21}$	13.62	1–159	38.61
8	Mal d 1	*Malus domestica*	Food allergen	CAA96534	159	47GDGGVG52 117TSHYHT122	$1.5e^{-30}$	12.67	1–159	53.16
				CAA96535	160	47GDGGVG52	$1.7e^{-28}$	13.39	1–158	54.43
				CAA96536	160	47GDGGVG52	$1.9e^{-28}$	13.34	1–158	53.80
				CAA96537	160	47GDGGVG52	$1.9e^{-28}$	13.22	1–158	54.43
9	Pru ar 1	*Prunus armeniaca*	Food allergen	O50001	160	47GDGGVG52 118TSHYHT123	$7.4e^{-31}$	13.12	1–158	53.80
10	Pru p 1.0101	*Prunus persica*	Food allergen and Pathogenesis related protein PR10	Q2I6V8	160	118TSHYHT123	$2.1e^{-29}$	13.38	1–158	51.90
11	Pru av 1	*Prunus avium*	Food allergen	O24248		118TSHYHT123	$5.5e^{-29}$	13.30	1–158	51.27
12	Bet v 1.1301	*Betula verrucosa*	Major pollen allergen	CAA54696	160	59FPEGSHFK67 131EEEIKAGK138	$3.9e^{-30}$	13.46	1–158	54.43
13	Cor a 1.0401	*Corylus avellana*	Food allergen and Bet v 1-related major hazelnut allergen	AAD48405	161	132EEEIKAGK139	$3.3e^{-26}$	14.31	1–161	49.37
	Cor a 1.0404	*Corylus avellana*		AAG40331	161	132EEEIKAGK139	$5.0e^{-26}$	14.25	1–161	48.73
	Cor a 1.0403	*Corylus avellana*		AAG40330	161	132EEEIKAGK139	$2.2e^{-26}$	14.34	1–161	50.00
	Cor a 1.0402	*Corylus avellana*		AAG40329	161	132EEEIKAGK139	$1.4e^{-26}$	13.56	1–161	50.00

[1]Structural database of allergenic proteins; [2]Property distance index; [3]Identity for two sequences.

```
Dau c 1.02    MGVQKTEVEAPSTVSAEKMYQGFLLDMDTVFPKVLPQLIKSVEILEGDGGVGTVRLVHLG 60
Api g 1.02    MGVQKTVVEAPSTVSAEKMYQGFLLDMDTVFPKVLPQLIKSVEILEGDGGVGTVKLVHLG 60
Pet c PR10    MGVQKSEVVITSSVPAAKLFKALCLDIDTLLPQVLPGAIKGGEILEGDGGVGTVKLVTLG 60
TcPR-10       MGVTTYTQEFTCSVAPARMFKALILDSDNLIPKLMPKSIKNVELIHGDGGVGSIKQTNFP 60
Que a 1.01    -GVFTHESQETSVIAPARLFKALFLDSDNLIQKVLPQAIKSTEIIEGNGGP--------- 50
Bet v 1.13    MGVFNYEDEATSVIAPARLFKSFVLDADNLIPKVAPENVSSAENIEGNGGPGTIKKITFP 60
Cor a 1.04    MGVFCYEDEATSVIPPARLFKSFVLDADNLIPKVAPQHFTSAENLEGNGGPGTIKKITFA 60
Pru p 1.01    MGVFTYESEFTSEIPPPRLFKAFVLDADNLVPKIAPQAIKHSEILEGDGGPGTIKKITFG 60
Pru av 1      MGVFTYESEFTSEIPPPRLFKAFVLDADNLVPKIAPQAIKHSEILEGDGGPGTIKKITFG 60
Rub i 1.01    ---------YTSVIPPPKLFKAFVLDADNLIPKIAPQAVKSVEIIEGDGGVGTVKKIHLG 51
Mad 1         MGVFNYETEFTSVIPPARLFNAFVLDADNLIPKIAPQAVKSAEILEGDGGVGTIKKINFG 60
Pru ar 1      MGVFTYETEFTSVIPPEKLFKAFILDADNLIPKVAPTAVKGTEILEGDGGVGTIKKVTFG 60
Act d 8.01    MGAITYDMEIPSSISAEKMFKAFVLDGDTIIPKALPHAITGVQTLEGDGGVGTIKLTTFG 60
Tar o RAP     --MAVAEFEITSSLSPSNIFKAFVIDFDTIAPKAEPETYKSIKTIEGDGGVGTIKSITYS 60
                     .. :.. .::::.: :* *.:  :   *    .   : :.*:**

Dau c 1.02    EATEYTTMKQKVDVIDKAGLGYTYTTIGGDILVEGLESVVNQFVVVP-TDGG-CIVKNTT 118
Api g 1.02    EATEYTTMKQKVDVIDKAGLAYTYTTIGGDILVDVLESVVNEFVVVP-TDGG-CIVKNTT 119
Pet c PR10    DASPYKTMKQKIDAIDKEAFTFSYSIIDGDILLGYIDSINNHLSFVPTADGG-CTATSTA 120
TcPR-10       EGSHFKYLKN-TDALDVDNCVCKYTTIEGDVIGDKLESISYELKFEAS--GAGCVCKMTS 118
Que a 1.01    ------------------------------------------------------------
Bet v 1.13    EGSHFKYMKHRVDEIDHANFKYCYSIIEGGPLGDTLEKISYEIKIVAAPGGG-SILKITS 119
Cor a 1.04    EGNEFKYMKHKVEEIDHANFKYCYSIIEGGPLGHTLEKISYEIKMAAAPHGGGSILKITS 120
Pru p 1.01    EGSQYGYVKHKIDSIDKENHSYSYTLIEGDALGDNLEKISYETKLVASPSGG-SIIKSTS 119
Pru av 1      EGSQYGYVKHKIDSIDKENYSYSYTLIEGDALGDTLEKISYETKLVASPSGG-SIIKSTS 119
Rub i 1.01    EGTEHSYVKHKIDGLDKVNFVYSYSITEGDALGDKIEKISYEIKLVASGRG--SIIKTTS 118
Mad 1         EGSTYSYVKHRIDGVDKENFVYKYSVIEGDAISETIEKISYETKLVASGSG--SVIKSTS 118
Pru ar 1      EGSQYAYVKHRVDGIDKDNLSYSYTLIEGDALSDVIENIAYDIKLVASPDGG-SIVKTTS 119
Act d 8.01    EGSVHKSVKHRIDGLDKENFTYSYSIIEGG-ALDVFESISYHIKIVATPDGG-CICKNRS 119
Tar o RAP     DGVPFTSSKHKVDAIDSNNFSISYTIFEGDVLMGIIESGTHHLKFLPSADGG-SVYKHSM 119

Dau c 1.02    IYNTKGDAVLPEDKVKEATEKSALAFKAVEAYLLAN----- 154
Api g 1.02    IYNTKGDAVLPEDKIKEATEKSALAFKAVEAYLLANLQFLA 159
Pet c PR10    VFNTKGDAVVPEENIKFANDQNNLIFKAVEAYLLAN----- 155
TcPR-10       HYHTKGDFVLKEEEIKAGKDQAVGMYKVVEEYLLANPNVYA 159
Que a 1.01    -----------------------------------------
Bet v 1.13    KYHTKGDISLNEEEIKAGKEKGAGLFKAVENYLVAHPNAYN 160
Cor a 1.04    KYHTKGNASINEEEIKAGKEKAAGLFKAVEAYLLAHPDAYC 161
Pru p 1.01    HYHTKGDVEIKEEHVKAGKEKASNLFKLIETYLKGHPDAYN 160
Pru av 1      HYHTKGNVEIKEEHVKAGKEKASNLFKLIETYLKGHPDAYN 160
Rub I 1.01    HYHCKGGAEIKEEQVKDGKERAAGLFKI------------- 137
Mad 1         HYHTKSDVEIKEEHVKAGKEKASHLFKLIENYLLAHSDAYN 159
Pru ar 1      HYHTKGDVEIKEEQVKAGKEKAAGLFKLVEAYLLANPDAYN 160
Act d 8.01    IYTPKCDAQVSEEEIKAGKERASGIFKKVEAYLLANPDC-- 157
Tar o RAP     VFKCKGDAKLTDENVSLMKEGLKKTFKAIETYVISHPEAC- 157
```

Figure 1. Amino acid sequence alignment of TcPR-10 with the allergens from the SDAP database (http://align.genome.jp/sit-bin/clustalw)**.** The three point mutations for TcPR-10 (T10P, I30V, H45S) are marked in sequence alignment and P-loop was underlined. The identical, highly conserved, and conserved amino acids among the sequences are denoted with (*), (:), and (.), respectively. Matching regions of contiguous amino acids are highlighted in black.

of 8 mg/mL, the wild TcPR-10 protein shows a 73% inhibition rate of growth for the fungus, and 61% for the mutant TcPR-10 protein, with no statistical difference between values ($p>0.05$;Tukey's test). Despite the fact that the wild-type protein shows a higher percentage of inhibition as compared with the mutant protein especially when the concentration increases to 10 μg/mL,

Table 2. Template obtained by PSI-Blast algorithm for modeling of proteins structures TcPR-10 wild and mutant.

	Template	Identify %	E-value	Organism	RMSD(Å)	Reference
TcPR-10 wild	1e09.pdb	51	$4e^{-43}$	*Prunus avium*	0.345	Neudecker et al., 2001
TcPR-10 Mutant	1e09.pdb	51	$2e^{-42}$	*Prunus avium*	0.351	Neudecker et al., 2001

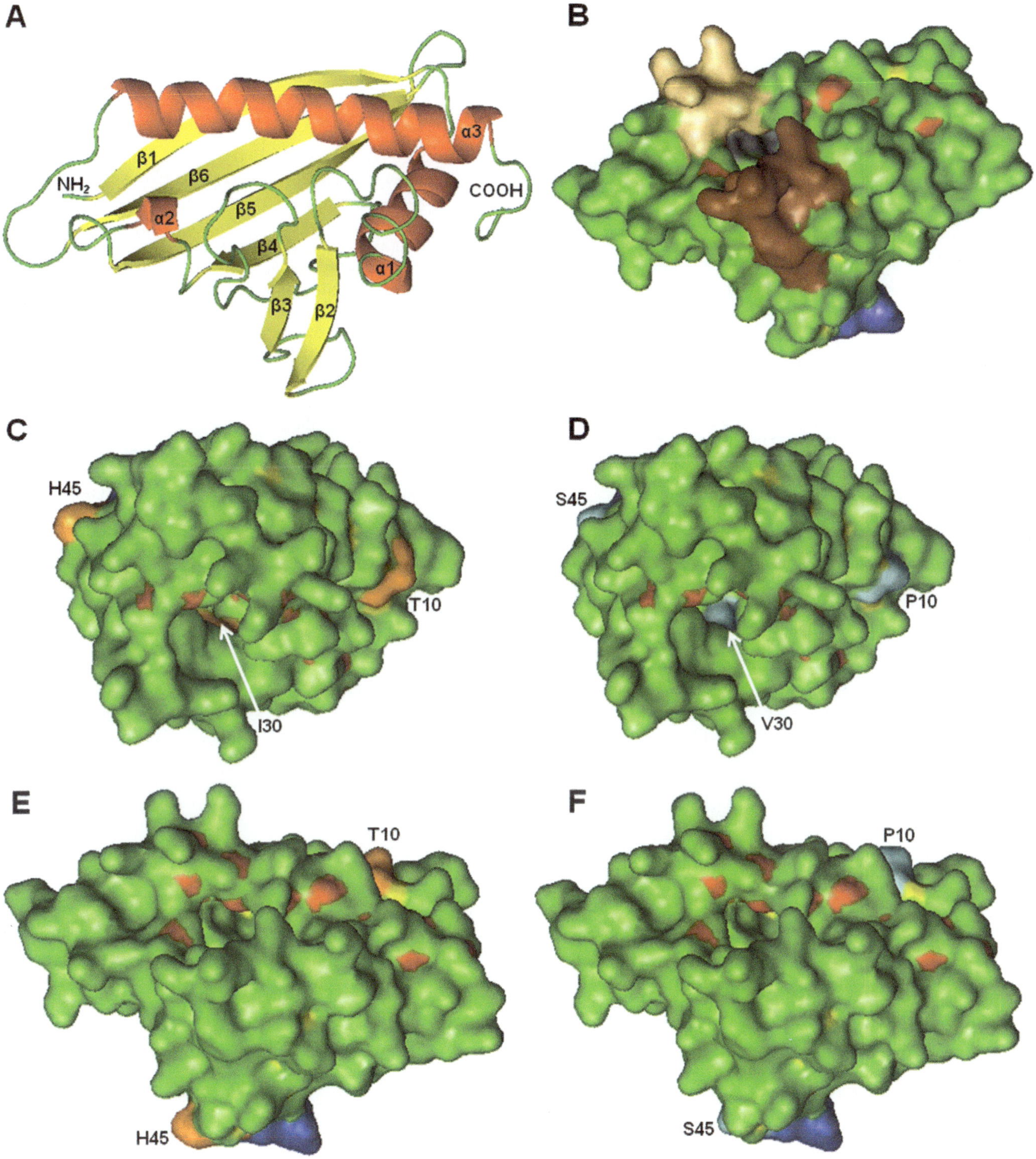

Figure 2. Three-dimensional structure of TcPR-10 obtained by homology modeling with Pru av1 (Protein Data Bank, 1e09_A) as template using SWISS-MODEL. A. The secondary structure elements are colored: alpha-helices in red, anti-parallel beta-sheets in yellow and P-loops in green. **B.** Molecular surface of TcPR-10 wild with matching regions of contiguous amino acids: 47GDGGVG52 in blue; 59FPEGSHFKY67 in brown; 116TSHYHT121 in gray; 129EEEIKAGK136 in peach. **C** e **E** Molecular surface of TcPR-10 wild type with amino acids for mutations highlighted in orangen (Thr10, Ile30, His45). **D e F.** TcPR-10 mutant type with point mutations in blue (Pro10, Val30, Ser45).

reducing the growth of the fungus by 91% - the mutant protein only reduces 56% - these values have not statistically differed ($p>0.05$, Tukey's test).

Immunological Response to *TcPR-10*

The production of immunoglobulin E (IgE) stimulated by an allergen usually triggers the typical symptoms of hypersensitivity

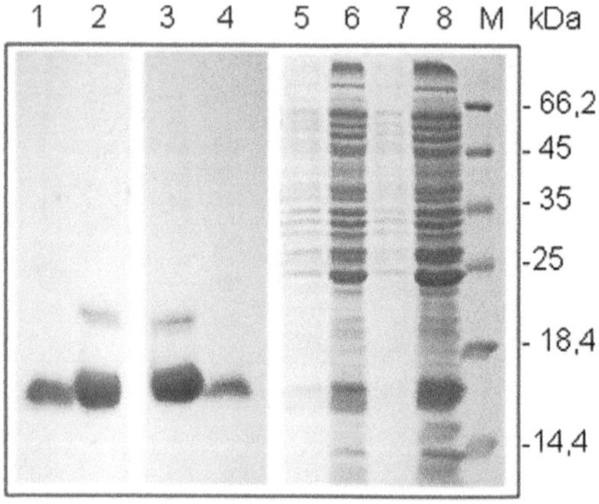

Figure 3. SDS-PAGE (15%) analysis of recombinants TcPR-10 Wild Types (wt) and Mutant (mut) proteins expressed in *E. coli* BL21(DE3). **1**– Soluble fraction TcPR-10 mut; **2**– Insoluble fraction TcPR10 mut; **3**– Soluble fraction TcPR-10 wt; **4**– Insoluble fraction TcPR10 wt; **5** - pET28a-TcPR-10 mut without induction; **6** - pET28a-TcPR-10 mut after induction; **7** - pET28a-TcPR-10 wt without induction; **8** - pET28a-TcPR-10 mut 3 h after induction; **M**- Protein molecular weight markers.

reactions. In order to evaluate the effect of wild and mutant TcPR-10 on airway inflammation, the IgE levels in serum and infiltration of inflammatory leukocytes in the lung have been examined. IgE levels in serum of animals challenged with the wild TcPR-10 protein has increased by 40% (M: 3.02; SD: +0.16) as compared to control animals (M: 1.8; SD: +0.32) ($p<0.001$; Tukey's test) (Figure 6A). On the other hand, those treated with mutant TcPR-10 have only increased by 17% (M: 2.18; SD: +0.34) ($p>0.05$; Tukey's Test) as compared to the control (Figure 6A). The IgE levels in animals treated with mutant protein is about 27% lower as compared with animals that received the wild-type TcPR-10, accordingly supporting the hypothesis that the insertion of mutations in TcPR-10 can reduce the allergenicability of this protein. The infiltration of inflammatory leukocytes was investigated by the following parameters: (i) total cell count in the BAL bronchoalveolar lavage fluid and (ii) analysis of histological sections. The total number of cells in BAL from animals treated with wild TcPR-10 protein (M: 12.95×104; D:+1.82×104) was higher than that present in the mutant and control groups, hence indicating increases of 62% (4.9×104+1.08×104) and 57% (M: 5.62×104; D: +1.81×104) ($p<0.001$, Tukey's test), respectively (Figure 6B).When comparing the mutant TcPR-10 protein with the control group, there was no significant difference but a 12.81% increase ($p>0.05$; Tukey's test). The histological analysis of lungs of mice treated with the wild-type TcPR-10 protein shows discrete cellular infiltrate in the peribronchiolar region and mild desquamation of the epithelium, with presence of mucus in the lumen of the bronchi (Figure 6D). These changes were not seen in the lungs of mice treated with the mutant protein (Figure 4E) and neither in the control animals (Figure 6C).

Discussion

The pathogenesis-related proteins (PR) involved in plant defense response against pathogens - including PR class 10 - are reported to be constitutively expressed in pollen, fruits and vegetables and may cause allergic reactions in humans [32,33,34]. The ribonuclease and antifungal activities of the heterologous protein TcPR-10 makes it important to the defense of *T. cacao* against *M. perniciosa*. This fact suggests that the *TcPR-10* gene can be used to increase the resistance of plants to pathogens [24] and is therefore subject of considerable biotechnological interest. Yet, despite the importance of biotechnology, the allergenicity potential of TcPR-10 had not been previously reported.

The identification of the allergenicity potential of proteins is usually conducted using bioinformatics tools and immunological assays [26,35,36]. In conjunction with the Food and Agriculture Organization of the United Nations [37], the World Health Organization has recommended two criteria using bioinformatics analysis to identify the allergenic potential of proteins, both based on sequence alignments: one that indicates identity greater than 35% in a window of 80 amino acids and another with 6 continuous amino acids between the sequence examined and those available in the databases and already reported to induce IgE production [38,39,40,41].

According to these parameters, the TcPR10 sequence showed similarity with thirteen allergenic sequences, and the region rich in glycine (P-loop motif 47GXGGXGXXK55) was highly conserved in all sequences (Table 1). Among the allergens that showed similarity with TcPR-10, Dau c 1, Pet c PR10, Tar o RAP, Api g 1, Mal d 1, Pruar 1, Pruav 1, Bet v 1 Cora 1 are reported as belonging to the family of pathogenesis-related proteins 10 - Bet v 1 (PF00407) [26]. The analysis of X-ray diffraction of protein Bet v 1 has identified several regions responsible for intermolecular contacts with the monoclonal Fab fragment of the IgG1 molecule (BV16), the region 42ENIEGNGGPGT52 (corresponding to the P-loop) identified as the main binding epitope [20]. Other sites of contact have been identified: R70, D72, H76, I86, E87 and K97 [20]. The TcPR-10 protein has the same amino acid residues at positions 72, 86 and 87, located near the conserved region 59FPEGSHFKY67, thus suggesting that these regions may act as binding sites for IgE. The crystalized structure of the Bet v 1-BV16 Fab complex demonstrated that the epitope formed by these amino acids, is clearly conformational [21], however, it is interesting to notice that the P-loop region is also a sequential

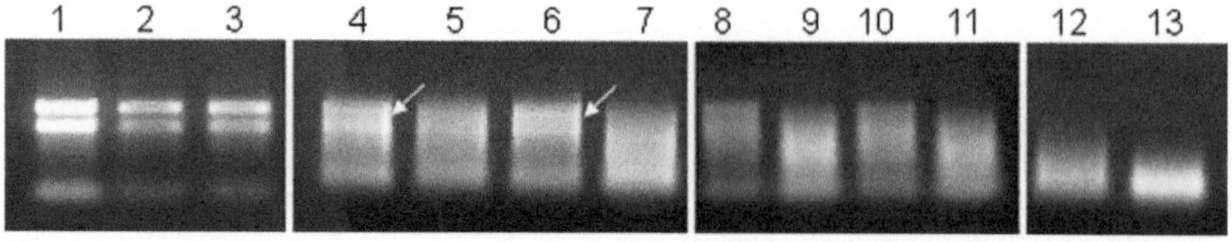

Figure 4. Ribonuclease activity of recombinant TcPR-10 Wild Types (wt) and Mutant visualized in 1% agarose gel. 1 μg RNA from *M. perniciosa* was incubated with 1 μg of recombinats proteins at 25°C at different times. Lane **1.** RNA without protein; Lane **2.** RNA with boiled TcPR10 mut 2 h incubation; Lane **3.** RNA with boiled TcPR10 wt 2 h incubation; Lane **4, 6, 8, 10** and **12** RNA incubated with TcPR10 mut by 10 min, 20 min, 1 h, 2 h and 3 h, respectively; Lane **5, 7, 9, 11** and **13** RNA incubated with TcPR10 wt by 10 min 20 min, 1 h, 2 h and 3 h, respectively. Arrows indicate RNA bands without degradation.

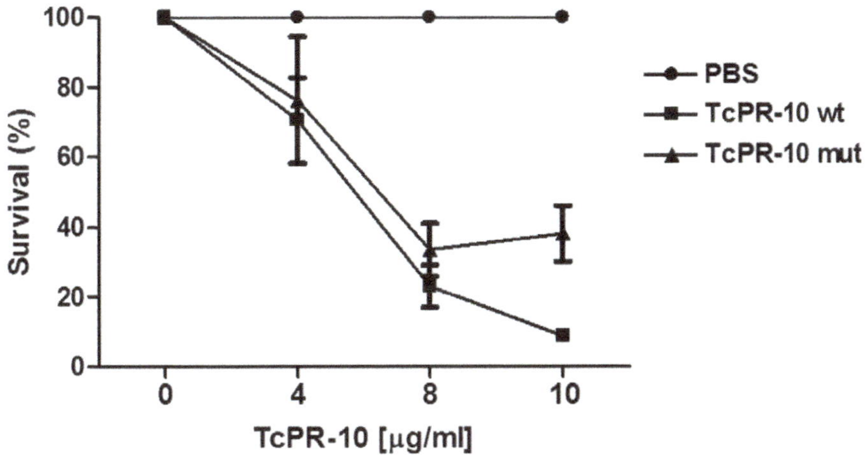

Figure 5. Survival of *M. perniciosa* dikaryotic broken hyphae incubated with different TcPR-10 wild and mutant type protein concentrations (4, 8 and 10 μg/ml).

motif [21]. The P-loop has been suggested as an important area of the epitope also in the ligation of IgE to Bet v 1. Mutations in the E45 residue, located in the middle of the BV16 epitope, was defined as the dominant epitope in the ligation of IgE in the serum of patients allergic to birch [21]. The residue of the amino acid 45, although not conserved in TcPR-10 (His-45), also is localized structurally in the superficial area which covers the location of the P-loop. In Pru av 1, the mutation in the E45W amino acid, also located in the P-loop region, does not alter the tertiary structure of the protein, but alters the biophysical properties of the lateral chain, and also reducing significantly the capacity of ligation to IgE for Pru av a in the serum of patients allergic to cherry [42]. In

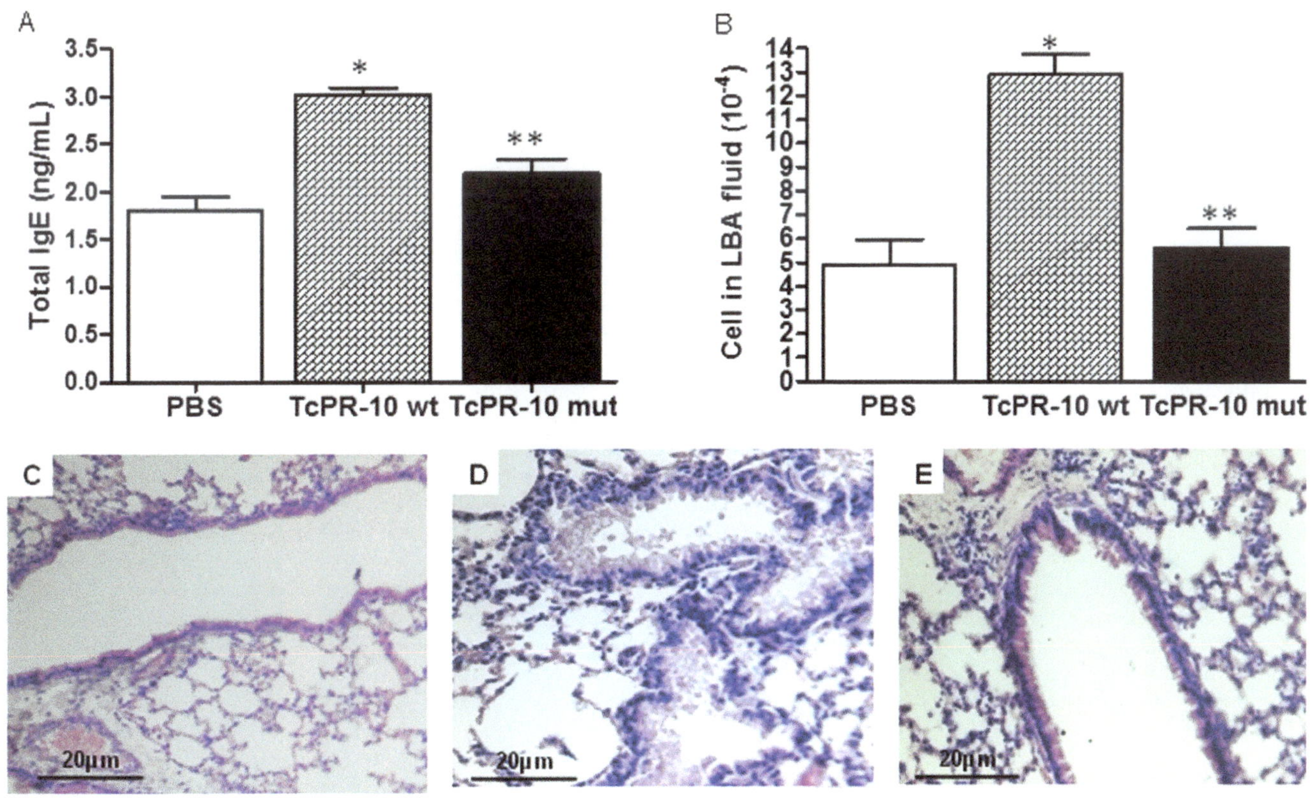

Figure 6. Quantification of polyclonal IgE, BAL total cell count and histological illustration of the lung of BALB/c mice. A. Quantification of polyclonal IgE antibody levels in serum of BALB/c mice. **B.** Cell counting in BAL fluid. The set average values *per se* quantification of antibodies and showed normal ($p<0,05$; Shapiro Wilk Test) using the comparison test of means the parametric Tukey Test ($\alpha = 0,05$). *Significantly high values compared to control. **Significantly reduced values compared to TcPR-10 wt. Horizontal bars represent the mean value of each group. C. Lung were removed twenty-four hours after the last challenge. Lung tissue was fixed, embedded, cut into slices and stained with hematoxylin e eosin (H&E) solution. **C:** Sections from control; **D:** wild TcPR-10; **E:** mutant TcPR-10.

Bet v 1, other residues such as Asn-28, Lys-32 and Pro-108, also had a significant contribution as to the ligation to IgE [21]. Residue 28 is also considered in Pru av 1 as a second region of the IgE epitope [42].

Conserved areas of the molecular surface are listed as probable IgE-binding epitopes [16]. The modeling of TcPR-10 protein shows that the conserved regions with allergens in SDAP 59FPEGSHFKY67, 116TSHYHT121 and 129EEEIKAGK136 are located near the hydrophobic cavity (Figure 2B); it is relevant to speculate whether these conserved areas indeed represent the IgE binding epitopes. The internal cavity present in the PR-10 protein is reported as a binding site or reservoir for hydrophobic ligands in the aqueous environment of the cell [3,12,43]. The location of these conserved regions close to the cavity enables one to underscore the importance of the cavity for the biological function of PR-10 proteins. Furthermore, this is a possible indicator of the location of epitopes binding to IgE; a fact that may hinder the application of *TcPR-10* gene in cocoa breeding.

The determination of three-dimensional structures of allergenic proteins allows to identify amino acids exposed on the molecular surface and that can act as IgE-binding epitopes [20]. Studies of structure analysis suggest the presence of common regions between Bet v 1, allergens, pollens, food, and PR proteins, therefore allowing the use of molecular modeling to predict protein structures. Using the SWISS-MODEL, the secondary structure of the protein TcPR-10 (Figure 2A) indicates a pattern similar to Bet v 1 and Pru av 1, differing by the presence of six β-sheets in TcPR-10 [12,44]. The TcPR-10 protein has high homology with pollen and food allergens showing possible IgE-binding epitopes (Table 1) - as Bet v 1 and Pru av 1, respectively - for those parameters, two questions are of great importance respecting the parameters analyzed: 1) Is TcPR10 capable of triggering IgE-dependent hypersensitivity? Is there a possible expression of a mutant from the TcPR10 protein that maintains antifungal and ribonuclease activities and reduces or eliminates the potential for IgE production? The modeling of TcPR-10 protein has allowed to select Thr10, Ile30 and His45 sites for insertion of mutations. The amino acid Thr10 in TcPR-10 belongs to the β1 chain (3–12) located on the exposed surface of the protein (Figure 2A and C) is not situated near the conserved areas identified via SDAP. In turn, the amino acid Ile30 located in loop L2 (27–39) is situated in the cavity of the protein and near the conserved region 25DSDNLI30. The T10P and I30V substitutions inserted in TcPR-10 have been demonstrated in other PR-10 proteins - as an example, Bet v 1 [45] e Mal d 1 [22] - and are involved in the formation of IgE epitopes. The substitution of histidine for serine at position 45, located on β2 (40–46), was introduced for it precedes the conserved region of P-loop 47GDGGVG52 from TcPR-10. In Bet v 1, the residue from glutamic acid (E) at position 45 is considered as crucial for the recognition of antibodies [20,21].

Analysis of the influence of site-directed mutations regarding the IgE binding capacity has demonstrated that the P-loop is not always involved in IgE binding and that similar amino acid substitutions in proteins with high identity not always result in loss of IgE binding capacity [22,23,46,47]. In Mal d 1, a single point mutation at position 111 replacing serine for proline was responsible for reducing allergenicity [48]. The ability of TcPR-10 wt and TcPR-10 mut proteins to modulate the production response of IgE was examined in a urine model. The elevation of serum IgE levels in animals subjected to systemic sensitization by subcutaneous injection followed by exposure of the airways to the wild TcPR-10 indicate that this protein can modulate the response of total IgE. In line with the high levels of IgE antibodies, the number of leukocytes present in the BAL fluid was also higher in the wild-type TcPR-10 experimental group (Figures 6A and B), thus indicating the potential of TcPR10 in recruiting inflammatory cells, especially polymorph nuclear cells (Figure 6D). Histological analysis of lung tissue has confirmed the presence of cellular infiltration detected in BAL fluid samples (Figure 6D). On the other hand, there was a more attenuated inflammatory response in mice challenged with the TcPR-10 mutant protein characterized by lower levels of IgE and total leukocytes present in BAL fluid (Figure 6E).

Interestingly, the insertion of mutations has not altered the characteristics of ribonuclease and antifungal activity of the TcPR-10 protein, which are crucial in the resistance of *T. cacao*; hence, the method of insertion is of interest in the genetic improvement of these plants. In AhPR10, isolated protein from *Arachis hypogaea*, mutations in the K54N residue of the P-loop region has led to complete loss of ribonuclease activity, while other points of substitutions such as F148S and H150Q have partially affected the catalytic activity, thus indicating that these residues are important for the RNase function of this protein [19]. The maintenance of catalytic activity in mutant TcPR-10 (Figure 4) suggests that the amino acids Thr10, Ile30 and His45 may not determine this function in protein, but influences the allergenic character, as observed in the modulation of IgE production and recruitment of inflammatory cells. Some authors suggest that ribonuclease is associated with the capacity to inhibit fungal growth [19,49]. The TcPR-10 mutant protein shows a small reduction in the time of degradation of RNA and also presents a reduction in the ability to inhibit fungal growth at a concentration of 10 μg/μl, as compared with the wild-type TcPR-10, thus indicating that these activities could be correlated. The presence of P-loop is also associated with the ribonuclease of PR-10 proteins. Site-directed mutations in three conserved amino acids (E95A, E147A, Y150A) and the construction of deletions in the P-loop protein SPE-16 isolated from *Pachyrrhizus erosus* seeds and classified as a member of the family PR-10 has shown different changes in ribonuclease activity [50]. In TcPR-10, the presence of conserved amino acid residues E97, E149 and Y151 is associated with ribonuclease activity [24].

The constitutive expression of genes in transgenic plants is the major concern about the allergenic potential of PR proteins. Sowoboda et al (1995) [51] emphasize that the conditions of pathogenic infections and stress can increase the level of expression of proteins homologous to Bet v 1 in pollens and other plant parts and thereby contribute to a significant increase in the incidence of type 1 hypersensitivity detected over the last years in industrialized countries. The overexpression of the *TcPR-10* gene in cocoa fruit should not be a critical factor limiting the genetic improvement of this species by transgenic techniques, since the processing of cocoa beans for chocolate production could reduce the possible allergenic activity of this protein. In addition, there are few reports of cases of clinical sensitivity to chocolate, what can be explained by the changes that proteins undergo as a result of the processing of cocoa beans [52]. Yet, the introduction of new forms of chocolate that are less processed, such as pieces of raw or toasted cocoa bean is a worrying concern, considering that the allergenicity and the importance of cross-reactivity of these products with other food allergens is unknown [53]. The possibility of a constitutive expression of the TcPR-10 protein in transgenic plants can become a public health problem, since the protein is expressed in pollen grains and could become a potential source of allergens triggering airway hypersensitivity, or the protein could show cross-reactivity with food allergens.

The experimental evidences generated from this study pave the way for the continuous use of the TcPR-10 protein as a potential antifungal agent that can be used in cocoa breeding through molecular engineering techniques. Besides maintaining the ribonuclease activity, the mutant TcPR-10 protein possibly modulates the immune response, showing characteristics that can be exploited in view of future applications in immunotherapies.

Materials and Methods

TcPR-10 Sequence

The *TcPR-10* gene (accession number ES439858) used in this study was identified from a cDNA library of cacao (cv. Catongo) inoculated by *M. perniciosa* [54]. Open reading frame (ORF) analysis of the nucleotide sequence obtained from the interaction cDNA library followed by homology search on BLAST [30] against sequences in the National Center for Biotechnology Information database identified a putative *PR-10* gene (insert size of 779 bp) with an ORF of 480 nucleotides encoding a protein of 159 amino acid residues. The *TcPR-10* gene was cloned into the pET28a (*Novagen*) expression vector as previously described [24].

Identification of Potential Allergenic TcPR-10 Proteins through Bioinformatics Analysis

The analysis of the potential allergenicity of the amino acid sequence of the TcPR-10 protein was done using Bioinformatics tools available in Structural Database of Allergenic Proteins (SDAP, http://fermi.utmb.edu/SDAP). The sequence of TcPR-10 underwent alignments based on identity more than 35% in the window of 80 amino acids and identity of six contiguous amino acids of the TcPR-10 protein in a known allergen available in Base SDAP. The similarity of TcPR-10 with sequence available in the SDAP allergens was done using the statistical E-value and the property distance index PD. A low E-value (e.g. less than 10^{-6}) indicates a high significance of the sequence match. The index PD values measure the similarity of two peptides based on five amino acid descriptors E1–E5 that were determined by a multidimensional scaling of 237 physicochemical properties of amino acids [55].

$$PD(A,B)=\frac{1}{N}\sum_{i=1}^{N}\left[\sum_{j=1}^{5}\lambda_j\left(E_j\left(A_i-E_j(B_i)\right)\right)^2\right]^{1/2}.$$

Where: λ_j is the eigenvalue of the j-th E component, $E_j(A_i)$ is the E_j value for the amino acid in the i-th position from sequence A, and $E_j(B_i)$ is the E_j value for the amino acid in the i-th position from sequence B.

Molecular Modeling

Comparative protein modeling was used to predict a structural model of TcPR-10 protein implemented by Swiss Pdb-Viewer v.3.7 accessible via the Expasy web Server (http://swissmodel.expasy.org/) [31,56]. The homology modeling of protein TcPR-10 was performed using as a template the three-dimensional structure of the major cherry allergen, Pru av 1 (pdb:1e09_A), in solution, resolved by heteronuclear multidimensional NMR spectroscopy [17]. The modeling procedure started with the choice of the template based on the alignment of the sequences of proteins TcPR-10 wild and mutant to be modeled using the PSI-BLAST [30] with known three-dimensional (3-D) proteins structures available in the Protein Data BankProtein (pdb) (http://www.pdb.org). After align primary target sequence with template was submitted to modeling request to the Swiss Model Server.

Validation of the secondary structure was performed using PsiPred (Protein struture prediction Server - http://bioinf.cs.ucl.ac.uk/psipred/) [57]. The stereochemical quality of structural models of TcPR-10 wild type and mutant proteins obtained by homology modeling with the protein structure Pru av 1 (SolutionNMR) was assessed using the programs PROCHECK 3.4 [58] and ANOLEA (Atomic Non-Local Environment Assessment) [59]. The Root Mean Square Deviation (RMSD) differences from ideal geometries for bond lengths and bond angles were calculated on Pymol 3.0.

Site-directed Mutagenesis

TcPR-10 inserted into the pET28a expression vector was modified by site-directed mutagenesis by overlap-extension based on polymerase chain reaction (PCR). Three oligonucleotide primer sets were constructed by site directed mutagenesis (Thr10Pro, Ile30Val, His45Ser) (Table 3). The PCR amplification was done at an annealing temperature of 50°C for 40 cycles of polymerization using *Taq* polymerase (Taq High Fidelity-*Fermentas*). The PCR product were digested with *Nde*I and *Sal*I and subcloned in expression vector pET28a (Novagen). The plasmid pET28a with TcPR-10 insert were transformed into *Escherichia coli* BL21(DE3) for protein expression. In the following TcPR-10 inserted into the pET28a without modification will be referred to as TcPR-10 wild type (TcPR-10 wt) and engineered mutant as TcPR-10 mutant (TcPR-10 mut).

Expression and Purification of Recombinants Wild and Mutant-type TcPR-10

The expression of recombinant proteins TcPR-10 wt and TcPR-10 mut was obtained by the induction of a colony transformant grown in LB medium (Luria-Bertani) containing Kanamycin (50 µg.mL^{-1}) and Chloramphenicol (34 µg.mL^{-1}) under constant shaking at 37°C until reaching an OD_{600} between 0.5 and 0.7. Expression of recombinant proteins was induced by 1 mM *Isopropyl-β-D-thio-galactoside* (IPTG) followed by 15 h incubation at 18°C. The cells were centrifuged (11000×*g*, 20 min, 4°C) and pellets suspended in lyses buffer (50 mM phosphate buffer [PB], 300 mM NaCl, 2% of Nonidet, lysozyme at 0.1 mg.mL^{-1}, pH 7.4) and sonicated by 4 min (30 s pulse/min, 75% output) (*Gex Ultrasonic processor 130, 130 W*). Subsequently, after centrifuged (11000×*g*, 20 minutos, 4°C) the samples were purified with TALON® Metal Affinity Resins (*Clontech Laboratories*) according to the manufacturer's instructions. Expression of recombinant proteins was induced and harvested as described previously [24]. Expression and purification of recombinants TcPR-10 wt and TcPR-10 mut were analyzed by 15% Sodium

Table 3. Primer sets used for mutation at positions Thr10Pro, Ile30Val and His45Ser in the *TcPR-10* gene.

Primers		Sequence (5′ to 3′)	Nucleotides
T10P	Forward	CAA GAG TTC <u>C**C**C</u> TGC TCA GTT G	22–43
	Reverse	C AAC TGA GCA <u>GG**G**</u> GAA CTC TTG	
I30V	Forward	C GAC AAC CTT <u>**G**TC</u> CCC AAA CTC	81–102
	Reverse	GAG TTT GGG <u>GA**C**</u> AAG GTT GTC G	
H45S	Forward	G GAG TTG ATT <u>**AG**T</u> GGA GAT GG	126–146
	Reverse	CC ATC TCC <u>**AC**T</u> AAT CAC CTC C	

The mutated codon is underlined and nucleotide substitution in bold.

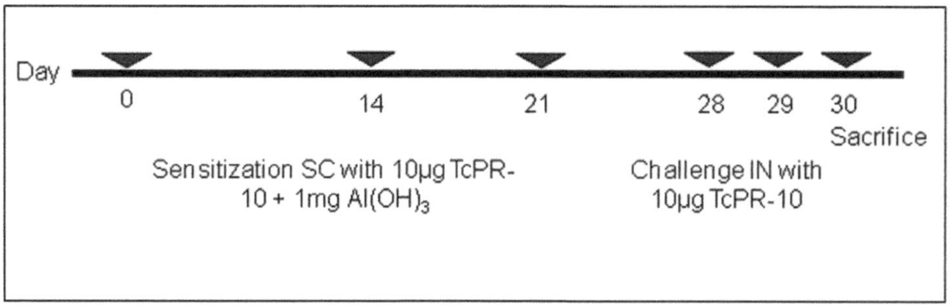

Figure 7. Experimental design of sensitization and challenge with TcPR-10 wild types and mutant.

dodecyl sulfate polyacrylamide gel electrophoresis (SDS-PAGE). Protein concentrations were determined by Bradford protein assay [60].

Ribonuclease and Antifungal Activity of Mutant-type TcPR-10

Ribonuclease and antifungal activity of TcPR-10 mut was verified according to Bantignies and associates (2000) [61] with suggested modifications by Pungartnik and associates (2009). The RNA from *M. perniciosa* (Cp 553CEPLAC), growing in complete medium CPD (2% glucose, 2% peptone, 2% agar added for solid media), was extracted using phenol–chloroform method followed by ethanol precipitation and analyzed by 1% agarose gel electrophoresis. One microgram of RNA was incubated with TcPR-10 mutant protein (1 µg) at 25°C at different times (10 min, 20 min, 1 h, 2 h and 3 h). Positive control used wild-type TcPR-10 previously characterized with ribonuclease activity. Ribonuclease activity was determined by degradation total of RNA observed in 1% agarose gel. Antifungal activities of TcPR-10 mut protein were determined by inhibiting growth of dikaryotic *M. perniciosa* broken hyphae in increasing concentrations of the recombinant protein (0, 4, 8 e 10 µg/plate) [62].

Allergen Sensitization and Challenge with Wild and Mutant-type TcPR-10

Female BALB/c mice, 8–10 weeks old, obtained from the Centro de Bioterismo (CEBIO) do Instituto de Ciências Biológicas da Universidade Federal de Minas Gerais, Brasil (UFMG) were used in this experiment. The animals were kept under conventionally standard housed conditions of the Instituto de Ciências Biológicas (ICB) of UFMG. This study, under the supervision of Dr. Abelmon da Silva Gesteira, was specifically approved by the Ethics Committee in Animal Experimentation (CEUA) of the Universidade Estadual de Santa Cruz (UESC) under protocol n. 001/09.

BALB/c mice were sensitized via subcutaneous (SC) in three time periods 0, 14 and 28 days, with the proteins and 1 mg Al(OH)3. For induction of allergic airway inflammation mice were challenged intranasal (IN) at 35 and 36 days as shown in Figure 7. The experiments were carried out in three experimental groups (n = 5): (i) 10 µg of TcPR10 wild protein [0.8 µg/µL], (ii) 10 µg of mutant [0.8 µg/µL] and (iii) control (PB, 300 mM NaCl).

Measurement of Total IgE

Mice were bled after 24 h of the last IN challenge to antibody detection IgE by Enzyme-Linked Immunosorbent Assay (ELISA). Blood samples were centrifuged (5000 ×*g*, 10 min, 4°C) and serum was collected. Plates were coated with a rat anti-mouse IgE antibodies (UNLB) diluted in Coating Buffer (pH 9.6) (1:250). Plates were incubated overnight in cold chamber at 4°C. Afterwards they were washed with PBS. The coated wells were blocked with PBS-Casein (50 mM phosphate buffer pH 7.2 with 0.25% of casein) for 1 h at room temperature. Detection of IgE was carried out using biotinylated rat antimouse IgE (1:500) incubated for 1 h at room temperature. Streptavidin-peroxidase (Sigma-Aldrich) was used as a second-step reagent, developed using H_2O_2 with Ortho-Phenylenediamine (OPD) solved in citrate buffer, pH 5 (4 mg de OPD com 2 µL de H_2O_2 a 30%). The reaction was blocked by adding sulfuric acid 2N. The reactions were read on microplates BioRad Model 450 at 492 nm.

Bronchoalveolar Lavage and Pulmonary Histopathology

For the determination of cellular infiltration in the lung, bronchoalveolar lavage fluids, were collected. After the sacrifice, lungs were washed with 1 mL of cold PBS containing bovine serum albumin (0.03%). Total number of cells was determined by counting in a Neubauer chamber. The count was done by two independent investigators under the optic microscope (OLYMPUS B12).

After the collection of the bronchoalveolar lavage the lungs were removed and fixed with 10% buffered formaldehyde (v/v) (0.1 M phosphate buffer, pH 7.4) and processed in a standard manner. For the histological examination, fixed embedded lungs were sectioned into 5 µm sections, deparaffinized with xylene and graded ethanol and stained with haematoxylin and eosin (H&E). For the morphological evaluation of lung tissues the preparations were carried out microscopically (OLYMPUS B12) and images captured in digital camera for evaluation of the symptons of the airway inflammation as expression of infiltration of inflammatory cells.

Statistical Analysis

Data were subjected to the Shapiro Wilk normality test followed by analysis of variance for parametric data with Tukey Test ($\alpha = 0.05$) to compare the means of experimental groups with control. For nonparametric data the Kruskal-Wallis test was used. Data are shown as mean (M) and standard deviation (SD). Differences were considered significant for p values <0,05. Analyses were carried out using the Bioestat v4.0 [63] and GraphPad PRISM v.4.0 [64].

Acknowledgments

We thank Claudia Fortes Ferreira (Embrapa, Brazil) for helpful advice and critical reading of the manuscript.

Author Contributions

Conceived and designed the experiments: ASG FM JLS. Performed the experiments: SPM THSC JLS FSMN ACA AMCF. Analyzed the data: ASG SPM JSL AMCF FM CPP. Contributed reagents/materials/analysis tools: ASG FM. Wrote the paper: ASG SPM JLS AMCF.

References

1. Van Montagu M (2011) It Is a Long Way to GM Agriculture. Annual Review of Plant Biology, Vol 62 62: 1–23.
2. Gallo M, Sayre R (2009) Removing allergens and reducing toxins from food crops. Current opinion in biotechnology 20: 191–196.
3. Bahramnejad B, Goodwin PH, Zhang J, Atnaseo C, Erickson LR (2010) A comparison of two class 10 pathogenesis-related genes from alfalfa and their activation by multiple stresses and stress-related signaling molecules. Plant cell reports 29: 1235–1250.
4. Gomez-Gomez L, Rubio-Moraga A, Ahrazem O (2011) Molecular cloning and characterisation of a pathogenesis-related protein CsPR10 from Crocus sativus. Plant biology 13: 297–303.
5. Lebel S, Schellenbaum P, Walter B, Maillot P (2010) Characterisation of the Vitis vinifera PR10 multigene family. BMC plant biology 10: 184.
6. Liu JJ, Ekramoddoullah AK, Piggott N, Zamani A (2005) Molecular cloning of a pathogen/wound-inducible PR10 promoter from Pinus monticola and characterization in transgenic Arabidopsis plants. Planta 221: 159–169.
7. Walter MH, Liu JW, Wunn J, Hess D (1996) Bean ribonuclease-like pathogenesis-related protein genes (Ypr10) display complex patterns of developmental, dark-induced and exogenous-stimulus-dependent expression. European Journal of Biochemistry 239: 281–293.
8. Ebner C, Hoffmann-Sommergruber K, Breiteneder H (2001) Plant food allergens homologous to pathogenesis-related proteins. Allergy 56: 43–44.
9. Hoffmann-Sommergruber K (2002) Pathogenesis-related (PR)-proteins identified as allergens. Biochemical Society Transactions 30: 930–935.
10. Midoro-Horiuti T, Brooks EG, Goldblum RM (2001) Pathogenesis-related proteins of plants as allergens. Annals of allergy, asthma & immunology : official publication of the American College of Allergy, Asthma, & Immunology 87: 261–271.
11. Salcedo G, Asensio T, Crespo JF, Sanchez-Monge R, Lopez-Torrejon G, et al. (2004) Novel plant pathogenesis-related protein family involved in food allergy. Journal of Allergy and Clinical Immunology 114: 896–899.
12. Gajhede M, Osmark P, Poulsen FM, Ipsen H, Larsen JN, et al. (1996) X-ray and NMR structure of Bet v 1, the origin of birch pollen allergy. Nature Structural Biology 3: 1040–1045.
13. Schenk MF, Gilissen LJWJ, Esselink GD, Smulders MJM (2006) Seven different genes encode a diverse mixture of isoforms of Bet v I, the major birch pollen allergen. BMC genomics 7.
14. Baraldi E, Zubini P, Zambelli B, Musiani F, Ciurli S, et al. (2009) The RNA Hydrolysis and the Cytokinin Binding Activities of PR-10 Proteins Are Differently Performed by Two Isoforms of the Pru p 1 Peach Major Allergen and Are Possibly Functionally Related. Plant physiology 150: 1235–1247.
15. Puehringer HM, Zinoecker I, Marzban G, Katinger H, Laimer M (2003) MdAP, a novel protein in apple, is associated with the major allergen Mal d 1. Gene 321: 173–183.
16. Wiche R, Gubesch M, Konig H, Fotisch K, Hoffmann A, et al. (2005) Molecular basis of pollen-related food allergy: identification of a second cross-reactive IgE epitope on Pru av 1, the major cherry (Prunes avium) allergen. Biochemical Journal 385: 319–327.
17. Neudecker P, Schweimer K, Nerkamp J, Scheurer S, Vieths S, et al. (2001) Allergic cross-reactivity made visible - Solution structure of the major cherry allergen Pru av 1. Journal of Biological Chemistry 276: 22756–22763.
18. Peters S, Imani J, Mahler V, Foetisch K, Kaul S, et al. (2011) Dau c 1.01 and Dau c 1.02-silenced transgenic carrot plants show reduced allergenicity to patients with carrot allergy. Transgenic research 20: 547–556.
19. Chadha P, Das RH (2006) A pathogenesis related protein, AhPR10 from peanut: an insight of its mode of antifungal activity. Planta 225: 213–222.
20. Mirza O, Henriksen A, Ipsen H, Larsen JN, Wissenbach M, et al. (2000) Dominant epitopes and allergic cross-reactivity: Complex formation between a Fab fragment of a monoclonal murine IgG antibody and the major allergen from birch pollen Bet v 1. Journal of Immunology 165: 331–338.
21. Spangfort MD, Mirza O, Ipsen H, van Neerven RJJ, Gajhede M, et al. (2003) Dominating IgE-binding epitope of Bet v 1, the major allergen of birch pollen, characterized by X-ray crystallography and site-directed mutagenesis. Journal of Immunology 171: 3084–3090.
22. Ma Y, Gadermaier G, Bohle B, Bolhaar S, Knulst A, et al. (2006) Mutational analysis of amino acid positions crucial for IgE-binding epitopes of the major apple (Malus domestica) allergen, Mal d 1. International Archives of Allergy and Immunology 139: 53–62.
23. Wangorsch A, Ballmer-Weber BK, Rosch P, Holzhauser T, Vieths S (2007) Mutational epitope analysis and cross-reactivity of two isoforms of Api g 1, the major celery allergen. Molecular immunology 44: 2518–2527.
24. Pungartnik C, da Silva AC, de Melo SA, Gramacho KP, de Mattos Cascardo JC, et al. (2009) High-affinity copper transport and Snq2 export permease of saccharomyces cerevisiae modulate cytotoxicity of PR-10 from Theobroma cacao. Molecular plant-microbe interactions : MPMI 22: 39–51.
25. Dearman RJ, Skinner RA, Herouet C, Labay K, Debruyne E, et al. (2003) Induction of IgE antibody responses by protein allergens: inter-laboratory comparisons. Food and chemical toxicology : an international journal published for the British Industrial Biological Research Association 41: 1509–1516.
26. Ivanciuc O, Garcia T, Torres M, Schein CH, Braun W (2009) Characteristic motifs for families of allergenic proteins. Molecular immunology 46: 559–568.
27. Selgrade MK, Bowman CC, Ladics GS, Privalle L, Laessig SA (2009) Safety assessment of biotechnology products for potential risk of food allergy: implications of new research. Toxicological sciences : an official journal of the Society of Toxicology 110: 31–39.
28. Ivanciuc O, Schein CH, Braun W (2003) SDAP: database and computational tools for allergenic proteins. Nucleic Acids Research 31: 359–362.
29. Ivanciuc O, Schein CH, Braun W (2002) Data mining of sequences and 3D structures of allergenic proteins. Bioinformatics 18: 1358–1364.
30. Altschul SF, Madden TL, Schaffer AA, Zhang J, Zhang Z, et al. (1997) Gapped BLAST and PSI-BLAST: a new generation of protein database search programs. Nucleic Acids Research 25: 3389–3402.
31. Guex N, Peitsch MC (1997) SWISS-MODEL and the Swiss-PdbViewer: An environment for comparative protein modeling. Electrophoresis 18: 2714–2723.
32. Veluthakkal R, Dasgupta MG (2010) Pathogenesis-related genes and proteins in forest tree species. Trees-Structure and Function 24: 993–1006.
33. van Loon LC, Rep M, Pieterse CMJ (2006) Significance of inducible defense-related proteins in infected plants. Annual review of phytopathology 44: 135–162.
34. Breiteneder H, Ebner C (2000) Molecular and biochemical classification of plant-derived food allergens. Journal of Allergy and Clinical Immunology 106: 27–36.
35. Thomas K, Herouet-Guicheney C, Ladics G, McClain S, MacIntosh S, et al. (2008) Current and future methods for evaluating the allergenic potential of proteins: international workshop report 23–25 October 2007. Food and chemical toxicology : an international journal published for the British Industrial Biological Research Association 46: 3219–3225.
36. Thomas WR (2011) The advent of recombinant allergens and allergen cloning. J Allergy Clin Immunol 127: 855–859.
37. WHO (2001) Evaluation of Allergenicity of Genetically Modified Foods Rome, Italy: Report of a Joint FAO/WHO Expert Consultation on Allergenicity of Foods Derived from Biotechnology. 30p.
38. Ivanciuc O, Schein CH, Garcia T, Oezguen N, Negi SS, et al. (2009) Structural analysis of linear and conformational epitopes of allergens. Regulatory toxicology and pharmacology : RTP 54: S11–19.
39. Breiteneder H, Mills ENC (2005) Plant food allergens - structural and functional aspects of allergenicity. Biotechnology advances 23: 395–399.
40. Silvanovich A, Bannon G, McClain S (2009) The use of E-scores to determine the quality of protein alignments. Regulatory Toxicology and Pharmacology 54: S26-S31.
41. Cressman RF, Ladics G (2009) Further evaluation of the utility of "Sliding Window" FASTA in predicting cross-reactivity with allergenic proteins. Regulatory Toxicology and Pharmacology 54: S20-S25.
42. Neudecker P, Lehmann K, Nerkamp J, Haase T, Wangorsch A, et al. (2003) Mutational epitope analysis of Pru av 1 and Api g 1, the major allergens of cherry (Prunus avium) and celery (Apium graveolens): correlating IgE reactivity with three-dimensional structure. Biochemical Journal 376: 97–107.
43. Fernandes H, Bujacz A, Bujacz G, Jelen F, Jasinski M, et al. (2009) Cytokinin-induced structural adaptability of a Lupinus luteus PR-10 protein. Febs Journal 276: 1596–1609.
44. Neudecker P, Schweimer K, Nerkamp J, Boehm M, Scheurer S, et al. (2000) Sequence-specific H-1, C-13 and N-15 resonance assignments of the major cherry allergen Pru a 1. Journal of Biomolecular Nmr 18: 71–72.
45. Ferreira F, Ebner C, Kramer B, Casari G, Briza P, et al. (1998) Modulation of IgE reactivity of allergens by site-directed mutagenesis: potential use of hypoallergenic variants for immunotherapy. Faseb Journal 12: 231–242.
46. Scheurer S, Son DY, Boehm M, Karamloo F, Franke S, et al. (1999) Cross-reactivity and epitope analysis of Pru a 1, the major cherry allergen. Molecular immunology 36: 155–167.
47. Midoro-Horiuti T, Brooks EG, Goldblum RM (2001) Pathogenesis-related proteins of plants as allergens. Annals of Allergy Asthma & Immunology 87: 261–271.
48. Son DY, Scheurer S, Hoffmann A, Haustein D, Vieths S (1999) Pollen-related food allergy: cloning and immunological analysis of isoforms and mutants of Mal d 1, the major apple allergen, and Bet v 1, the major birch pollen allergen. European Journal of Nutrition 38: 201–215.
49. Xie YR, Chen ZY, Brown RL, Bhatnagar D (2010) Expression and functional characterization of two pathogenesis-related protein 10 genes from Zea mays. Journal of plant physiology 167: 121–130.
50. Wu F, Yan M, Li YK, Chang SJ, Song XM, et al. (2003) cDNA cloning, expression, and mutagenesis of a PR-10 protein SPE-16 from the seeds of

Pachyrrhizus erosus. Biochemical and biophysical research communications 312: 761–766.
51. Swoboda I, Scheiner O, Heberlebors E, Vicente O (1995) Cdna Cloning and Characterization of 3 Genes in the Bet-V-1 Gene Family That Encode Pathogenesis-Related Proteins. Plant Cell and Environment 18: 865–874.
52. Chapman JA, Bernstein IL, Lee RE, Oppenheimer J, Nicklas RA, et al. (2006) Food allergy: a practice parameter. Annals of Allergy Asthma & Immunology 96: S1-S68.
53. Chapman HD (2000) Practical use of vaccines for the control of coccidiosis in the chicken. Worlds Poultry Science Journal 56: 7–20.
54. Gesteira AS, Micheli F, Carels N, Da Silva AC, Gramacho KP, et al. (2007) Comparative analysis of expressed genes from cacao meristems infected by Moniliophthora perniciosa. Annals of botany 100: 129–140.
55. Venkatarajan MS, Braun W (2001) New quantitative descriptors of amino acids based on multidimensional scaling of a large number of physical-chemical properties. Journal of Molecular Modeling 7: 445–453.
56. Guex N, Peitsch MC, Schwede T (2009) Automated comparative protein structure modeling with SWISS-MODEL and Swiss-PdbViewer: A historical perspective. Electrophoresis 30: S162-S173.
57. Jones DT (1999) Protein secondary structure prediction based on position-specific scoring matrices. Journal of molecular biology 292: 195–202.
58. Laskowski RA, Chistyakov VV, Thornton JM (2005) PDBsum more: new summaries and analyses of the known 3D structures of proteins and nucleic acids. Nucleic Acids Research 33: D266-D268.
59. Melo F, Feytmans E (1998) Assessing protein structures with a non-local atomic interaction energy. Journal of molecular biology 277: 1141–1152.
60. Bradford MM (1976) A rapid and sensitive method for the quantitation of microgram quantities of protein utilizing the principle of protein-dye binding. Analytical biochemistry 72: 248–254.
61. Bantignies B, Seguin J, Muzac I, Dedaldechamp F, Gulick P, et al. (2000) Direct evidence for ribonucleolytic activity of a PR-10-like protein from white lupin roots. Plant molecular biology 42: 871–881.
62. Filho DF, Pungartnik C, Cascardo JC, Brendel M (2006) Broken hyphae of the basidiomycete Crinipellis perniciosa allow quantitative assay of toxicity. Current microbiology 52: 407–412.
63. Ayres M, Jr MA, Ayres DL, Santos ASd (2005) BioEstat. Aplicações estatísticas nas áreas das ciências biológicas e médicas. Belém - Pará - Brasil: Sociedade Civil Mamirauá. 323p p.
64. Motulsky HJ (2003) Prism 4 Statistics Guide - Statistical analyses for laboratory and clinical researchers. San Diego CA: GraphPad Software Inc. www.graphpad.com.

Citrus Allergy from Pollen to Clinical Symptoms

Rosa Anna Iorio[1], Stefano Del Duca[1]*, Elisabetta Calamelli[2], Chiara Pula[2], Magda Lodolini[3], Fortuna Scamardella[3], Andrea Pession[2], Giampaolo Ricci[2]

1 Department of Biological, Earth and Environmental Sciences, University of Bologna, Bologna, Italy, **2** Department of Pediatric Allergology of the Women's, Children's and Adolescents' Health Gozzadini Children's Hospital Sant'Orsola-Malpighi, University of Bologna, Bologna, Italy, **3** Laboratory Analysis Unit. Maggiore Hospital, Bologna, Italy

Abstract

Allergy to citrus fruits is often associated with pollinosis and sensitization to other plants due to a phenomenon of cross-reactivity. The aims of the present study were to highlight the cross-reactivity among citrus and the major allergenic pollens/fruits, throughout clinical and molecular investigations, and to evaluate the sensitization frequency to citrus fruits in a population of children and adults with pollinosis. We found a relevant percentage of sensitisation (39%) to citrus fruits in the patients recruited and in all of them the IgE-mediated mechanism has been confirmed by the positive response to the prick-to-prick test. RT-PCR experiments showed the expression of Cit s 1, Cit s 3 and a profilin isoform, already described in apple, also in *Citrus clementine* pollen. Data of multiple sequence alignments demonstrated that *Citrus* allergens shared high percentage identity values with other clinically relevant species (i.e. *Triticum aestivum, Malus domestica*), confirming the possible cross-allergenicity citrus/grasses and citrus/apple. Finally, a novelty of the present work has been the expression of two phospholipaseA2 isoforms (PLA2 α and β) in *Citrus* as well as in *Triticum* pollens; being PLA2 able to generate pro-inflammatory factors, this enzyme could participate in the activation of the allergenic inflammatory cascade.

Editor: Phillip A. Stumbles, Murdoch University, Australia

Funding: This work was supported by the Programma Operativo Regionale (POR FESR 2007-2013) of Regione Calabria "My Darling Clementine": un prodotto salutistico nuovo e innovativo dalle clementine e dal limone di Calabria". The funders had no role in study design, data collection and analysis, decision to publish, or preparation of the manuscript.

Competing Interests: The authors have declared that no competing interests exist.

* E-mail: stefano.delduca@unibo.it

Introduction

The regular consumption of fruit and vegetables is generally encouraged also by the European Community as the basis of a daily diet healthy and able to improve human health and prevent some diseases: there are many data that confirm the direct correlation between the consumption of fresh fruit and the reduction in the incidence of cardio-vascular disease, asthma, diabetes and cancer [1,2]. The benefit derives not only from their nutritional properties in terms of vitamins, minerals and fibres, but also from the "non-nutritional" component, such as the high content in secondary metabolites (phenols, flavonoids, carotenoids) that play an important antioxidant role.

Unfortunately, about 1/5 of the population in Western countries suffer from respiratory allergies [3]. Recent epidemiological studies estimate that food allergies are increasing and affecting millions of people (1–2% of world population), as to consider them as the epidemic of the XXI century [4]. Nearly 4% of the US populations are afflicted with food allergies, a prevalence much higher than appreciated in the past. In addition, the frequency of food hypersensitivities is greater in the first few years of life, affecting about 6% of infants less than 3 years of age and decreasing over the first decade [5].

For food allergies there is still no effective treatment and, consequently, up to now the only therapy is still the avoidance of fruits that cause allergy [6] and, considering that a regular consumption of fruits is reported to enhance human health and prevent various diseases, it is easy to understand that allergy can significantly affect the quality of life of allergic patients in a profoundly negative way [7]. The problem is compounded by the fact that food allergy may also arise as a result of cross-pollen allergy [8].

Oranges (*Citrus sinensis*) are largely consumed worldwide and commonly included in the population's diet in many countries, both as fresh fruit or derived beverages (juices) and foods (jams) [9,10]. This fact has probably led to point to orange among the main allergenic plant food in a public perception survey of food allergies [11]. Although in the daily clinical practice orange allergy is obviously rarely observed in Central Europe, some early studies suggested oranges being an important allergenic food, as for other foods and pollens such as kiwi, strawberry, peach, banana, grasses (www.foodallergyitalia.org) [12]. However, allergy to oranges or other citrus fruits has been scarcely investigated [10]; when present, it is often associated with pollinosis and sensitization to other plants [10] due to a phenomenon of cross-reactivity, whereby the pollen would be the cause of a sensitization by the respiratory way that could predispose to allergy towards foods that contain homologous proteins to those in sensitizing pollen. In an English study on 67 asthmatic children which compared a multiple food specific IgE antibodies (sIgE) test to parental perception of food allergy, oranges resulted implicated in the 15% of patients [13]. Another study reported a frequency of 17% of adverse food reactions after eating oranges in a population of 100 adults suffering from oral allergy syndrome (OAS) as common manifestations of allergy to oranges [14]. Previous studies indicated mild local reactions and described subjects affected from orange-dependent exercise-induced anaphylaxis after eating oranges [12].

The three major orange allergens that have been recently identified and characterized are Cit s 1, a germin-like protein (GLP) [14,15], Cit s 2, a profilin [9,10] and Cit s 3, a new member of the lipid transfer protein pan-allergen family (LTP) [9]. Cit s 1 is a glycoprotein of 24 kDa recognized by patients' sera IgE recently described by Ibáñez et al. [15] and Pignataro et al. in lemon fruit flavedo [16]; its biological activity in fruit need to be clarified, but it is considered one of the major orange allergen [12] displaying an high *in vitro* reactivity with its glycans constituting the major IgE epitopes [9]. Moreover, the protein could be present in different isoforms ranging from 20 to 120 kDa [16]. Cit s 2 represents the other major allergen according to its *in vitro* and *in vivo* reactivity in patients with allergy to this fruit [10]. Its biological activity is associated to the structural organization of actin filament; in particular it is believed to be involved in the transition between G- and F-actin, playing a very important role for pollen germination and indeed for plant fertilization [17]; its reactivity with patient-s'sera is associated to plan pollen allergy [18]. Cit s 3 behaves as a minor allergen (approximately 35% prevalence) [9], contrary to the fact that LTPs are considered in general the major fruit allergen in the Mediterranean area [12]. Cit s 3 is present in pulp, but in lower amount comparing to flavedo, so the moderate IgE reactivity observed might be explained by the low nsLTP concentration in the orange pulp [19]. LTP role in plant is believed to be related to the defence mechanisms and in the control of pathogen attack responses. Moreover, a role in transporting lipid molecules to the outer layers of plant organs, in embryogenesis and in abiotic stress response has been also proposed [20]. The multiple function of LTPs is also supported by the presence of isoforms showing moderate levels of amino acid sequence identity and different gene expression patterns [21].

Ahrazem et al. [19] sought to identify and isolated citrus fruit LTPs and to explore their relevance in orange allergy in 27 patients with OAS after orange ingestion and with positive skin-prick test (SPT) as well as prick-to-prick test (PPT) responses and sIgE levels to orange. This study showed that members of the LTP allergen family are involved in orange's allergy, displaying positive *in vivo* and *in vitro* tests in 30–50% of the subjects studied. Furthermore, both orange and lemon allergens showed cross-reactivity with the major peach LTP allergen Pru p 3: the recombinant orange isoform (rCit s 3) presented 67% sequence identity with rPru p 3 [19].

Crespo et al. [12] documented a statistically significant correlation between the presence of IgE mediated sensitization to the two orange major allergens, Cit s 1 and Cit s 2 and the positive response to Skin-Prick test (SPT) respectively to olive and cypress (Cit s 1) and to platanus (Cit s 2) in 56 patients with self-reported adverse reactions to oranges.

The purposes of the present study were to i) deeply investigate the cross-reactivity among citrus and the major allergenic pollens and fruits, either under clinical and molecular points of view, and to ii) evaluate the frequency of sensitization and/or allergy to citrus fruits (oranges, lemons and clementines) in a population of children and young adults with pollinosis (allergic hay fever and/or asthma) recruited for this monocentric observational study.

The cross-reactivity aspect has focused on the analysis of i) the sIgE levels in patients serum in order to determine the major citrus allergens levels by the use of the recombinant molecules Pru p 3 (LTP protein homolog to Cit s 3), r Phl p 12 (profilin homolog to Cit s 2) and MuxF3-CCD, marker of sensitization for Cross-reactive carbohydrate determinants (CCD) and of ii) allergens expression (Cit s 1, Cit s 2, Cit s 3) in *Citrus clementine* pollen, in order to assess its potential allergenicity and cross-reactivity with other pollens, especially *Triticum aestivum*, whose allergens sequences are conserved in the *poaceae* family. The three important citrus allergens reported above were also analyzed in citrus pollen because of the possible cross-reactivity between pollen and fruits, as documented for apple [22]. *Citrus clementine* pollen can be potentially important from the allergenic point of view because present in some foods as marmalade and honey and for farmers cultivating citrus fields.

The research for sensitizing agents in pollen continued with the evaluation of the expression of two isoforms of secretory phospholipase (PLA2 α and β), key enzymes in the synthesis of pro-inflammatory eicosanoids that may have a key role in raising sensitization and allergic reaction [23,24].

Materials and Methods

Chemicals and Antibodies

All chemicals (unless otherwise indicated) were obtained from Sigma-Aldrich (Milan, Italy).

Plant material

Mature pollen of clementine (*Citrus clementine* Hort. Ex Tan. cv. Comune) was collected from flowers kindly donated by Professor S. Mazzucca, University of Calabria (Dipartimento di Ecologia), and pollen of *Triticum aestivum* (wheat) was kindly donated by Azienda Agricola Rondinini (Faenza, Ra). Handling and storage were performed as reported by Bagni et al. [25], stored at $-20°C$ with NaOH pellets to maintain it dry.

Fruits of oranges, clementines and lemons have been provided by Azienda Agricola "San Mauro" di Minisci Edmondo (Corigliano Calabro, Cosenza) within the project "My Darling Clementine": un prodotto salutistico nuovo e innovativo dalle clementine e dal limone di Calabria" (POR FESR 2007–2013).

In vitro germination

Pollen was hydrated at 20°C-100% rHu for 1 h and allowed to germinate (1 mg/mL in germination medium: 15% sucrose, 324 μM boric acid, 2% agar) 13 h (overnight, o/n) into glass Petri dishes at 20°C-100% rHu.

Total RNA isolation and cDNA synthesis

Total RNA was extracted from 30 mg of frozen ungerminated (UGP) and germinated (GP) *Citrus c.* and *Triticum a.* pollens following the basic protocol for phenol/SDS method [26] with minor modifications as published by Paris et al. [27]. The purity and concentration of the extracted RNAs were evaluated by measuring the absorbance at 260 and 280 nm wavelengths using a NanoDrop Spectrophotometer ND-1000 (EuroClone S.p.A., Italy). RNA was considered pure if the A260/280 ratio was grater than 1.8 and A260/230 ratio higher than 2. First-strand cDNA was synthesized following the instruction from Stratagene (Agilent Technologies, USA), starting from 1 μg DNA-free RNA, and 2 μl was used for the semi-quantitative PCR analyses.

Primer design

Specific primer pairs (Table 1 and Table 2) were designed on the basis of the sequences obtained from National Center for Biotechnology Information (NCBI) Reference Sequence database (http://www.ncbi.nlm.nih.gov) with the software Primer3 version 0.4.0 (http://frodo.wi.mit.edu/primer3) and further tested with the software PrimerSelect® v8.0-MegAlign for the formation of primer homo and heterodimers. As endogenous control the EF1-α gene of *Citrus sinensis* (GenBank ID AY498567) and the UBQ10 (GenBank ID CB322134.1) genes were used.

Table 1. Primer sequences and amplicon characteristics for *Citrus sinensis* genes used in semi-quantitative and qRT-PCR.

Gene	GeneBank accession number	Sequence 5′-3′	Product size (bp)	Ta (°C)	qRT-PCR Efficiency *	R^2*
UB10	CB322134.1	GATCCCACCAGACCAGCAA	105	60	1,953	1
		ACCAAATGAAGGGTTGATTCCTT				
EF1	AY498567.1	ATTGACAAGCGTGTGATTGAGC	132	60	1,948	0,999
		TCCACAAGGCAATATCAATGGTA				
Cit s 1	UniProt P84159	CATTCCAGTTGGACCCAAAG	191	60	1,961	1
		CAGTCAGCCTGGAGAGAGGT				
Cit s 2	AJ865015.1	CTTTCCTGCGTTTAGGCTTG	189	60	n.d.	n.d.
		AGGGCCTGATTGGTCTTCTT				
Cit s 3	AJ783335.1	CCCTATACCTGTGCCATGCT	199	60	1,902	1
		GCAGTCAGTGGAGATGCTGA				
PLA2 α	GU075396	GCCATAGCCCATGTTTTCAT	184	60	1,89	1
		CACTGTACAGCAGCCCACAG				
PLA2 β	GU075398	GTATCTCTGCAAGCGCACTG	180	60	1,961	1
		TGCCATGTCCATACCCTGTA				

*The qRT-PCR efficiency and correlations; R^2 were determined with LinRegPCR software.

Allergen gene expression analysis by semi-quantitative PCR

The PCR reactions were performed in a 15 µl reaction containing 2 µl cDNA, 0.1 µM specific primers (Table 1 and Table 2), 1.5 mM MgCl2, 100 µM dNTPs, 0.5 Unit Taq DNA Polymerase (Fermentas, M-Medical, Italy) and 1X reaction buffer. The reaction included an initial 5 min denaturation step at 94°C, followed by 40 PCR cycles at 94°C 30 s, the optimised annealing temperature for 45 s and 1 min at 72°C.

The number of amplification cycles was chosen to be in the exponential phase of amplification. The amplicons were visualised with a transilluminator (Vilber Lournet, Genenco) at 302 nm after electrophoresis in 2% (w/v) agarose gels in TAE 1X Buffer, containing 0.5 µg/ml ethidium bromide, and photographed (Nikon E5400 Coolpix). The experiment was repeated twice.

Real-time PCR (qRT-PCR) analysis

The transcript levels were determined by real-time quantitative RT-PCR (qRT-PCR) using a StepOnePlus^{TM} Real Time PCR System (Applied Biosystems, USA) and the Power SYBR Green PCR Master Mix (Applied Biosystems, USA) as recommended by the manufacturer. PCR reactions were carried out in 96-well plates (10 µl per well) in a buffer containing SYBR Green (including Taq polymerase, dNTPs, SYBR Green dye) and 200 nM of each primer (forward and reverse, Table 1). After denaturing at 95°C for 10 min, a two-step amplification occurred: 15 s of denaturation at 95°C and 1 min of annealing/extension at 60°C, with a total of 40 cycles. The melting curves were analyzed at 60°C-95°C after 40 cycles to ensure that the resulting fluorescence originated from a single PCR product did not represent primer-dimers formed during the PCR or a nonspecific product. Each qRT-PCR analysis was performed in triplicate. Negative controls without cDNA were routinely included.

qRT-PCR results were analyzed with the sequence detection software SDS version 1.1 (Applied Biosystems, USA). The SYBR green fluorescent signal was standardized to a passive reference dye (ROX) included in the PCR master mix. Direct detection of the PCR product was measured by monitoring the increase in

Table 2. Primer sequences and amplicon characteristics of *Triticum aestivum* (wheat) and *Malus domestica* (apple) cross-allergens.

Gene	GeneBank accession number	Sequence 5′-3′	Product size (bp)	Ta (°C)
Tri a 12	X89827.1	CCTTGCACCAACTGGTCTTT	162	60
		CCAGGAGTCATGGGTTCATC		
Tri a 14	AJ784902.1	GGCGTCAAGAACCTCCATAA	177	60
		GCTGCAGTCGATGTTGAGAC		
Mal d 3.02	AY572532.1	TGGCCAGGTGAGCTCCAA	247	60
		TGGTGGAGGTGCTGATCTTG		
Mal d 4.02	AY792613.1	GTGTTACTTGTCAAGAAGAGCACAA	126	58
		GCTCAATGAGATAATCCGCA		
PLA 2.23	EEF48118.1	TGGGAAGTATTGTGGGCTTT	259	52
		AGCAACTAAAGCAGCCTCCA		

fluorescence caused by the binding of SYBR green dye to double-stranded DNA.

To estimate the expression variation levels of the eight candidate genes, geNorm software package for Microsoft Excel (http://medgen.ugent.be/*jvdesomp/genorm/) [28] was applied to analyze the data obtained from the samples of citrus pollen [29]. The PCR efficiency was calculated for each gene with LinRegPCR program [30] from raw fluorescence data taken from the Applied Biosystems detection system. Results from the LinRegPCR software were imported into Microsoft Excel, transformed to relative quantities using the comparative Ct (ΔΔCt) method, and taken into account the different amplification efficiencies for the different genes (just replace value 2 with the actual efficiency of the gene (e.g. 1.95 for 95%) in the formula of ΔCt [31]. Data have been normalized to the geometric mean of two housekeeping genes (EF-1 and UBQ 10), chosen according to the geNorm software.

Multiple sequence alignments

The multiple sequence alignments of the sensitizing factors annotated in the UniProtKB database (http://www.ebi.ac.uk/uniprot/) has been performed through ClustalΩ tool (http://www.ebi.ac.uk/Tools/msa/clustalo/) to find sequence homology among *Citrus sinensis* and *Triticum aestivum, Phleum pratense, Cynodon dactylon, Betula pendula, Artemisia vulgaris, Parietaria judaica, Malus domestica, Corylus avellana, Olea europaea, Arachis hypogaea.*

Study population for clinical trials

This monocentric observational study enrolled all caucasian children and young adults affected from pollinosis [allergic rhino-conjunctivitis (RC) and/or asthma] consecutively referred to the Allergologic Center of the Paediatric Department of Bologna University (Northern Italy) from December 2011 to May 2012.

The criteria for study inclusion were:

- aged between 4 and 22 years;
- diagnosis of allergic RC and/or asthma with or without sensitization/allergy to oranges;
- Written informed consent from all patients (or from parents for patients younger than 18 years old).

The criteria for study exclusion were:

- Children with height or weight less than 3rd centile;
- Patient affected from systemic disease (different from allergy or asthma) including: gastro-esophageal reflux disease under medical treatment, epilepsy, severe neurological or neurodevelopmental disorders, tuberculosis, previous thoracic surgery, major congenital malformations, heart diseases (with the exception of atrial sept defect without hemodynamic significance and ventricular sept defect), primary or secondary immunodeficiencies.

Allergometric assays

In each patient, the presence of symptoms of food allergy and/or OAS to oranges and other citrus fruits was investigated. Skin-Prick test (SPT) with commercial extracts (Lofarma, Milano) of pollens (grass, composites, parietaria) were performed as well as prick-by-prick test (PPT) with fresh fruit pulp of oranges, lemons and clementines. A SPT result was considered positive when elicited a wheal at least greater than half of histamine control.

In the patients with a positive PPT with citrus fruits pulp, the levels of specific IgE were determined to a panel of the main pollens (*Phleum p., Parietaria j., Olea e., Betula v., Corylus a.*), recombinant allergens (rPhl p 1, rPhl p 12, rBet v 2, rPru p 3), fruit extracts (orange, apple, peanut, wheat) and MuxF3-CCD, a marker of sensitization for cross-reactive carbohydrate determinants (CCD) (ImmunoCAP 1000 FEIA, ThermoFisher-Sweden). In addition, the choice of determining the sIgE levels for rPhl p 12 and rPru p 3 has been made on the base of the high degree of homology with orange profilin Cit s 2 (almost 75%) [32] and orange LTP Cit s 3 (almost 67%) [18] respectively. Levels of sIgE greater than 0.35 kU/L were considered positive.

Data and Statistics

The values reported are expressed as mean ± SD; they have been calculated on the basis of the data obtained from three independent experiments run separately and each sample was undertaken in triplicate (total nine replicates for each determination). Differences between sample sets were determined by the Student's *t*-test with 95% confidence limits. When indicated statistical analysis was performed using GraphPad Prism (version 5.03 Windows GraphPad Software Inc., La Jolla, CA, USA).

Ethic Statement

The research was conducted according to the principles expressed in the Declaration of Helsinki, and approved by Ethic Committee of Bologna University, S. Orsola-Malpighi Hospital (protocol name: OrangeAllergy; number: 108/2011/U/Oss.). Written informed consent was obtained from all the parents or guardians of the minors involved in the study.

Results

Clinical results

We have recruited 72 children and young adults (50 males, 69% and 22 females, 31%) with mean age of 12,3 years (range 6–22 years) and clinical history of pollinosis, who presented a positive reactions to SPT with grass pollen extract.

Forty-seven patients (65%) had symptoms of allergic RC, 25 (35%) presented both RC and asthma. Nine patients (12%) referred systemic symptoms after ingesting the following foods (alone or in combination): 6 to nuts (2 to hazelnut, 1 to peanut, 1 to walnut, and 2 to a not specified nut), 2 to citrus fruits (1 to orange and 1 to clementine), 1 to kiwi, 1 to apple, 1 to tomato, 1 to egg, 1 to fish and 1 to milk. Four patients (6%) presented symptoms of OAS to the following plant-derived foods (alone or in combination): 2 to kiwi, 2 to melon, 1 to orange, 1 to strawberry and 1 to peanut. Overall three out of patients (4%) showed symptoms after ingestion of citrus fruits (2 systemic food allergy – 1 to orange and 1 to clementine – and 1 OAS to orange). The patient with systemic orange allergy showed a severe reaction with urticaria and vomiting immediately after ingestion of orange, otherwise the other patient with systemic citrus allergy presented abdominal pain and diarrhea after the assumption of a clementine. The case of OAS due to citrus fruits was elicited by the contact with an orange. The clinical features and allergological assays of the three patients with documented citrus fruits allergy are reported in Table 3.

PPT with the pulp of fresh orange, lemon and clementine resulted positive in 28 patients (39%): 24 (33%) to orange (mean wheal diameter = 2.8 mm, range: 2–7 mm), 16 (22%) to lemon (mean wheal diameter = 2.8 mm, range: 2–6 mm) and 12 (17%) to clementine (mean wheal diameter = 2,9 mm, range 2–6 mm).

Fourteen out of the 28 patients with a positive PPT performed with fresh citrus fruit accepted to perform blood test: the mean values of sIgE against orange and the main pollens and plant

Table 3. Clinical features of the three patients with citrus fruit allergy.

PATIENT DATA	Patient	**1**	**2**	**3**
	Sex	F	M	M
	Age yrs	20	20	12
	Respiratory disease (A/RC)	A, RC	A, RC	RC
	Symptoms with citrus fruits	Urticaria Vomiting (Orange)	OAS (Orange)	Abdominal pain Diarrhoea (clementine)
	Food Allergy/ OAS to other foods	apple, nuts, tomato	kiwy, melon, strawberry	kiwy
PRICK-TO-PRICK WITH FRUIT PULP *Mean wheal diameter (mm)*	*Orange*	7	4	0
	Clementine	6	3	3
	Lemon	6	0	0
SPECIFIC IGE (KU/L)	*Orange*	39.2	<0.10	4.3
	Wheat	14.3	<0.10	6.5
	Apple	45.7	<0.10	24.4
	Peanut	47.8	<0.10	13.1
	Phleum p.	87.8	14.3	83.9
	Olea e.	56.8	0.8	33.3
	Betula v.	>100	<0.10	57.3
	Corylus a.	92.7	0.4	59
	r Phl p 1	41	15.1	71.2
	r Phl p 12	34.2	0.31	4
	r Bet v 2	47	<0.10	7.1
	r Pru p 3	19.7	<0.10	16.6
	MuxF3-CCD	1.23	<0.10	0.74

Patient data, results of prick-to-prick (PPT) with fresh citrus fruit pulp and specific IgE (sIgE) against the main pollens, (*Phleum p., Olea e., Betula v., Corylus a.*), fruit extracts (orange, apple, peanut, wheat), recombinant allergens (rPhl p 1, rPhl p 12, rBet v 2, rPru p 3) and MuxF3-CCD.
A: Asthma; OAS: oral allergy syndrome; RC: rhino-conjunctivitis; yrs: years.

derived foods are reported in Table 4; the geometric mean value of sIgE for orange was 3.5 kU/L (range: 0.85–39,2 kU/L). A direct correlation seems to exist between the high level of sIgE for the rPhl p12 and rPru p 3, homolog to the two orange allergens Cit s 2 and Cit s 3 respectively, and the generalized clinical symptoms (vomiting and urticaria, abdominal pain and diarrhoea) as reported in Table 3 for the patient 1 (sIgE = 34.2 and 19.7 for rPhl p 12 and rPur p 3 respectively) and patient 3 (sIgE = 4 and 16.6 for rPhl p 12 and rPur p 3 respectively).

Expression analysis of sensitizing factors in citrus pollen

The gene expression analysis were conducted in order to study which allergens and other sensitizing factors were actually expressed even in the pollen, after the recently identification and characterization of the three major orange allergens in fruits [9,10,12,15,16]: transcripts for Germin-like proteins (GLP, Cit s 1), profilins (Cit s 2), non specific Lipid Transfer Proteins (nsLTP, Cit s 3) and two isoforms of secretory phospholipase A2 (PLA2 α and PLA2 β) were tested in ungerminated (UGP) and germinated (GP) pollen of *Citrus clementine* (Cit UGP and Cit GP) and *Triticum aestivum* (Tri UGP and Tri GP) through either semi-quantitative RT-PCR (Figure 1A) and qRT-PCR (Figure 1D). The evaluation of the expression profile of the *Cit s* 1–3 allergens by semi-quantitative RT-PCR (Figure 1A) allowed to verify the presence of Cit s 1 (GLP) and Cit s 3 (nsLTP) transcripts even in the citrus pollen with a different pattern of expression than those observed in the literature for the orange fruits [12]: for the citrus pollen the two major allergens are the Cit s 1 and Cit s 3, whereas the expression of Cit s 2 is not detectable according to the experimental conditions described in Material and Methods section. The densitometry analysis (Figure 1B) performed on the semi-quantitative RT-PCR shown in Figure 1A, confirmed differences in the expression profile between Cit UGP and Cit GP: Cit s 1 and Cit s 3 are both expressed almost with the same intensity in UGP, whereas in GP Cit s 1 showed an higher expression signal (about 2.5 fold) when compared to Cit s 3 (1,55±0,08 Cit s 1 *vs* 0,58±0,05 Cit s 3); as concerning PLA2 isoforms, both enzymes were expressed more in Cit GP (1,3±0,03 PLA2 α *vs* 1,25±0,03 PLA2 β) compared to Cit UGP (1±0,03 PLA2 α *vs* 1,16±0,03 PLA2 β).

Since clinical data reported in literature [12] often shown that allergic patients to citrus fruits also manifest sensitization to grass pollens, expression analysis of *Cit s* 1–3 and grass specific allergens has been assessed to confirm cross-reactivity between pollens; among grass allergens have been chosen those from *Triticum aestivum* (wheat) pollen (Figure 1A and Figure 1B): Tri a 12.0103 (GenBank ID X89827.1), a profilin, and Tri a 14.0101 (GenBank ID AJ784902), a nsLTP. They represented conserved allergens among the most allergenic species of the *poaceae* family (i.e. *Triticum aestivum, Cynodon dactylon* and *Phelum pratense*) as shown by the

Table 4. Pollinosis patients' clinical features.

ALLERGENS	n of positive/14 (≥ 0.35 kU/L)	g mean sIgE (kU/L)°	range (kU/L)°
Orange	9	3.5	0.85–39.2
Phleum p.	14	52.0	1.5–>100
Betula v.	13	8.2	0.4–>100
Corylus a.	14	7.0	0.4–92.7
Olea e.	13	7.5	0.8–70.8
Parietaria j.	13	5.2	0.36–43.2
r Phl p 1	12	49.2	15.1–>100
r Phl p 12	11	2	0.35–34.2
r Bet v 2	4	9.6	2.38–47
r Pru p 3	5	4.83	1.07–19.7
MuxF3-CCD	5	1.14	0.42–6.43
CITRUS FRUITS	**N of positive PPT (%)**§		**PPT** Mean wheal diameter mm (range) §
Orange	**24/72 (33)**		2.8 (2–7)
Lemon	**16/72 (22)**		2.8 (2–6)
Clementine	**12/72 (17)**		(2–6)

Levels of specific IgE (sIgE) against the main pollens (*Phleum p., Parietaria j., Olea e., Betula v., Corylus a.*), fruit extracts (orange, apple, peanut, wheat), recombinant allergens (rPhl p 1, rPhl p 12, rBet v 2, rPru p 3) and MuxF3-CCD in children and young adults with pollinosis. The geometric mean values of sIgE were calculated on the 14 out of the 28 patients with a positive reaction to prick-to-prick (PPT) with fresh citrus fruit pulp who accepted to perform blood test.
g mean: geometric mean; N: number; sIgE: specific IgE; PPT: prick-to-prick test.
§Calculated on the 72 patients enrolled in the study.
° Calculated on the 14 patients who perform blood test.

multiple sequence alignments performed with ClustalΩ for profilin proteins, that shared identity values in the range between 76–82% (Figure 2A); on the contrary only isoforms for *Triticum a.* nsLTP proteins were annotated in the UniProtKB database, while sequences for *Cynodon d.* and *Phelum p.* were not yet present. Since one of the aims of the present study was to investigate on molecules involved in the cross-allergenicity citrus *vs* grass pollens, we have chosen that of *Triticum aestivum* as model.

The expression profiles performed through semi-quantitative RT-PCR (Figure 1A) and the densitometry analysis reported in Figure 1B showed that wheat allergens were remarkably expressed in *Triticum a.* pollen, with significantly differences between Tri UGP and Tri GP: GP showed the highest expression levels of both allergens with Tri a 12 more expressed than Tri a 14; the difference between Tri a 12 and Tri a 14 is higher in Tri UGP, where Tri a 12 showed an almost double fold expression level than Tri a 14. Moreover, we observed a faint signal for Cit s 1 and Cit s 2 allergens and PLA2 α enzyme also in wheat pollen grain (Figure 1A), with Cit s 1 expressed only in Tri GP and Cit s 2 and PLA2 α in both Tri UGP and Tri GP, emphasizing the cross-sensitization between citrus and grass pollens. Finally, it should be noted as the Tri a 14 is also expressed in *Citrus c.* pollen, both Cit UGP and Cit GP, emphasizing the pan-allergenic nature of nsLTPs.

Unexpectedly, the presence of allergens with common sequence has been observed also between *Citrus c.* and *Malus domestica* pollens. Among all the apple allergen sequences tested (known to be present also in apple fruits), it has been obtained signal for two specific allergen isoforms (Mal d 3.02, an nsLTP and Mal d 4.02, a profilin) and for potential sensitizing factors, PLA2 (isoform 23): in fact, these three pairs of primers were able to generate transcripts in *Citrus c.* both Cit UGP and Cit GP (Figure 1C) with different expression profile as Mal d 3.02 and PLA 2.23 showed an higher signal in UGP when compared to GP. These data were confirmed by the multiple sequence alignments for *Citrus c.* and *Malus d.* proteins, which shared values of 69% identity Mal d 3 *vs* Cit s 3, 90% identity Mal d 4 *vs* Cit s 2 and 77% identity PLA 2.23 *vs* PLA2 β.

To confirm previous results and to obtained quantitative data about allergens expression, the qRT-PCR methodology was followed and data are shown in Figure 1D. The technique of qRT-PCR combined with the use of highly specific primers designed for each allergen allowed to test in a precise, accurate and sensitive manner the gene expression at the level of messenger RNA. The selection of the optimal reference target has been performed by geNorm software [28]: in this experimental situation the optimal number of housekeeping genes was 2, represented by EF1 and UBQ10 (geNorm V <0.15 when comparing a normalization factor based on the 2 or 3 most stable targets). As shown in Figure 1D, Cit s 2 was not detected even after 40 cycles; Cit s 1 was higher expressed in Cit GP when compared to Cit UGP (2,03±0,02 in Cit GP *vs* 1,53±0,1 in Cit UGP), whereas Cit s 3 expression was higher in Cit UGP (2,24±0,1) than in Cit GP (1,08±0,14), being also the allergen with the highest level detected in *Citrus c.* pollen. As described before and confirmed also by qRT-PCR for Cit GP, Cit s 1 showed an expression signal double higher than Cit s 3. The two isoforms of PLA2 (PLA2 α and PLA2 β), were differentially expressed in Cit UGP and Cit GP with a stronger signal for PLA2 β in respect to PLA2 α, showing the same trend reported for the densitometry analysis (Figure 1B): an higher signal in Cit GP (1,61±0,34 PLA2 α *vs* 1,81±0,18 PLA2 β) when compared to Cit UGP (1,14±0,18 PLA2 α *vs* 1,65±0,15 PLA2 β) for both PLA enzyme isoforms.

According to the World Health Organization (WHO), two proteins can be considered cross-allergens if they share 35% identity on 80 residues and have an exact match of 6–8 residues

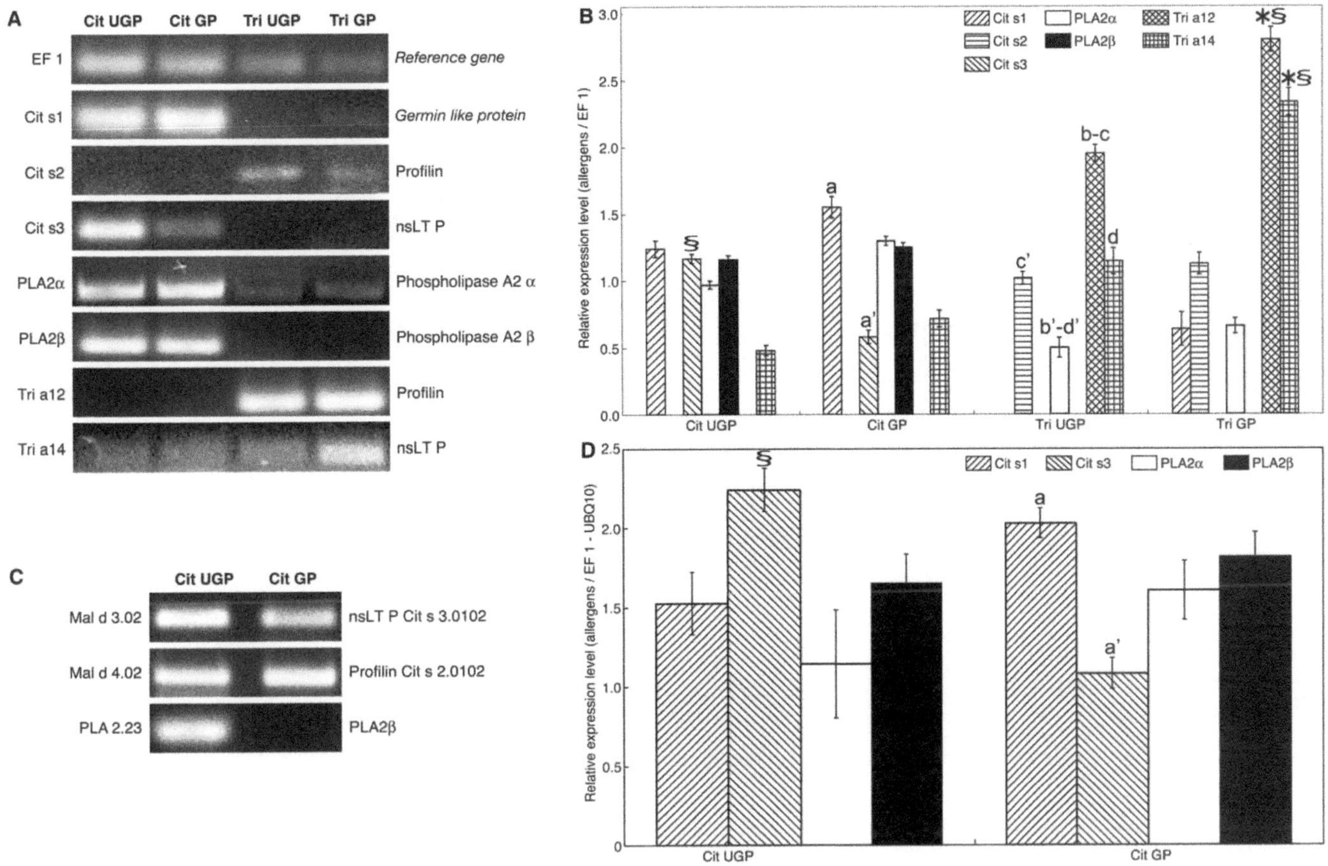

Figure 1. Allergens and phospholipase expression analysis in *Citrus clementine* and *Triticum aestivum* pollens. The cDNAs obtained from mRNA of *Citrus c.* (Cit) and *Triticum a.* (Tri) pollens ungerminated (UGP) and germinated (GP) have been tested for the different allergens (Cit s 1, Cit s 2, Cit s 3, Tri a 12 and Tri a 14) and phospholipase isoforms (PLA2 α and PLA2 β) through semi-quantitative RT-PCR after 40 cycles. EF-1 expression was used as reference gene (**A**). Lanes: *Citrus clementine* pollen ungerminated: Cit UGP; *Citrus clementine* pollen germinated: Cit GP; *Triticum aestivum* pollen ungerminated: Tri UGP; *Triticum aestivum* pollen germinated: Tri GP. Densitometries of the PCR bands revealed through semi-quantitative RT-PCR (**B**). Data are expressed as allergen/reference gene ratio ± SD. EF-1 expression was used as reference gene. The cDNAs of *Citrus clementine* UGP and GP have been tested for two different apple allergens (Mal d 3.02 and Mal d 4.02), and one isoform of apple secretory phospholipase (PLA 2.23) through semi-quantitative RT-PCR after 40 cycles (**C**). Logarithmic histogram (LOG10) of the expression levels of the different allergens (Cit s 1, Cit s 2, Cit s 3) and phospholipase isoforms (PLA2 α and PLA2 β) obtained through qRT-PCR in samples of *Citrus c.* pollen (Cit UGP and Cit GP) after 40 cycles of reaction (**D**). Data were calculated on the basis of the quantitative-comparative Ct (ΔΔCt) method normalized to the geometric mean of two housekeeping genes (EF-1 and UBQ 10), chosen according to the geNorm software. Values are the mean (n = 9) ± SD. Different letters (a–a′, b–b′, c–c′, d–d′) indicate means that are significantly different in allergens pairwise comparison (between bars marked by the same letter, i.e. a and a′, b and b′ etc.); * Statistical significance compared different allergens in the same sample (Tri GP); § Statistical significance compared the same allergen among the different samples (p≤0.05 with the Student's *t*-test [two-tailed distribution, two-sample equal variance]).

on a single peptide (http://www.codexalimenatarius.net) [32]. On these basis and according to the data reported both in literature [12,33,34] and in the clinical results section about cross-allergenicity, we performed a bioinformatics approach based on the ClustalΩ multiple sequence alignments to find sequence homologies among the three main allergens in *Citrus sinensis* (Cit s 1, Cit s 2 and Cit s 3) and the same class of proteins, that may be present in the well known allergenic plant species considered in the clinical trials (i.e. *Triticum aestivum, Phleum pratense, Cynodon dactylon, Betula pendula, Artemisia vulgaris, Parietaria judaica, Malus domestica, Corylus avellana, Olea europaea, Arachis hypogaea*). As reported in Figure 2B, profilin proteins were the most conserved and with the highest identity percentage values (70–90%); on the contrary, nsLTP sequence identity values were lower in the range between 23% Cit s 3 *vs Parietaria judaica* to 69% Cit s 3 *vs Malus domestica*; as regards GLP, the identity values didn't exceed the percentages of 35% to consider them cross-allergens (it was in the range 12–32%).

Discussion

Pollen allergens studies and sensitization patients' analysis to plant allergens describe a picture in which allergies to citrus fruit and cross-allergies with other pollen/fruit proteins could play an important role in the insurgence of sensitization and/or allergy reactions.

The allergy to citrus fruits is not clinically relevant as other foods and pollens (www.foodallergyitalia.org), even if some early studies suggested oranges being an important allergenic food [9,10,12,35]. This is possibly due to the fact that a very high percentage of sensitization to citrus is not accompanied by clinical reactivity to these fruit, because only one third of self-reported reactions were confirmed by oral provocations [12]; it is also evident that clinical orange allergy exists and confirmed by challenge tests [10,15].

As in literature few data are reported about allergy to citrus fruits, above all in paediatric population, the aim of this study was to investigate this topic in a population of children and young

A

Poaceae **PROFILIN**	Identity (%) PROF_WHEAT	PROF_PHLPR	PROF_CYNDA
PROF_WHEAT	89 - 98	76 - 80	77 - 79
PROF_PHLPR	76 - 80	96 - 99	82
PROF_CYNDA	77 - 79	82	100

B

GLP	Identity (%)	**PROFILIN**	Identity (%)	**nsLTP**	Identity (%)
GLP_CITSI	100	PROF_CITSI	100	NLTP_CITSI	100
GER_WHEAT	20 - 32	PROF_WHEAT	75 - 76	NLTP_WHEAT	36 - 47
GLP_BETPN	12 - 18	PROF_PHLPR	70 - 73	NLTP_ARTVU	43 - 54
		PROF_CYNDA	78	NLTP_PARJU	23 - 27
		PROF_ARTVU	71 - 72	NLTP_OLEEU	55
		PROF_BETPN	74 - 75	NLTP_ARAHY	61
		PROF_PARJU	74	NLTP_MALDO	69
		PROF_OLEEU	79 - 80	NLTP_CORAV	59
		PROF_ARAHY	73 - 78		
		PROF_MALDO	75 - 91		
		PROF_CORAV	76 - 81		

Figure 2. ClustalΩ multiple sequence alignments of allergen sequences annotated in UniProtKB database. Identity degree values expressed as multiple sequence alignment percentages of *Triticum aestivum* (PROF_WHEAT, Uniprot ID P49232-34, B6EF35), *Phleum pratense* (PROF_PHLPR, Uniprot ID P35079, O24650, O24282) and *Cynodon dactylon* (PROF_CYNDA, Uniprot ID O04725) profilin proteins (**A**). Identity percentages obtained from *Citrus sinensis* Cit s 1 (GLP), Cit s 2 (PROFILIN) and Cit s 3 (nsLTP) multiple sequence alignments (**B**). First column: *Citrus sinensis* GLP (GLP_CITSI, Uniprot ID P84159) with those for *Triticum aestivum* (GER_WHEAT, Uniprot ID P15290, B9VR55, C3UZE8, P26759, Q9SM34, Q9LD27, Q70PK0) and *Betula pendula* (GLP_BETPN, Uniprot ID P85352-54, P85336). Second column: *Citrus sinensis* PROFILIN (PROF_CITSI, Uniprot ID P84177) with those of *Triticum aestivum* (PROF_WHEAT, Uniprot ID P49232-34, B6EF35), *Phleum pratense* (PROF_PHLPR, Uniprot ID P35079, O24650, O24282), *Cynodon dactylon* (PROF_CYNDA, Uniprot ID O04725), *Artemisia vulgaris* (PROF_ARTVU, Uniprot ID Q8H2C8-9), *Betula pendula* (PROF_BETPN, Uniprot ID A4K9Z8, P25816), *Parietaria judaica* (PROF_PARJU, Uniprot ID Q9XG85, Q9T0M8), *Olea europaea* (PROF_OLEEU, Uniprot ID O24169-71), *Arachis hypogaea* (PROF_ARAHY, Uniprot ID Q9SQI9, Q5XXQ5, D3K177), *Malus domestica* (PROF_MALDO, Uniprot ID Q9XF40-42), *Corylus avellana* (PROF_CORAV, Uniprot ID A4KA40-45, Q9AXH4-5). Third column: *Citrus sinensis* nsLTP (NLTP_CITSI, Uniprot ID Q8L5S8, Q6EV47) with those of *Triticum aestivum* (NLTP_WHEAT, Uniprot ID Q5NE27-31, Q2PCB0, Q2PCB7-8, Q2PCD1-2, Q84N29), *Artemisia vulgaris* (NLTP_ARTVU, Uniprot ID P0C088, C4MGH0-2, C4MGG9), *Parietaria judaica* (NLTP_PARJU, Uniprot ID P43217, P55958, O04403-4, Q40905), *Olea europaea* (NLTP_OLEEU, Uniprot ID B2BGS3), *Arachis hypogaea* (NLTP_ARAHY, Uniprot ID B6CEX8, B6CG41), *Malus domestica* (NLTP_MALDO, Uniprot ID Q5GLH0, Q9M5X7, Q5J026), *Corylus avellana* (NLTP_CORAV, Uniprot ID Q9ATH2). Data are presented as range of percentage identity values as it has been considered all the allergen isoforms annotated and reviewed in UniProtKB database.

adults with pollinosis. Interestingly, we found a relevant percentage of sensitisation (39%) to citrus fruits in the population of pollen allergic patients recruited. Moreover, three out of the 72 pollen allergic patients (4%) presented adverse reactions after the ingestion of orange (2 patients) and clementine (1 patient) and in all of them the IgE- mediated mechanism has been confirmed by the positive response to the PPT with the fresh citrus fruit pulp. In a previous study, Kumar et al. [36] described a lower percentage (9.2%) of citrus fruit sensitization in 216 Indian children and adults affected from asthma. Asero et al. [37] reported that out of 200 children and adults with pollen allergy, 7 (3.5%) presented adverse reactions to a citrus fruit (orange, tangerine) with a similar percentage obtained also for the present study. Moreover, the present data reported that 2 out of 3 citrus allergic patients presented systemic reactions (urticaria, gastrointestinal symptoms) and 1 patient OAS after the ingestion of citrus fruits. The 2 patients with the generalized clinical symptoms showed high level of sIgE for the rPhl p12 and rPru p 3, homolog to the two orange allergens Cit s 2 and Cit s 3 respectively, emphasizing a direct correlation between sensitization/specific antibodies levels and the allergenic symptomatology. In particular, profilin are mainly involved in local symptoms (i.e. OAS) [15] contrary to systemic symptomatology mainly due to a sensitization towards nsLTPs, as highlighted by our clinical data.

The other patient with OAS has clear skin sensitization but not significant positivity to profilins and nsLTPs: probably other allergenic molecules are implied for such symptoms.

As suggested from previous works [38,39], patients allergic to pollen may present different kinds of symptoms after eating several plant foods due to the cross-reactivity of pollen allergen specific IgE that reacts with homologous plant food proteins. Examples for such cross-reactive allergens are profilins as Phl p 12 or Bet v 2, which are recognised by IgE from 10% to 20% of pollen-allergic patients [40] and cause IgE cross-reactivity among botanically unrelated pollen and between pollen and food [41,42]. In a previous study [15] about the evaluation of different pattern of allergen recognition in 6 orange allergic children, all the patients with isolated OAS presented sensitization to a profilin (Bet v 2), and the 2 patients with systemic reactions (general discomfort, urticaria) were Bet v 2 negative. In contrast, in the present study the patients recruited with generalized symptoms were all Bet v 2 positive and the one with OAS resulted Bet v 2 negative.

Moreover all patients who presented a positive PPT reactions to citrus fruit, included the three patients with citrus fruit allergy, presented a positive response to SPT with grass pollen extract and/or the presence of sIgE against *Phleum p.*, which belongs as *Triticum a.* to *poaceae* family. The presence of cross-reactivity between grass and citrus pollen has been described even by El-Qutob Lòpez et al. [43], who reported a case of systemic reaction (urticaria and angioedema) after ingestion of orange blossom pollen in a woman sensitized to several pollens included the grass one. In conclusion the present clinical data confirm a relevant prevalence of citrus fruit sensitization and show that orange and clementine allergy is not a so rare condition in pollen sensitized patients.

The molecular characterization of citrus pollen and cross-allergenicity was aimed to verify whether some important citrus allergen genes (Cit s 1, Cit s 2 and Cit s 3), known to be expressed in the fruit and to provoke allergic reactions after ingestion [12] were also expressed in pollen.

In the international allergen database (http://www.allergen.org/index.php) a single GLP, a single profilin and two nsLTPs were listed as allergens in sweet orange (*Citrus sinensis*). We demonstrated the expression of these allergens also in *Citrus clementine* pollen and in particular, Cit s 1 and Cit s 3 represent the two allergens commonly expressed in fruit and pollen, whereas Cit s 2 is present in citrus fruit and not detectable in citrus pollen. Hyun and Kim [44] reported the genomic identification of putative members of *Citrus c.* allergens, five different isoforms of nsLTP (Cit c 3) and three different isoforms of profilin (Cit c 2) annotated on Phytozome (http://www.phytozome.net/) and the Citrus Genome Database (http://www.citrusgenomedb.org/); the molecular data presented in this study demonstrated the presence of a GLP also in clementine pollen.

About profilin, when the RT-PCR was performed with the primers for a profilin isoform of *Malus domestica* fruit, the *Citrus c.* pollen showed a clear band either in Cit UGP and Cit GP; however, this result was not obtained when the RT-PCR was assessed with primers specific for the *Citrus sinensis* profilin. The data could mean that the isoform of *Citrus sinensis* annotated in UniProtKB database is not present in clementine pollen. Interestingly, the Cit s 2 isoform present in citrus fruit is also present in *Triticum a.* pollen, supporting the hypothesis of a cross-sensitization between *poaceae* pollen and citrus fruits. On the other hand, the Tri a 14, the nsLTP specific of *Triticum a.* is present in citrus pollen both Cit UGP and Cit GP, emphasizing the pan-allergenic nature of nsLTPs. As *Triticum a.* profilin and nsLTP protein sequences are annotated in UniProtKB database, we verified their homology sequences among the well known species of *poaceae* family considered allergenic (i.e. *Phleum pratense* and *Cynodon dactylon*) to assessed the degree of sequences identity and the possible cross-allergenicity between citrus and grass pollens. From the bioinformatics data, we showed that profilin were the most conserved proteins and with the highest identity percentage values, whereas nsLTP sequence identity values were lower; on the contrary, GLP cannot be considered involved in the cross-allergenicity, being the identity values lower than 35%.

Interestingly, we demonstrated both through clinical data and molecular approaches that *Citrus c.* and *Malus d.* specific allergen isoforms (Mal d 3.02, an nsLTP and Mal d 4.02, a profilin) shared high percentage identity values, confirming the possible cross-allergenicity citrus/apple.

The presence of phospholipase A2 (PLA2) in pollen of *Arabidopsis thaliana* has been reported only recently [45]; although the proven involvement of plant PLA2s in many biological functions, including i.e. senescence, wounding and stress responses, relatively little is known about plant PLA2s, and their genes essentially remain uncharacterized. In *Arabidopsis t.* three of four PLA2 paralogs (PLA2 β, γ and δ) have been characterized and found to be expressed in pollen, localized to the endoplasmic reticulum and/or Golgi, and playing critical roles in pollen development and tube growth.

A novelty of the present work is the finding of the PLA2 α and β in *Citrus c.* pollen, either UGP and GP, as in fruits, as well as the presence of PLA2 α also in *Triticum a.*; being PLA2 able to generate pro-inflammatory factors as eicosanoid substances, this enzyme could represent a key factor in the inflammatory response to allergens possibly activating the inflammatory cascade. From the apple genome database (http://genomics.research.iasma.it), we found that the apple PLA2.23 is conserved also in Cit UGP as shown by the semi-quantitative RT-PCR; the sequence alignments of PLA2.23 with PLA2 β from citrus fruit showed that the two sequences are very conserved [identities =116/150 (77%), positives =129/150 (86%)].

In conclusion, according to the molecular analysis performed in this work, Cit s 1 and Cit s 3, but also profilin, even if a different isoform from that expressed in orange fruit, and two isoforms of PLA2 enzyme (PLA2 α and PLA2 β) were identified as important allergens and sensitizing factors in *Citrus c.* pollen UGP and GP. As consequence, data obtained support the evidences that cross-sensitization among citrus and other plant homolog allergens, could play an important role in inflammatory response to citrus proteins and emphasize that citrus allergy can be considered a relevant food related allergy in pollen sensitizing patients.

Finally, we can hypothesize that allergy to oranges can occur mainly through local symptoms (i.e OAS and erythema) unlike other food allergy, such as apple or peach, characterized with more generalized symptoms such as vomiting, diarrhea and abdominal pain. The clinical data presented support the hypothesis that a sensitization towards nsLTPs mainly cause a systemic symptomatology and the relevant high percentages (39%) of children and young adults sensitized to citrus fruits recruited for our monocentric observational study suggest that there is a risk to develop an allergenic symptomatology in the future.

Acknowledgments

We thank the project "My Darling Clementine": un prodotto salutistico nuovo e innovativo dalle clementine e dal limone di Calabria"(POR FESR 2007-2013)", Prof. Mazzucca who kindly donated pollen of *Citrus clementine* and Mr. Rondinini for the pollen of *Triticum aestivum*.

We thank Mr. N. Mele for the image elaboration.

Author Contributions

Conceived and designed the experiments: SDD GR AP. Performed the experiments: RI CP EC ML FS. Analyzed the data: SDD RI GR AP. Contributed reagents/materials/analysis tools: SDD GR AP. Wrote the paper: SDD RI GR CP EC. Designed the pollen molecular investigation: SDD. Designed the clinical investigation: GR AP. Performed the molecular biology experiments: RI. Performed the clinical observational studies: CP EC. Performed the immunological tests of sera against Phl p12: ML FS.

References

1. Knekt P, Isotupa S, Rissanen H, Heliövaara M, Järvinen R, et al. (2000) Quercetin intake and the incidence of cerebrovascular disease. Eur J Clin Nutr 54: 415–417.
2. Le Marchand L, Murphy SP, Hankin JH, Wilkens LR, Kolonel LN (2000) Intake of flavonoids and lung cancer. J Natl Cancer Inst 92: 154–160.
3. D'Amato G, Cecchi L, D'Amato M, Liccardi G (2010) Urban air pollution and climate change as environmental risk factors of respiratory allergy: an update. J Investig Allergol Clin Immunol 20: 95–102.
4. Sampson HA (1999) Food allergy. Part 1: Immunopathogenesis and clinical disorders. J Allergy Clin Immun 103: 717–728.
5. Sampson HA (2004) Update on food allergy. J Allergy Clin Immun 113: 805–819.
6. Bolhaar ST, van de Weg WE, van Ree R, Gonzalez-Mancebo E, Zuidmee L, et al. (2005) In vivo assessment with prick-to-prick testing and double-blind, placebo-controlled food challenge of allergenicity of apple cultivars. J Allergy Clin Immun 116: 1080–1086.
7. Mills EN, Mackie AR, Burney P, Beyer K, Frewer L, et al. (2007) The prevalence, cost and basis of food allergy across Europe. Allergy 62: 717–722.
8. Marzban G, Puehringer H, Dey R, Brynda S, Ma Y, et al. (2005) Localisation and distribution of the major allergens in apple fruits. Plant Sci 169: 387–394.
9. Ahrazem O, Ibàñez MD, Lòpez-Torrejòn G, Sánchez-Monge R, Sastre J, et al. (2006) Orange Germin-Like Glycoprotein Cit s 1: An Equivocal Allergen. Int Arch Allergy Immunol 139: 96–103.
10. Lòpez-Torrejòn G, Ibàñez MD, Ahrazem O, Sánchez-Monge R, Sastre J, et al. (2005) Isolation, cloning and allergenic reactivity of natural profilin Cit s 2, a major orange allergen. Allergy 60: 1424–1429.
11. Sloan AE, Powers ME (1986) A perspective on popular perceptions of adverse reactions to food. J Allergy Clin Immun 78: 127–132.
12. Crespo JF, Retzek M, Foetish K, Sierra Maestro E, Cid-Sanchez AB, et al. (2006) Germin-like protein Cit s 1 and profilin Cit s 2 are major allergen in orange (*Citrus sinensis*) fruits. Mol Nutr Food Res 50: 282–290.
13. Adler BR, Assadullahi T, Warner JA, Warner JO (1991) Evaluation of a multiple food specific IgE antibody test compared to parental perception, allergy skin tests and RAST. Clin Exp Allergy 21: 683–688.
14. Ortolani C, Ispano M, Pastorello EA, Ansaloni R, Magri GC (1989) Comparison of results of skin prick tests (with fresh foods and commercial food extracts) and RAST in 100 patients with oral allergy syndrome. J Allergy Clin Immunl 83: 683–690.
15. Ibañez MD, Sastre J, Martinez SAN Ireneo M, Laso MT, et al. (2004) Differents patterns of allergen recognition in children allergic to orange. J Allergy Clin Immun 113: 175–177.
16. Pignataro V, Canton C, Spadafora A, Mazzuca S (2010) Proteome from lemon fruit flavedo reveals that this tissue produces high amounts of the Cit s1 germin-like isoforms. J Agric Food Chem 58: 7239–7244.
17. Krishnan K, Moens PDJ (2009) Structure and functions of profilins. Biophys Rev 1: 71–81.
18. Enrique E, Alonso R, Bartolome B, San Miguel-Moncin M, Bartra J, et al. (2004) IgE reactivity to profilin in Platanus acerifolia pollen-sensitized subjects with plant-derived food allergy J Investig Allergol Clin Immunol 14: 335 – 342.
19. Ahrazem O, Ibanez MD, Lopez-Torrejon G, Sanchez- Monge R, Sastre J, et al. (2005) Lipid transfer proteins and allergy to oranges. Int Arch Allergy Immunol 137: 201–210.
20. Kader JC (1996) Lipid-transfer proteins in plants. Annu Rev Plant Physiol Plant Mol Biol 47: 627–654.
21. Botton A, Begheldo M, Rasori A, Bonghi C, Tonutti P (2002) Differential expression of two lipid transfer protein genes in reproductive organs of peach (Prunus persica L. Batsch). Plant Sci 163: 993–1000.
22. Iorio RA, Di Sandro A, Paris R, Pagliarani G, Tartarini S, et al. (2012) Simulated environmental criticalities affect transglutaminase of *Malus* and *Corylus* pollens having different allergenic potential. Amino Acids 42: 1007–1024.
23. Behrendt H, Kasche A, Ebner von Eschenbach C, Risse U, Huss-Marp J, et al. (2001) Secretion of proinflammatory eicosanoid-like substances precedes allergen release from pollen grains in the initiation of allergic sensitization. Int Arch Allergy Immunol 124: 121–125.
24. Gunawan H, Takai T, Kamijo S, Wang XL, Ikeda S, et al. (2008) Characterization of proteases, proteins, and eicosanoid-like substances in soluble extracts from allergenic pollen grains. Int Arch Allergy Immunol 147: 276–288.
25. Bagni N, Adamo P, Serafini-Fracassini D, Villanueva VR (1981) RNA, proteins and polyamines during tube growth in germinating apple pollen. Plant Physiol 68: 727–730.
26. Wilkins TA, Smart LB (1996) Isolation of RNA from plant tissue – A laboratory guide to RNA: isolation, analysis, and synthesis. In: Krieg PA, editor. New York: Wiley-Liss. 21–42.
27. Paris R, Cova V, Pagliarani G, Tartarini S, Komjanc M, et al. (2009) Expression profiling in *HcrVf2*-transformed apple plants in response to *Venturia inaequalis*. Tree Genetics & Genomes 5: 81–91.
28. Vandesompele J, De Preter K, Pattyn F, Poppe B, Van Roy N, et al. (2002) Accurate normalization of real-time quantitative RT-PCR by geometric averaging of multiple internal control genes. Genome Biol 3: RESEARCH0034.
29. Yan J, Yuan F, Long G, Qin L, Deng Z (2012) Selection of reference genes for quantitative real-time PCR analysis in citrus. Mol Biol Rep 39: 1831–1838.
30. Ramakers C, Ruijter JM, Deprez RH, Moorman AF (2003) Assumption-free analysis of quantitative real-time polymerase chain reaction (PCR) data. Neurosci Lett 339: 62–66.
31. Livak KJ, Schmittgen TD (2001) Analysis of relative gene expression data using real-time quantitative PCR and the 2-ΔΔCT method. Methods 25: 402–408.
32. Garcia BE, Lizaso MT (2011) Cross-reactivity Syndromes in Food Allergy. J Investig Allergol Clin Immunol 21: 162–170.
33. Eriksson NE, Werner S, Foucard T, Möller C, Berg T, et al. (2003) Self-reported hypersensitivity to exotic fruit in birch pollen-allergic patients. Allergol Int 52: 199–206.
34. Glaspole IN, de Leon MP, Rolland JM, O'Hehir R (2007) Anaphylaxis to lemon soap: citrus seed and peanut allergen cross-reactivity. Ann Allergy Asthma Immunol 98: 286–289.
35. Ebo DG, Ahrazem O, Lopez-Torrejon G, Bridts CH, Salcedo G, et al. (2007) Anaphylaxis from mandarin (Citrus reticulata): identification of potential responsible allergens. Int Arch Allergy Immunol 144: 39–41.
36. Kumar R, Singh BP, Srivastava P, Sridhara S, Arora N, et al. (2006) Relevance of serum IgE estimation in allergic bronchial asthma with special reference to food allergy. Asian Pac J Allergy Immunol 24: 191–199.
37. Asero R, Monsalve R, Barber D (2008) Profilin sensitization detected in the office by skin prick test: a study of prevalence and clinical relevance of profilin as a plant food allergen. Clin Exp Allergy 38: 1033–1037.
38. Ricci G, Righetti F, Menna G, Bellini F, Miniaci A, et al. (2005) Relationship between Bet v 1 and Bet v 2 specific IgE and food allergy in children with grass pollen respiratory allergy. Mol Immunol 42: 1251–1257.
39. Bohle B (2007) The impact of pollen-related food allergens on pollen allergy. Allergy 63: 3–10.
40. Radauer C, Hoffmann-Sommergruber K (2004) Profilins. Plant food allergens. In: Mills ENC, Shewry PR, editors. Oxford: Blackwell Publishing. 105–124.
41. Mari A (2001) Multiple pollen sensitization: a molecular approach to the diagnosis. Int Arch Allergy Immunol 125: 57–65.
42. van Ree R, Voitenko V, van Leeuwen WA, Aalberse RC (1992) Profilin is a cross-reactive allergen in pollen and vegetable foods. Int Arch Allergy Immunol 98: 97–104.
43. El-Qutob López D, Morales Rubio C, Cervera Aznar R, Pelaez Hernández A (2006) Allergic reaction after ingestion of orange blossom pollen. J Investig Allergol Clin Immunol 16: 140–141.
44. Hyun KT, Kim J (2011) Genomic identification of putative allergen genes in woodland strawberry (*Fragaria vesca*) and mandarin orange (*Citrus clementina*). Plant Omics J 4: 428–434.
45. Kim HJ, Ok SH, Bahn SC, Jang J, Oh SA, et al. (2011) Endoplasmic Reticulum– and Golgi-Localized Phospholipase A2 Plays Critical Roles in Arabidopsis Pollen Development and Germination. The Plant Cell 23: 94–110.

Heat-Induced Structural Changes Affect OVA-Antigen Processing and Reduce Allergic Response in Mouse Model of Food Allergy

Jaroslav Golias[1,9], Martin Schwarzer[2*,9], Michael Wallner[3], Miloslav Kverka[1], Hana Kozakova[2], Dagmar Srutkova[2], Klara Klimesova[1], Petr Sotkovsky[1], Lenka Palova-Jelinkova[1], Fatima Ferreira[3], Ludmila Tuckova[1]

1 Department of Immunology and Gnotobiology, Institute of Microbiology, v.v.i., Academy of Sciences of the Czech Republic, Prague, Czech Republic, **2** Department of Immunology and Gnotobiology, Institute of Microbiology, v.v.i., Academy of Sciences of the Czech Republic, Novy Hradek, Czech Republic, **3** Christian Doppler Laboratory for Allergy Diagnosis and Therapy, Department of Molecular Biology, University of Salzburg, Salzburg, Austria

Abstract

Background and Aims: The egg protein ovalbumin (OVA) belongs to six most frequent food allergens. We investigated how thermal processing influences its ability to induce allergic symptoms and immune responses in mouse model of food allergy.

Methodology/Principal Findings: Effect of increased temperature (70°C and 95°C) on OVA secondary structure was characterized by circular dichroism and by the kinetics of pepsin digestion with subsequent HPLC. BALB/c mice were sensitized intraperitoneally and challenged with repeated gavages of OVA or OVA heated to 70°C (h-OVA). Levels of allergen-specific serum antibodies were determined by ELISA (IgA and IgGs) or by β-hexosaminidase release test (IgE). Specific activities of digestive enzymes were determined in brush border membrane vesicles of jejunal enterocytes. Cytokine production and changes in regulatory T cells in mesenteric lymph nodes and spleen were assessed by ELISA and FACS. Heating of OVA to 70°C caused mild irreversible changes in secondary structure compared to boiling to 95°C (b-OVA), but both OVA treatments led to markedly different digestion kinetics and Tregs induction ability in vitro, compared to native OVA. Heating of OVA significantly decreased clinical symptoms (allergic diarrhea) and immune allergic response on the level of IgE, IL-4, IL-5, IL-13. Furthermore, h-OVA induced lower activities of serum mast cell protease-1 and enterocyte brush border membrane alkaline phosphatase as compared to native OVA. On the other hand h-OVA stimulated higher IgG2a in sera and IFN-γ secretion by splenocytes.

Conclusions: Minor irreversible changes in OVA secondary structure caused by thermal processing changes both its digestion and antigenic epitopes formation, which leads to activation of different T cell subpopulations, induces shift towards Th1 response and ultimately reduces its allergenicity.

Editor: Lucienne Chatenoud, Université Paris Descartes, France

Funding: This work was supported by grants from the Czech Science Foundation (GA310/07/0414, 310/08/H077 and 310/08/H077), http://www.gacr.cz/; Synlab (http:www.synlab.cz), the Academy of Sciences of the Czech Republic (IAA500200801, IAA500200710 and KJB500200904), http://www.gaav.cz/; the Czech Ministry of Education, Youth and Sports (2B06155 and LC07017), http://www.msmt.cz; and by Institutional Research Concept Grant AV0Z50200510, http://www.isvav.cz. The funders had no role in study design, data collection and analysis, decision to publish, or preparation of the manuscript.

Competing Interests: The authors have declared that no competing interests exist.

* E-mail: schwarzer@biomed.cas.cz

9 These authors contributed equally to this work.

Introduction

Food allergy is a serious health concern affecting 6–8% of young children and about 2–4% of adults. Allergies to eggs, milk and peanut are currently the most frequent food allergies and their prevalence, severity and persistence has been increasing during the last decades. Food allergy is considered mainly as an IgE-mediated type I hypersensitivity, characterized by an increased production of IgE antibodies and Th2 cytokines, common markers found both in human disease and in experimental models [1–4].

Depending on the route of exposure, dose of allergen and the presence of suitable adjuvant, the immune response can result in either sensitization or oral (mucosal) tolerance induction [4–6]. In mouse models of food allergy, oral administration of allergen usually results in oral tolerance induction, but its co-administration with strong mucosal adjuvant such as cholera toxin or with anti acid drugs (increasing gastric pH) could be used for allergic sensitization [7–10]. Another reliable and effective approach to overcome the oral tolerance induction is pretreatment of mice by systemic intraperitoneal (*i.p.*) administration of allergen with aluminum hydroxide (alum) as adjuvant followed by repeated intra-gastric treatments. This experimental model mimics a mild form of human allergy with IgE–mediated mast cell degranulation causing increased small intestine permeability [2,11,12] with diarrhea as one of the symptoms of anaphylaxis. Histological examination of small intestine reveals changes of epithelium, *e.g.* alteration in number of goblet cells and mucin production and the damage of tips of villi, as well as changes of lamina propria, *e.g.* increased cell infiltration and/or activation [13–15].

The mucosa of small intestine is an actively metabolizing, rapidly proliferating, absorptive epithelium with nutritional and homeostatic functions. The activity of brush border enzymes is sensitive marker of intestinal cell differentiation and postnatal development, reflecting both dietary changes and microbial colonization [16–18]. Partial and subtotal atrophy of the villous apparatus was shown to correlate with the activity and expression of alkaline phosphatase [19]. Moreover, this enzyme may be also involved in host's defense against pathological stress-induced damage, such as during inflammation and infection [20].

Egg white contains several allergens such as ovalbumin (OVA), ovomucoid, ovotransferin and lysozyme. Forming approximately 60% of the total egg white protein, OVA is by far the most abundant of them [21]. Like the majority of food allergens OVA is consumed after thermal processing and it has been shown that after heating its molecular structure as well as allergenicity is altered [22,23]. However, it should be considered that egg allergens are processed at different temperatures (baked, scrambled or soft/hard boiled eggs or even native as whipped egg white) and these processing conditions can have a major impact on the secondary structure, susceptibility to enzymatic digestion in the gastrointestinal tract and allergenicity. Partial decrease of IgE binding after OVA thermal processing suggested that both linear and conformational epitopes participate in the OVA-IgE specific interactions [22–24]. Moreover, heating of allergens can lead to their aggregation, which reduces their absorption and transport through epithelial layer and thus decreases their allergenicity [25]. However, the impact of different temperature treatment on the changes in the secondary structure of OVA and on its ability to induce clinical symptoms of food allergy hasn't been studied in detail.

In the present study we show that heating of hen egg allergen OVA to 70°C has only minor effect on its secondary structure. However, these minor changes lead to different kinetics and occurrence of fragments after digestion. This result in activation of different T cell subpopulations and changes in both cytokine production and specific antibody formation, which leads to significant reduction of egg allergy symptoms.

Materials and Methods

Ethics Statement

All animal experiments were approved by the Laboratory Animal Care and Use Committee of the Institute of Microbiology v.v.i., Academy of Sciences of the Czech Republic, approval ID: 94/2006 and 244/2009.

Animals

Two month-old female BALB/c mice (*H-2b*) (Animal facility of the Institute of Physiology ASCR, Czech Republic) were kept under standard conditions, fed by OVA-free diet and water *ad libitum*.

Ovalbumin Preparation

For *i.p.* sensitization, OVA (Worthington, Lakewood, NJ, USA) and heated OVA (h-OVA; prepared by exposure of OVA to 70°C for 10 minutes, enabling accurate and reproducible dosing) were dissolved in phosphate-buffer saline (PBS) to a final concentration of 300 μg/ml containing 5 mg/ml of alum adjuvant (Sigma, Steinheim, Germany). For oral administration, OVA and h-OVA were dissolved in PBS to a final concentration of 100 mg/ml. For *in vitro* studies boiled OVA (b-OVA) was prepared by exposure of OVA to 95°C for 10 minutes. EndoGrade® Ovalbumin (Hyglos GmbH, Germany) with endotoxin content <1 EU/mg was used for enzymatic digestion and *in vitro* stimulation.

Circular Dichroism

Protein secondary structure elements were determined by CD spectroscopy. Spectra were recorded in 5 mM sodium phosphate buffer (pH 7.4) with a JASCO J-815 spectropolarimeter fitted with a PTC-423S Peltier single position cell holder (Jasco, Tokyo, Japan). All spectra are baseline-corrected and presented as mean residue molar ellipticity $[\Theta]_{MRW}$ at a given wavelength. Thermal denaturation of proteins was monitored from 20°C to 70°C or from 20°C to 95°C at the fixed wavelength of 222 nm with a temperature slope of 1°C/min. The melting point (Tm) was calculated from the inflection point of the resulting sigmoid curve [26].

Enzymatic Digestion and HPLC Separation of Ovalbumin Fragments

Peptides of OVA, h-OVA or b-OVA were prepared using pepsin-agarose gel similarly as described previously [27]. Briefly, digestion of proteins was stopped after 20, 40, or 60 minutes by removing the pepsin-agarose gel by centrifugation (10 min; 1500 g) and by neutralization with 1 M NaOH to final pH 7. Digested or undigested proteins were separated using SP 250/10 NUCLEOSIL 300-7 C18 column (Macherey-Nagel, Düren, Germany) on the HPLC system Gold 125NM Solvent Module (Beckman Coulter, Miami, FL, USA). Samples were applied on columns and separated as described previously [27]. For *in vitro* stimulations, digests were dissolved in complete RPMI-1640 (Sigma-Aldrich, St. Louis, MO, USA) to a final concentration of 500 μg/ml.

Experimental Protocol

Mice were divided into the three groups according to the treatment – OVA, h-OVA and PBS (controls). Mice were sensitized *i.p.*, with a two week interval, with 60 μg of either OVA or h-OVA together with 1 mg of alum in a final volume of 200 μl PBS on day 1 and 14. Control mice received only 200 μl PBS containing 1 mg of alum. Two weeks later, the mice were challenged 10 times at 2–3 days intervals by *i.g.* gavages of 15 mg of OVA in a final volume of 150 μl PBS. Diarrhea was assessed visually by monitoring mice for 30 minutes after each *i.g.* exposure. Body weight was recorded before gavage and rectal temperature both before and 30 minutes after each *i.g.* exposure.

Quantification of OVA-specific Antibodies and Mast Cell Protease-1

Blood samples were collected before the first *i.p.* injection, during the experiment and at sacrifice. Allergen-specific serum IgG1, IgG2a and IgA levels were determined by ELISA [28]. Briefly, 96-well microtiter plates were coated either with OVA, h-OVA or b-OVA (5 μg/ml). Serum samples were diluted 1/10000 for IgG1, 1/100 for IgG2a and 1/10 for IgA. Rat anti-mouse IgG1, IgG2a and IgA antibodies (Abs) (1 μg/ml Pharmingen, San Diego, CA, USA) were applied, followed by peroxidase-conjugated mouse anti-rat IgG Abs (1/1000; Jackson, Immuno Labs., West

Grove, PA, USA) for detection. Antibody levels were reported as optical density (OD). As it was shown that allergen-specific IgG interferes with allergen-specific IgE detection [29], allergen-specific IgE levels in sera were quantified by degranulation of rat basophil leukemia (RBL-2H3) cells (originally described by [30], kindly provided by prof. Ursula Wiedermann). RBL-2H3 cells were plated in 96-well tissue culture plates (4×10^4 cells/per well) and passively sensitized by incubation with mouse sera in a final dilution of 1/90 for 2 hours. After washing, OVA, h-OVA or b-OVA (0.6 μg/ml) were added for 30 min at 37°C to induce degranulation. Supernatants were incubated with 4-methylumbelliferyl-N-acetyl-β-D-glucosaminide (Sigma-Aldrich, St. Louis, MO, USA) for analysis of β-hexosaminidase using a fluorescence microplate reader (λ_{ex}:360 nm/λ_{em}:465 nm) Infinite M200 (Tecan Group Ltd., Grödig, Austria). Results are reported as percentage of total β-hexosaminidase release from cells after disruption with 1% Triton X-100.

Levels of serum mouse mast cell protease-1 (MMCP-1) enzyme were determined by commercial kit (eBioscience, San Diego, USA) according to manufacturer's instructions. Sacrifice sera were diluted 1/250 and the MMCP-1 levels are reported as ng/ml.

Cell Culture and Cytokine Evaluation

Mesenteric lymph nodes (MLN) and spleens were removed at sacrifice. Single-cell suspensions were prepared in RPMI-1640 containing 10% fetal bovine serum (BioClot GmbH, Aidenbach, Germany) and 1% Antibiotic-Antimycotic solution (Sigma-Aldrich). Cells (6×10^5/well) were cultured in a flat-bottom 96-well plate (TPP, Trasadingen, Switzerland) without any stimuli or in the presence of either OVA or h-OVA (100 μg/well) for 72 hours (37°C, 5% CO_2). Supernatants were collected and stored at −40°C until analyses. IL-4, IL-5, IL-6, IL-10, IL-13, IL-17, INF-γ and TNF-α were determined by the MILLIPLEX MAP Mouse Cytokine/Chemokine Magnetic Panel (Millipore, Billerica, USA) according to manufacturer's instructions and analyzed with the Bio-Plex System (Bio-Rad Laboratories, Hercules, USA) with sensitivities <0.3 pg/ml for IL-4, <0.8 pg/ml for IL-5, <2.1 pg/ml for IL-6, <2.6 pg/ml for IL-10, <12.4 pg/ml for IL-13, <0.7 pg/ml for IL-17, <1.1 pg/ml for IFN-γ and <3.1 pg/ml for TNF-α. Values are reported in pg/ml after subtraction of baseline levels of non-stimulated cultures. Values below assay sensitivity were considered non-detectable (n.d.). In order to measure the capacities of OVA, h-OVA and b-OVA and their peptic digests (100 μg/well) to induce Tregs, we cultivated them with naïve mouse splenocytes for 48 hours.

Flow Cytometry Analysis

Single-cell suspensions of spleens or MLN were stained for regulatory T cells using Foxp3 Staining Buffer Set (eBioscience, San Diego, CA, USA) with fluorochrome labeled anti-mouse monoclonal Abs: CD3e-Fluorescein isothiocyanate (eBioscience; clone 145-2C11), CD4-Qdot® 605 (Invitrogen, clone RM4-5), CD25-Alexa Fluor® 700 (eBioscience; clone PC61.5) and Foxp3-phycoerythrin (eBioscience; clone FJK-16s) according to the manufacturer's recommendation. Flow cytometric analysis was performed on LSRII (BD Biosciences, San Jose, CA, USA) and data were analyzed using FlowJo software (Tree Star, Ashland, OR, USA).

Determination of Enterocyte Brush-border Enzyme Activities

Jejunum was removed, washed with cold saline and brush border membrane vesicles (BBMV) were prepared from jejunal scrapings as described by Kessler *et al.* [31]. Protein concentration in BBMV was determined by the method of Lowry *et al.* [32] using bovine serum albumin, fraction V (Serva, Heidelberg, Germany) as standard. The activity of alkaline phosphatase (EC 3.1.3.1), γ-glutamyltranspeptidase (EC 2.3.2.2), dipeptidyl peptidase IV (EC 3.4.14.5), lactase (EC 3.2.1.23/62/108) and sucrase (EC 3.2.1.48/10) were determined as described previously [33]. Enzyme activities were expressed in nkat/mg protein, 1 nkat being the amount of the enzyme that converts 1 nmol of substrate per second under the given conditions.

Histology and Morphometry

Intestinal tissue sections were fixed immediately in 4% formalin. The fixed tissues were cut and processed using routine methods. Paraffin sections (5 μm) were deparaffinized in xylene, rehydrated through an ethanol gradient to water and stained by hematoxylin-eosin. Villus height was evaluated under the Olympus BX 40 microscope equipped with Photo camera DP 70 using program QuickPhoto Micro 23 program (Olympus, Japan). The mean height of 20–30 villi ± SEM was calculated.

Statistical Analysis

Differences between multiple experimental groups were evaluated by one-way analysis of variance (ANOVA) with Tukey's multiple comparison test, and differences between two groups were evaluated using unpaired two-tailed Student's *t*-test. Data were expressed as the mean ± SEM unless otherwise stated. GraphPad Prism statistical software (version 5.03 GraphPad Software, La Jolla, CA, USA) was used for analyses.

Results

The Effect of Thermal Processing on OVA Secondary Structure and Enzymatic Digestion

Since eggs could be consumed after various kinds of processing, we analyzed the effect of different temperatures on the secondary structure of OVA allergen. Employing the circular dichroism technique, we found that heating to 70°C or 95°C causes irreversible changes in secondary structure of OVA allergen (Fig. 1). The structural changes induced by heating were accompanied by different susceptibility to pepsin digestion. HPLC elution profiles of pepsin-digested OVA, h-OVA or b-OVA were documented after 20 and 40 minutes (Fig. 2). The majority of native OVA was split to fragments after 20 min, while the majority of both forms of heated OVA remained undigested. However, while both h-OVA and b-OVA had similar peptide profiles after 20 or 40 min of digestion, these were both quite different from those of untreated OVA (Fig. 2). The profiles after 40 min of digestion remained almost unchanged after 60 min of digestion (data not shown).

Experimental Allergic Diarrhea Induced by OVA and Heated-OVA

Allergic diarrhea appeared in about 70% of mice already after the 5th *i.g.* dose of OVA, but only in 20% of those fed with h-OVA. After 7 *i.g.* doses, the disease symptoms were found in more than 90% of OVA fed animals, but only in 35% of those fed with h-OVA. At the end of the experiment (10 *i.g.* doses), the diarrhea was found in all mice fed with OVA, but only in 70% of mice fed with h-OVA (Fig. 3a, b). There were small, non-significant differences in body weight and in rectal temperature after each *i.g.* dose of either OVA or h-OVA and PBS control group (data not shown). Morphometry analysis of histological

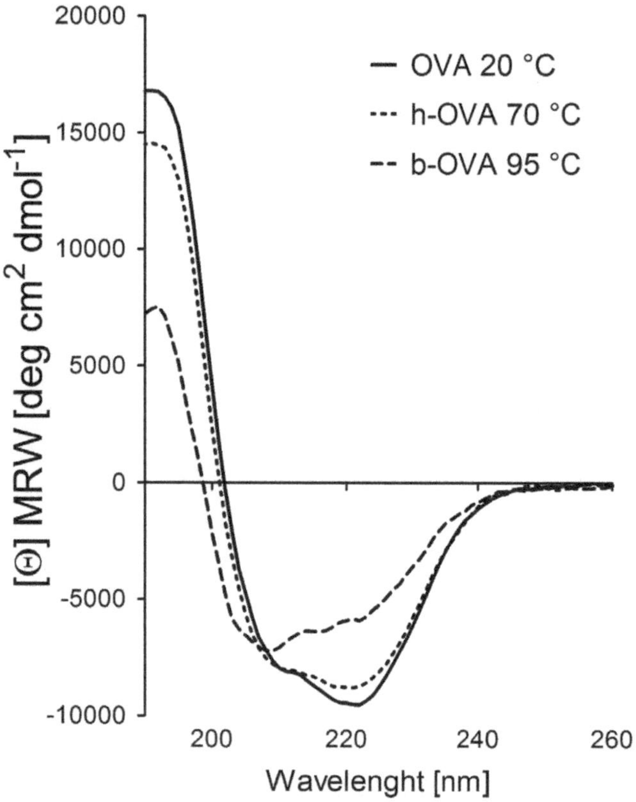

Figure 1. Circular dichroism spectra of native and heated-OVA. Circular dichroism spectra showed only minor irreversible structural changes of hen egg ovalbumin-OVA heated for 10 minutes at 70°C (h-OVA, dotted line) as compared to OVA heated at 95°C (b-OVA, dashed line). Spectra were taken after renaturation at 20°C, native conformation of OVA at 20°C is shown as control (solid line).

pictures documented shortening of villi in mice treated with either form of OVA, as compared to PBS-treated controls (PBS 190.2±5.1 μm, OVA 157.7±14.0* μm, h-OVA 161.4±6.0** μm).

OVA and h-OVA Treatment Changes Activity of Brush-border Hydrolases

The brush-border membrane hydrolases are enzymes involved in the final steps of digestion processes. We tested if these enzymes are involved in small intestine homeostasis and could be therefore considered as new markers in food allergy. We determined their activities in the jejunum of OVA-, h-OVA- and PBS-treated mice (Table 1). We found that the specific activity of alkaline phosphatase was significantly higher in mice treated with native OVA but only slightly increased in those exposed to h-OVA, as compared with PBS-treated mice. On the other hand, as compared to PBS-treated controls, both OVA and h-OVA treatments significantly decreased the specific activity of dipeptidyl peptidase IV. We did not observe any significant changes among the three experimental groups in the levels of glutamyl transpeptidase, lactase or sucrase (Table 1).

Thermal Processing of OVA Changes the Kinetics of OVA-specific Antibody Responses and the Levels of Serum MMCP-1

To determine the effect of thermal processing of the allergen on the level and specificity of anti-OVA antibodies, the serum levels of IgE, IgG1, IgG2a and IgA against either OVA or h-OVA were determined in the course of the experiment. As shown in Fig. 3c the level of IgE anti-OVA Abs was higher in response to native OVA than to h-OVA. In contrast, OVA-specific IgG2a was significantly higher after h-OVA feeding. The levels of the other two isotypes (IgG1 and IgA) were increased compared to controls but the differences corresponding to the two OVA forms were diminished towards the end of experiment. At the end of the

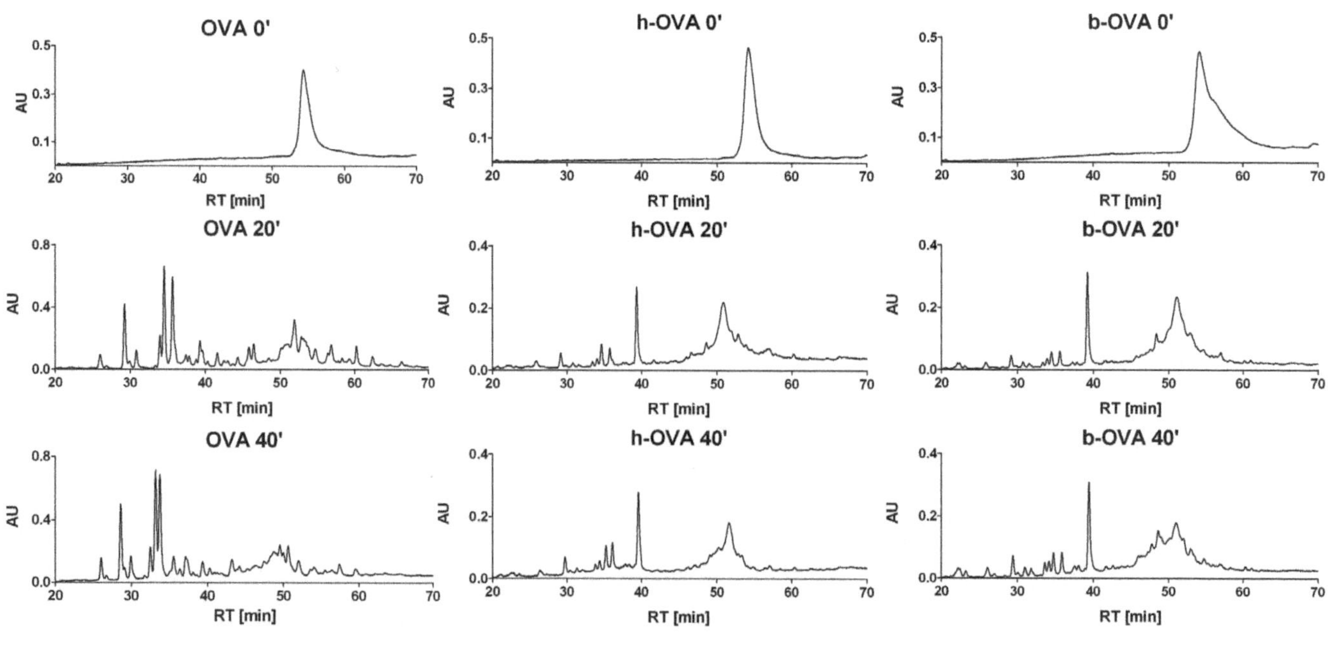

Figure 2. RP-HPLC separation profile of native-OVA and heated-OVA peptic digests. RP-HPLC separation profile monitored at 280 nm corresponds to OVA and OVA heated at 70°C (h)-OVA or boiled at 95°C (b)-OVA undigested (0′) and after 20 (20′) and 40 minutes (40′) of digestion by pepsin. RT – retention time.

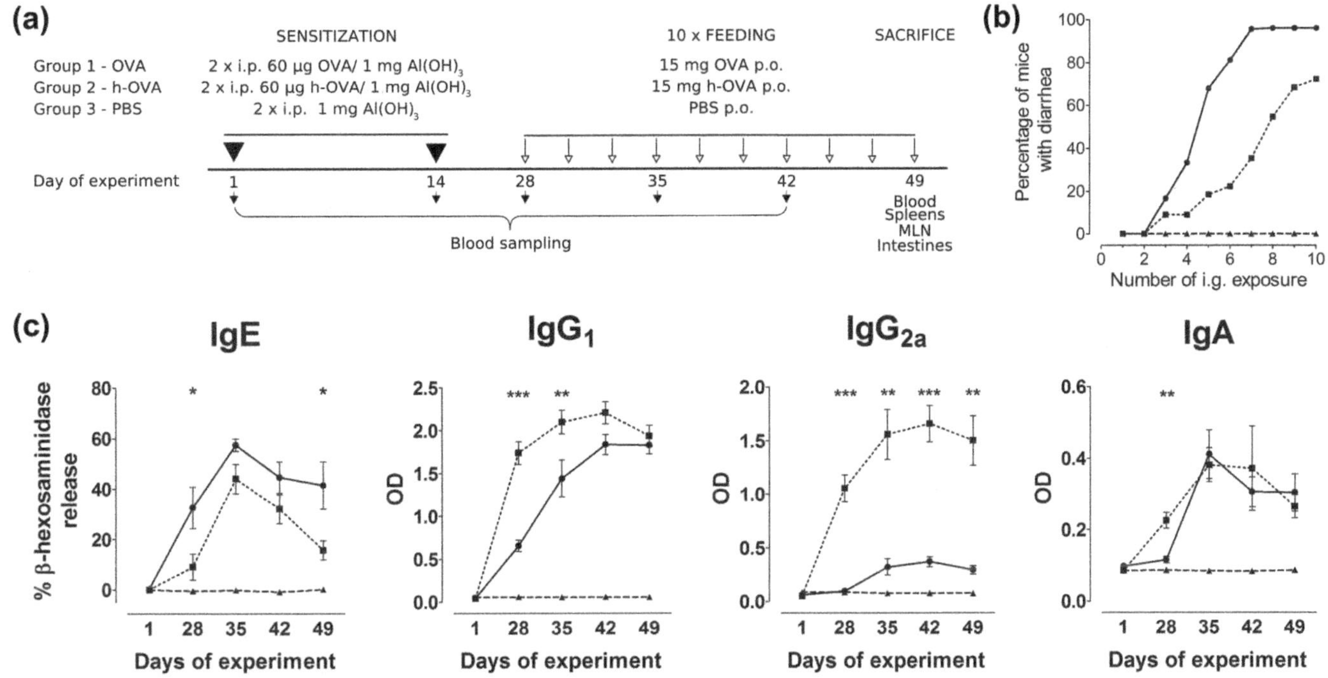

Figure 3. Impact of heating on OVA-induced allergic response. Experimental design (a). Mice were sensitized twice intraperitoneally (*i.p.*) with OVA/Al(OH)3, heated OVA (h-OVA)/Al(OH)3 or PBS/Al(OH)3 alone and subsequently challenged with ten doses of OVA, h-OVA or PBS by intragastric tubing (*i.g.*). Blood samples were taken at indicated time points for antibody analysis. At the end of the experiment, spleens and mesenteric lymph nodes were taken for FACS and cytokine assays, small intestine for histology and enterocyte brush border for enzyme activity analysis. **Occurrence of allergic diarrhea (b)**. Occurrence of allergic diarrhea in OVA (solid line) or h-OVA (dotted line) challenged mice, data pooled from three independent experiments. PBS controls are shown as dashed line. **The kinetics of specific Abs formation (c)**. Levels of specific antibodies in sera from mice exposed to OVA (solid line), h-OVA (dotted line) or PBS (dashed line) were detected by ELISA (IgA, IgG1and IgG2a) or by β-hexosaminidase release assay (IgE). Data are represented as mean ± SEM (n = 10 mice/group), representative data from one out of three independent experiments. *P≤0.05, **P≤0.01, ***P≤0.001.

experiment, we characterized the specificity and the degree of cross-reactivity of anti-OVA antibodies using ELISA with OVA, h-OVA or b-OVA bound as an antigen (Fig. S1). The levels of OVA-specific antibodies remained unchanged, when we used h-OVA or OVA as a coating antigen, except for IgG1, which levels were significantly higher, when h-OVA instead of OVA was used. When b-OVA was used as coating antigen, the response of both OVA- and h-OVA treated mice decreased significantly in all measured isotypes.

Table 1. Specific activities of enterocyte brush-border enzymes (nkat/mg protein) in jejunum of treated mice.

Enzyme (nkat/mg protein)	OVA	h-OVA	PBS
Alkaline phosphatase	14.26±1.09***	10.08±0.84#	8.27±0.29
GGT	10.79±3.33	8.64±1.59	9.74±2.02
DPP IV	4.61±0.50**	5.39±0.45*	7.39±0.77
Lactase	9.19±0.63	8.37±0.59	9.99±1.61
Sucrase	32.16±8.04	36.00±4.10	27.30±4.24

GGT – gamma-glutamyltranspeptidase, DPP IV – Dipeptidyl peptidase IV. Values are expressed as the mean ± SEM.
*$P<0.05$ ovalbumin-treated group (OVA) *vs.* PBS-treated group.
**$P<0.01$ ovalbumin-treated group (OVA) *vs.* PBS-treated group.
***$P<0.001$ ovalbumin-treated group (OVA) *vs.* PBS-treated group.
#$P<0.05$ heated-ovalbumin-treated group (h-OVA) *vs.* ovalbumin-treated group (OVA).

Increase of allergen specific IgE is essential for mast cell activation and development of allergic diarrhea symptoms. We determined the level of MMCP-1 enzyme as the marker of mast cell activation and degranulation. In this case, the reducing effect of thermal processing was clearly demonstrated; the h-OVA induced only half the level of serum MMCP-1 compared to the native OVA (Fig. 4).

Ex vivo Cytokine Production by MLN and Splenocytes Induced by OVA Allergens

Local and systemic cell responses to OVA and h-OVA were evaluated in all three groups of animals as *in vitro* cytokine production by MLN and splenocytes after exposure to corresponding allergens. Cytokine production from controls (PBS group) was low or not detectable and did not change after exposure to either form of OVA (data not shown). As shown in Fig. 5a, the levels of TNF-α, IL-4, IL-5, IL-10 and IL-13 were higher in culture media obtained from MLN exposed to native OVA. The differences in cytokine secretion were less pronounced in the experiments with splenocytes cultures (Fig. 5b). Only the production of IFN-γ was higher after exposure to h-OVA as compared to OVA. Levels of IL-6 and IL-17 didn't differ among the groups neither in MLN nor in spleen (data not shown).

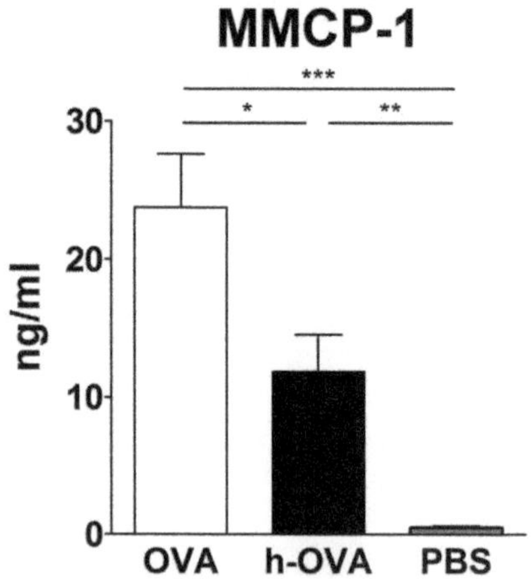

Figure 4. Decreased mast cell protease induction by heated-OVA. Heated OVA (h-OVA, black bar) induced significantly lower amounts of mast cell protease (MMCP-1), the marker of mast cell activation, compared to mice fed with native OVA (white bar). Data are represented as mean ± SEM (n = 10 mice/group), representative data from one out of three independent experiments. *P≤0.05, **P≤0.01, ***P≤0.001.

Differentiation of CD4+CD25+Foxp3+ T Cells in OVA and h-OVA Fed BALB/c Mice

Since regulatory T cells (Tregs) are known to be crucial for induction of oral tolerance to protein antigens [34], we analyzed the changes in Tregs in spleen and MLNs of OVA-, h-OVA- and PBS-treated mice at the end of the experiment. In spleen we observed a decrease in Tregs in h-OVA treated mice, as compared to OVA- and PBS-treated mice (Fig. 6). Only a non-significant increase was found in MLNs of h-OVA treated mice.

Induction of CD4+Foxp3+ T Cells by h-OVA and b-OVA in vitro is Increased After a 20-min Pepsin Digestion

To characterize the effect of heating and enzymatic digestion on T cell subpopulations, especially on regulatory T cell differentiation in more detail, splenocytes from naïve (untreated) BALB/c mice were cultured *in vitro* either with OVA, h-OVA or b-OVA as well as with their peptic digests. As shown in Fig. 7, the *in vitro* stimulation of splenocytes with undigested heated proteins led to a slight increase in proportion of CD4+Foxp3+ Treg cells compared to native form of OVA. Interestingly, 20 min peptic digests of heated forms of OVA induced increased proportion of Tregs, but this ability decreased again after 40 min of digestion. In contrast the pepsin digestion did not change the ability of OVA to slightly increase the proportion of Tregs as compared to undigested OVA.

Discussion

In this study, we showed that small irreversible changes in secondary structure of egg allergen OVA caused by thermal processing significantly affect its digestion by gut enzymes and decrease its allergenicity in the mouse model of food allergy. While both heated and native OVA induced allergic diarrhea in BALB/c mice, the disease symptoms appeared much earlier and with a higher frequency in OVA fed mice than in those fed with h-OVA. As compared to OVA-treated group, the sera of h-OVA-treated mice contained also significantly lower levels of specific IgE and MMCP-1, known markers of mast cell activation and degranulation [35]. It seems that even slight changes in the secondary structure elements have a high impact on the immunological behavior of the allergen. This could be explained by differences either in allergen absorption, which could lead to a decrease in allergen exposure, or in allergen digestion, which leads to production of peptides with different allergenicity and to a partial loss of conformational epitopes and/or exposure of new linear epitopes to immune cells.

The small intestine is noted for its plasticity in response to various dietary changes, which may be reflected in activation of enterocyte brush-border enzymes. Here we demonstrated for the first time that alkaline phosphatase (ALP) can be used as a new marker in food allergy, because its specific activity was significantly increased in OVA-treated group compared to controls. This is in line with the recent findings that ALP has a crucial role in regeneration of enterocytes and that its activity correlates with villous atrophy [19,36]. We can speculate that the increased level of ALP contributes to restoration of homeostasis in the enterocyte membranes after long-term stimulation with OVA allergens. On the contrary, dipeptidyl peptidase IV (CD26 - that cleaves L-alanine or L-proline residues in the penultimate N-terminal position) was significantly reduced in both OVA- and h-OVA-treated groups, as compared to PBS controls. Interestingly, a decrease in CD26 was found in patients with celiac disease induced by gluten, which belongs to wheat components responsible for food- or wheat-dependent exercise-induced allergy and for occupational asthma [37,38].

The changes in secondary structure by heating could influence antibody response *in vivo*. Here we report that OVA induced significantly higher levels of OVA-specific IgE and lower levels of IgG2a, as compared to h-OVA. High levels of potentially "blocking" IgG2a (mouse homolog of human IgG4) may compete for allergen [22]. The ability of heat-denatured allergens to induce Th1 associated IgG2a was also shown for other allergens, such as bee venom or birch pollen [39]. However, the effect cannot be generalized, because in a recent study by van der Ventel [15] a higher sensitizing potential was shown for cooked fish proteins. Surprisingly, when we changed the coupling allergen (h-OVA was used for OVA sensitized sera and vice versa) the binding of specific Abs was retained. Moreover, the binding was significantly higher when h-OVA antigen was used for specific IgG1 antibody determination. We assume that this is caused by heating-uncovered linear epitopes (supplementing the loss of the conformational ones), which are then presented after processing by antigen-presenting cells to T and B lymphocytes. On the other hand, when the extensively heated b-OVA was used, we observed a strong drop in the signal in all OVA-specific antibodies, which correlated with observed circular dichroism structural changes, and suggested the importance of structural epitopes in specific antibody formation.

Next, we addressed the question if the differences in OVA and h-OVA-specific antibody responses are also associated with cytokine milieu. On the local level in MLNs, we found a significantly higher production of Th2 cytokines in the OVA-treated mice, accompanied by proinflammatory TNF-α production after an *in vitro* exposure to OVA. Surprisingly, we determined an up-regulation of regulatory cytokine IL-10, which could be a result of a biological feedback aimed at dampening down the local inflammation, similar to chronic experimental colitis [40]. OVA-treatment did not significantly influence cytokine production in splenocytes, except for IFN-γ, which was produced predominantly by h-OVA stimulated splenocytes. The same observation was recently made by van der Ventel [15], who showed an increased IFN-γ production by splenocytes of mice challenged with heated fish extract. Our findings suggest that heating of OVA induces

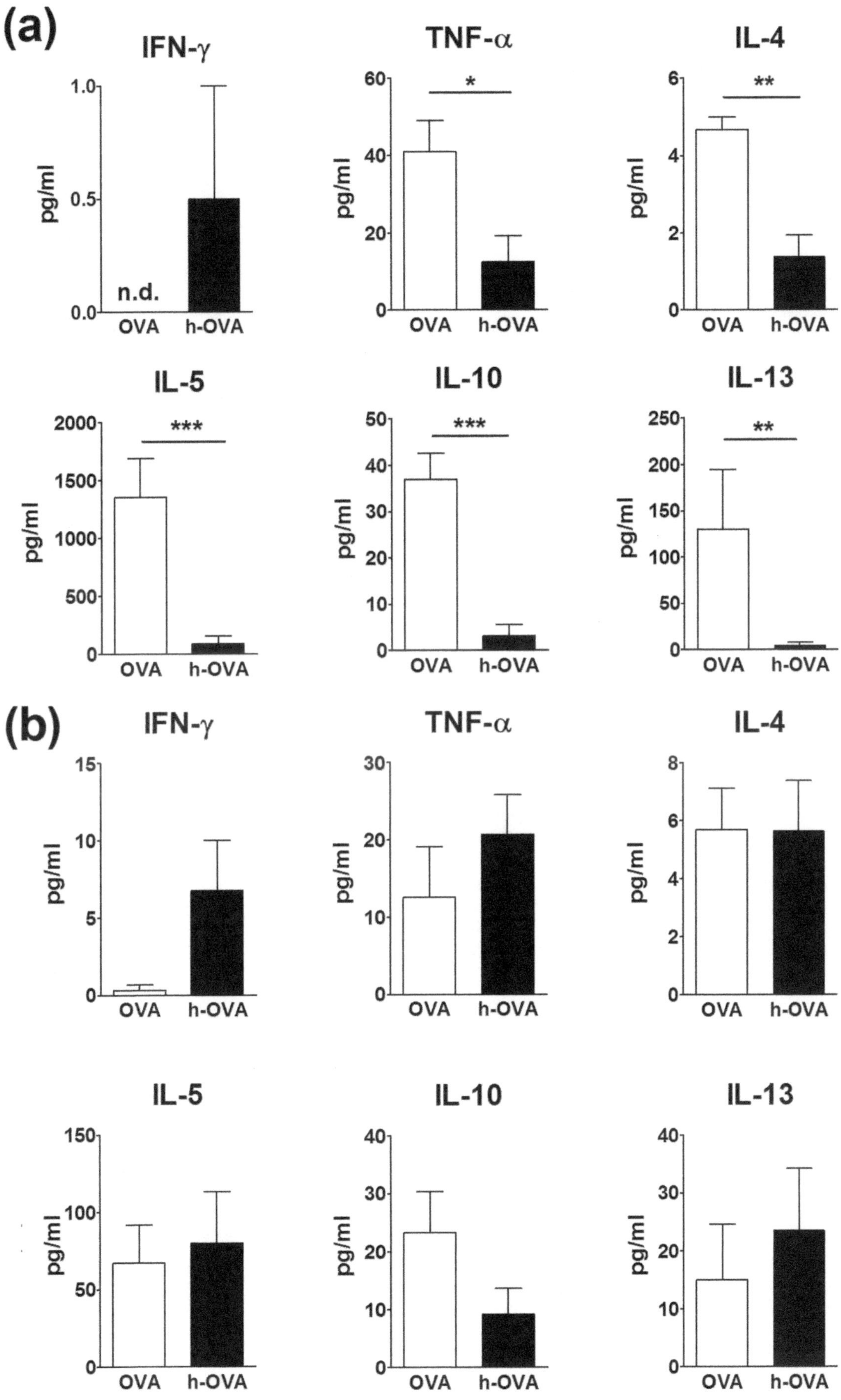
(a)
IFN-γ
TNF-α
IL-4
IL-5
IL-10
IL-13
pg/ml
n.d.
OVA
h-OVA
*
**
***
(b)
IFN-γ
TNF-α
IL-4
IL-5
IL-10
IL-13

Figure 5. Cytokine production after *in vitro* restimulation with OVA. The cytokine production from mesenteric lymph nodes (a) and splenocytes (b) of BALB/c mice fed with OVA (white bars) or h-OVA (black bars) and stimulated *in vitro* with appropriate allergen. Cytokine levels are expressed after subtraction of base line levels of unstimulated lymph node cells or splenocytes. Data shown are mean values ± SEM (n = 4–7 mice/group), representative data from one out of three independent experiments. *P≤0.05, **P≤0.01, ***P≤0.001, n.d. = not detectable.

changes in its digestion and processing by immune cells that lead to changes in the local cytokine environment ultimately leading to a shift from Th2- toward Th1-type response, reduction in the level of specific IgE and an increased production of blocking IgG2a antibodies [22]. These data fit well with clinical symptoms observed in allergic subjects in response to heated egg allergens [5,24].

Moreover, our results support recent data showing that thermal processing interferes with OVA stability [23]. Here, we show that h-OVA and b-OVA are initially (at 20 min) more resistant to proteolysis than native OVA. The difference in degradation kinetics could be explained by partial aggregation of heated forms of OVA, which makes the target structures less accessible for the enzyme. Nevertheless, after 40 min digestion the number of h-OVA and b-OVA fragments was even higher and their spectrum differed from those obtained from OVA. However, the spectra of h-OVA and b-OVA fragmented peptides were similar, differing only in the region corresponding to retention time of 50 min. Surprisingly, when we stimulated splenocytes from naïve mice *in vitro* we found an increase in the percentage of regulatory T cells in response to h-OVA and b-OVA. The capacity of both heated forms of OVA to induce Tregs was increased after 20 min of pepsin digestion and decreased again after 40 min digestion. The prolonged digestion had no effect on Treg inducing capacity of

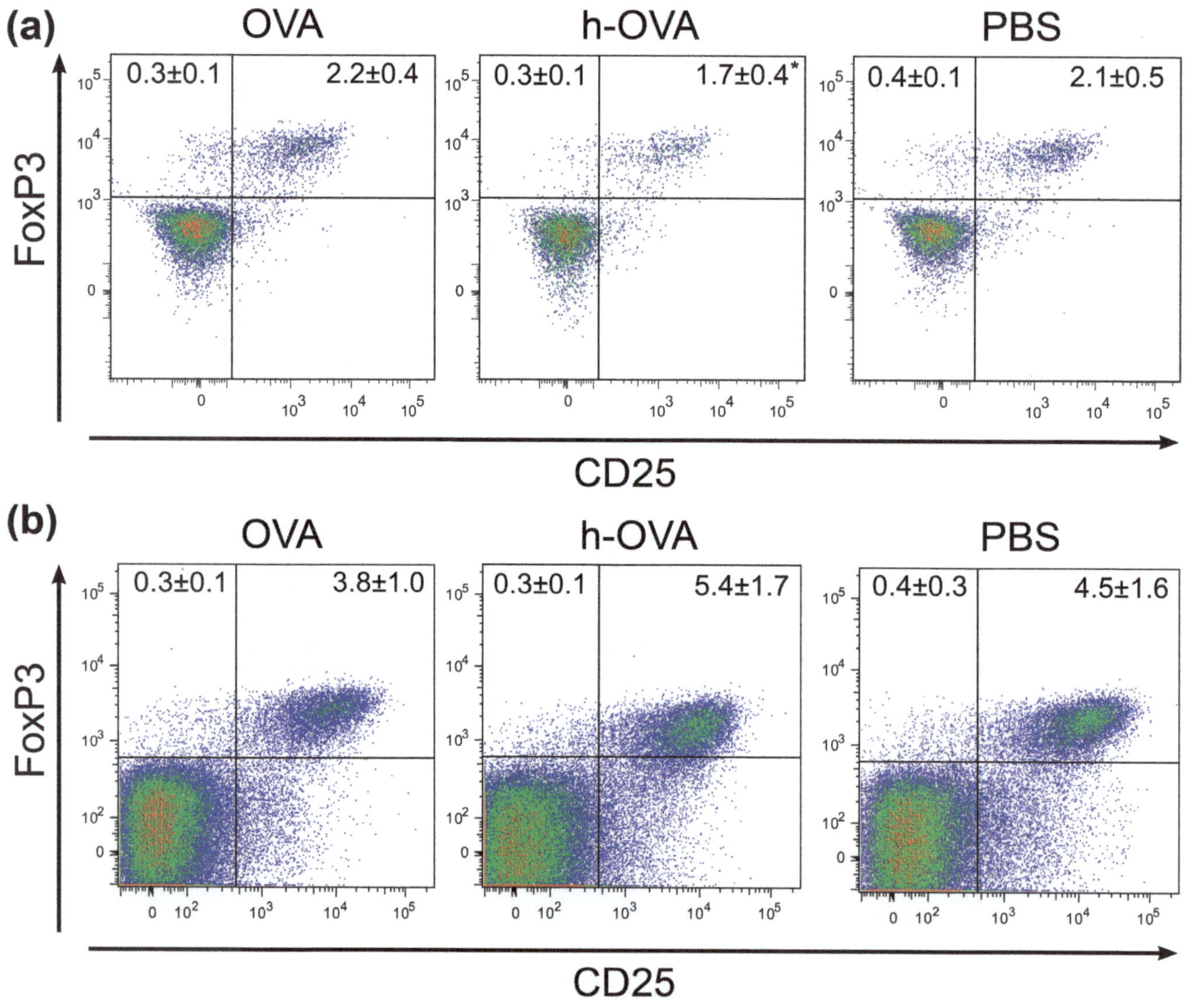

Figure 6. Numbers of Tregs in splenocytes and mesenteric lymph nodes of OVA treated mice. Typical plots depicting numbers of Tregs in mouse splenocytes (a) and mesenteric lymph node (b) in gated CD3+CD4+CD8– T helper cells after feeding with OVA, h-OVA or PBS, respectively. Numbers in upper quadrants shows proportions (mean ± SD) of either CD25–Foxp3+ or CD25+Foxp3+ Th cells out of all cells. Representative data from one out of three independent experiments. *P≤0.05.

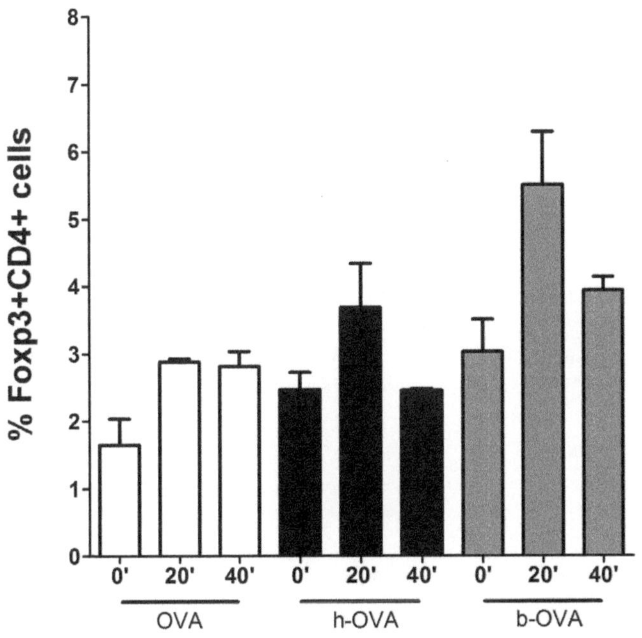

Figure 7. Number of Tregs in spleen cell suspensions co-cultured *in vitro* with OVA digests. The percentage of Tregs in cell suspension isolated from spleens of non-stimulated (naïve) BALB/c mice cultured *in vitro* for 48 hours with undigested (0′) and after 20 (20′) and 40 minutes (40′) peptic digest of OVA (white bars), h-OVA (black bars) or b-OVA (grey bars). The data represent the percentage of CD4+Foxp3+ cells out of all live cells as measured by FACS. Representative data from one out of three independent experiments are shown. Data are represented as mean ± SEM.

native (heat untreated) OVA digests. These data are supported by recent evidence in experimental mouse model of suppressive effects of some OVA T cell epitope peptides on allergic immune responses via Foxp3+ T cell generation [41].

A direct continuation of the study would be the analysis of intestinal DC subsets and goblet cells [42–44] in initial steps of allergen sensitization in our model, which should contribute to understanding how the tolerance or allergic response is achieved. The analysis of the role of enzymes in brush-border membrane of epithelial cells (activated after OVA gavages) will shed light on allergen digestion and immunogenicity of fragments (esp. dipeptidases) and on regeneration of gut epithelium (ALP). Moreover, it would be of great importance to apply this model for verification of hygiene hypothesis using animals kept under conventional and/or germ-free condition and subsequently colonized with various bacterial strains.

In conclusion, we showed that even a mild change in the secondary structure of OVA after thermal processing has far-reaching consequences concerning its antigenic properties. After digestion of h-OVA, fragments with different immunogenic properties are formed leading to the shift from Th2 to Th1-type response as compared to native OVA. Nevertheless, the h-OVA fragments still have the ability to induce allergic symptoms, but these are less pronounced and need longer time to develop.

Supporting Information

Figure S1 Cross-reactivity of anti-OVA specific antibodies. At the end of the experiment we determined the levels of OVA-specific antibodies in OVA and heated (h)-OVA treated mice against OVA, h-OVA (70°C) and boiled (b)-OVA (95°C). The levels were retained for IgE, IgG2a and IgA (a, c, d) when we used OVA as coating antigen for h-OVA-treated mice or h-OVA as coating antigen for OVA treated mice. In case of IgG1 (b) the levels were significantly higher when we used h-OVA as coating antigen for either OVA- or h-OVA- treated mice. When we used b-OVA we observed a significant drop in the signal for all measured antibodies. Representative data from one out of three experiments (n = 8). Repeated measures ANOVA with Tukey's multiple comparison test was used for analysis of differences between antibody levels of the same sample measured either against OVA, h-OVA and b-OVA antigen. n.s. non-significant, *P≤0.05, **P≤0.01, ***P≤0.001.
(TIF)

Acknowledgments

The authors thank Jana Cinová for her help with cell cultivation, Alena Smolová for excellent technical assistance and Anna Koffer for language revision.

Author Contributions

Conceived and designed the experiments: JG LT FF MS HK. Performed the experiments: JG MS MK DS HK MW KK PS. Analyzed the data: MS JG MK DS LT HK MW KK PS LP-J. Contributed reagents/materials/analysis tools: LT MW HK FF. Wrote the paper: LT MS JG MK MW HK PS. Obtained permission for use of animal model: LT.

References

1. Savage JH, Matsui EC, Skripak JM, Wood RA (2007) The natural history of egg allergy. J Allergy Clin Immunol 120: 1413–1417.
2. Herouet-Guicheney C, Aldemir H, Bars R, de Barbeyrac D, Kennel P, et al. (2009) Inter-laboratory comparisons of assessment of the allergenic potential of proteins in mice. J Appl Toxicol 29: 141–148.
3. Sicherer SH, Wood RA, Stablein D, Burks AW, Liu AH, et al. (2010) Immunologic features of infants with milk or egg allergy enrolled in an observational study (Consortium of Food Allergy Research) of food allergy. J Allergy Clin Immunol 125: 1077–1083.
4. Perrier C, Thierry AC, Mercenier A, Corthésy B (2010) Allergen-specific antibody and cytokine responses, mast cell reactivity and intestinal permeability upon oral challenge of sensitized and tolerized mice. Clin Exp Allergy 40: 153–162.
5. Mine Y, Yang M (2007) Epitope characterization of ovalbumin in BALB/c mice using different entry routes. Biochim Biophys Acta 1774: 200–212.
6. Repa A, Kozakova H, Hudcovic T, Stepankova R, Hrncir T, et al. (2008) Susceptibility to nasal and oral tolerance induction to the major birch pollen allergen Bet v 1 is not dependent on the presence of the microflora. Immunol Lett 117: 50–56.
7. Lee SY, Huang CK, Zhang TF, Schofield BH, Burks AW, et al. (2001) Oral administration of IL-12 suppresses anaphylactic reactions in a murine model of peanut hypersensitivity. Clin Immunol 101: 220–228.
8. Diesner SC, Knittelfelder R, Krishnamurthy D, Pali-Schöll I, Gajdzik L, et al. (2008) Dose-dependent food allergy induction against ovalbumin under acid-suppression: A murine food allergy model. Immunol Lett 121: 45–51.
9. Brunner R, Wallmann J, Szalai K, Karagiannis P, Altmeppen H, et al. (2009) Aluminium *per se* and in the anti-acid drug sucralfate promotes sensitization via the oral route. Allergy 64: 890–897.
10. Pali-Schöll I, Herzog R, Wallmann J, Szalai K, Brunner R, et al. (2010) Antacids and dietary supplements with an influence on the gastric pH increase the risk for food sensitization. Clin Exp Allergy 40: 1091–1098.
11. Dearman RJ, Kimber I (2007) A mouse model for food allergy using intraperitoneal sensitization. Methods 41: 91–98.
12. Brandt EB, Munitz A, Orekov T, Mingler MK, McBride M, et al. (2009) Targeting IL-4/IL-13 signaling to alleviate oral allergen-induced diarrhea. J Allergy Clin Immunol 123: 53–58.
13. Li X, Schofield BH, Huang CK, Kleiner GI, Sampson HA (1999) A murine model of IgE-mediated cow's milk hypersensitivity. J Allergy Clin Immunol 103: 206–214.

14. Saldanha JCS, Gargiulo DL, Silva SS, Carmo-Pinto FH, Andrade MC, et al. (2004) A model of chronic IgE-mediated food allergy in ovalbumin-sensitized mice. Braz J Med Biol Res 37: 809–816.
15. van der Ventel ML, Nieuwenhuizen NE, Kirstein F, Hikuam C, Jeebhay MF, et al. (2011) Differential responses to natural and recombinant allergens in a murine model of fish allergy. Mol Immunol 48: 637–646.
16. Simon PM, Kedinger M, Raul F, Grenier JF, Haffen K (1979) Developmental pattern of rat intestinal brush-border enzymic proteins along the villus-crypt axis. Biochem J 178: 407–413.
17. Kozáková H, Reháková Z, Kolínská J (2001) Bifidobacterium bifidum monoassociation of gnotobiotic mice: effect on enterocyte brush-border enzymes. Folia Microbiol 46: 573–576.
18. Hudcovic T, Kozáková H, Kolínská J, Stepánková R, Hrncír T, et al. (2009) Monocolonization with Bacteroides ovatus protects immunodeficient SCID mice from mortality in chronic intestinal inflammation caused by long-lasting dextran sodium sulfate treatment. Physiol Res 58: 101–110.
19. Lallès JP (2010) Intestinal alkaline phosphatase: multiple biological roles in maintenance of intestinal homeostasis and modulation by diet. Nutr Rev 68: 323–332.
20. Harada T, Koyama I, Kasahara T, Alpers DH, Komoda T (2003) Heat shock induces intestinal-type alkaline phosphatase in rat IEC-18 cells. Am J Physiol Gastrointest Liver Physiol. 284: G255–G262.
21. Huntington JA, Stein PE (2001) Structure and properties of ovalbumin. J Chromatogr B Biomed Sci Appl. 756(1–2): 189–198.
22. Lemon-Mulé H, Sampson HA, Sicherer SH, Shreffler WG, Noone S, et al. (2008) Immunologic changes in children with egg allergy ingesting extensively heated egg. J Allergy Clin Immunol 122: 977–983.
23. Martos G, Lopez-Exposito I, Bencharitiwong R, Berin MC, Nowak-Węgrzyn A (2011) Mechanisms underlying differential food allergy response to heated egg. J Allergy Clin Immunol 127: 990–997.
24. Nowak-Węgrzyn A, Sampson HA (2011) Future therapies for food allergies. J Allergy Clin Immunol 127: 558–573.
25. Roth-Walter F, Berin MC, Arnaboldi P, Escalante CR, Dahan S, et al. (2008) Pasteurization of milk proteins promotes allergic sensitization by enhancing uptake through Peyer's patches. Allergy 63: 882–890.
26. Himly M, Nony E, Chabre H, Van Overtvelt L, Neubauer A, et al. (2009) Standardization of allergen products: 1. Detailed characterization of GMP-produced recombinant Bet v 1.0101 as biological reference preparation. Allergy 64: 1038–1045.
27. Tučková L, Novotná J, Novák P, Flegelová Z, Květoň T, et al. (2002) Activation of macrophages by gliadin fragments: isolation and characterization of active peptide. J Leukoc Biol 71: 625–631.
28. Wiedermann U, Jahn-Schmid B, Bohle B, Repa A, Renz H, et al. (1999) Suppression of antigen-specific T- and B-cell responses by intranasal or oral administration of recombinant bet v 1, the major birch pollen allergen, in a murine model of type I allergy. J Allergy Clin Immunol 103: 1202–1210.
29. Lehrer SB, Reish R, Fernandes J, Gaudry P, Dai G, et al. (2004) Enhancement of murine IgE antibody detection by IgG removal. J Immunol Methods 284: 1–6.
30. Barsumian EL, Isersky C, Petrino MG, Siraganian (1981) IgE-induced histamine release from rat basophilic leukemia cell lines: isolation of releasing and nonreleasing clones. Eur J Immunol 11: 317–323.
31. Kessler M, Acuto O, Storelli C, Murer H, Müller M, et al. (1978) A modified procedure for the rapid preparation of efficiently transporting vesicles from small intestinal brush border membranes. Their use in investigating some properties of D-glucose and choline transport systems. Biochim Biophys Acta 506: 136–154.
32. Lowry OH, Rosebrough NJ, Farr Al, Randall RJ (1951) Protein measurement with the Folin phenol reagent. J Biol Chem 193: 265–275.
33. Kozakova H, Kolinska J, Lojda Z, Rehakova Z, Sinkora J, et al. (2006) Effect of bacterial monoassociation on brush-border enzyme activities in ex-germ-free piglets: comparison of commensal and pathogenic *Escherichia coli* strains. Microbes Infect 8: 2629–2639.
34. Whitacre CC, Gienapp IE, Orosz CG, Bitar DM (1991) Oral tolerance in experimental autoimmune encephalomyelitis. III. Evidence for clonal anergy. J Immunol 147: 2155–2163.
35. Vaali K, Puumalainen TJ, Lehto M, Wolff H, Rita H (2006) Murine model of food allergy after epicutaneous sensitization: role of mucosal mast cell protease-1. Scand J Gastroenterol 41: 1405–1413.
36. Lynes MD, Widmaier EP (2011) Involvement of CD36 and intestinal alkaline phosphatases in fatty acid transport in enterocytes, and the response to a high-fat diet. Life Sci 88: 384–391.
37. Smith MW, Phillips AD (1990) Abnormal expression of dipeptidylpeptidase IV activity in enterocytes brush-border membranes of children suffering from coeliac disease. Exp Physiol 75: 613–616.
38. Detel D, Persić M, Varljen J (2007) Serum and intestinal dipeptidyl peptidase IV (DPP IV/CD26) activity in children with celiac disease. J Pediatr Gastroenterol. Nutr 45: 65–70.
39. Johansen P, Senti G, Gómez JMM, Wüthrich B, Bot A, et al. (2005) Heat denaturation, a simple method to improve the immunotherapeutic potential of allergens. Eur J Immunol 35: 3591–3598.
40. Alex P, Zachos NC, Nguyen T, Gonzales L, Chen TE, et al. (2009) Distinct cytokine patterns identified from multiplex profiles of murine DSS and TNBS-induced colitis. Inflamm Bowel Dis 15: 341–352.
41. Yang M, Yang C, Mine Y (2010) Multiple T cell epitope peptides suppress allergic responses in an egg allergy mouse model by the elicitation of forkhead box transcription factor 3- and transforming growth factor-β-associated mechanisms. Clin Exp Allergy 40: 668–678.
42. Viney JL, Mowat AM, O'Malley JM, Williamson E, Fanger NA (1998) Expanding dendritic cells in vivo enhances the induction of oral tolerance. J Immunol 160: 5815–5825.
43. Lied GA, Vogelsang P, Berstad A, Appel S (2011) Dendritic cell populations in patients with self-reported food hypersensitivity. Int J Gener Med 4: 389–396.
44. McDole JR, Wheeler LW, McDonald KG, Wang B, Konjufca V, et al. (2012) Goblet cells deliver luminal antigen to CD103+ dendritic cells in the small intestine. Nature 483: 345–349.

Natural History of Perceived Food Hypersensitivity and IgE Sensitisation to Food Allergens in a Cohort of Adults

Antonios Patelis[1]*, Maria Gunnbjörnsdottir[1], Magnus P. Borres[2,6], Peter Burney[7], Thorarinn Gislason[3], Kjell Torén[4], Bertil Forsberg[5], Kjell Alving[6], Andrei Malinovschi[8], Christer Janson[1]

1 Department of Medical Sciences: Respiratory Medicine and Allergology, Uppsala University, Uppsala, Sweden, 2 Immunodiagnostics, Thermo Fischer Scientific, Uppsala, Sweden, 3 University of Iceland, Medical Faculty and Department of Respiratory Medicine and Sleep, Landspitali University Hospital, Reykjavik, Iceland, 4 Section of Occupational and Environmental Medicine, Institute of Medicine, University of Gothenburg, Gothenburg, Sweden, 5 Division of Occupational and Environmental Medicine, Umeå University, Umeå, Sweden, 6 Department of Women's and Children's Health, Uppsala University, Uppsala, Sweden, 7 Respiratory Epidemiology and Public Health, Imperial College, London, United Kingdom, 8 Department of Medical Sciences: Clinical Physiology, Uppsala University, Uppsala, Sweden

Abstract

Background: No longitudinal studies exist on the natural history of food hypersensitivity and IgE sensitisation to food allergens in adults.

Objective: To examine the natural history of food hypersensitivity, the natural history of IgE sensitisation to food allergens and to investigate the risk factors for new onset food hypersensitivity.

Methods: Food hypersensitivity was questionnaire-assessed in 2307 individuals (aged 20–45 years) from Iceland and Sweden during the European Community Respiratory Health Survey both at baseline and follow-up 9 years later. IgE food and aeroallergen sensitisation were assessed in a subgroup of these individuals (n = 807). Values of 0.35 kU/L and above were regarded as positive sensitisation.

Results: Food hypersensitivity was reported by 21% of the subjects and this proportion remained unchanged at follow-up ($p = 0.58$). Fruits, nuts and vegetables were the three most common causes of food hypersensitivity, with a similar prevalence at baseline and follow-up. The prevalence IgE sensitisation to food allergens decreased in general by 56% ($p < 0.001$) and IgE sensitisation to peanut decreased in particular by 67% ($p = 0.003$). The prevalence of timothy grass IgE sensitisation decreased by 15% ($p = 0.003$) while cat, mite and birch IgE sensitisation did not decrease significantly. Female sex, rhinitis, eczema and presence of IgE sensitisation to aeroallergens were independently associated with new onset food hypersensitivity.

Conclusion: The prevalence of food hypersensitivity remained unchanged while the prevalence of IgE sensitisation to food allergens decreased in adults over a 9-year follow-up period. The decrease in prevalence of IgE sensitisation to food allergens was considerably larger than the change in prevalence of IgE sensitisation to aeroallergens.

Editor: Giuseppe Remuzzi, Mario Negri Institute for Pharmacological Research and Azienda Ospedaliera Ospedali Riuniti di Bergamo, Italy

Funding: This study was supported financially by the Swedish Heart and Lung Foundation, the Vårdal Foundation for Health Care Science and Allergy Research, the Swedish Association against Asthma and Allergy, Agnes and Mac Rudberg's Foundation and the Bror Hjerpstedt Foundation. The funders had no role in study design, data collection and analysis, decision to publish, or preparation of the manuscript.

Competing Interests: Kjell Alving is an employee and minority shareholder of Aerocrine AB and has received funds for research from the same company. Magnus Borres is an employee of ThermoFisher Scientific (which manufactures kits to measure IgE antibodies against allergens). This does not alter the authors' adherence to all the PLOS ONE policies on sharing data and materials.

* E-mail: antonios.patelis@medsci.uu.se

These authors contributed equally to this work.

Introduction

Several population surveys in the 1990s have estimated the prevalence of perceived food hypersensitivity, e.g. self-reported adverse reactions after food ingestion, regardless of the underlying mechanism [1], at 12% to 20% in adults [2–4]. The majority of adverse reactions to food are not IgE-mediated [5] and there is limited information on the prevalence and distribution of IgE food sensitisation. About 15% to 20% of the population has IgE to at least one food allergen over the detection limit [6,7] e.g. food IgE sensitisation. However, only a small fraction of subjects with IgE antibodies against food allergens have clinical IgE-mediated food allergy. As an example, Liu et al [7] reported that the prevalence of food IgE sensitisation was 15% whereas the prevalence of IgE-mediated food allergy was only 2%.

Aeroallergen IgE sensitisation, especially against perennial allergens, is linked to asthma and airway inflammation [8–11]. The natural history of prevalence of aeroallergen IgE sensitisation has been examined in longitudinal studies in adults [12–18], but the results are contradictory and show the prevalence decreasing

[15,18], remaining stable [12,19] or increasing [13,14,16,17] over time.

To the best of our knowledge, no study exists about the natural history of food hypersensitivity and IgE sensitisation to food allergens in adults. Another reason for studying IgE sensitisation to food allergens and IgE-mediated food allergy is that not only aeroallergen sensitisation, but also food IgE sensitisation, is linked to increased exhaled nitric oxide levels and increased risk for asthma [6,7,20].

The aim of this study was to examine the natural history food hypersensitivity symptoms and IgE sensitisation to food allergens and to investigate the risk factors for new onset food hypersensitivity and sensitisation.

Methods

Population

The study was based on the European Community Respiratory Health Survey (ECRHS) I (1991–92) and II (2000–01) [21] from four participating centres (Reykjavík, Uppsala, Gothenburg and Umeå). Each participant in ECRHS I was sent a brief questionnaire (Stage 1) and among those who responded, both a random and a "symptomatic" sample (consisting of subjects with symptoms of asthma or asthma medication), were invited to undergo a more detailed clinical examination (Stage 2). Subjects from Stage 2 of ECRHS I were invited to participate in the follow-up study, ECRHS II, and answered a standardized questionnaire and underwent a clinical visit [21]. A total of 2,307 individuals answered questions about food hypersensitivity symptoms both at ECRHS I and II. No difference in age, sex, BMI, prevalence of asthma, rhinitis, total IgE, food IgE sensitisation, aeroallergen IgE sensitisation and smoking history were found between subjects with and without follow-up data about food hypersensitivity symptoms (all $p>0.05$). A subgroup of ECRHS participants in Iceland (Reykjavík) and Sweden (Uppsala, Gothenburg and Umeå) from the random sample ($n = 807$) was examined against IgE to food allergens at ECRHS I [22] [23] and ECRHS II (Figure 1).

Questionnaires

The main questionnaire used in ECRHS I and II http://www.ecrhs.org [24] gathered information about respiratory symptoms, exposure to investigated allergens, and smoking history.

Diagnosis of asthma

A person was defined as asthmatic if he/she had ever been diagnosed with asthma and had an asthma attack or one of the following symptoms: nocturnal chest tightness, attack of shortness of breath, chest wheezing or whistling during the last 12 months [25].

Definition of food hypersensitivity

An individual was considered having food hypersensitivity [1] if he/she answered yes to the following questions "Have you ever had an illness or trouble caused by eating a particular food or foods?" and if so, "Have you nearly always had the same illness or trouble after eating this type of food?" Respondents were then asked to list the food(s) and symptoms [2].

Measurements of IgE to aeroallergens and food allergens and total IgE

Venous blood samples were drawn from all participants in the clinical visits and frozen at $-20°C$ for measurement of total serum IgE (total IgE) and serum IgE antibodies to cat, *D. pteronyssinus*, timothy grass, birch, and *Cladosporium*, as part of the ECRHS I and II protocol [21]. Measurement of IgE antibodies against birch was performed in all centres in the ECRHS I and in the Uppsala centre in ECRHS II. In addition, IgE antibodies to a mix of food allergens (containing egg white, milk, cod fish, wheat, peanut, and soybean) were measured in the subgroup of ECRHS participants in Iceland (Reykjavík) and Sweden (Uppsala, Gothenburg and Umeå) from the random sample by same technique and reagents at ECRHS I and II (Pharmacia CAP System, MultiCap fx5, Thermo Fisher Scientific, Uppsala, Sweden). Serum with a positive reaction to the food panel (fx5) was further analysed for the single allergens in the panel. The results are presented in kU/L, and values of 0.35 kU/L and above were regarded as positive sensitisation [26]. A titre below the detection level (<0.35 kU/L) was arbitrarily given the value 0.17 kU/L). All samples from ECRHS I from Reykjavík, Uppsala, Gothenburg and Umeå were analysed in Uppsala, as previously described [22] while samples from the random sample of ECRHS II (depending on availability of residual samples) were analysed within the frame of Euro-PREVALL in Manchester, as described elsewhere [27].

Statistics

Statistical analyses were performed using STATA 12.1 software (Stata Corp., 2011, Texas, USA). IgE titres (both total and specific) were log transformed before analysis. Mc Nemar's test was used to compare prevalence of food hypersensitivity, various food related symptoms and IgE sensitisation in ECRHS I and II. Chi-squared test (for categorical variables) and unpaired t-test (for numerical variables) were used to compare individuals with new onset and no food hypersensitivity and prevalence of IgE sensitisation to food, cat/mite and timothy grass allergens. Chi-squared test was also used to compare prevalence of IgE sensitisation to food in subjects according to age (< or > median age). Paired t-test was used to compare levels of IgE to specific allergens between ECRHS I and II in subjects sensitised to each respective allergen at either ECRHS I or II and unpaired t-test was used to compare levels of IgE against food allergens at ECRHS I in subjects with persistence and remission of IgE sensitisation to food allergens. Multiple logistic regression models were used when examining predictors for new onset food hypersensitivity, and persistent food sensitisation. These models always included age, gender, body mass index, rhinitis, current asthma, total IgE, IgE against food allergens, sample and IgE against aeroallergens. A p–value of <0.05 was considered statistically significant.

Ethics

All subjects consented to the utilization of personal data for the purpose of this study. The study was approved by the Ethics Committee at the Medical Faculty at Uppsala University and University of Iceland.

Results

The study population comprised of 2,307 individuals who answered questions about food hypersensitivity symptoms in both ECRHS I and II. Of these, 53% were women. The group characteristics of the participants are presented in Table 1.

Natural history of food hypersensitivity symptoms

Around 21% of the interviewed subjects reported food hypersensitivity symptoms in both ECRHS I and II (Table 2). The most common foods related to these symptoms were fruits followed by nuts and then vegetables. The prevalence of food

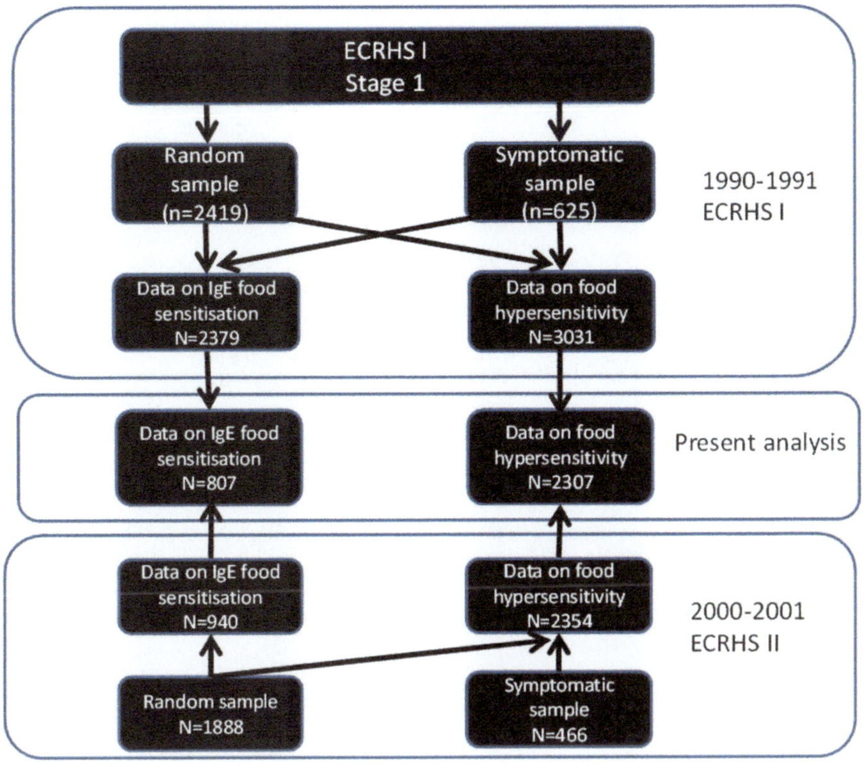

Figure 1. Flow chart explaining the selection of the studied population.

hypersensitivity in relation to ingestion of fish (including seafood and shellfish) increased significantly from ECRHS I to II and become, together with vegetables, the fourth most common cause of food hypersensitivity. Food hypersensitivity symptoms due to dairy products, wheat products (gluten, cereal and wheat) and spices (herbs, chili, and garlic) also increased significantly from ECRHS I to II (Table 2).

Skin reactions were the most common reported symptoms both at baseline and follow-up (Table 3). No significant change in the prevalence of the different symptoms was found during the 9-year period between ECRHS I and II.

Table 1. Characteristics of the participants (n = 2,307; mean ± SD and n (%)).

	ECRHS I 1991–92	ECRHS II 2000–01	p value
Age	33.6 ±7.3	42.4 ±7.2	<0.001
BMI	23.8 ±3.6	25.7 ±4.2	<0.001
Current asthma	314 (13.4)	428 (18.3)	<0.001
Rhinitis	783 (33.3)	904 (38.5)	<0.001
Smoking history			<0.001
Never	1093 (46.6)	1044 (45.9)	
Ex	54 (23.1)	730 (32.2)	
Current	711 (30.3)	497 (21.9)	

Natural history of prevalence of IgE sensitisation to food and aeroallergens

Prevalence of IgE sensitisation to at least one food allergen decreased by 56% during the study (Figure 2A). Prevalence of peanut IgE-sensitisation was the highest among food allergens and decreased by 67%. The prevalence of soy IgE sensitisation decreased significantly between ECRHS I and II, whereas similar prevalence of IgE sensitisation to wheat, milk, egg and fish was found at both time points (Figure 2B). No significant change of prevalence of cat, birch and mite IgE sensitisation was found, whereas prevalence of timothy grass IgE sensitisation decreased by 15% (from 17% to 15%) (Figure 2A).

The prevalence of IgE sensitisation to food allergens decreased from ECRHS I to ECRHS II by 63% (from 6% to 2%) ($p<0.001$) in subjects younger than 31 years and by 44% (from 4% to 2%) ($p<0.001$) in subjects older than 31 years (median age of cohort in ECRHS I).

Changes over time of levels of IgE against food- and aeroallergens and total IgE

Significant decreases of IgE antibodies against peanut ($p<0.001$, Figure 3a) and soy ($p<0.001$ Figure 3b), but not against wheat ($p = 0.12$, Figure 3c), milk ($p = 0.9$), egg ($p = 0.4$) were found between ECRHS I and II among individuals who were IgE-sensitised to the respective allergen either at baseline or follow-up.

Similarly, among the aeroallergens, the levels of IgE antibodies against timothy grass decreased ($p<0.001$) whereas levels of IgE against cat ($p = 0.18$), birch ($p = 0.43$) and mite ($p = 0.12$) remained stable between ECRHS I and II among individuals who were IgE-sensitised to the respective allergen either at baseline or follow-up.

Table 2. Prevalence (n (%)) of type of food reported as cause of food hypersensitivity (n = 2,307).

	ECRHS I 1991–92	ECRHS II 2000–01	p value
Any food	496 (21.5)	508 (22.0)	0.58
Fruits	195 (8.5)	215 (9.3)	0.19
Nuts	126 (5.5)	135 (5.9)	0.47
Vegetables	78 (3.4)	97 (4.2)	0.11
Fish, seafood, shellfish	56 (2.4)	97 (4.2)	<0.001
Chocolate	27 (1.2)	23 (1.0)	0.65
Egg	24 (1.0)	19 (0.8)	0.34
Milk and dairy products	22 (1.0)	57 (2.5)	<0.001
Meat	11 (0.4)	19 (0.8)	0.14
Herbs, chilli, garlic	9 (0.3)	20 (0.9)	0.004
Gluten, cereal, wheat products	5 (0.3)	14 (0.6)	0.049

Total IgE increased between ECHRS I and II (17.7 (16.0, 19.7) vs. 25.7 (23.4, 28.2) kU/L (geometric mean) (p<0.001)).

Incidence of food hypersensitivity

The incidence of food hypersensitivity was 11.7% during this 9-year study. The incidence in the symptomatic sample was higher than the random sample (20.6% vs. 9.9%, p<0.001). Female sex, rhinitis, eczema, asthma and presence of IgE sensitisation to aeroallergens were associated with new onset food hypersensitivity (Table 4) and these associations were consistent in a multiple logistic regression model (Figure 4).

Incidence and persistence of IgE sensitisation to food allergens

New onset IgE food sensitisation (n = 8) was not associated with age, gender, BMI, current rhinitis, current asthma, current smoking and IgE sensitisation to aeroallergens (data not shown). Persistent IgE food sensitisation was associated with higher total IgE levels at baseline (Table 5) and this association remained significant also after adjusting for age, gender, BMI, current rhinitis, current asthma, current smoking and IgE sensitisation to aeroallergens (OR (95% CI) = 9.8 (1.6, 60.5) per unit of natural logarithm-transformed total IgE). No relation between persistence of IgE sensitisation to food allergens and specific IgE levels to food allergens or aeroallergens or prevalence of IgE sensitisation to aeroallergens at baseline was found (Table 5).

Discussion

The main findings in the present investigation are that one in five adults reported food hypersensitivity symptoms after food intake and this proportion remained unchanged during this 9-year longitudinal study. The prevalence of IgE-sensitisation to food allergens decreased during that 9-year period whereas the prevalence of sensitisation to aeroallergens remained relatively unchanged.

To our knowledge this is the first study that analysed longitudinal changes of perceived self-reported food hypersensitivity in adults. The prevalence of food hypersensitivity reported here is in line with reports from previous cross-sectional studies [2–4,28]. Our results showing an unchanged prevalence of food hypersensitivity over time are opposite to what is known about the

Table 3. Prevalence (n (%)) of symptoms reported after food intake (n = 2,307).

	ECRHS I 1991–92	ECRHS II 2000–01	p value
Rash or itchy skin	101 (4.4)	112 (4.9)	0.39
Diarrhoea or vomiting	40 (1.7)	47 (2.0)	0.26
Runny or stuffy nose	42 (1.8)	48 (2.1)	0.42
Severe headache	18 (0.8)	25 (1.1)	0.21
Breathlessness	54 (2.3)	56 (2.4)	0.87
Other	131 (5.7)	149 (6.5)	0.047

natural history of food hypersensitivity in children, where major remission of symptoms has been reported [29–31].

The two most common reported symptoms of food hypersensitivity were skin reactions and gastrointestinal reactions. Reactions occurring at the skin or mucosa were also the most prevalent in a previous study [4]. Fruits, nuts and vegetables were the three

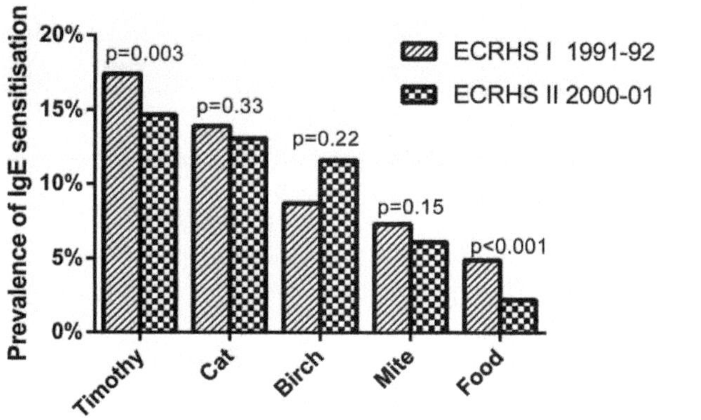

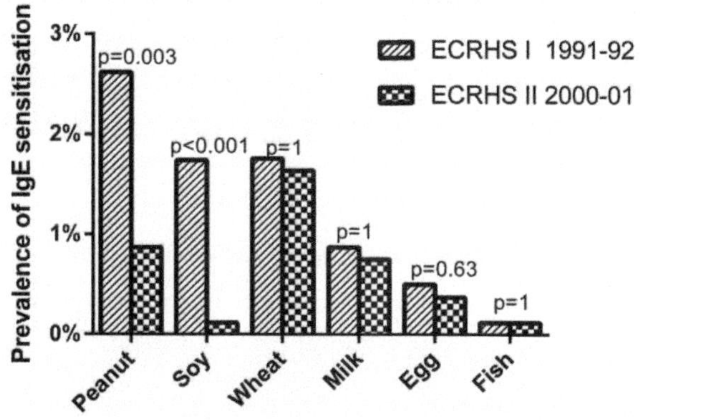

Figure 2. Prevalence (number of individuals of the study population who have IgE for respective allergen ≥0.35 KU/L) of sensitisation to food (n = 807) and aeroallergens (n = 804) (upper panel) and prevalence (number of individuals of the study population who have IgE for respective allergen ≥0.35 KU/L) of IgE sensitisation to individual food allergens (lower panel) in ECRHS I and II. Birch pollen was measured only in Uppsala (n = 138).

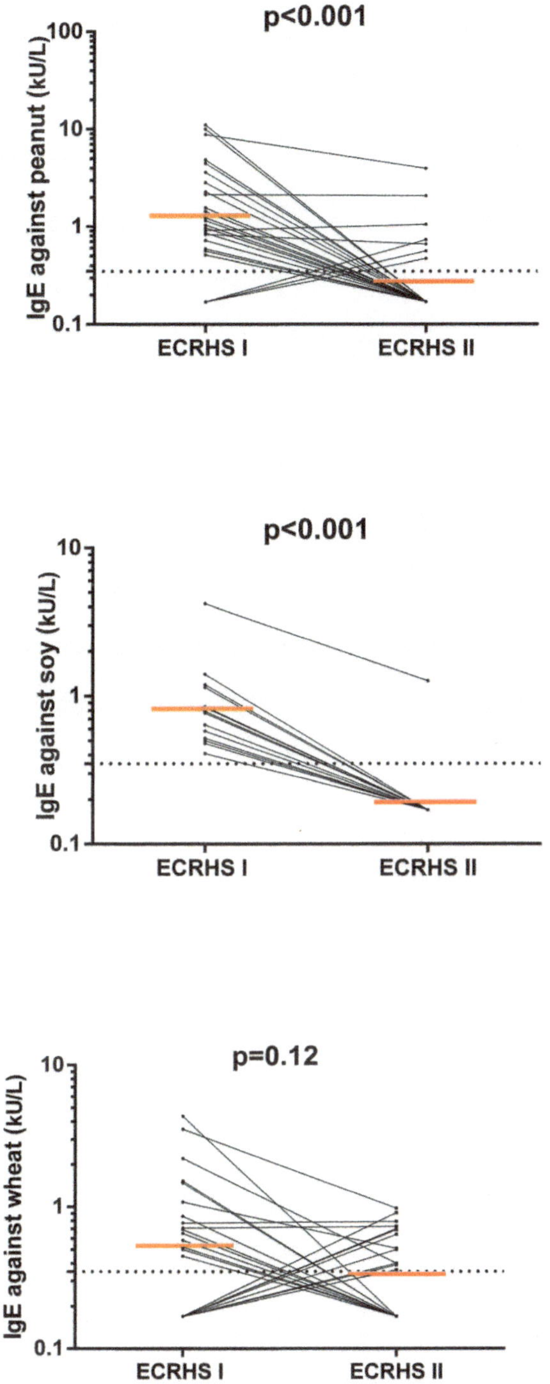

Figure 3. Change in levels of specific IgE against peanut (n = 24), soy (n = 14) and wheat (n = 22) between baseline and follow-up in subjects sensitised either at baseline or at follow-up. (The dotted line corresponds to the detection limit of 0.35 kU/L and the red lines correspond to the geometrical mean of levels of specific IgE against each respective allergen).

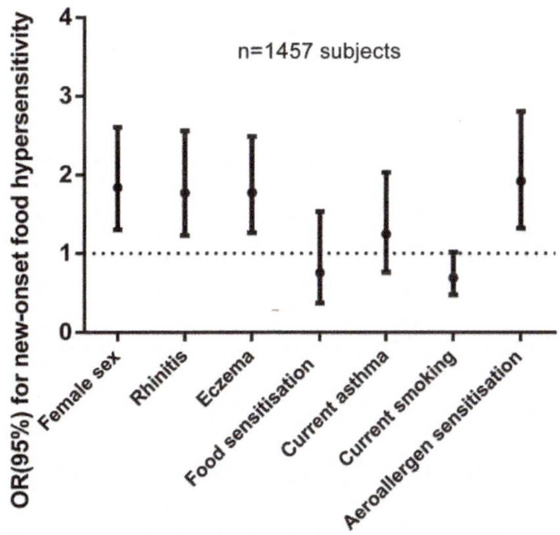

Figure 4. Risk factors (Odds Ratios (95%CI)) for new onset food hypersensitivity. Odds ratios are adjusted for the variables in the figure and age, body mass index, current smoking, sample and total IgE.

most common causes of food hypersensitivity in our population, with a similar prevalence at baseline and follow-up. A previous study [4] showed the same major causes of adverse reactions to foods.

The risk factors for new onset food hypersensitivity in the present study were female sex, rhinitis, eczema, asthma and presence of IgE sensitisation to aeroallergens. Thus, incidence of food hypersensitivity seems to be related to the atopic trait of an individual. We are not aware of any published longitudinal study to compare our results with. However, there are cross-sectional studies showing that food hypersensitivity in adults is often associated with concomitant sensitisation to aeroallergens [4], IgE sensitisation to food allergens [32] and other manifestations of atopy, especially rhinitis [4].

A novel finding of the study was the marked reduction of prevalence of IgE sensitisation to food allergens over time in adults. The natural history of prevalence of IgE sensitisation to food allergens has previously been studied only in children [33] where sensitisation rates to food allergens remained stable during the first 6 years of life (10%). The majority of children outgrow their allergies to milk, soy, egg, and wheat, and some to peanut also [34]. The decrease in the prevalence of IgE sensitisation to food allergens does not appear to be related to the initial age of the subjects, which tends to preclude the possibility that the effect is related to a specific birth cohort. Reductions of similar size could be observed in both younger and older subjects. This probably signals that the decreasing prevalence is somehow related to aging. Previous longitudinal studies [12,14,16,17] on the prevalence of IgE sensitisation to aeroallergens in relation to age report inconsistent results.

In the present study the prevalence of sensitisation to aeroallergens decreased to a much lesser extent than sensitisation to food allergens. However, the levels of IgE antibodies decreased during the 9-year follow-up period for both food and aeroallergens, whereas the levels of total IgE increased. Most of the longitudinal studies have analysed changes in the prevalence of IgE sensitisation without reporting changes in the degree of IgE sensitisation. A decrease of IgE titres to mite in a long-term follow-up of subjects with house-dust allergic asthma has been reported [35]. Karakaya and Kalyoncu [18] reported that the wheal diameter in response to skin prick test decreased under a two-year period for two of the studied allergens, timothy grass and mite. The reason why specific IgE decreased and total IgE increased in the present study is unclear. However our finding of increase total IgE is consistent with an increase of total IgE in all ECRHS centres [36] even if other longitudinal studies reported stable levels

Table 4. Population characteristics in different population strata, subdivided according to presence/absence of food hypersensitivity at ECRHS I and II.

	No food hypersensitivity (n = 1601)	New-onset food hypersensitivity (n = 211)	p value*
Age (years)	33.8±7.3	33.4±7.3	0.35
Female sex	48.8	61.6	<0.001
BMI (kg/m²)	23.7±3.3	23.5±3.4	0.43
Current smoker	31.6	26.5	0.133
Rhinitis	23.0	43.1	<0.001
Eczema	46.6	62.6	<0.001
Asthma	8.8	16.1	0.001
Total IgE (kU/L)	19.0 (18–20)	23.0 (18–29)	0.09
IgE sensitisation to food allergen	5.0	6.8	0.32
IgE sensitisation to aeroallergens	26.5	46	<0.001

Results presented as either prevalence (%), mean±SD or geometric mean (95% CI).
*p-value for comparison new-onset food hypersensitivity vs. no food hypersensitivity

over time [17], [37]. The total IgE levels reflect more than the sum of specific IgE towards a broad panel of allergens [38]. Moreover the fraction of total IgE not-related to specific sensitisations was not related to the specific IgE fraction of total IgE [38]. The factors that control the fraction of total IgE that are not related to specific IgE sensitisation are not fully understood.

Subjects with higher total IgE levels at baseline were more likely to have persistent sensitisation to food allergens in our study. Increased levels of total IgE have been reported to predict the development of IgE sensitisation to aeroallergens and asthma symptoms in children [39]. As far as we know, no study has analysed the relation between baseline total IgE levels and persistence of IgE sensitisation to food allergens, whereas increased total IgE at baseline related [37] to persistence of aeroallergen IgE sensitisation in previous longitudinal studies.

The strength of this study is the population setting and the long follow-up period. This is the first study to our knowledge assessing food hypersensitivity and IgE levels against food allergens in a longitudinal setting. A weakness of the present study is that we were not able to assess the persistence/remission of food hypersensitivity as the questions refer to ever having food hypersensitivity. A limitation is the fairly limited number of participants for whom we had data from repeated measurements of IgE against food allergens. Another limitation is that several of the most common food allergens in adulthood, such as hazelnut, shrimp, peach and apple [27], were not analysed at both time points. The different freezing times before analysis of IgE for samples from ECRHS I and II and that measurements were performed in different laboratories (Uppsala for ECRHS I and Manchester for ECRHS II) does not appear to influence the measured IgE levels [40,41]. Cross reactivity with IgE antibodies against birch or timothy grass can influence the measured IgE sensitisation to food allergens, and the lower prevalence of IgE sensitisation to food allergens at follow-up could have been due to a reduced prevalence of IgE sensitisation to birch at the follow-up. However, the prevalence of IgE sensitisation to birch did not decrease in the present study while the prevalence of IgE sensitisation to timothy grass decreased to a much lesser degree than IgE sensitisation to food allergens.

In conclusion, the prevalence of food hypersensitivity remained unchanged while IgE sensitisation to food allergens decreased in this 9 year follow up study performed in adults. The prevalence of IgE sensitisation towards food allergens decreased to a larger extent than the prevalence and persistence of IgE sensitisation to

Table 5. Baseline characteristic of subjects with persistent IgE food sensitisation compared to those with remission.

	Persistent IgE food sensitisation (n = 10)	Remission of IgE food sensitisation (n = 30)	p value*
Female sex	60.0	43.0	0.36
Age (years)	29.7 ±1.9	30.3 ±0.8	0.74
BMI (kg/m²)	23.2 ±1	24 ±0.6	0.55
Smoking	20.0	17.0	0.81
Rhinitis	50.0	80.0	0.07
Asthma	10.0	23.0	0.36
Food hypersensitivity	44.4	40.0	0.81
Total IgE (kU/L)	370 (110–1242)	106 (72–155)	0.008
IgE sensitisation to aeroallergens	9.0 (90)	24.0 (80)	0.47

Results presented as either prevalence (%), mean ± SD or geometric mean (95% CI).
*p-value for comparison persistent IgE food sensitisation and remission of IgE food sensitisation

aeroallergens. The biological explanation for the high prevalence of food hypersensitivity should be further investigated.

Acknowledgments

We would like to acknowledge Colin Summers for his contribution to EuroPrevall.

Author Contributions

Conceived and designed the experiments: AP CJ AM. Performed the experiments: CJ PB TG KT BF MG. Analyzed the data: AP CJ AM. Contributed reagents/materials/analysis tools: CJ MB KA. Wrote the paper: AP AM CJ. Revised critically: AP MG MB PB TG KT BF KA AM CJ. Final approval: AP MG MB PB TG KT BF KA AM CJ.

References

1. Johansson SG, Bieber T, Dahl R, Friedmann PS, Lanier BQ, et al. (2004) Revised nomenclature for allergy for global use: Report of the Nomenclature Review Committee of the World Allergy Organization, October 2003. J Allergy Clin Immunol 113: 832–836.
2. Woods RK, Abramson M, Bailey M, Walters EH (2001) International prevalences of reported food allergies and intolerances. Comparisons arising from the European Community Respiratory Health Survey (ECRHS) 1991–1994. Eur J Clin Nutr 55: 298–304.
3. Altman DR, Chiaramonte LT (1996) Public perception of food allergy. Journal of Allergy and Clinical Immunology 97: 1247–1251.
4. Schafer T, Bohler E, Ruhdorfer S, Weigl L, Wessner D, et al. (2001) Epidemiology of food allergy/food intolerance in adults: associations with other manifestations of atopy. Allergy 56: 1172–1179.
5. Taylor SL (1986) Food allergies and sensitivities. J Am Diet Assoc 86: 599–600.
6. Patelis A, Gunnbjornsdottir M, Malinovschi A, Matsson P, Onell A, et al. (2012) Population-based study of multiplexed IgE sensitization in relation to asthma, exhaled nitric oxide, and bronchial responsiveness. J Allergy Clin Immunol 130: 397–402 e392.
7. Liu AH, Jaramillo R, Sicherer SH, Wood RA, Bock SA, et al. (2010) National prevalence and risk factors for food allergy and relationship to asthma: results from the National Health and Nutrition Examination Survey 2005–2006. J Allergy Clin Immunol 126: 798–806 e713.
8. Sears MR, Herbison GP, Holdaway MD, Hewitt CJ, Flannery EM, et al. (1989) The relative risks of sensitivity to grass pollen, house dust mite and cat dander in the development of childhood asthma. Clin Exp Allergy 19: 419–424.
9. Malinovschi A, Janson C, Holmkvist T, Norback D, Merilainen P, et al. (2006) IgE sensitisation in relation to flow-independent nitric oxide exchange parameters. Respir Res 7: 92.
10. Sporik R, Ingram J, Price W, Sussman J, Honsinger R, et al. (1995) Association of asthma with serum IgE and skin test reactivity to allergens among children living at high altitude. Tickling the dragon's breath. Am J Respir Crit Care Med 151: 1388–1392.
11. Peat JK, Tovey E, Toelle BG, Haby MM, Gray EJ, et al. (1996) House dust mite allergens. A major risk factor for childhood asthma in Australia. Am J Respir Crit Care Med 153: 141–146.
12. Jarvis D, Luczynska C, Chinn S, Potts J, Sunyer J, et al. (2005) Change in prevalence of IgE sensitization and mean total IgE with age and cohort. J Allergy Clin Immunol 116: 675–682.
13. Barbee RA, Kaltenborn W, Lebowitz MD, Burrows B (1987) Longitudinal changes in allergen skin test reactivity in a community population sample. J Allergy Clin Immunol 79: 16–24.
14. Linneberg A, Nielsen NH, Madsen F, Frolund L, Dirksen A, et al. (2002) Is the increase in allergic respiratory disease caused by a cohort effect? Clin Exp Allergy 32: 1702–1705.
15. Warm K, Backman H, Lindberg A, Lundback B, Ronmark E (2012) Low incidence and high remission of allergic sensitization among adults. J Allergy Clin Immunol 129: 136–142.
16. Broadfield E, McKeever TM, Scrivener S, Venn A, Lewis SA, et al. (2002) Increase in the prevalence of allergen skin sensitization in successive birth cohorts. J Allergy Clin Immunol 109: 969–974.
17. Oryszczyn MP, Annesi I, Neukirch F, Dore MF, Kauffmann F (1995) Longitudinal observations of serum IgE and skin prick test response. Am J Respir Crit Care Med 151: 663–668.
18. Karakaya G, Kalyoncu AF (2006) The natural course of atopy determined by skin prick tests in patients with bronchial asthma and/or rhinitis. Allergol Immunopathol (Madr) 34: 257–262.
19. Linneberg A, Friedrich N, Husemoen LL, Thuesen B, Gonzalez-Quintela A, et al. (2010) Incidence and remission of specific IgE aeroallergen sensitization from age of 40 to 60 years, and association with alcohol consumption. Int Arch Allergy Immunol 151: 142–148.
20. Hughes JL, Brown T, Edgar JD, Shields MD (2010) Peanut allergy and allergic airways inflammation. Pediatr Allergy Immunol 21: 1107–1113.
21. Burney PG, Luczynska C, Chinn S, Jarvis D (1994) The European Community Respiratory Health Survey. Eur Respir J 7: 954–960.
22. Bjornsson E, Janson C, Plaschke P, Norrman E, Sjoberg O (1996) Prevalence of sensitization to food allergens in adult Swedes. Ann Allergy Asthma Immunol 77: 327–332.
23. Gislason D, Bjornsson E, Gislason T, Janson C, Sjoberg O, et al. (1999) Sensitization to airborne and food allergens in Reykjavik (Iceland) and Uppsala (Sweden) - a comparative study. Allergy 54: 1160–1167.
24. (2002) The European Community Respiratory Health Survey II. Eur Respir J 20: 1071–1079.
25. Olafsdottir IS, Gislason T, Thjodleifsson B, Olafsson I, Gislason D, et al. (2005) C reactive protein levels are increased in non-allergic but not allergic asthma: a multicentre epidemiological study. Thorax 60: 451–454.
26. Bousquet J, Chanez P, Chanal I, Michel FB (1990) Comparison between RAST and Pharmacia CAP system: a new automated specific IgE assay. J Allergy Clin Immunol 85: 1039–1043.
27. Burney P, Summers C, Chinn S, Hooper R, van Ree R, et al. (2010) Prevalence and distribution of sensitization to foods in the European Community Respiratory Health Survey: a EuroPrevall analysis. Allergy 65: 1182–1188.
28. Young E, Stoneham MD, Petruckevitch A, Barton J, Rona R (1994) A population study of food intolerance. The Lancet 343: 1127–1130.
29. Sampson HA (1996) Epidemiology of food allergy. Pediatr Allergy Immunol 7: 42–50.
30. Eggesbo M, Halvorsen R, Tambs K, Botten G (1999) Prevalence of parentally perceived adverse reactions to food in young children. Pediatr Allergy Immunol 10: 122–132.
31. Sicherer SH, Leung DY (2013) Advances in allergic skin disease, anaphylaxis, and hypersensitivity reactions to foods, drugs, and insects in 2012. J Allergy Clin Immunol 131: 55–66.
32. Skypala I (2011) Adverse food reactions–an emerging issue for adults. J Am Diet Assoc 111: 1877–1891.
33. Kulig M, Bergmann R, Klettke U, Wahn V, Tacke U, et al. (1999) Natural course of sensitization to food and inhalant allergens during the first 6 years of life. J Allergy Clin Immunol 103: 1173–1179.
34. Ramesh S (2008) Food allergy overview in children. Clin Rev Allergy Immunol 34: 217–230.
35. Rawle FC, Burr ML, Platts-Mills TA (1983) Long-term falls in antibodies to dust mite and pollen allergens in patients with asthma or hay fever. Clin Allergy 13: 409–417.
36. Carsin AE, Zock JP, Jarvis D, Basagana X, Heinrich J, et al. (2013) Serum total immunoglobulin E is a surrogate of atopy in adult-onset asthma: a longitudinal study. Int Arch Allergy Immunol 160: 387–392.
37. Barbee RA, Halonen M, Kaltenborn W, Lebowitz M, Burrows B (1987) A longitudinal study of serum IgE in a community cohort: correlations with age, sex, smoking, and atopic status. J Allergy Clin Immunol 79: 919–927.
38. Jackola DR, Blumenthal MN, Rosenberg A (2004) Evidence for two independent distributions of serum immunoglobulin E in atopic families: cognate and non-cognate IgE. Hum Immunol 65: 20–30.
39. Sherrill DL, Stein R, Halonen M, Holberg CJ, Wright A, et al. (1999) Total serum IgE and its association with asthma symptoms and allergic sensitization among children. J Allergy Clin Immunol 104: 28–36.
40. Linneberg A, Nielsen NH, Madsen F, Frolund L, Dirksen A, et al. (2000) Increasing prevalence of specific IgE to aeroallergens in an adult population: two cross-sectional surveys 8 years apart: the Copenhagen Allergy Study. J Allergy Clin Immunol 106: 247–252.
41. Paganelli R, Ansotegui IJ, Sastre J, Lange CE, Roovers MH, et al. (1998) Specific IgE antibodies in the diagnosis of atopic disease. Clinical evaluation of a new in vitro test system, UniCAP, in six European allergy clinics. Allergy 53: 763–768.

Anti-Allergic Role of Cholinergic Neuronal Pathway via α7 Nicotinic ACh Receptors on Mucosal Mast Cells in a Murine Food Allergy Model

Takeshi Yamamoto[1], Toshihisa Kodama[1], Jaemin Lee[1], Naho Utsunomiya[1], Shusaku Hayashi[1], Hiroshi Sakamoto[2], Hirofumi Kuramoto[3], Makoto Kadowaki[1]*

1 Division of Gastrointestinal Pathophysiology, Institute of Natural Medicine, University of Toyama, Toyama, Toyama, Japan, **2** Department of Physical Therapy, Health Science University, Fujikawaguchiko, Yamanashi, Japan, **3** Department of Applied Biology, Kyoto Institute of Technology, Kyoto, Kyoto, Japan

Abstract

The prevalence of food allergy (FA) has increased in developed countries over the past few decades. However, no effective drug therapies are currently available. Therefore, we investigated cholinergic anti-inflammatory pathway as a regulatory system to ameliorate disrupted mucosal immune homeostasis in the gut based on the pathophysiological elucidation of mucosal mast cells (MMCs) in a murine FA model. BALB/c mice sensitized with ovalbumin received repeated oral ovalbumin for the development of FA. FA mice developed severe allergic diarrhea and exhibited enhanced type 2 helper T (Th2) cell immune responses in both systemic immunity and mucosal immunity, along with MMCs hyperplasia in the colon. MMCs were localized primarily in the strategic position of the mucosal epithelium. Furthermore, the allergic symptoms did not develop in p85α disrupted phosphoinositide-3 kinase-deficient mice that lacked mast cells in the gut. Vagal stimulation by 2-deoxy-D-glucose and drug treatment with nicotinic ACh receptor (nAChR) agonists (nicotine and α7 nAChR agonist GTS-21) alleviated the allergic symptoms in the FA mice. Nicotine treatment suppressed MMCs hyperplasia, enhanced MPO and upregulated mRNA expression of Th1 and Th2 cytokines in the FA mice colon. MMCs, which are negatively regulated by α7 nAChRs, were often located in close proximity to cholinergic CGRP-immunoreactive nerve fibers in the FA mice colon. The present results reveal that the cholinergic neuroimmune interaction via α7 nAChRs on MMCs is largely involved in maintaining intestinal immune homeostasis and can be a target for a new therapy against mucosal immune diseases with homeostatic disturbances such as FA.

Editor: Kenji Hashimoto, Chiba University Center for Forensic Mental Health, Japan

Funding: This research was supported by a Grant-in-Aid for Scientific Research from the Ministry of Education, Culture, Sports, Science and Technology of Japan (http://www.jsps.go.jp/j-grantsinaid/index.html) to T. Yamamoto (No. 25460891) and M. Kadowaki (No. 24590879). The funders had no role in study design, data collection and analysis, decision to publish, or preparation of the manuscript.

Competing Interests: The authors have declared that no competing interests exist.

* E-mail: makotok@inm.u-toyama.ac.jp

Introduction

Food allergy (FA) is an abnormal immunologic reaction to food proteins, and its prevalence has increased in developed countries over the past few decades. However, the pathogenic mechanisms underlying FA are not fully understood, and no effective drug therapies are yet available. The only way to avoid allergic reactions to food is to avoid the foods that trigger these responses [1].

It is well known that type 2 helper T (Th2) cell-biased immune responses are responsible for allergic diseases. There is a growing body of work that has examined the interaction between T cells and mast cells and how these relationships might alter immunity to foreign antigens [2]. Th2 cell-associated cytokines, such as IL-4, IL-5, IL-9 and IL-13, are involved in B cell class switching to IgE and in the differentiation and maturation of mast cells and Th2 cells [3,4,5].

In the pathological Th2 cell-biased immunological environment, mast cells are usually positioned close to the external environment to respond to the pathogens, and mast cells play a central role as an effector cell and a conductor cell in the pathogenesis of various allergic diseases [5,6]. The activation of mast cells results in the release of various inflammatory mediators, such as proteases, eicosanoids, biogenic amines, cytokines and chemokines [2]. Despite their strategic location in the mucosa of the intestinal microenvironment, the role of mast cells in FA has not been well investigated.

We previously demonstrated that the number of mucosal mast cells (MMCs) is greatly increased in the colonic mucosa of ovalbumin (OVA)-induced FA mice [7]. Mast cells are classified as MMCs or connective tissue mast cells (CTMCs). Considerable evidence has demonstrated that MMCs are morphologically, biochemically and functionally distinct from CTMCs [2]. CTMCs reside in connective tissues, such as the skin, whereas MMC progenitors migrate to intestinal or bronchial mucosal tissues, where MMCs are able to mature following antigen exposure. CTMCs contain high concentrations of histamine in their granules and mainly contribute to allergic symptoms, such as congestion, itch, urticaria and anaphylaxis, whereas MMCs contain low concentrations of histamine [8]. Consequently, anti-histamine agents have no effect on FA. Furthermore, CTMC stabilizers (e.g., tranilast, ketotifen, and cromolyn) are frequently used for the treatment of various allergic disorders, while these stabilizers fail to exert therapeutic effects on FA, which is supported by our finding that these stabilizers are not able to suppress MMC activation [9].

Recent advances in neuroscience and immunology have revealed a bidirectional interaction between the nervous and immune systems. Therefore, the function of the intestine may be modulated by neuro-immune interactions, but this interaction is not fully understood. Mast cells are ubiquitous in the body, and these cells are often found in close proximity to nerve fibers in various tissues, including the lamina propria of the intestine [3,4,10,11]. Mast cells and nerves are assumed to communicate bilaterally to modulate neuro-physiological effects and mast cell functions [12], which suggests that the neuro-immune interaction may be involved in the pathology of allergic diseases.

Until now, findings on the cholinergic regulation of immune responses have been accumulated in various inflammatory experimental models [13,14,15,16], while there has been little information obtained on the cholinergic control in allergic models, especially in FA models. We have already shown that nicotine exerts an inhibitory effect on antigen-induced degranulation in mucosal-type murine bone marrow-derived mast cells (mBMMCs) through α7 nicotinic ACh receptors (nAChRs), which is reversed by the α7 nAChR antagonist methyllycaconitine [17].

Therefore, an elucidation of the cholinergic regulatory pathway has provided new concepts in understanding and treating FA.

Materials and Methods

Ethics statement

This study was carried out in strict accordance with the recommendations in the Guide for the Care and Use of Laboratory Animals of the National Institutes of Health. The Animal Experiment Committee at the University of Toyama approved all of the animal care procedures and experiments (authorization no. S-2009 INM-9).

Animals

Male BALB/c mice, C57BL/6 mice and BALB/c nude (nu/nu) mice (5 weeks old) were purchased from Japan SLC (Shizuoka, Japan). BALB/c background p85α subunit-disrupted class Ia phosphoinositide-3 kinase (PI3K)-deficient ($PI3K^{-/-}$) mice were gifted from Drs. Shigeo Koyasu (Keio University, Tokyo, Japan) and Takashi Kadowaki (the University of Tokyo, Tokyo, Japan). All mice were housed in the experimental animal facility at the University of Toyama and were provided free access to food and water.

Induction of food allergy

The murine model of FA was initiated as described previously.8 Briefly, male BALB/c mice (5 weeks old) were sensitized twice at 2-week intervals using an intraperitoneal injection of 50 μg OVA (fraction V; Sigma-Aldrich, St. Louis, MO) in the presence of 1.3 mg/100 μl aluminium hydroxide gel adjuvant (Sigma-Aldrich). Two weeks after systemic priming, the mice received repeated oral administrations of 50 mg/0.3 ml OVA every other day. Diarrhea resulting from FA was assessed by visual monitoring for up to 1 hour following oral challenge. Profuse liquid stool was detected as allergic diarrhea, and the diarrhea-presenting mice were considered to be FA mice.

For the pharmacological evaluation of an activation of nicotinic AChRs (nAChRs) in the FA model, a non-selective nAChR agonist nicotine (Sigma-Aldrich) or a selective α7 nAChR agonist GTS-21 (10 mg/kg, Taiho, Tokushima, Japan) was subcutaneously administered to mice 1 hour before the oral OVA challenges. A central vagal stimulant 2-deoxy-D-glucose (2-DG, 200 mg/kg, Sigma-Aldrich) was intraperitoneally administered 30 minutes before OVA challenges. Furthermore, hexamethonium (C6, 100 mg/kg, Sigma-Aldrich) as a non-selective nAChR antagonist was intraperitoneally administered 30 minutes before 2-DG administration. A CTMC stabilizer disodium cromoglycate (cromolyn, 100 mg/g, Sigma-Aldrich), a CTMC and MMC stabilizer doxantrazole (10 mg/kg, Sigma-Aldrich) or an anti-inflammatory drug prednisolone (10 mg/kg, Sigma-Aldrich) was administered 1 hour before OVA challenges.

One hour after the 6th oral OVA challenge, the proximal colon and spleen were used for morphological and biological analyses, and plasma was for measurement of OVA-specific IgE and mouse mast cell protease (mMCP)-1 (a marker of mouse MMCs) levels. Plasma OVA-specific IgE level was measured using an ELISA kit (DS Pharma Biomedical, Osaka, Japan). Plasma mMCP-1 level was measured using an ELISA kit (Moredun Scientific). These measurements were performed according to the manufacturers' instructions.

Measurement of myeloperoxidase activity

One hour after the 6th oral OVA challenge, the entire colon of each mouse was excised. Each colon was weighed and cut into small pieces. The colon was homogenized on ice in 1 ml of 0.5% hexadecyltrimethylammonium bromide in 50 mM potassium phosphate buffer (pH 6.0) using a Polytron homogenizer (Kinematica, Littau, Switzerland) and fortified with an additional quantity of the same buffer to 100 mg of the colon in 1 ml. The homogenate was frozen and thawed three times and then was vortex-mixed. The suspension was centrifuged at 15,000×*g* for 20 minutes at 4°C. Myeloperoxidase (MPO) activity of the resulting supernatant was measured. The supernatant (100 μl) was vortex-mixed with 2.87 ml of 0.5 mM *o*-dianisidine in 50 mM potassium phosphate buffer (pH 6.0) and 30 μl of 0.05% hydrogen peroxide. The mixture was measured spectrophotometrically at 460 nm for 4 minutes of incubation. MPO activity is expressed as units per wet weight of the colon in grams (gwwt).

Expression of cytokine mRNA

One hour after the 6th oral OVA challenge, 2 cm of the proximal colon and spleen were excised. Total RNA was extracted from the tissues using Sepasol Super (Nacalai Tesque, Kyoto, Japan) according to the manufacturer's instructions. Reverse transcription was performed using the Exscript RT reagent kit (Takara Bio, Ohtsu, Japan) and random primers, followed by real-time PCR. Real-time PCR amplification of IL-4, IL-5, IFN-γ and GAPDH was performed using SYBR Premix Ex Taq (Takara Bio). The following primer pairs were used:

IL-4, forward 5′-GGTCTCAACCCCCAGCTAGT-3′ and reverse 5′-GCCGATGATCTCTCTCAAGTGAT-3′;

IL-5, forward 5′-GAAGTGTGGCGAGGAGAGAC-3′ and reverse 5′-GCACAGTTTTGTGGGGTTTT-3′;

IFN-γ, forward 5′-CGGCACAGTCATTGAAAGCCTA-3′ and reverse 5′-GTTGCTGATGGCCTGATTGTC-3′;

GAPDH, forward 5′-TGACCACAGTCCATGCCATC-3′ and reverse 5′-GACGGACACATTGGGGGTAG-3′.

The PCR reaction conditions consisted of 10 seconds at 95°C followed by 40 cycles of 5 seconds at 95°C and 20 seconds at 63°C. Target mRNA levels were normalized to those of GAPDH as an internal control in each sample. The results are expressed as the ratio relative to the naïve group average.

Morphological analysis

One hour after the 6th oral OVA challenge, the proximal colon was excised. The proximal colon was fixed with 4% paraformaldehyde (w/v) in 0.1 M sodium phosphate buffer (PB; pH 7.3) and immersed for 12–18 hours at 4°C. The tissue was washed with 0.01 M phosphate-buffered saline (PBS; pH 7.3), cryoprotected with 30% sucrose in 0.01 M PBS and embedded in OCT compound. Frozen sections (25 μm) were cut at −20°C using a cryostat microtome (Leica Microsystems, Nussloch, Germany). The sections were soaked for 12–18 hours in 0.01 M PBS containing 0.3% Triton X-100 to increase permeability, and they were then exposed to normal donkey serum (1:10; Jackson Immunoresearch Laboratories, West Grove, PA) for 30 minutes to reduce the nonspecific binding of antisera and washed in 0.01 M PBS. The sections were exposed to each primary antibody for 12–18 hours, washed with 0.01 M PBS and incubated with the appropriate secondary antibody for 2 hours. All incubations were performed at room temperature. The following primary antibodies were used: goat anti-choline acetyltransferase (ChAT) (1:200; Chemicon, Temecula, CA), sheep anti-mouse mast cell protease (mMCP)-1 (1:5,000; Moredun Scientific, Midlothian, UK) and rabbit anti- CGRP (1:10,000; Chemicon). Cy3-conjugated donkey anti-sheep IgG (1:200; Jackson Immunoresearch Laboratories, West Grove, PA) and Alexa 488-conjugated donkey anti-rabbit IgG (1:200; Jackson Immunoresearch Laboratories) were used as secondary antibodies. The preparations were examined using a fluorescence microscope (IX71 system; Olympus, Tokyo, Japan) with a U-MWIG3 filter set (Olympus) and photographed using an Olympus digital camera (DP70; Olympus). The preparations were also observed using confocal laser-scanning microscopy (LSM700; Carl Zeiss, Oberkochen, Germany) to examine the proximity between mMCP-1-positive cells and CGRP-immunoreactive (IR) nerve fibers in the colonic mucosa of the FA mice. Stacks of confocal sections were three-dimensionally reconstructed and observed using Imaris software (Bitplane, Zurich, Switzerland). Surface rendering of each channel was performed in an optimal intensity threshold setting. The intensity threshold setting was optimized by visual comparison between the original and the three-dimensional rendered result.

Furthermore, a segment of the proximal colon was opened along the mesenteric border and fixed with 4% paraformaldehyde. The whole-mount preparation of longitudinal muscle with adherent enteric plexus was dissected from the proximal colon, and the aforementioned immunohistochemical procedures were performed to examine the ChAT and CGRP immunoreactivities in nerve cell bodies of the enteric neurons.

Sections (1 μm thick) of the fixed colon embedded in LR white resin (Sigma-Aldrich) were stained with 1% toluidine blue and observed with light microscopy for the analysis of mast cells.

The brightness and contrast of the images were modified using Adobe Photoshop Elements 2.0 (Adobe Systems, San Jose, CA).

Electron microscopy

For electron microscopy, the FA mice were perfusion-fixed with 2% paraformaldehyde and 2.5% glutaraldehyde in 0.1 M PB and the proximal colon was removed. The colon was transversely sectioned into 0.5–1.0 mm thick sections with a razor blade. The sections were post-fixed for 1 hour by 1% OsO_4 in 0.1 M PB, dehydrated in graded ethanol and embedded in EPON 812 (Shell Chemical, Houston, Tex). Ultrathin sections were cut using an LKB 2088-V ultramicrotome (LKB, Bromma, Sweden). The ultrathin sections were collected on copper grids, stained with lead citrate and uranyl acetate and examined with an electron microscope (H-7500, Hitachi, Tokyo, Japan).

Statistical analysis

The data are expressed as the means ±SE. The statistical comparisons were performed using Student's unpaired *t*-test, the chi-squared test and one-way repeated measures ANOVA followed by Tukey's HSD. A significant difference was defined as $P<0.05$.

Results

Induction of food allergy in mice

Repeated oral OVA challenges to systemically OVA primed mice produced FA associated with allergic diarrhea in Th2-prone BALB/c mice (FA mice, $n=5–7$), but not in Th1-prone C57BL/6 mice ($n=8$) (Figure 1A). The occurrence of allergic diarrhea reached about 80.0% after the 6th OVA challenge. However, repeated OVA challenges without systemic OVA priming did not induce allergic diarrhea in BALB/c mice ($n=5$) (Figure 1A).

The plasma level of OVA-specific IgE was elevated after the systemic OVA priming, and subsequent repeated oral OVA challenges caused a remarkable elevation of the OVA-specific IgE level (naïve mice 0.0±0.0 μg/ml, OVA primed mice

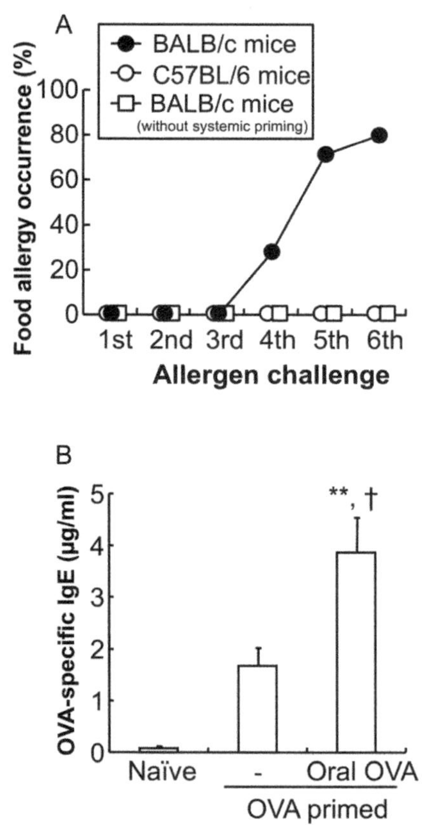

Figure 1. Induction of Th2-mediated food allergy. The allergic responses were induced by two instances of systemic OVA priming and repeated oral OVA (50 mg) challenges. *A*: Systemically primed BALB/c mice (closed circle) and C57BL/6 mice (open circle) and non-systemically primed BALB/c mice (open square) were subjected to food allergy (FA)-inducing oral OVA challenges ($n=5–8$ mice per group). *B*: The level of OVA-specific IgE in the plasma of naïve mice, systemically primed mice, and systemically primed and repeated oral OVA challenged mice is shown. The level of OVA-specific IgE in the plasma was determined using an ELISA kit. Data are expressed as means ±SE. $^{**}P<0.01$ vs. naïve mice. $^{†}P<0.05$ vs. systemically primed mice ($n=5$ mice per group).

1.7±0.2 μg/ml, oral OVA challenged OVA primed mice 3.8±0.7 μg/ml; $^{**}P<0.01$ vs. naïve mice, †$P<0.05$ vs. OVA primed mice; $n=5$ mice per group) (Figure 1B).

Systemic and mucosal immune responses in food allergy mice

The expression of Th1 and Th2 cytokine mRNA was measured using real-time PCR. In systemic immunity (spleen, Figure 2A), mRNA levels of Th2 cytokines (IL-4 and IL-5) were significantly increased in the FA mice (IL-4: naïve mice 1.0±0.2, FA mice 3.7±0.8, $^{*}P<0.05$ vs. naïve mice; IL-5: naïve mice 1.0±0.4, FA mice 3.2±0.9, $^{*}P<0.05$ vs. naïve mice; $n=5$–6 mice per group), whereas the Th1 cytokine (IFN-γ) mRNA level was significantly decreased in the FA mice (naïve mice 1.0±0.1, FA mice 0.5±0.1; $^{**}P<0.01$ vs. naïve mice; $n=6$ mice per group). On the other hand, in mucosal immunity (proximal colon, Figure 2B), Th2 cytokine (IL-4 and IL-5) mRNA levels were significantly increased in the FA mice (IL-4: naïve mice 1.0±0.7, FA mice 2.9±0.6, $^{*}P<0.05$ vs. naïve mice; IL-5: naïve mice 1.0±0.2, FA mice 11.3±1.4, $^{**}P<0.01$ vs. naïve mice; $n=4$ mice per group), and the Th1 cytokine (IFN-γ) mRNA level exhibited a tendency to be increased in the FA mice (naïve mice 1.0±0.3, FA mice 2.4±0.8; $n=5$–8 mice per group).

Mucosal mast cell hyperplasia in the colon of food allergy mice

We investigated mucosal mast cells in the proximal colon by immunohistochemistry. As shown in Figure 3A, very few MMCs (mMCP-1-positive cells) were scattered in the lamina propria and submucosal layer of the mice colon two weeks after twice systemic OVA priming. The distribution of MMCs was similar to that in the proximal colon of the vehicle-treated control mice. MMCs began to occur in the mucosal epithelium of the primed mice proximal colon two days after the second oral OVA administration, and the number of MMCs was dramatically elevated in the mucosal epithelium of the primed mice colon in proportion to the OVA challenge time. MMCs were localized primarily in the mucosal epithelium of the upper half of the crypts throughout the primed mice colon two days after the fifth oral OVA administration.

To investigate the degranulation of mucosal mast cells, we measured the concentration of plasma mMCP-1 by ELISA (Figure 3B). There was no detectable plasma mMCP-1 in naïve mice. In contrast, the repeated OVA challenges resulted in a dramatic increase in the plasma mMCP-1 level (naïve mice 0.0±0.0 μg/ml, FA mice 29.0±8.0 μg/ml; $^{**}P<0.01$ vs. naïve mice; $n=5$ mice per group).

Involvement of T cell in the development of food allergy in mice

In the FA mouse model, we used BALB/c nude mice that lack functional T cells due to their thymus deficiency. The nude mice did not exhibit any sign of allergic responses following exposure to

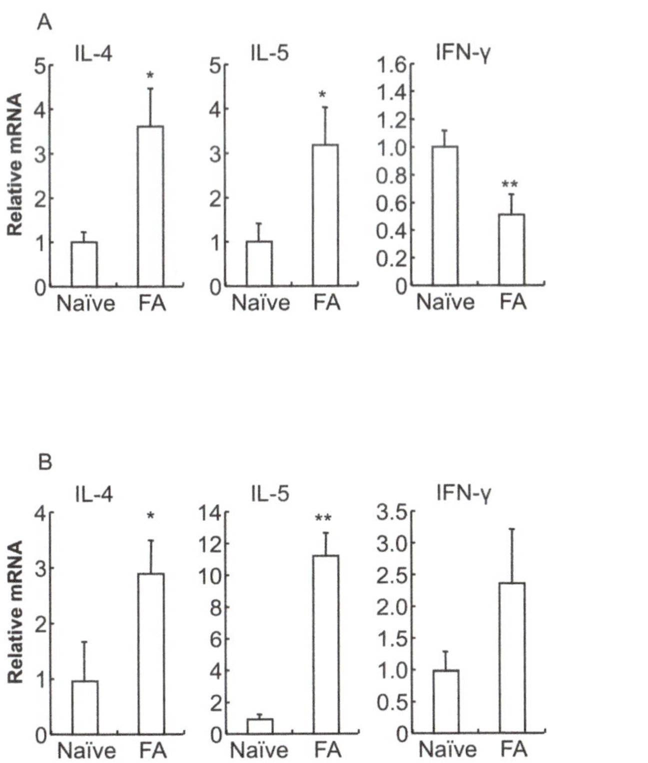

Figure 2. Induction of predominant Th2 cytokine responses in food allergy mice. IL-4, IL-5 and IFN-γ cytokine mRNA expression in the spleen (*A*) and proximal colon (*B*) from naïve mice and FA mice were measured by real-time PCR. Relative mRNA levels of cytokines were normalized to GAPDH expression. Data are expressed as means ±SE. $^{*}P<0.05$, $^{**}P<0.01$ vs. naïve mice ($n=4$–8 mice per group).

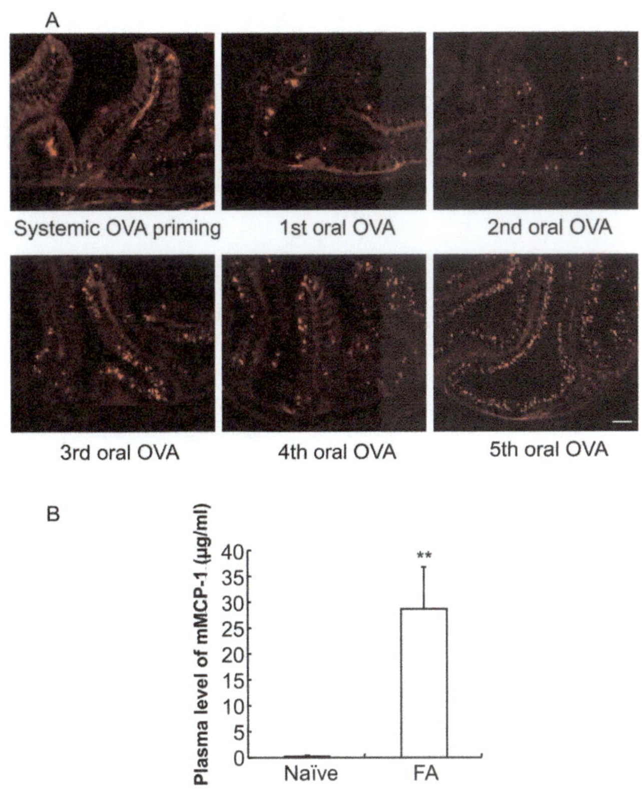

Figure 3. Mucosal mast cell hyperplasia and degranulation in the colon of food allergy mice. *A*: The proximal colons of systemically OVA primed mice and oral OVA-challenged mice after each oral OVA challenge were stained with anti-mouse mast cell protease-1 (mMCP-1) antibodies. Scale bar represents 200 μm. *B*: The concentration of mMCP-1 in the plasma of naïve mice and FA mice is shown. The concentration of mMCP-1 in the plasma was determined using an ELISA kit. Data are expressed as means ±SE. $^{**}P<0.01$ vs. naïve mice ($n=5$ mice per group).

repeated oral allergen challenges (Figure 4A, $n = 5$ mice per group) and that OVA-specific IgE and mMCP-1 were not detected in the plasma of nude naïve mice and nude FA mice (Figure 4B: **$P<$ 0.01 vs. wild-type (WT) naïve mice, ††$P<0.01$ vs. WT FA mice: $n = 3$–5 mice per group; Figure 4C: *$P<0.05$ vs. WT naïve mice, ††$P<0.01$ vs. WT FA mice: $n = 3$–5 mice per group). Furthermore, no increase of mucosal mast cells was observed in the mucosal layer of the proximal colons of nude FA mice as compared to those of WT mice in the FA model (Figure 4D).

Characteristics of mast cells in the colon of food allergy mice

Mast cells were observed in the proximal colon of the FA mice and contained many granules intensely stained with toluidine blue (Figure 5A). Only a few mast cells were observed in the lamina propria. These mast cells contained numerous granules in the cytoplasm, most of which exhibited reddish violet metachromasia with toluidine blue (Figure 5B), indicating that these mast cells exhibit properties of CTMCs because in rodents, CTMC granules stain purple, and MMC granules stain blue with toluidine blue [18]. However, a few granules in these mast cells in the lamina

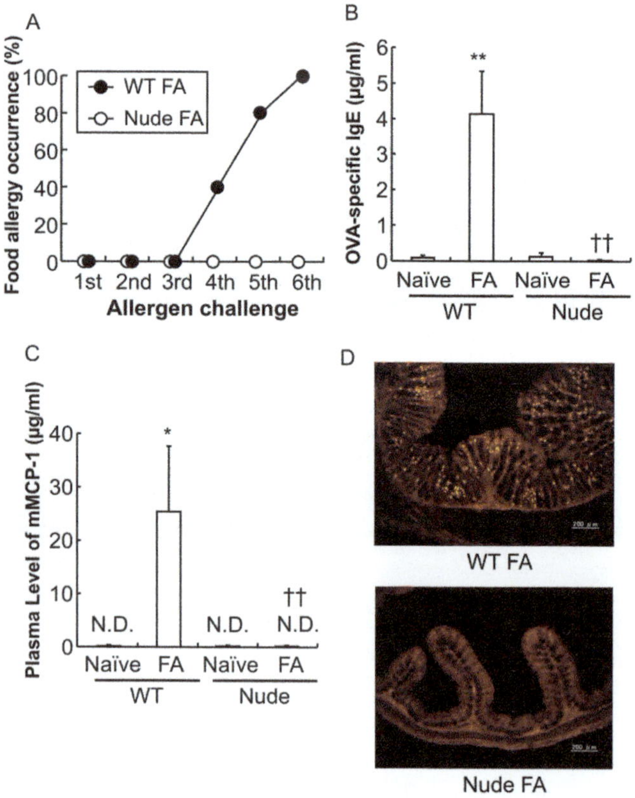

Figure 4. Induction of food allergy in athymic nude mice. *A*: The occurrence of allergic diarrhea in wild-type (WT) FA mice and nude FA mice after each oral OVA challenge is shown (n = 5 mice per group). *B*: The level of OVA-specific IgE in the plasma of WT naïve mice, WT FA mice, nude naïve mice and nude FA mice is shown. The level of OVA-specific IgE in the plasma was determined using an ELISA kit. **$P<0.01$ vs. WT naïve mice, ††$P<0.01$ vs. WT FA mice ($n = 3$–5 mice per group). *C*: The level of mMCP-1 in the plasma of WT naïve mice, WT FA mice, nude naïve mice and nude FA mice is shown. The level of mMCP-1 in the plasma was determined using an ELISA kit. *$P<0.05$ vs. WT naïve mice, ††$P<0.01$ vs. WT FA mice ($n = 3$–5 mice per group). *D*: The proximal colon of WT FA mice and nude FA mice after the 6th oral OVA challenge was stained with anti-mMCP-1 antibodies. Scale bars represent 200 µm.

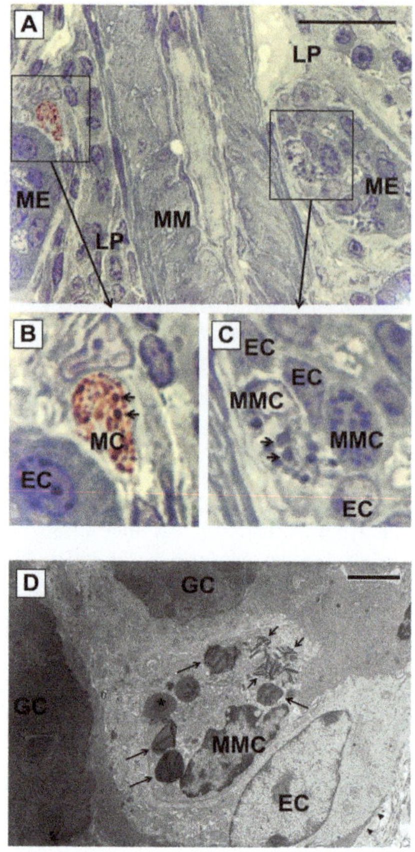

Figure 5. Morphology of mast cells in the colon of food allergy mice. Sections (1 µm thick) of the fixed colon embedded in resin were stained with 1% toluidine blue and were observed with light microscopy for the analysis of mast cells. *A*: On the left hand side of the picture, a mast cell (surrounded by a square) with metachromatic granules was observed in the lamina propria. On the other side, two mast cells (surrounded with another square) with nonmetachromatic granules were localized in the mucosal epithelium. ME: mucosal epithelium, LP: lamina propria, MM: muscularis mucosa. Scale bar represents 50 µm. *B*: An image of higher magnification of the mast cell in the lamina propria. Most of granules of the mast cell exhibited metachromasia, but a few granules (arrows) were nonmetachromatic. MC: mast cell, EC: epithelial cell. *C*: An image of higher magnification of mucosal mast cells (MMCs) in the mucosal epithelium. The granules in MMCs did not exhibit metachromasia and some of the granules were polymorphic in shape (arrows). MMC: mucosal mast cell. *D*: Electron microscopic analysis of mucosal mast cells in the proximal colon of food allergy mice. A variety of morphologies of granules was seen in a MMC: one (asterisk) showed amorphous inner structure, some (long arrows) showed crystals with amorphous matrix and others (short arrows) seemed to be occupied by the crystalline structure. Arrowheads indicate basement membrane. GC: goblet cell. Scale bar represents 4 µm.

propria were nonmetachromatic and were larger than metachromatic granules (Figure 5B; arrows).

Many MMCs were observed in the mucosal epithelium, and the majority of MMC granules were larger (Figure 5C) and were spherical or polymorphic in shape (Figure 5C; arrows). In addition, these MMC granules, which exhibited nonmetachromasia, were strongly stained with toluidine blue, but some were weakly stained.

Ultrastructural characteristics of mucosal mast cells in food allergy mice

MMCs in the mucosal epithelium of the FA mice proximal colon have been examined with the electron microscope (Figure 5D). Many MMCs were observed within the mucosal epithelium, and they were characterized by the presence of peculiar large granules (0.5–2.5 μm) in the cytoplasm. MMCs had specific granules of varying size, shape and electron-density. Many of the granules (Figure 5D, long arrows) contained crystalline inclusions with cylindrical shape and had irregular contours and showed polymorphic shapes. Other granules seemed to be occupied by crystalline structures (Figure 5D, short arrows). Some of the granules had relatively homogeneous matrix with round or oval contours without the crystalline inclusion (Figure 5D, asterisk).

Critical involvement of mast cells in the pathogenesis of food allergy in mice

Mice that specifically lack only mast cells have not been reported/generated; two mouse strains, WBB6F1/J-Kit^{W}/Kit^{W-v} and C57BL/6-Kit^{W-sh}/Kit^{W-sh} are profoundly deficient in mast cells. These mice are most frequently used to analyze the *in vivo* functions of mast cells, but we could not employ these strains to examine the role of mast cells in the induction of FA because the genetic background of these mice is not BALB/c and these mice have other phenotypic abnormalities, such as gastric ulcer and intestinal motility disorder.

Therefore, in this study, we employed PI3K$^{-/-}$ mice with a BALB/c genetic background that exhibit a selective loss of gastrointestinal mast cells [19]. As a result, PI3K$^{-/-}$ mice failed to develop allergic diarrhea (PI3K$^{-/-}$ FA mice) (Figure 6A, $n = 5$ mice per group). As shown in Figure 6B, immunohistochemical staining with the mMCP-1 antibody revealed that MMCs were dramatically increased in the proximal colon of WT FA mice, whereas only a few mast cells were observed in the mucosal layer of PI3K$^{-/-}$ FA mice. Plasma mMCP-1 was almost undetectable in PI3K$^{-/-}$ naïve mice and PI3K$^{-/-}$ FA mice (Figure 6C: $^{**}P<0.01$ vs. WT naïve mice, ††$P<0.01$ vs. WT FA mice; $n = 3–5$ mice per group).

Furthermore, in systemic immunity (spleen, Figure 6D), mRNA levels of Th2 cytokines (IL-4 and IL-5) were increased in PI3K$^{-/-}$ FA mice as compared to PI3K$^{-/-}$ naïve mice (IL-4: $^{*}P<0.05$ vs. WT naïve mice, $^{**}P<0.01$ vs. PI3K$^{-/-}$ naïve mice; IL-5: $^{**}P<0.01$ vs. WT naïve mice; $n = 4–7$ mice per group), which is similar to those in WT FA mice. On the other hand, in mucosal immunity (proximal colon, Figure 6E, lower expression of mRNA for Th2 cytokines was found in PI3K$^{-/-}$ FA mice as compared to WT FA mice (IL-4: $^{*}P<0.05$ vs. WT naïve mice, ††$P<0.01$ vs. WT FA mice; IL-5: $^{*}P<0.05$ vs. WT naïve mice; $n = 4–7$ mice per group).

Effect of mast cell stabilizers on the induction of food allergy in mice

The critical involvement of MMCs in the pathogenesis of FA was pharmacologically investigated in the FA model. The subcutaneous administration of a CTMC and MMC dual stabilizer doxantrazole (10 mg/kg) completely prevented the allergic responses following exposure to repeated oral allergen challenges, whereas the oral treatment with cromolyn (100 mg/kg), a CTMC stabilizer failed to suppress these responses (Figure 7: $^{**}P<0.01$ vs. FA mice; $n = 10–15$ mice per group). In addition, mice treated with an anti-inflammatory drug prednisolone (10 mg/kg) did not exhibit any sign of allergic diarrhea in the FA model.

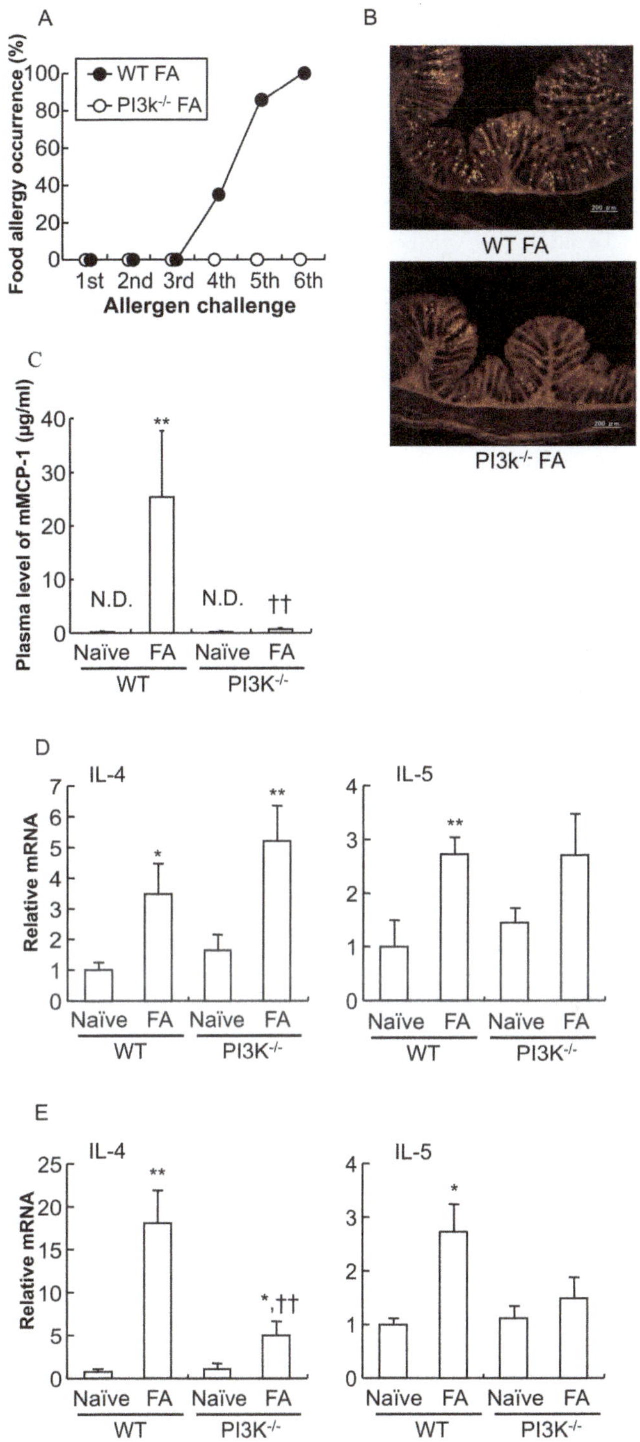

Figure 6. Induction of food allergy in PI3K-deficient mice. PI3K$^{-/-}$ mice as a gastrointestinal mast cell-deficient murine model were subjected to FA-inducing oral OVA challenges. *A*: The occurrence of allergic diarrhea in WT mice (WT FA mice) and PI3K$^{-/-}$ mice (PI3K$^{-/-}$ FA mice) after each oral OVA challenge is shown ($n = 5$ mice per group). *B*: The proximal colon of FA-induced PI3K$^{-/-}$ mice after oral OVA challenge was stained with anti- mMCP-1 antibodies. Scale bars represent 200 μm. *C*: The level of mMCP-1 in the plasma of PI3K$^{-/-}$ naïve mice and PI3K$^{-/-}$ FA mice is shown. The level of mMCP-1 in the plasma was determined using an ELISA kit. Data are expressed as means ±SE. $^{**}P<0.01$ vs. WT naïve mice, ††$P<0.01$ vs. WT FA mice ($n = 3–5$ mice per group). IL-4 and IL-5 cytokine mRNA expression in the spleen (*D*) and proximal colon (*E*) from WT naïve mice, WT FA mice, PI3K$^{-/-}$

naïve mice and PI3K$^{-/-}$ FA mice were measured by real-time PCR. Relative mRNA levels of cytokines were normalized to GAPDH expression. *$P<0.05$, **$P<0.01$ vs. each naïve mice, ††$P<0.01$ vs. WT FA mice ($n=4$–7 mice per group).

Cholinergic anti-inflammatory pathway in food allergy mice

To investigate whether vagal activity influences the development of FA, we examined the effect of 2-deoxy-D-glucose (2-DG), a central vagal stimulant on the FA model. Intraperitoneal injection of 2-DG (200 mg/kg) significantly ameliorated allergic diarrhea. After the 6th OVA challenge, the occurrence of allergic diarrhea was significantly decreased from 100.0% to 54.5% (Figure 8A: *$P<0.05$ vs. vehicle, $n=11$–18 mice per group). The therapeutic effect of 2-DG was significantly blocked by the subcutaneous injection of the non-selective nAChR antagonist hexamethonium (C6) at 32 mg/kg (Figure 8A: †$P<0.05$ vs. 2-DG, $n=11$ mice per group).

We next examined the therapeutic effect of nAChR activation on the development of FA. The subcutaneous injection of nicotine attenuated the induction of allergic diarrhea at 1 and 3.2 mg/kg (Figure 8B: *$P<0.05$, **$P<0.01$ vs. FA mice, $n=10$–74 mice per group). The selective α7 nAChR agonist GTS-21 was used to determine whether α7 nAChR mediated the therapeutic effect of nicotine. The subcutaneous injection of GTS-21 (10 mg/kg) resulted in a significant suppression of allergic diarrhea (Figure 8C: *$P<0.05$, **$P<0.01$ vs. FA mice, $n=23$–40 mice per group).

Effect of nicotine treatment on the systemic and mucosal immune responses in food allergy mice

The number of MMCs that was dramatically increased in the proximal colon of the FA mice was significantly decreased in that of nicotine-treated FA mice (Figure 9A).

MPO activity in the colon of the FA mice was significantly increased approximately 2.5-fold compared to that in the naïve mice colon, and the subcutaneous injection of nicotine significantly suppressed the increment of MPO activity in the FA mice (Figure 9B: naïve mice 534.8±56.5 units/gwwt, FA mice 1285.7±123.5 units/gwwt, nicotine-treated FA mice 740.5±138.4 units/gwwt; *$P<0.05$ vs. naïve mice, †$P<0.05$ vs. FA mice; $n=3$–10 mice per group).

In contrast, the plasma level of OVA-specific IgE remained unchanged in nicotine-treated FA mice compared to the FA mice (Figure 9C: naïve mice 0.1±0.0 μg/ml, FA mice 3.8±0.7 μg/ml, nicotine-treated FA mice 4.3±0.4 μg/ml; **$P<0.01$ vs. naïve mice; $n=5$ mice per group).

To investigate the effects of nicotine treatment on the cytokine profile in the FA mice, cytokine mRNA expression was detected by real-time PCR. In systemic immunity (spleen), the upregulated Th2 cytokine (IL-4 and IL-5) mRNA expression observed in the FA mice was not significantly changed by nicotine treatment (Figure 9D: $n=6$ mice per group), which is almost consistent with no effect of nicotine on the enhanced plasma OVA-specific IgE level in the FA mice (Figure 9C). In contrast, the downregulated Th1 cytokine (IFN-γ) mRNA expression observed in the FA mice was significantly increased in nicotine-treated FA mice (Figure 9D: *$P<0.01$ vs. FA mice, $n=6$ mice per group). On the other hand, in mucosal immunity (proximal colon), the upregulated mRNA expression of both Th1 (IFN-γ) and Th2 (IL-4 and IL-5) cytokines was significantly suppressed in nicotine-treated FA mice (Figure 9E: *$P<0.05$, **$P<0.01$ vs. FA mice, $n=3$–6 mice per group).

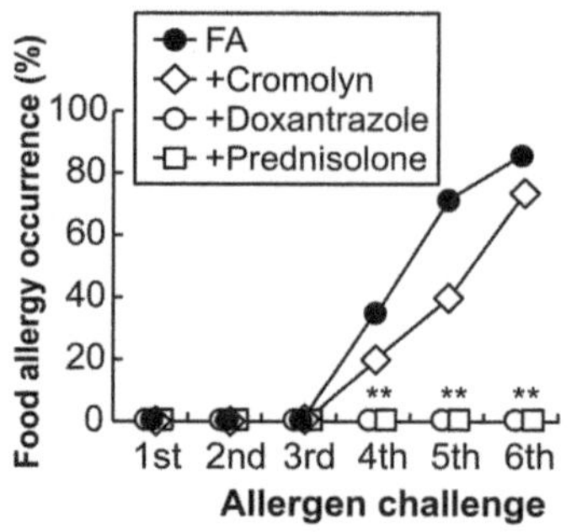

Figure 7. Effect of mast cell stabilizers on the induction of food allergy in mice. The occurrence of allergic diarrhea in FA mice (closed circle) and cromolyn-treated mice (open diamond) after each oral OVA challenge is shown ($n=14$–15 mice per group). In addition, mice treated with the subcutaneous administration of doxantrazole (open circle, 10 mg/kg) or the oral administration of prednisolone (open square, 10 mg/kg) did not exhibit any sign of allergic responses in the FA model. **$P<0.01$ vs. FA mice ($n=10$ mice per each group).

Morphological analysis of mucosal mast cell–cholinergic nerve interactions in the colon of food allergy mice

We have demonstrated that α7 nAChRs are expressed in mBMMCs and that the stimulation of α7 nAChRs can negatively regulate the activation of mBMMCs [17]. Therefore, we investigated the morphological interaction of MMCs and cholinergic nerve fibers in the lamina propria of the FA mouse proximal colon. It was difficult to investigate the morphological interaction of MMCs and cholinergic nerve fibers using two-dimensional images with fine-resolution in the colon. Therefore, digital images acquired by confocal laser-scanning microscopy were three-dimensionally reconstructed and observed using Imaris software (Figure 10A). The majority of mMCP-1-positive MMCs (green) were located in close vicinity of the CGRP-IR cholinergic nerve fibers (red) in the FA mouse proximal colon (Figure 10B, C, D: arrows). Furthermore, we verified that CGRP-IR neurons (Figure 10E: arrows) exhibited ChAT immunoreactivities in the myenteric and submucosal neurons of the mouse enteric nervous system.

Discussion

In this study, we provide evidence that MMCs are primarily responsible for the pathology of the FA model and that the cholinergic neuro-immune interaction via α7 nAChRs on MMCs play a crucial role in controlling pathological immune activation to restore the homeostasis in the intestine.

The neuro-immune interaction can be targeted for the design of novel therapeutic agents for the treatment of intestinal immune diseases.

Our murine FA model exhibited various features of type 1 hypersensitive allergic reactions, such as allergic diarrhea within 1 hour after oral antigen exposure, antigen-specific IgE hyperproduction and MMC hyperplasia and degranulation. In addition, Th1-prone C57BL/6 mice did not develop the allergic diarrhea.

Taken together, these data suggest that enhanced Th2-mediated immune responses are responsible for the pathology of our murine FA model.

In the mRNA analysis of cytokines, the FA mice exhibited Th2-biased immune responses in systemic immunity. On the other hand, in mucosal immunity, Th2 immune responses were significantly enhanced, whereas Th1 immune responses were not decreased, but rather increased, indicating that there is a

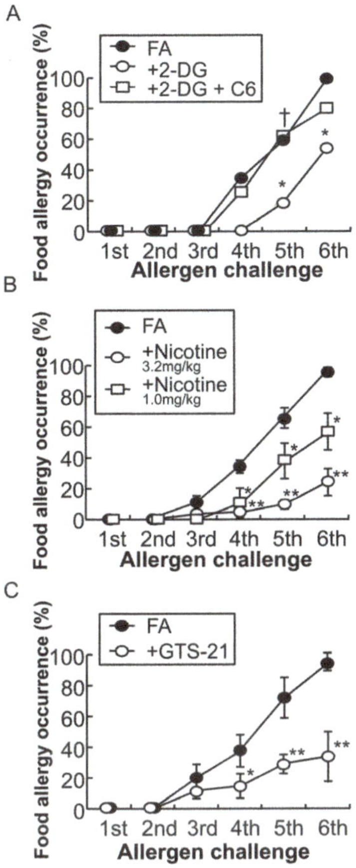

Figure 8. Cholinergic control of food allergy in mice. *A*: The occurrence of allergic diarrhea in FA mice (closed circle), 2-deoxy-d-glucose (2-DG)-treated mice (open circle) and hexamethonium (C6)-treated mice prior to 2-DG administration (open square) after each oral OVA challenge is shown. *$P<0.05$ vs. FA mice. †$P<0.05$ vs. 2-DG mice ($n = 11$–18 mice per group). *B*: The occurrence of allergic diarrhea in FA mice (closed circle) and nicotine-treated mice (3.2 mg/kg; open circle, 1.0 mg/kg; open square, and 0.32 mg/kg; open diamond) after each oral OVA challenge is shown. *$P<0.05$, **$P<0.01$ vs. FA mice ($n = 10$–74 mice per group). *C*: The occurrence of allergic diarrhea in FA mice (closed circle) and GTS-21-treated mice (open circle) after each oral OVA challenge is shown. *$P<0.05$, **$P<0.01$ vs. FA mice ($n = 23$–40 mice per group).

difference between the systemic immune responses and the mucosal immune responses in the FA mice. Furthermore, these enhanced Th2 responses were almost consistent with those observed in other murine OVA-induced FA models, but Th1 responses in the mucosal immunity were different from those in the other models [20,21]. Kweon et al. observed increased IFN-γ production in the spleen and no IFN-γ production in the colon using ELISA in another murine FA model with allergic diarrhea [21], and Brandt et al. reported no change of IFN-γ mRNA expression in the jejunum of their FA mice with allergic diarrhea [20]. These discrepancies may be due to differences in immunization protocols, cytokine measurement methods and tissue segments. Thus, our murine FA model is characterized by the activation of not only Th2 but also Th1 immune responses in the mucosal immunity of the FA mice colon [7].

Furthermore, to determine whether T cells have a pathological role in the development of FA, we examined whether food allergic diarrhea was induced in nude mice that lack functional T cells due

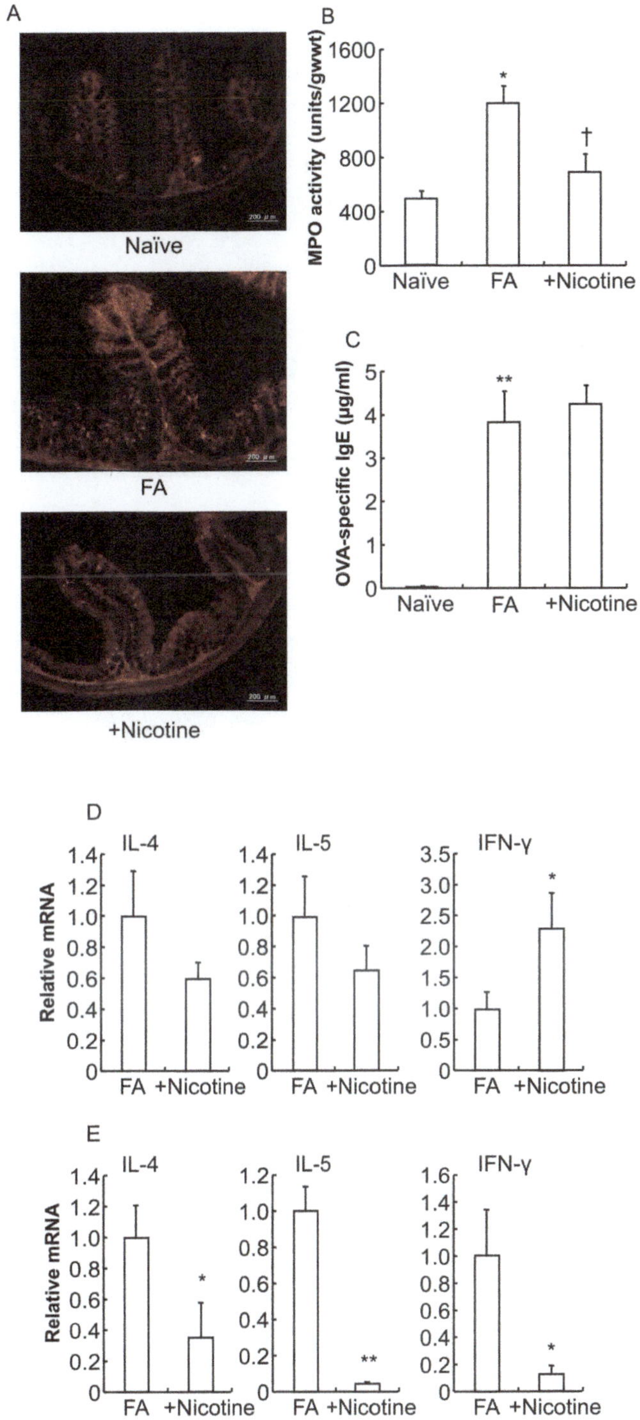

Figure 9. Effect of nicotine on the pathology of food allergy in mice. *A*: The proximal colons of naïve mice, FA mice, and mice treated with the subcutaneous administration of nicotine were stained with mMCP-1 antibodies. Scale bars represent 200 μm. *B*: MPO activity was measured in the colon of naïve mice, FA mice and nicotine-treated FA mice. *$P<0.01$ vs. naïve mice. †$P<0.05$ vs. FA mice ($n = 3$–10 mice per group). *C*: The level of OVA-specific IgE in the plasma of naïve mice, FA mice and nicotine-treated FA mice is shown. The level of OVA-specific IgE in the plasma was determined using an ELISA kit. **$P<0.01$ vs. naïve mice ($n = 5$ mice per group). IL-4, IL-5 and IFN-γ cytokine mRNA expression in the spleen (*D*) and proximal colon (*E*) from FA mice and nicotine-treated FA mice were measured by real-time PCR. Relative mRNA levels of cytokines were normalized to GAPDH expression. *$P<0.05$, **$P<0.01$ vs. FA mice ($n = 3$–6 mice per group).

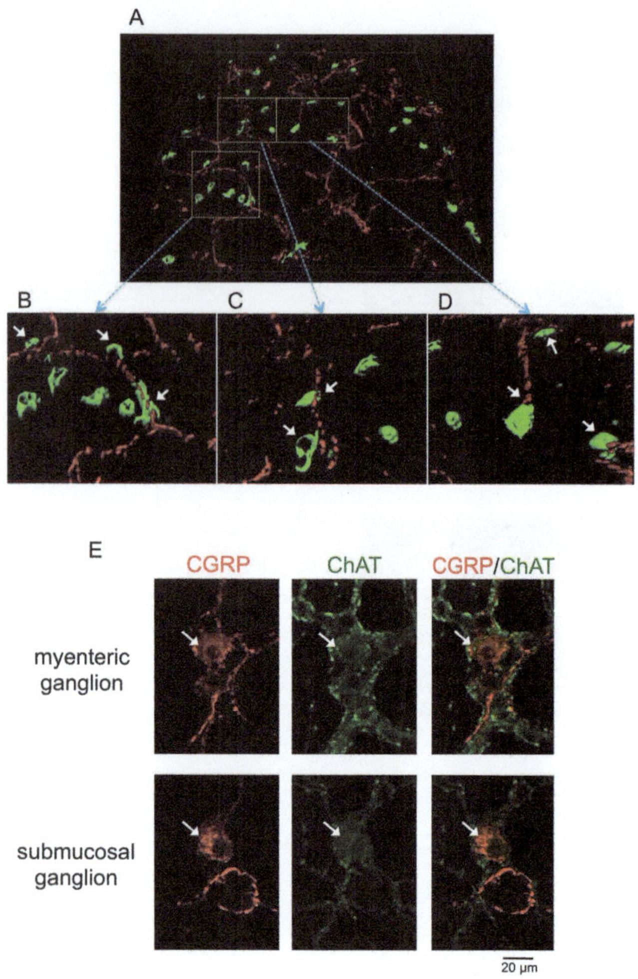

Figure 10. Spatial relationship of mucosal mast cells and cholinergic nerve fibers in the FA mouse colon. *A*: Three-dimensional reconstruction of the confocal images reveals the morphological interaction of mMCP-1-positive MMCs (green) and cholinergic CGRP- immunoreactive nerve fibers (red). Major grid space represents 20 μm. *B–D*: High-magnification images of three boxed regions in (*A*). *E*: CGRP- immunoreactive neurons (arrows) exhibited ChAT immunoreactivities in the myenteric and submucosal ganglion of the mouse enteric nervous system. Scale bar represents 20 μm.

to their thymus deficiency. We found that nude mice failed to exhibit allergic responses in the FA mouse model and that increased OVA-specific IgE and mMCP-1 levels in the plasma and mastocytosis in the mucosa of the proximal colon were not detected in nude naïve mice and nude FA mice. In addition, in this study, OVA-challenged mice without systemic priming failed to exhibit allergic diarrhea. Thus, these results indicate that the T-cell-mediated immune responses in the systemic immunity are essentially required for the development of the allergic responses in our FA model.

This study revealed that mMCP-1 immunoreactive MMCs increased in the mucosal epithelium of the FA mice colon, which is similar to previous reports on the appearance of mast cells in the jejunal mucosa of oral allergen–induced diarrhea mice [20] and parasite-infected mice [22,23]. Thus, these findings suggest that MMCs are localized in the strategic position to enhance a rapid expulsion of food antigens or parasites from the gut by bioactive products released from MMCs.

The toluidine blue staining revealed a difference between mast cells in the lamina propria and MMCs in the mucosal epithelium of the FA mice colon. Most of the granules of mast cells in the lamina propria, but not MMCs exhibited metachromasia presumably caused by sulfate radicals of proteoglycan such as heparin, suggesting that the difference results from chemical properties of substances contained in the granules of mast cells and that the granules of MMCs in the mucosal epithelium have depleted the reactive substances.

In the previous studies with mMCP-1-deficient mice in the parasite infection model, the light microscopic analysis reveals that MMCs in the jejunal mucosa of the deficient mice have smaller, less intensely toluidine blue-positive granules than those in WT mice and that the granules of MMCs in the deficient mice are uniformly round, whereas those in WT mice are irregularly shaped [23]. Furthermore, previous ultrastructural analysis demonstrates that crystalline inclusions with a cylindrical shape abundantly exist in the irregularly shaped granules of MMCs in the jejunal mucosa of the murine parasite infection model [23], which is consistent with the present findings using the electron microscopy in the granules of MMCs in the mucosal epithelium of the FA mice colon. However, in the mMCP-1 deficient mice, the shapes of MMC granules are regular and oval, and no crystalline structures are observed within the granules in the parasite infection model [23]. Taken all together, it is suggested that the disappearance of matrix constituents such as chondroitin sulfate in the granules of mast cells may be related to the formation of crystalline structures of chymases such as mMCP-1.

The PI3K family is involved in signal transduction that regulates cell proliferation, survival and differentiation. In particular, PI3K is involved in many functions of immune cells [24], and in mast cells, the activation of class Ia PI3K is required in the downstream signaling cascades initiated by the stimulation of high-affinity IgE receptor FcεRI. $PI3K^{-/-}$ mice are observed to be deficient in gastrointestinal mast cells but still have abundant dermal mast cells [19], indicating that the p85α subunit of PI3K is required for the development of gastrointestinal mast cells, but not dermal mast cells.

$PI3K^{-/-}$ mice failed to develop FA in our FA model, which were attributed to a deficiency of mast cells in the intestine, because: 1) mast cells can promote T-cell migration by producing chemokines [25,26], 2) mast cell products can promote dendritic cells to acquire a Th2 cell-inducing phenotype [2,27], and 3) mast cells themselves can produce Th2 cytokines, such as IL-4, 5 and 13 [2,25].

Furthermore, despite our finding that nicotine treatment atteuated allergic diarrhea in the FA mouse model, nicotine had no effect on the enhanced plasma IgE level.

Thus, these data suggest that the pathogenesis of FA is mainly attributed to mast cell hyperplasia in the intestine, but not antigen-specific IgE hyperproduction. Taken all together, our results indicate that MMCs critically contribute to the development of FA through orchestrating Th2 immune responses in the mucosal immunity of the FA mice.

The cross-talk between the autonomic nervous system and immune system is becoming increasingly elucidated to be of great importance for the maintenance of immune homeostasis. Several lines of evidence indicate that parasympathetic vagus nerve, through release of acetylcholine, plays a counter-regulatory role to restore immune homeostasis in diverse inflammatory disease models, such as ischemia-reperfusion injury [28], pancreatitis [29], peritonitis [30], DSS-induced colitis [31] and postoperative ileus [32,33]. The anti-inflammatory properties of the vagus nerve in these mouse models are primarily attributed to the suppression of macrophage activation that leads to the induction of inflammation through the release of the central inflammatory mediator TNF-α. Recently, it has become clear that nAChRs are expressed in various immune cells [14,32] as well as macrophages [34]. However, it still remains unclear whether the stimulation of nAChRs on these immune cells ameliorates diverse inflammatory diseases. In particular, it is worth noting that it is unknown whether cholinergic activation via nAChRs serves as an anti-inflammatory pathway in Th2-related diseases, especially allergic diseases.

In this FA study, vagal stimulation with 2-DG ameliorated the development of FA, which was reversed by the nAChR antagonist C6, indicating that vagus nerves exhibit anti-allergic properties via nAChRs. The therapeutic potential of the cholinergic agonist nicotine in inflammatory diseases has recently been demonstrated. In fact, nicotine has been shown to suppress inflammatory responses in various clinical studies, animal models and in vitro studies [12,35,36,37]. Notably, in a randomized double-blind study, nicotine patches in combination with conventional therapy have ameliorated ulcerative colitis, in which Th2-mediated phenomena tend to predominate, as compared to placebo patches and conventional therapy; however, nicotine patch treatment has caused adverse side effects, such as nausea, dizziness, headache and addiction due to non-selectivity of nicotine for subtypes of nAChRs [38].

In this study, nicotine treatment significantly ameliorated FA, mainly due to the suppression of upregulated mucosal immune responses via α7 nAChRs on immune cells. Therefore, the therapeutic effects of nicotine and GTS-21 on the FA model raise the possibility that a strategy for drug discovery against FA by targeting α7 nAChRs could potentially have therapeutic benefits.

Moreover, we have demonstrated that mBMMCs express α7 nAChRs and that their activation exerts inhibitory effects on antigen-IgE-mediated degranulation in mBMMCs [17]. In addition, our results in this study reveal that MMCs can orchestrate the allergic and inflammatory responses in the mucosal immune environment of the FA mice colon. Therefore, it is suggested that nicotine treatment suppresses the activation of MMCs through α7 nAChRs on MMCs, thereby reducing the number of MMCs and the plasma mMPC-1 level, which results in the significant amelioration of FA.

Furthermore, to examine whether the cholinergic anti-allergic pathway is a hard-wired connection between the immune and nervous systems closely interacting to regulate FA, we undertook morphological analysis in the mucosa of the FA mouse colon. Previous reports and this study demonstrate that in the mouse enteric nervous system, CGRP is exclusively contained in intrinsic primary afferent neurons that are immunoreactive for choline acetyltransferase [39,40], indicating that CGRP-IR neurons contain ACh as a neurotransmitter in the mouse colon. Our morphological findings of the close proximity between MMCs and CGRP-IR cholinergic nerve fibers in the colonic mucosa of the FA mice imply that the neural cholinergic regulation of immune responses occurs via nAChRs on immune cells, which is consistent with previous reports [14,32]. Collectively, it is suggested that cholinergic nerve fibers closely communicate with MMCs to regulate mast cell functions in the FA mice colon.

Further investigation of this cholinergic counter-regulatory nerve-immune interactions in the intestine will provide new insights to elucidate FA. In addition, new strategies for drug discovery that target the hard-wired connection via α7 nAChRs can lead to novel drug therapies against diverse intestinal immune diseases.

Supporting Information

Figure S1 α7 nAChR-mediated control of food allergy in mice. The occurrence of allergic diarrhea in FA mice (closed circle), GTS-21-treated mice (open circle; 10 mg/kg, p.o.) and MLA-treated mice prior to GTS-21 administration (open square; 1 mg/kg, s.c.) after each oral OVA challenge is shown. $^{*}P<0.05$, $^{**}P<0.01$ vs. FA mice. $^{\dagger}P<0.05$ vs. GST-21-treated mice ($n=6$–18 mice per group).
(DOCX)

Author Contributions

Conceived and designed the experiments: MK. Performed the experiments: TY TK JL NU SH HS HK MK. Analyzed the data: JL TY. Contributed reagents/materials/analysis tools: TY JL HS HK. Wrote the paper: MK JL TY.

References

1. Sicherer SH, Sampson HA (2010) Food allergy. J Allergy Clin Immunol 125: S116–125.
2. Abraham SN, St John AL (2010) Mast cell-orchestrated immunity to pathogens. Nat Rev Immunol 10: 440–452.
3. Eigenmann PA, Frossard CP (2003) The T lymphocyte in food-allergy disorders. Curr Opin Allergy Clin Immunol 3: 199–203.
4. MacDonald TT, Di Sabatino A (2009) The immunologic basis for gastrointestinal food allergy. Curr Opin Gastroenterol 25: 521–526.
5. Paul WE, Zhu J (2010) How are T(H)2-type immune responses initiated and amplified? Nat Rev Immunol 10: 225–235.
6. Dawicki W, Marshall JS (2007) New and emerging roles for mast cells in host defence. Curr Opin Immunol 19: 31–38.
7. Yamamoto T, Fujiwara K, Yoshida M, Kageyama-Yahara N, Kuramoto H, et al. (2009) Therapeutic effect of kakkonto in a mouse model of food allergy with gastrointestinal symptoms. Int Arch Allergy Immunol 148: 175–185.
8. Metcalfe DD, Baram D, Mekori YA (1997) Mast cells. Physiol Rev 77: 1033–1079.
9. Kageyama-Yahara N, Suehiro Y, Maeda F, Kageyama S, Fukuoka J, et al. (2010) Pentagalloylglucose down-regulates mast cell surface FcepsilonRI expression in vitro and in vivo. FEBS Lett 584: 111–118.
10. Bienenstock J, Goetzl EJ, Blennerhassett MG (2003) Autonomic neuroimmunology. London: CRC Press. 392 p.
11. van Diest SA, Stanisor OI, Boeckxstaens GE, de Jonge WJ, van den Wijngaard RM (2012) Relevance of mast cell-nerve interactions in intestinal nociception. Biochim Biophys Acta 1822: 74–84.
12. Bauer O, Razin E (2000) Mast Cell-Nerve Interactions. News Physiol Sci 15: 213–218.
13. de Jonge WJ, Ulloa L (2007) The alpha7 nicotinic acetylcholine receptor as a pharmacological target for inflammation. Br J Pharmacol 151: 915–929.
14. Rosas-Ballina M, Tracey KJ (2009) Cholinergic control of inflammation. J Intern Med 265: 663–679.
15. Tracey KJ (2009) Reflex control of immunity. Nat Rev Immunol 9: 418–428.
16. van Der Zanden EP, Boeckxstaens GE, de Jonge WJ (2009) The vagus nerve as a modulator of intestinal inflammation. Neurogastroenterol Motil 21: 6–17.
17. Kageyama-Yahara N, Suehiro Y, Yamamoto T, Kadowaki M (2008) IgE-induced degranulation of mucosal mast cells is negatively regulated via nicotinic acetylcholine receptors. Biochem Biophys Res Commun 377: 321–325.
18. Miller HR, Walshaw R (1972) Immune reactions in mucous membranes. IV. Histochemistry of intestinal mast cells during helminth expulsion in the rat. Am J Pathol 69: 195–208.
19. Fukao T, Yamada T, Tanabe M, Terauchi Y, Ota T, et al. (2002) Selective loss of gastrointestinal mast cells and impaired immunity in PI3K-deficient mice. Nat Immunol 3: 295–304.
20. Brandt EB, Strait RT, Hershko D, Wang Q, Muntel EE, et al. (2003) Mast cells are required for experimental oral allergen-induced diarrhea. J Clin Invest 112: 1666–1677.
21. Kweon MN, Yamamoto M, Kajiki M, Takahashi I, Kiyono H (2000) Systemically derived large intestinal CD4(+) Th2 cells play a central role in STAT6-mediated allergic diarrhea. J Clin Invest 106: 199–206.
22. Friend DS, Ghildyal N, Austen KF, Gurish MF, Matsumoto R, et al. (1996) Mast cells that reside at different locations in the jejunum of mice infected with Trichinella spiralis exhibit sequential changes in their granule ultrastructure and chymase phenotype. J Cell Biol 135: 279–290.

23. Wastling JM, Knight P, Ure J, Wright S, Thornton EM, et al. (1998) Histochemical and ultrastructural modification of mucosal mast cell granules in parasitized mice lacking the beta-chymase, mouse mast cell protease-1. Am J Pathol 153: 491–504.
24. Koyasu S (2003) The role of PI3K in immune cells. Nat Immunol 4: 313–319.
25. Galli SJ, Nakae S, Tsai M (2005) Mast cells in the development of adaptive immune responses. Nat Immunol 6: 135–142.
26. Nakajima T, Inagaki N, Tanaka H, Tanaka A, Yoshikawa M, et al. (2002) Marked increase in CC chemokine gene expression in both human and mouse mast cell transcriptomes following Fcepsilon receptor I cross-linking: an interspecies comparison. Blood 100: 3861–3868.
27. Mazzoni A, Siraganian RP, Leifer CA, Segal DM (2006) Dendritic cell modulation by mast cells controls the Th1/Th2 balance in responding T cells. J Immunol 177: 3577–3581.
28. Bernik TR, Friedman SG, Ochani M, DiRaimo R, Ulloa L, et al. (2002) Pharmacological stimulation of the cholinergic antiinflammatory pathway. J Exp Med 195: 781–788.
29. van Westerloo DJ, Giebelen IA, Florquin S, Bruno MJ, Larosa GJ, et al. (2006) The vagus nerve and nicotinic receptors modulate experimental pancreatitis severity in mice. Gastroenterology 130: 1822–1830.
30. van Westerloo DJ, Giebelen IA, Florquin S, Daalhuisen J, Bruno MJ, et al. (2005) The cholinergic anti-inflammatory pathway regulates the host response during septic peritonitis. J Infect Dis 191: 2138–2148.
31. Ghia JE, Blennerhassett P, Kumar-Ondiveeran H, Verdu EF, Collins SM (2006) The vagus nerve: a tonic inhibitory influence associated with inflammatory bowel disease in a murine model. Gastroenterology 131: 1122–1130.
32. Dhawan S, Cailotto C, Harthoorn LF, de Jonge WJ (2012) Cholinergic signalling in gut immunity. Life Sci 91: 1038–1042.
33. The FO, Boeckxstaens GE, Snoek SA, Cash JL, Bennink R, et al. (2007) Activation of the cholinergic anti-inflammatory pathway ameliorates postoperative ileus in mice. Gastroenterology 133: 1219–1228.
34. Wang H, Yu M, Ochani M, Amella CA, Tanovic M, et al. (2003) Nicotinic acetylcholine receptor alpha7 subunit is an essential regulator of inflammation. Nature 421: 384–388.
35. Andersson U, Tracey KJ (2012) Reflex principles of immunological homeostasis. Annu Rev Immunol 30: 313–335.
36. Lakhan SE, Kirchgessner A (2011) Anti-inflammatory effects of nicotine in obesity and ulcerative colitis. J Transl Med 9: 129.
37. Yoshikawa H, Kurokawa M, Ozaki N, Nara K, Atou K, et al. (2006) Nicotine inhibits the production of proinflammatory mediators in human monocytes by suppression of I-kappaB phosphorylation and nuclear factor-kappaB transcriptional activity through nicotinic acetylcholine receptor alpha7. Clin Exp Immunol 146: 116–123.
38. Pullan RD, Rhodes J, Ganesh S, Mani V, Morris JS, et al. (1994) Transdermal nicotine for active ulcerative colitis. N Engl J Med 330: 811–815.
39. Furness JB, Robbins HL, Xiao J, Stebbing MJ, Nurgali K (2004) Projections and chemistry of Dogiel type II neurons in the mouse colon. Cell Tissue Res 317: 1–12.
40. Qu ZD, Thacker M, Castelucci P, Bagyanszki M, Epstein ML, et al. (2008) Immunohistochemical analysis of neuron types in the mouse small intestine. Cell Tissue Res 334: 147–161.

23

Assessment of the Sensitizing Potential of Processed Peanut Proteins in Brown Norway Rats: Roasting Does Not Enhance Allergenicity

Stine Kroghsbo[1¤a], Neil M. Rigby[2], Philip E. Johnson[2¤b], Karine Adel-Patient[3], Katrine L. Bøgh[1], Louise J. Salt[2], E. N. Clare Mills[2¤b], Charlotte B. Madsen[1]*

1 National Food Institute, Technical University of Denmark, Søborg, Denmark, **2** Institute of Food Research, Norwich Research Park, Colney, Norwich, United Kingdom, **3** INRA, UR496, Unité d'Immuno-Allergie Alimentaire, Jouy-en-Josas, France

Abstract

Background: IgE-binding of process-modified foods or proteins is the most common method for examination of how food processing affects allergenicity of food allergens. How processing affects sensitization capacity is generally studied by administration of purified food proteins or food extracts and not allergens present in their natural food matrix.

Objectives: The aim was to investigate if thermal processing increases sensitization potential of whole peanuts via the oral route. In parallel, the effect of heating on sensitization potential of the major peanut allergen Ara h 1 was assessed via the intraperitoneal route.

Methods: Sensitization potential of processed peanut products and Ara h 1 was examined in Brown Norway (BN) rats by oral administration of blanched or oil-roasted peanuts or peanut butter or by intraperitoneal immunization of purified native (N-), heated (H-) or heat glycated (G-)Ara h 1. Levels of specific IgG and IgE were determined by ELISA and IgE functionality was examined by rat basophilic leukemia (RBL) cell assay.

Results: In rats dosed orally, roasted peanuts induced significant higher levels of specific IgE to NAra h 1 and 2 than blanched peanuts or peanut butter but with the lowest level of RBL degranulation. However, extract from roasted peanuts was found to be a superior elicitor of RBL degranulation. Process-modified Ara h 1 had similar sensitizing capacity as NAra h 1 but specific IgE reacted more readily with process-modified Ara h 1 than with native.

Conclusions: Peanut products induce functional specific IgE when dosed orally to BN rats. Roasted peanuts do not have a higher sensitizing capacity than blanched peanuts. In spite of this, extract from roasted peanuts is a superior elicitor of RBL cell degranulation irrespectively of the peanut product used for sensitization. The results also suggest that new epitopes are formed or disclosed by heating Ara h 1 without glucose.

Editor: Kottarappat N. Dileepan, University of Kansas Medical Center, United States of America

Funding: This work was funded by the EU through the project EuroPrevall (FP6-FOOD-CT-2005-514000). The funders had no role in study design, data collection and analysis, decision to publish, or preparation of the manuscript.

Competing Interests: The authors have declared that no competing interests exist.

* E-mail: charm@food.dtu.dk

¤a Current address: Unisensor A/S, Allerød, Denmark
¤b Current address: Manchester Interdisciplinary Biocentre, University of Manchester, Manchester, United Kingdom

Introduction

Food allergy is an adverse reaction to an otherwise harmless food or food component that involves an abnormal response of the immune system to specific proteins in foods. It is an allergen-specific immunologic response mediated by IgE. One of the major unanswered questions in food allergy research is what makes some foods and food proteins more allergenic than others. Seeking such answer is difficult since the proteins involved in sensitizing or eliciting allergic reactions may have undergone extensive modifications during food processing or be presented within complex food matrices. Certainly, both food processing and structure of the food matrix may impact allergenicity of food allergens [1–4].

Food processing may involve many different and complex physicochemical changes of the food which make it difficult to study and predict how processing affects the allergenic potential of a food protein. Moreover, alterations induced by processing may change the way in which a food protein is digested, influence allergen release from the food matrix or affect the form in which it is taken up across the epithelial barrier and presented to the immune system. Hence, the impact of processing on allergenicity of a food protein may be different from food to food or protein to protein. It is important to notice that the majority of proteins within foods may become insoluble after food processing. By this way, only a small part of proteins in processed foods are examined for changes in allergenicity by most serological and clinical analyses, as they are usually performed with food proteins extracted by simple salt solutions [2,5–7]. Different processing methods may impact the allergenic potential of foods or proteins, but there is no general rule on how different allergenic foods or proteins respond to physical, chemical or biochemical exposures during processing [7]. Allergenicity in the terms of IgE-binding may be decreased, unaltered or increased [2,6–8] and may be influenced by food processing conditions, variability in the allergen composition of the whole food, food matrix structure, multiplicity and types of IgE epitopes, thermodynamics of the allergen, and stability of the scaffold [7,8]. The most common types of modifications that food proteins undergo during processing include protein unfolding and aggregation, in addition to chemical modification, thus both the secondary and tertiary structure of native proteins can be altered as a consequence of processing [2,9].

Thermal processing is one of the most commonly used methods in food processing and depending on the time and temperature, thermal processing may alter protein structure and thereby the allergenicity of food proteins [8]. One of the most important chemical modifications occurring in foods during thermal processing is the reaction between free amino groups (generally lysine residues) of proteins and the aldehyde and ketone groups of sugars known as the Maillard reaction (non-enzymatic browning). This complex reaction occurs during heating of proteins leading to formation of a variety of poorly characterized molecules responsible for different odors and flavors [10]. The extent of glycation depends on different factors such as heating temperature and duration, and the concentration of reducing sugars [10,11]. The impact of Maillard reaction on IgE-binding has been studied for food allergens from milk [10]; peanut [11–17]; buckwheat [18]; scallop [19]; squid [20]; cherry [21]; apple [22]; and hazelnut [23]. Results from these studies are ambiguous and show that glycation can both increase and decrease IgE-binding. In spite of these studies it has not been possible to set up a general rule on how non-enzymatic glycation affects allergenicity of food proteins.

Peanuts are easy and cheap to produce and are consumed worldwide and one of the most widely processed food products in the western world. The majority of peanuts consumed in westernized countries have been processed by roasting whereas boiling is the preferred processing method in Asia and Africa [24]. Peanut seems to have an increased IgE-binding after dry-roasting as a whole food [11,12] compared to cooked or fried peanut [13,17]. However when looking at the two major peanut allergens, Ara h 1 and Ara h 2 they seem to be affected in different ways [16]. Furthermore there is no general consensus on how IgE-binding is affected by different forms of thermal processing for the two individual allergens [11,14–17,25–29] suggesting that the type of parameters such as allergen, food structure, and thermal processing may be of great importance when studying the impact of processing on food allergenicity. Moreover, the impact of food processing and food matrix on the sensitization capacity of peanut food allergens has only been rarely studied [30,31].

It has been shown that roasting of peanuts increases IgE-binding. This has been interpreted as roasting increases allergenicity of peanut proteins. To investigate if roasting increases sensitization capacity of peanut proteins, blanched (mildly heated) peanut, oil-roasted peanut and peanut butter were examined in an oral Brown Norway rat model for food allergy. In addition, process-modified purified Ara h 1 was used to study the impact of heating and heat-induced glycation on sensitization potential of a well-characterized major peanut allergen.

Materials and Methods

Ethics Statement

Animal experiments were carried out at the DTU Food (Mørkhøj, Denmark) facilities. Ethical approval was given by the Danish Animal Experiments Inspectorate. The authorization number given: 2004/561-917. The experiments were overseen by the National Food Institutes in-house Animal Welfare Committee for animal care and use.

Purification and Processing of Peanut Proteins

Native Ara h 1 and Ara h 2 were purified from peeled raw red shelled peanuts (obtained from a local supplier, UK). Ara h 1 was purified as described previously by Marsh *et al.* [32] and Ara h 2 was purified as described by Johnson *et al.* [33]. Concentrations of purified native and process-modified peanut proteins were determined by amino acid analysis [34].

Heating and glycation of native Ara h 1. Native (NAra h 1) and processed (HAra h 1, GAra h 1) peanut proteins were obtained as described in Blanc *et al.* [17]. Heating of Ara h 1 induced hydrolysis, partial loss of secondary structure and aggregation regardless of whether glucose was present. Heating alone (HAra h 1) resulted in formation of aggregates comprised of lower M_r polypeptides (~6–67 kDa) whereas aggregates of higher M_r polypeptides (>200 kDa) were formed by heating in the presence of glucose (GAra h 1) [17]. Samples were kept at −70°C in aliquots until use for animal experiments and immunochemical analysis.

Preparation of Peanut-water Mixtures for Use in Oral Sensitization Studies

Blanched and oil-roasted peanuts were kindly provided by Kraft Foods Norway (Runners peanuts grown in Argentina). Blanched peanuts were steam blanched at 120–130°C for 10–15 min to remove skin and prevent microbial growth. Oil-roasted peanuts were pretreated by blanching before oil roasting in a continuous roaster (150–160°C for 3–5 min). Peanut butter was purchased from a local retail outlet (Sunpat peanut butter, smooth; produced from roasted peanuts, 48.9% fat, 25.0% protein; UK). For oral dosing of rats by gavage, blanched or roasted peanuts or peanut butter were milled in a food processor together with water to obtain nut-water mixtures. Samples of peanut-water mixtures were stored at −20°C until use for animal experiments.

Preparation of Peanut Product Extracts for Analysis of Antibody Response

For immunochemical analysis of rat sera, peanut protein extracts were prepared from each of the peanut-water mixtures by addition of 5 mL carbonate buffer (20 mM, pH 9.6) per 2 g of peanut-water mixture before homogenization using an Ultraturrhax (15,000–20,000 rpm; IKA Werke GmbH & Co, Staufen, Germany). Then carbonate buffer was added to obtain a final volume of 40 mL, incubated overnight under agitation at 4°C followed by centrifugation (6000×*g*, 45 min, 4°C) and collection of supernatant containing peanut protein extract. Protein concentrations in extracts were estimated by the method of bicinchoninic acid (Pierce BCA Protein Assay Kit; Thermo Fisher Scientific Inc., Rockford, IL, USA) according to manufacturer's instructions. The yield of protein extraction was calculated to be 7.6 mg/mL (blanched peanuts), 3.6 mg/mL (roasted peanuts) and 4.4 mg/mL (peanut butter).

The presence of Ara h 1, Ara h 2 and other relevant peanut proteins in the peanut product extracts was confirmed by SDS-

PAGE under reducing conditions (Figure 1). SDS-PAGE was performed using NuPAGE 4–12% Bis-Tris gels (Invitrogen, Paisley, UK) with MES running buffer according to manufacturer's instructions. Mark12 MW Standard (Invitrogen) was used as molecular mass standards and gels were stained using a Coomassie-based stain (SimplyBlue SafeStain; Invitrogen). After destaining, gels were scanned using Pharos FX plus Imager and analyzed using Quantity One software v4.6.1 (BioRad, Hertfordshire, UK).

Animals

Inbred high IgE-responder Brown Norway (BN) rats were from our in-house colony at the DTU Food (Denmark). Rats were weaned at three weeks of age. Rats, 4–6 weeks of age, were randomized into groups. Randomization was done to ensure that animals from the same litter were distributed as evenly as possible in different groups and that the age distribution in the groups was comparable. Animals were housed in macrolon cages (two/cage) at 22±1°C, relative humidity 55 ± 5%, air change 10 times/h, and electric light from 9.00 am – 9.00 pm. Animals had hidings and a wooden block. Diet and acidified water (pH 3.5) were given *ad libitum*. Animals were inspected twice daily and body weights recorded weekly. To avoid tolerization against peanut proteins, animals were bred for at least three generations on a diet without *leguminosa* developed and produced at the DTU Food (Denmark) [35]. Diet samples were analyzed using Peanut Assay Kit (Neogen Europe, Flintshire, UK) and Soy Residue kit (Elisa Systems, Queensland, Australia) to ensure that the diet was not contaminated with minor amounts of peanut or cross-reacting soy proteins. Assay procedure and detection limits were as described previously [35]. At termination of sensitization experiments all animals were anaesthetized by carbon dioxide inhalation and killed by exsanguinations.

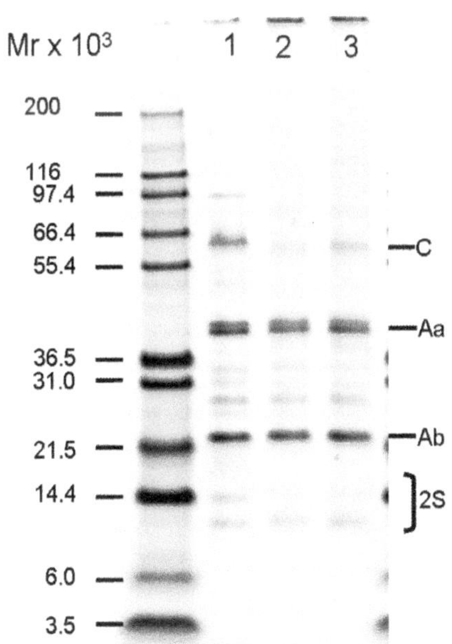

Figure 1. Identification of soluble peanut allergens in peanut product extracts. Extracts of blanched peanuts (lane 1), roasted peanuts (lane 2) and peanut butter (lane 3) were analyzed by SDS-PAGE under reducing conditions. Mark12 MW Standard (Invitrogen) was used as molecular mass standard and the gel was stained using a Coomassie-based stain (SimplyBlue SafeStain; Invitrogen). Calculated protein loading per lane is 0.65 µg based on determination of protein concentration by BCA assay. Protein Identification: C (Conarachin, 7S globulin), Aa (Arachin acidic subunits, 11S globulin), Ab (Arachin basic subunits, 11S globulin), 2S (2S albumins).

Animal Sensitization Studies

Positive control sera for native Ara h 1 and Ara h 2 were produced by intraperitoneal (i.p.) immunization with 50 µg of peanut antigen absorbed on 12 mg $Al(OH)_3$ per rat at day 1 and 10 µg antigen per rat at day 21, 35 and 49. Blood was collected at sacrifice (day 56). In all experiments sera were obtained from blood samples and stored at −20°C until analysis.

Sensitization capacity of peanut products and native and processed Ara h 1 was examined in two different rat models. Peanut products were studied using an oral model (intra-gastric dosing of rats) to mimic human intake whereas an i.p. model was used for studies of native and processed Ara h 1 because of the lower amounts of purified protein required compared to the oral model.

Dosing or blood drawing of animals did not result in any adverse events.

Feeding study with peanut products. Groups of 16 BN rats (8 per sex) were dosed by gavage each day for 42 days with 0.5 mL per rat per day of peanut-water mixtures of blanched or roasted peanuts or peanut butter to study whether food processing influences the oral sensitization capacity of Ara h 1 in its natural matrix. Peanut-water mixtures were prepared and adjusted so rats were dosed with ~2 mg Ara h 1 and ~1 mg Ara h 2 per rat per day. Concentrations of Ara h 1 and Ara h 2 in peanut products were estimated based on data from 'The official Danish Food Composition Database version 7.01' [www.foodcomp.dk/v7; Technical University of Denmark) and personal communication [Neil M Rigby; IFR, Norwich, UK]. Dosing regime and concentration of Ara h 1 and Ara h 2 were chosen based on results obtained in a preliminary study (data not shown). A group of 16 untreated BN rats was included as control. Blood was collected under Hypnorm/Dormicum anesthesia before study initiation and one week after the last dosing.

I.p. study with native, heated and glycated Ara h 1. To examine whether heating and glycation affects the sensitization capacity of purified native Ara h 1, groups of 12 BN rats (6 per sex) were immunized i.p. three times (day 0, 14 and 28) with none (control) or 200 µg of NAra h 1, HAra h 1 or GAra h 1 in 0.5 mL PBS (pH 7.2) per rat per immunization. Blood was collected before study initiation and one week after the last immunization.

All dosing and handling of animals were done in the animal room by experienced animal technicians having an education approved by the Danish Animal Experiments Inspectorate.

Enzyme-Linked ImmunoSorbent Assay (ELISA)

Measurement of specific IgG1, IgG2a and IgE against native Ara h 1 (NAra h 1) was performed as described previously [35]. For details about washing procedures, development of enzymatic reaction and calculation of titer values see Kroghsbo *et al.* [35,36].

ELISAs for detection of specific IgG1 and IgG2a. For measurement of the specific IgG1 and IgG2a response plates (96-well, MaxiSorp; Nunc, Roskilde, Denmark) were coated overnight at 4°C with 0.5 µg/mL of Ara h 2 or 1.0 µg/mL of HAra h 1, GAra h 1 or peanut product extract in carbonate buffer (pH 9.6; 15 mM Na_2CO_3, 35 mM $NaHCO_3$). For detection of specific IgG1 and IgG2a against HAra h 1 and GAra h 1, plates were blocked for 1 h at 37°C with 200 µL/well of 1% BSA in PBS/Tween buffer (PBS-T, 0.05% Tween 20). A blocking step was not performed for plates used for detection of specific IgG1 and IgG2a against Ara h 2 or peanut product extracts as optimization procedures showed no effect of blocking on background absorbance values. Then, plates were incubated with serially diluted rat sera in PBS-T for 1 h at RT before incubation with horseradish peroxidase (HRP)-labeled mouse anti-rat IgG1 or IgG2a (1:2000; Zymed, San Francisco, CA, USA) in PBS-T for 1 h at RT followed by development with TMB-one (Kem-En-Tec, Copenhagen, Denmark) for 10 min in the dark. Detection limits were calculated to an absorbance value of 0.1 for all IgG1 assays and 0.2 for all IgG2a assays.

Inhibition ELISAs for examination of binding capacity of specific IgG1. Assay procedures were as described for measurement of specific IgG1 except that sera were preincubated with inhibitor solutions. Serum pools were diluted to reach an OD between 0.8 and 1.0 and preincubated (1 h at RT) with serial tenfold dilutions of NAra h 1, HAra h 1 or GAra h 1 (0.1 ng/mL–100 μg/mL) or peanut product extracts (1 ng/mL–1000 μg/mL) before triplicates of serum/inhibitor mix (and sera with no inhibitor as a control) were added to the wells. Results were expressed as B/B_0 where B corresponds to the specific IgG1-binding to immobilized protein when a known concentration of inhibitor is present and B_0 corresponds to the binding in the absence of inhibitor. For each serum pool the concentration of inhibitor that inhibits 50% of the binding to the coated antigen/extract (IC_{50}) was determined, where an increase in IC_{50} value is correlated to a lower IgG reactivity of the product used as inhibitor. Analysis of inhibition curves by GraphPad Prism (GraphPad Software, San Diego, CA, USA) showed that inhibition curves were parallel (slopes were not significantly different) which is important for appropriately comparison of IC_{50} values.

Antibody-capture ELISAs for detection of specific IgE. To avoid the interference of the much higher level of IgG than IgE, assays based on selective IgE capture was established for detection of antigen-specific IgE responses. Specific IgE against Ara h 2 or processed Ara h 1 was measured by coating plates overnight at 4°C with 0.5 μg/mL of mouse anti-rat IgE (HPMAB-123 HybriDomus, Cytotech, Hellebæk, Denmark) in carbonate buffer. After blocking of remaining active sites overnight at 4°C with PBS-T containing 1% rat serum from naïve rats, plates were incubated for 1 h at RT with serially diluted rat sera and then for 1 h with digoxigenin (DIG)-coupled antigen diluted to 0.2 μg/mL (10:1, DIG-Ara h 2) or 0.8 μg/mL (3.5:1; DIG-HAra h 1, DIG-GAra h 1) in PBS-T containing 3% rabbit serum. After washing, plates were incubated with HRP-labeled sheep anti-DIG (1:1000; Roche, Mannheim, Germany) before development for 20–30 min in the dark. Detection limits were calculated to an absorbance value of 0.1. Native Ara h 1 (NAra h 1) and Ara h 2 were coupled using a DIG protein-labeling kit from Roche whereas HAra h 1 and GAra h 1 were coupled using Chromalink digoxigenin one-shot antibody labeling kit (SoluLink, San Diego, CA, USA) as the kit from Roche was no longer available.

Sandwich ELISA for measurement of total IgE. Total IgE responses were measured for serum pools by coating plates overnight at 4°C with 0.5 μg/mL of mouse anti-rat IgE (HPMAB-123 HybriDomus, Cytotech) in carbonate buffer. After blocking of remaining active sites for 1 h at 37°C with PBS-T, plates were incubated for 1 h at RT with serially diluted rat sera (starting at 1:20) and rat IgE standard (Rat Myeloma IgE, 02-9788, Zymed). After washing, plates were incubated with HRP-labeled mouse anti-rat IgE (1:2000; MCA193P, AbD Serotec, Düsseldorf, Germany) for 1 h at RT before development for 20 min in the dark.

Concentrations of total IgE in serum samples were interpolated from the linear part of the standard curve for purified IgE (three-parameter analysis, KC4 version 2.7). The average concentration of at least two serum dilutions was used for final calculation.

Rat Basophilic Leukemia (RBL) Assay

Sera were examined by RBL assay using RBL-2H3 cells (DSMZ, Braunschweig, Germany). Cells were cultured, harvested and plated in flat-bottomed cell culture microtitre plates (Nunc) for attachment as described in Kroghsbo *et al.* [35] (1.5×10^5 cells/well). Attached cells were sensitized passively with 50 μL/well of serum pools from i.p. sensitization study (diluted 1:2) or feeding studies (undiluted), then washed twice before incubation with 100 μL/well of ten-fold diluted purified antigen solutions (0.01–100 μg/mL) or four-fold diluted peanut extract solutions (0.06–1000 μg/mL) for cross-linking. After incubation for 1 h plates were centrifuged and 25 μL supernatant (*Specific release*) was transferred to a microtitre plate (Nunc). Enzymatic activity in supernatants was detected by hydrolysis of the substrate *p*-nitrophenyl-*N*-acetyl β-D-glucosamimide (PNAG; N9376, Sigma, Saint Louis, MO, USA) by addition of 100 μL/well and incubation for 90 min at 37°C. Reaction was terminated by addition of 100 μL/well of 0.2 M glycine solution, pH 10.7 (G7126, Sigma). *β*-hexosaminidase release was quantitatively measured spectrophotometrically at 405 nm with a reference wavelength of 630 nm using a microplate reader (BioTek Instruments Inc.). Total release from remaining intact cells was measured for each well by addition of detergent (80 μL/well of 0.2% Triton X-100; X100, Sigma), incubated for 30 min before centrifugation and transfer of 25 μL supernatant (*Total release*) to a second microtitre plate.

For control of IgE-mediated degranulation (*Total IgE release*), serum-sensitized cells were stimulated with 1.25 μg mouse anti-rat IgE/mL (553914, BD Pharmingen, San Diego, CA, USA) found to be the optimal concentration for biological release in initial optimization studies. Negative controls (non-sensitized cells or cells sensitized with naïve sera stimulated with peanut extracts) were added to each plate to measure spontaneous release.

For each serum sample *β*-hexosaminidase release was calculated according to the following equation:

$$\%\textit{Specific release} = \frac{\text{Specific release (stimulated with antigen solution or peanut product extracts)}}{\text{Total release (lysed with detergent)}} \times 100\%$$

As total release was 30–40% for all serum pools and no statistically significant difference was found between groups, results are expressed as percent of maximum biological release:

$$\beta-\textit{hexosamindase release}(\%) = \frac{\%\text{Specific release}}{\%\text{Total IgE release}} \times 100\%$$

Statistical Analysis

All statistical calculations on data were carried out using GraphPad Prism version 4.00 for Windows (GraphPad Software). ELISA results expressed as antibody titers were examined using non-parametric statistical analysis because data was not normally distributed for all experimental groups. Results from inhibition ELISAs were analyzed by one-way ANOVA followed by Tukey's multiple comparison test. The Kruskal–Wallis test followed by

Dunn's multiple comparison test was used for comparison of more than three groups, RBL results were examined using a two-way ANOVA.

Differences between experimental groups were regarded as significant when $p \leq 0.05$.

Results

Dosing or blood drawing of animals did not result in any adverse events.

Protein Profiles of Peanut Product Extracts Differ in Solubility of Peanut Allergens

Ara h 1 and Ara h 2 monomers content in extracts of roasted peanuts and peanut butter was estimated to be decreased 7.1–11.5 fold for Ara h 1 and 1.3–2.5 fold for Ara h 2/6 compared to the content in the blanched peanut extract reflecting formation of insoluble aggregates during roasting (Figure 1, Table 1).

Ara h 1 and Ara h 2 Induce More Specific IgE when Present in Roasted Peanuts Compared to Blanched Peanuts and Peanut Butter

To examine whether processing and food matrix influence sensitization potential of peanut allergens, rats were dosed orally by gavage with water mixtures of blanched or roasted peanuts or peanut butter. As shown in Figure 2 all three peanut products induced a statistically significant IgG1 response against whole extracts (Figure 2A) and against Ara h 1 and Ara h 2, purified from raw peanuts (Figure 2B). Although not statistically significant, blanched and roasted peanuts had a tendency to induce more anti-Ara h 1 and anti-Ara h 2 IgG1 antibodies than peanut butter (Figure 2B). The Ara h 1- and Ara h 2-specific IgG2a response resembled the corresponding specific IgG1 response for all groups (data not shown) for which reason only results for specific IgG1 are shown.

Only oral dosing with roasted peanuts induced a statistically significant IgE response against Ara h 1 and Ara h 2 (Figure 2B). Specific IgE against peanut extracts was not assayed because coupling of peanut extracts to digoxigenin (DIG) most likely would result in ratios of coupled peanut proteins and peptides not resembling the actual ratios present in the extracts. Moreover specific IgE against extracts was not measured by direct ELISAs as the presence of a manifold higher concentration of IgG in the serum samples competes with IgE and dramatically lower assay sensitivity. No difference in total IgE was found between dosed groups or for the control group compared to dosed groups (data not shown).

Extract from Roasted Peanuts is a Superior Elicitor in RBL Assay, but the Biological Functionality does not Reflect Specific IgE Titers

Biological functionality of the specific IgE responses, i.e. whether it may induce elicitation of an allergic reaction, was analyzed using RBL assay by sensitizing cells with serum pools from each group of rats before stimulating with peanut product extracts (Figure 3). Regardless of the peanut product used for sensitization by gavage, extract from roasted peanut induced a statistically significant higher degranulation of sera-sensitized RBL cells compared to blanched peanut extract whereas no elicitation was observed for stimulation with peanut butter extract. While ELISA analysis showed the highest Ara h 1- and Ara h 2-specific IgE response induced by oral dosing with roasted peanuts (Figure 2B) examination of the same sera by RBL assay using extracts for stimulation showed a higher biological activity of specific IgE when rats were dosed with blanched peanuts or peanut butter compared to dosing with roasted peanuts (Figure 3).

It was not possible to detect any significant degranulation of RBL cells when sensitized cells were stimulated with purified native or processed Ara h 1 or purified native Ara h 2 (data not shown).

Heating and Heat Glycation Change the Immune Response to Ara h 1

Analysis of sera from rats immunized i.p. with native (NAra h 1) or processed Ara h 1 (HAra h 1 or GAra h 1) by ELISA showed that all three Ara h 1 products had sensitizing potential and induced a statistically significant specific IgG1 (Figure 4) and IgG2a (data not shown) response. No significant difference in IgG1 response to NAra h 1 was seen between groups. Animals immunized with HAra h 1 had a statistically significant higher IgG1 response against HAra h 1 and GAra h 1 compared to animals sensitized with NAra h 1 or GAra h 1. The same pattern was found for specific IgE responses (Figure 4) suggesting that new epitopes are formed or disclosed by heating without glucose. Because of the nature of the IgE ELISA where process modification may influence the DIG coupling, we have not tried to compare IgE ELISA results between N-, H- or GAra h 1. It may be more relevant to compare the biologic activity of IgE responses i.e. the degranulation of RBL cells sensitized with IgE against N-, H- or GAra h 1 and degranulated with the respective allergen. RBL results showed that sensitization to NAra h 1 and HAra h 1 induced comparable functional IgE responses at high stimulation concentrations whereas GAra h 1 induced a slightly lower response (Figure 5A). GAra h 1 seemed the least efficient in degranulating cells irrespective of IgE specificity. HAra h 1 was

Table 1. Composition of peanut extracts determined by densitometric analysis of lanes from SDS PAGE gel.

	Proteins %		
	Blanched PE*	**Roasted PE**	**PB extract**
7S (Ara h 1)	19	1.6	2.6
11S (Ara h 3/4)	57	86	85
2S (Ara h 2/6)	7.2	3.1	2.9

*PE: peanut extract, PB: peanut butter.

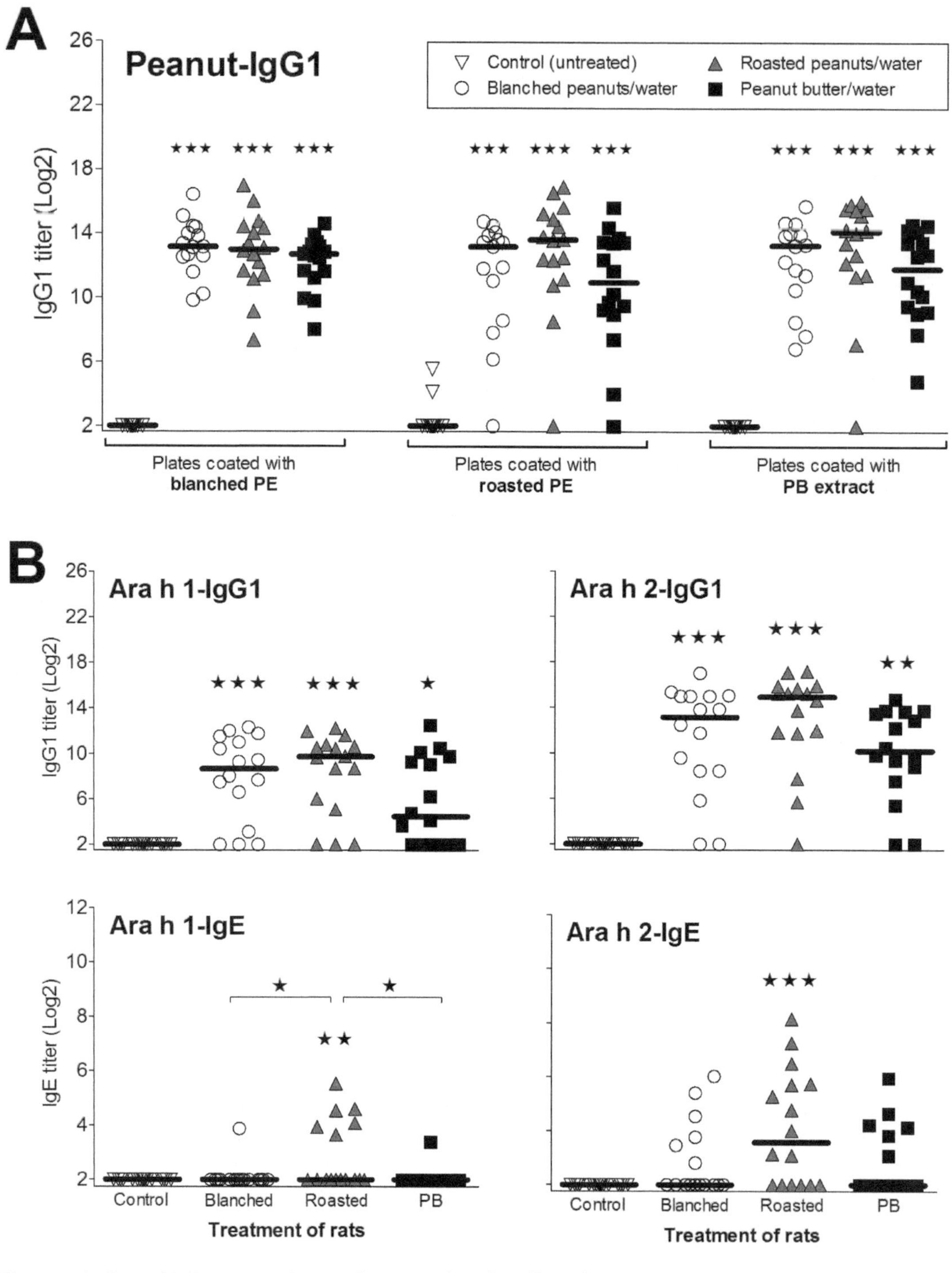

Figure 2. IgG1 and IgE response in sera from rats dosed orally with peanut products. Groups of BN rats were dosed for 42 days (day 1–42) with peanut-water mixtures prepared with blanched peanuts (open circles), roasted peanuts (grey triangles) or peanut butter (black squares) corresponding to approximately 2 mg Ara h 1 and 1 mg Ara h 2 per rat per day. Groups of untreated rats were included as controls (open triangles). Serum samples were obtained at sacrifice (day 49) and analyzed by ELISA. Sera were analyzed for specific IgG1 response against extracts of peanut-water mixtures (A) and against Ara h 1 and Ara h 2 purified from raw peanuts (B). Each symbol represents an animal. Horizontal bars indicate median values. Data were analyzed by non-parametrical test. Asterisks indicate statistically significant difference of a dosed group compared to the corresponding control group. Asterisks over a horizontal line indicate statistically significant difference between the two given groups. *: $p \leq 0.05$; **: $p \leq 0.01$; ***: $p \leq 0.001$.

found to be the most efficient degranulator of RBL cells sensitized with IgE against HAra h 1, whereas IgE induced by NAra h 1 reacted equally well with native and processed Ara h 1 (Figure 5A). This is in accordance with the ELISA results where IgE titers to NAra h 1 were comparable, whereas the IgE titer to HAra h 1 was highest in animals sensitized with HAra h 1.

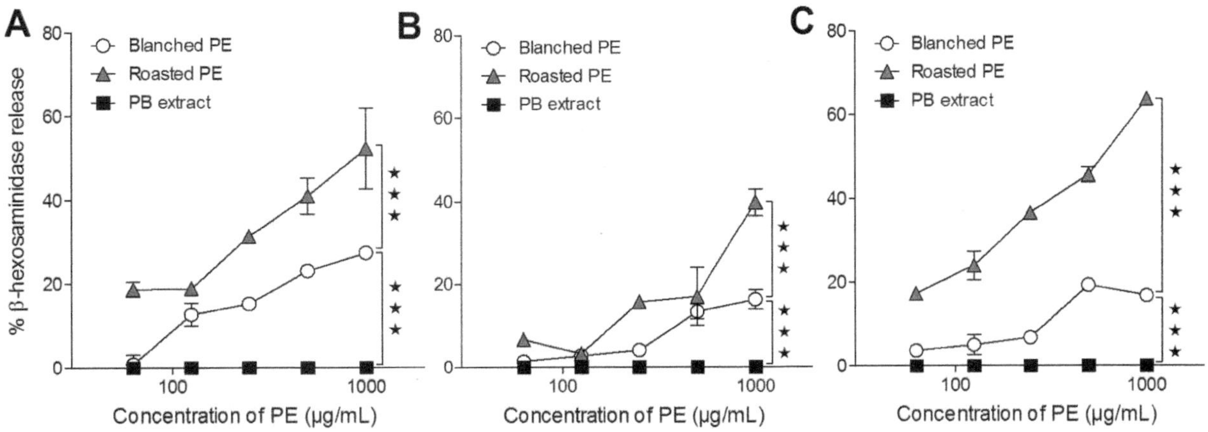

Figure 3. Allergen-specific degranulation of RBL cells sensitized with sera from rats dosed orally with peanut products. RBL cells were passively sensitized with serum pools (undiluted) from groups of BN rats dosed orally by gavage for 42 days with with blanched peanuts (**A**), roasted peanuts (**B**) and peanut butter (**C**) corresponding to approximately 2 mg Ara h 1 per rat per day. Peanut-water mixtures were prepared using blanched or roasted peanuts or peanut butter. For degranulation, cells were stimulated with dilutions of extracts of peanut-water mixtures (blanched PE, roasted PE or PB extract). Data are presented as percentage β–hexosaminidase release of total biological release induced by stimulation with 125 ng/well of anti-rat IgE. Symbols represent mean values ± SD for each serum pool. It was not possible to detect any degranulation of RBL cells when sensitized cells were stimulated with native or processed Ara h 1. The experiment was performed twice. Data were analyzed by two-way ANOVA. Statistical difference between extracts to induce allergen-specific degranulation is only indicated for least significant lines; ***: $p \leq 0.001$. RBL: rat basophilic leukemia, PE: peanut extract, PB: peanut butter.

Taking account of the difference in Ara h 1 content of the extracts, extracts from the roasted products are overall more efficient elicitors of degranulation irrespective of the specificity of the IgE (Figure 5B).

IgG1-binding Capacity of Sera Reflects whether Animals are Sensitized to Native or Processed Ara h 1 or Dosed with Blanched or Roasted Peanut Products

Results obtained by inhibition ELISAs showed that processed Ara h 1 (HAra h 1 and GAra h 1) were better inhibitors of IgG1-binding using sera from animals immunized with processed Ara h 1 compared to NAra h 1 (Figure 6). Also extracts of roasted peanuts and peanut butter showed higher IgG1-binding capacity than blanched peanut extract for groups immunized with processed Ara h 1 even though the Ara h 1 content of these extracts are much lower than that of the blanched peanut extract. IgG1-binding capacities of NAra h 1 and blanched peanut extracts were higher in rats sensitized with NAra h 1 (Figure 6).

Discussion

It has been suggested that the worldwide variation in peanut allergy prevalence may be caused by differences in peanut processing rather than being caused by differences in consumption. In China where peanuts are used as stable foods and boiled or fried, the peanut prevalence seems to be lower than in countries where peanuts are being consumed roasted as snack or in peanut butter [13,24]. This has been supported by studies showing that roasting increases IgE-binding [11,12] and that boiling or frying [13] reduces IgE-binding. Mondoulet *et al.* [14] was not able to confirm that roasting increases IgE-binding when analyzing whole peanut protein extracts but found that boiling released low-molecular weight allergens into the boiling water, explaining the lower IgE-binding of boiled peanuts. Recently, Blanc *et al.* [17] showed that IgE-binding capacity of roasted Ara h 1 was similar to native Ara h 1 whereas boiling of purified Ara h 1 reduced IgE-binding irrespective of the presence or absence of glucose during heating. The authors suggest that the difference in IgE-binding may be explained by formation of distinct morphological aggregates; roasted Ara h 1 comprised of compact globular aggregates with a higher content of native-like β-sheet structures compared to the more 'rod-like' branched aggregates induced by boiling.

We have used the well described BN rat as model for sensitization as it is very difficult to study sensitization in humans, because it is nearly impossible to know the exact exposure. We study the functionality of the response using an *in vitro* assay rather than burden the animals by challenge. This would also include the use of adjuvants in the sensitization process, which we avoid.

Only few studies have examined the sensitization potential of whole foods and to our knowledge the results presented herein are the first comparing how processing affects sensitization potential of whole foods and also the first study to examine sensitization potential of processed Ara h 1. As peanut processing decreases protein solubility [[37,38]; dosing with food extract (comprising of only soluble proteins) may bias result interpretation. On the other hand, at the moment the only way to perform *in vitro* analysis of the functionality of specific IgE and determination of specific IgE-binding is by the use of extracted soluble proteins.

Allergenicity in the terms of IgE-binding and mediator release assays have been used for examination of how different processing methods affect the allergenicity of peanut allergens. Nevertheless, these assays only reveal something about elicitation and not sensitization potential of food allergens.

We found that oral dosing of rats with roasted peanuts induced significant anti-Ara h 1 and anti–Ara h 2 IgE responses when measured by ELISA. In rats dosed with blanched peanuts or peanut butter a significant number of rats (5 out of 16 rats per group) developed IgE to Ara h 2, but not to Ara h 1 (1 out of 16). This difference in IgE titer to Ara h 1 and 2 is not reflected in the results of the RBL assay showing that sera from rats dosed with roasted peanuts induced a lower functional IgE response compared to sera from rats dosed with blanched peanuts and peanut butter when degranulation was induced by stimulation with the roasted peanut extract. In a previous study [35], we

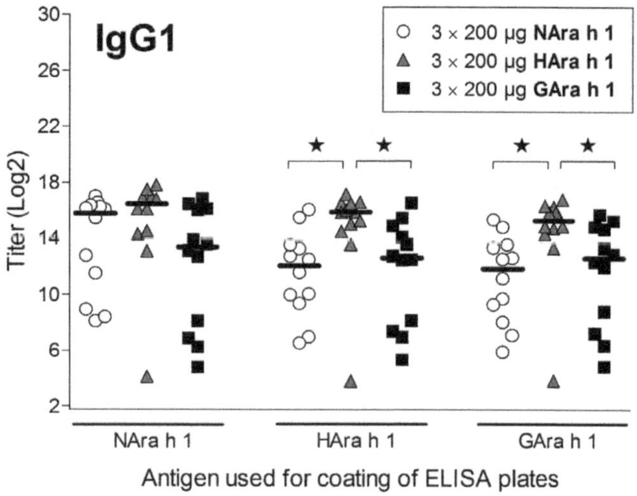

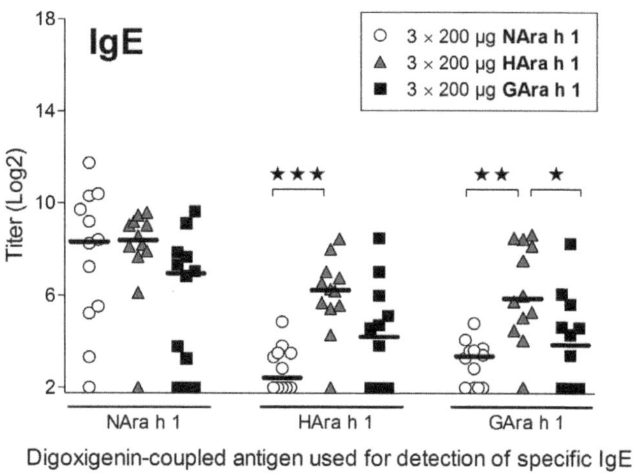

Figure 4. Specific IgG1 and IgE response in sera from rats immunized i.p. with native or processed Ara h 1. Groups of BN rats were immunized on day 0, 14 and 28 with 200 µg of NAra h 1 (open circles), HAra h 1 (grey triangles) or GAra h 1 (black squares). Serum samples were obtained at sacrifice (day 35) and analyzed by ELISA for specific IgG1 and IgE against native and processed Ara h 1. No allergen-specific IgG1 or IgE was detected for control animals (data not shown). Each symbol represents an animal. Horizontal bars indicate median values. Data were analyzed by non-parametrical test. Asterisks over a horizontal line indicate statistically significant difference between the two given groups. *: $p \leq 0.05$; **: $p \leq 0.01$; ***: $p \leq 0.001$.

showed that IgE titer may not always predict IgE functionality in BN rats which is supported by the findings that heated Ara h 1 possessed increased capacity to elicit mediator release although IgE-binding was reduced [16,17]. Weighting functionality based on whole peanut extracts higher than IgE titer against Ara h 1 and 2, our results show that roasted peanuts as such or in peanut butter are not more efficient to sensitize compared to blanched peanuts and that blanched peanuts and peanut butter (produced from roasted peanuts) are equally good as sensitizers. However, these results may be biased as it cannot be excluded that allergen(s) efficient for degranulation was altered through processing or not extracted from the peanut matrices.

Roasting of peanuts results in a significant decrease in protein solubility that may influence digestibility. How this exactly influences the ability to sensitize is difficult to predict as the solubility increases dramatically at pH 2 [37]. Ara h 2 from roasted peanuts has been found to possess increased trypsin inhibitory activity suggesting its role as a protector of other peanut proteins to proteolytic digestion [38]. We have previously shown that digested Ara h 1 has both sensitizing and eliciting properties [39]. To our knowledge, no previous study of peanut and peanut extract has compared sensitization to different peanut products. Sensitization potential of ground (presumably roasted) peanuts [30] and peanut extracts (probably from raw peanuts) with and without fat [31] have been studied in mice using oral dosing with cholera toxin as mucosal adjuvant showing that both peanut products were able to induce specific IgE. The fat content did not influence sensitization [31]. In summary, based on available information, we are not able to explain why oral sensitization to roasted peanuts induce a less functional IgE response than peanut butter and blanched peanuts.

Furthermore, the RBL assay also showed that irrespective of the peanut product used for sensitization, extract from roasted peanuts is a far better elicitor than extract from blanched peanuts and peanut butter. This may be explained by the fact that roasting increases aggregation of proteins [25,37] and that aggregates may be better elicitors of basophil degranulation.

Extracting proteins from processed peanuts may be difficult as the protein solubility is decreased by processing [25,37,40–42]. In this study the concentration of proteins extracted from blanched peanuts was nearly twofold higher compared to roasted peanuts and peanut butter. The extracts were therefore adjusted with respect to protein concentration [37].

The Ara h 1 and Ara h 2 content in extracts from roasted peanuts and peanut butter was lower than in the blanched peanut extract indicating that roasting decreases solubility of these proteins, in particularly Ara h 1. As total protein concentration was adjusted and the Ara h 1 and Ara h 2 content of processed peanuts was lower, the relative concentration of the other allergens has been higher in the roasted peanut extract compared to the blanched peanut extract.

In this way, the more efficient elicitation mediated by the roasted peanut extract may be a true difference but could also reflect dissimilarity in protein distribution as a consequence of difference in solubility. Ara h 2/6 has been reported to be much more potent elicitors of basophil degranulation compared to Ara h 1. Also Ara h 3 has been reported to be a more potent allergen than Ara h 1 [16,43]. It is not possible to elucidate how the decrease in Ara h 1 and 2 and increase in Ara h 3/4 may have influenced the RBL result. Unfortunately there are no clinical challenge studies in peanut allergic patients comparing raw, blanched or roasted peanuts so the possible clinical implication of the superior elicitation caused by roasted peanut extract remains unknown.

Examination of sensitization capacity of purified proteins can be difficult or in some cases impossible to perform in an oral model because of the amount of protein required. For this reason we chose to study heated and glycated Ara h 1 using i.p. immunization. The disadvantage of this model is that it bypasses the proteolytic environment of the gastrointestinal tract. As heating and glycation of Ara h 1 did not change *in vitro* digestibility (unpublished data) we found it justified comparing the sensitizing potential of native and process-modified Ara h 1 using the i.p. model.

Processing did not increase or decrease the sensitizing capacity of purified Ara h 1. However ELISA results showed differences in reactivity especially between IgG1 antibodies to NAra h 1 and HAra h 1 suggesting that new epitopes are formed or disclosed by

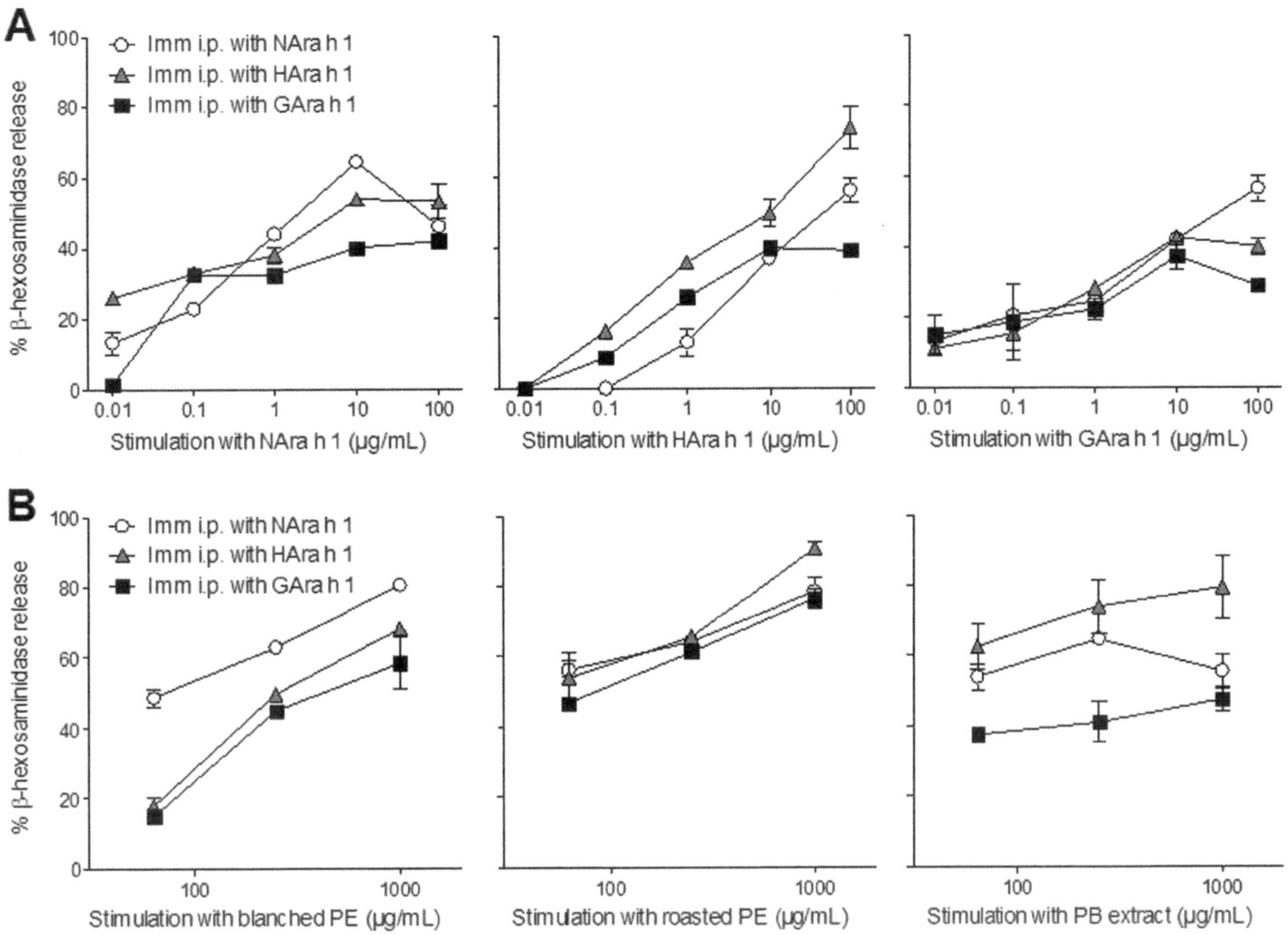

Figure 5. Allergen-specific degranulation of RBL cells sensitized with sera from i.p. study with Ara h 1. RBL cells were passively sensitized with serum pools (diluted 1:2) from groups immunized i.p. three times with 200 μg of NAra h 1 (open circles), HAra h 1 (grey triangles) or GAra h 1 (black squares). For degranulation cells were stimulated with dilutions of native or processed Ara h 1 (A) or extracts of peanut-water mixtures (B). Data are presented as percentage β–hexosaminidase release of total biological release induced by stimulation with 125 ng/well of anti-rat IgE. Symbols represent mean values ± SD for each serum pool. RBL: rat basophilic leukemia, Imm: immunization, PE: peanut extract, PB: peanut butter.

heating and to a lesser degree by glycation. This is also reflected in the inhibition ELISA results where NAra h 1 is a better inhibitor for sera raised against NAra h 1 and HAra h 1 is a better inhibitor for sera raised against HAra h 1 or GAra h 1. The same pattern was seen when extracts were used as inhibitor. Here blanched peanut extract was a very week inhibitor for sera raised against HAra h 1 or GAra h 1 although the Ara h 1 content is much higher than in the extracts from roasted peanut products. Together, the results obtained by RBL assay and inhibition ELISA indicate that the process modification of purified Ara h 1 caused by heating with or without glucose actually resembles what goes on in the peanut during the roasting procedure. Extract from roasted peanuts is a better elicitor and inhibitor of sera against HAra h 1 and GAra h 1 compared to extract from blanched peanuts especially when the higher Ara h 1 content in the blanched peanut extract is taken into account. This is in accordance with the finding that Ara h 1 purified from (dry-)roasted peanuts has similar IgE-binding capacity as native Ara h 1 despite being denatured and highly aggregated while boiling of Ara h 1 reduced IgE-binding capacity [17]. In contrary, other studies have shown increased IgE-binding of Ara h 1 after processing [12,14].

In addition, it seems that blanching for up to 15 min at 120–130°C induces much less protein change compared to roasting, as proteins are readily extracted and the distribution of allergens resembles the allergen content of peanuts reported in the literature [43]. Extract from blanched peanuts is a better elicitor and inhibitor of sera against NAra h 1 (from raw peanut) compared to extract from roasted peanuts even when the difference in Ara h 1 content is taken into account.

We have shown that IgE from animals sensitized with heated Ara h 1 has higher binding capacity to heated Ara h 1 compared to Ara h 1 from blanched peanuts. It is worth noting that studies comparing IgE-binding capacity of heat modified peanut allergens or products have used sera from patients that most probably have been sensitized to roasted peanuts either as such or in peanut butter [12–14]. In the light of our findings, the differences in IgE-binding of processed peanuts or processed peanut allergens using human sera may also be influenced by the initial sensitization.

In conclusion our results show that peanut products may sensitize BN rats and induce a functional specific IgE response

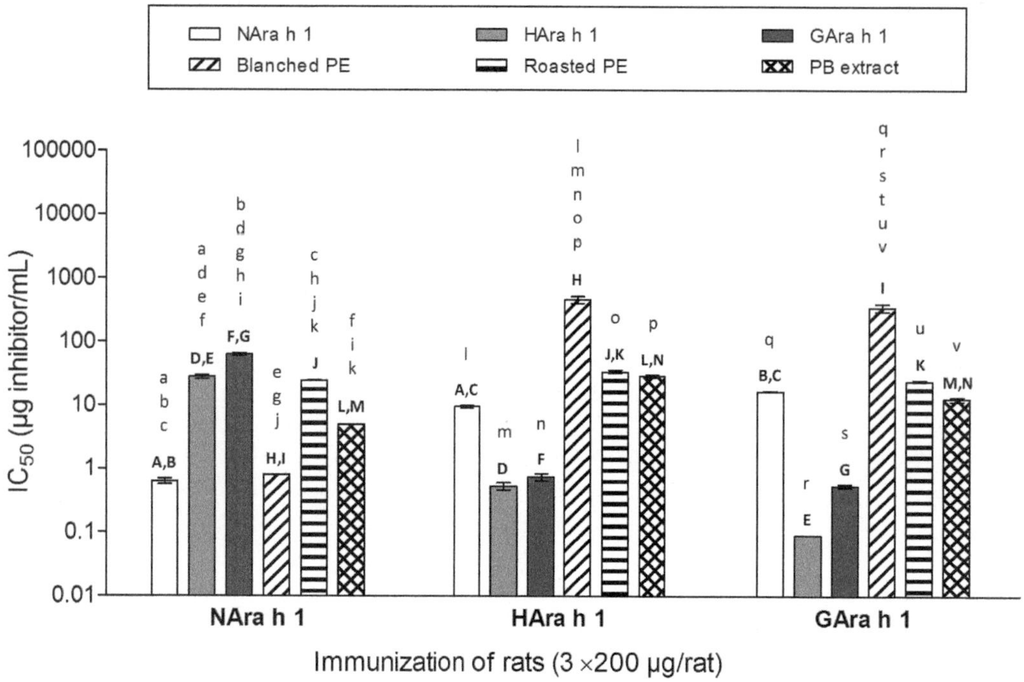

Figure 6. IgG1-binding capacity of sera from i.p. study with native and processed Ara h 1. Groups of rats were dosed i.p. on day 0, 14 and 28 with 200 µg of NAra h 1, HAra h 1 or GAra h 1. Serum pools obtained at sacrifice were preincubated with tenfold dilutions of native or processed Ara h 1 (0.0001 µg/mL–100 µg/mL) or peanut product extracts (0.001 µg/mL–1000 µg/mL) before measurement of IgG1-binding capacity by addition to ELISA plates coated with the antigen (N-, H- or GAra h 1) the group was sensitized against. Each bar represents IC_{50} mean values ± SD for a serum pool for each group of rats. Mean values were calculated as average of three measurements (each representing triplicate pipettings of the same serum/inhibitor mix) performed within one month. Data were analyzed by one-way ANOVA followed by Tukey's multiple comparison test. Statistically significant difference ($p \leq 0.05$) is shown by letters where two groups with the same letter are significant different (lower case letters: intragroup analysis, upper case letters: intergroup analysis). PE: peanut extract, PB: peanut butter.

when dosed orally without adjuvant. Roasted peanuts, either as such or as peanut butter, induced higher IgE anti-Ara h 1 and anti-Ara h 2 titers than blanched peanuts but these IgE showed low functionality in our cellular test. This is supported by the finding that process-modified Ara h 1 has a similar sensitizing capacity as native Ara h 1. On the other hand we found that irrespective of the peanut product used for sensitization, extract from roasted peanuts is a better elicitor than extract from blanched peanuts.

Acknowledgments

The authors thank Nehad Moradian, Dorte Lykkegaard Korsbech, Anne Ørngreen, Eva Ferdinansen, Elise Navntoft, Eigil Frank, Sarah Simonsen, Maja Danielsen and Kenneth Worm (DTU Food, Denmark) for excellent technical assistance and Anne Blicher and Vibeke Barkholt (DTU Systems Biology, Denmark) for performing amino acid analysis. We also wish to thank Marianne Lindblom and Oeivind Sagen (Kraft Foods, Oslo, Norway) for providing blanched and oil-roasted peanuts.

Author Contributions

Conceived and designed the experiments: SK CBM ENCM. Performed the experiments: SK PJ NR LS. Analyzed the data: SK KAP CBM KLB. Contributed reagents/materials/analysis tools: NR PJ LS KAP. Wrote the paper: SK KALB CBM ENCM.

References

1. Breiteneder H, Mills ENC (2005) Molecular properties of food allergens. J Allergy Clin Immunol 115: 14–23.
2. Mills ENC, Sancho AI, Rigby NM, Jenkins JA, Mackie AR (2009) Impact of food processing on the structure and allergenic properties of food allergens. Mol Nutr Res 53: 963–969.
3. Nowak-Wegrzyn A, Fiocchi A (2009) Rare, medium, or well done? The effect of heating and food matrix on food protein allergenicity. Curr Opin Allergy Clin Immunol 9: 234–237.
4. Grimshaw KEC, King RM, Nordlee JA, Hefle SL, Warner JO, et al. (2003) Presentation of allergen in different food preparations affects the nature of the allergic reaction – a case series. Clin Exp Allergy 33: 1581–1585.
5. Paschke A (2009) Aspects of food processing and its effect on allergen structure. Mol Nutr Food Res 53: 959–962.
6. Mills ENC, Mackie AR (2008) The impact of processing on allergenicity of food. Curr Opin Allergy Clin Immunol 8: 249–253.
7. Ladics GS (2009) Food Processing and Allergenicity. Mol Nutr Food Res 53: 945.
8. Sathe SK, Sharma GM (2009) Effects of food processing on food allergens. Mol Food Res 53: 970–978.
9. Davis PJ, Williams SC (1998) Protein modification by thermal processing. Allergy 53: 102–105.
10. Taheri-Kafrani A, Gaudin J-C, Rabesona H, Nioi C, Agarwal D, et al. (2009) Effects of heating and glycation of β-lactoglobulin on its recognition by IgE of sera from cow milk allergy patients. J Agric Food Chem 57: 4974–4982.
11. Chung S-Y, Champagne ET (2001) Association of end-product adducts with increased IgE binding of roasted peanuts. J Agric Food Chem 49: 3911–3916.
12. Maleki MJ, Chung S-Y, Champagne ET, Raufman J-P (2000) The effects of roasting on the allergenic properties of peanut proteins. J Allergy Clin Immunol 106: 763–768.
13. Beyer K, Morrow E, Li X-M, Bardina L, Bannon GA, et al. (2001) Effects of cooking methods on peanut allergenicity. J Allergy Clin Immunol 107: 1077–1081.

14. Mondoulet L, Paty E, Drumare MF, Ah-Leung S, Scheinmann P, et al. (2005) Influence of thermal processing on the allergenicity of peanut proteins. J Agric Food Chem 53: 4547–4553.
15. Vissers YM, Blanc F, Skov PS, Johnson PE, Rigby NM, et al. (2011) Effect of Heating and Glycation on the Allergenicity of 2S Albumins (Ara h 2/6) from peanut. PLoS ONE 6(8): e23998. doi:10.1371/journal.pone.0023998.
16. Vissers YM, Iwan M, Adel-Patient K, Stahl Skov P, Rigby NM, et al. (2011) Effect of roasting on the allergenicity of major peanut allergens Ara h 1 and Ara h 2/6: the necessity of degranulation assays. Clin Exp Allergy 41: 1631–1642.
17. Blanc F, Vissers YM, Adel-Patient K, Rigby NM, Mackie AR, et al. (2011) Boiling peanut Ara h 1 results in the formation of aggregates with reduced allergenicity. Mol Nutr Food Res 55: 1887–1894.
18. Nakamura S, Suzuki Y, Ishikawa E, Yakushi T, Jing H, et al. (2008) Reduction of in vitro allergenicity of buckwheat Fag e 1 through the Maillard-type glycosylation with polysaccharides. Food Chem 109: 538–545.
19. Nakamura A, Watanabe K, Ojima T, Ahn D-H, Saeki H (2005) Effects of Maillard reaction on allergenicity of scallop tropomyosin. J Agric Food Chem 53: 7559–7564.
20. Nakamura A, Sasaki F, Watanabe K, Ojima T, Ahn D-H, et al. (2006) Changes in allergenicity and digestibility of squid tropomyosin during the Maillard reaction with ribose. J Agric Food Chem 54: 9529–9534.
21. Gruber P, Vieths S, Wangorsch A, Nerkamp J Hofmann T (2004) Maillard reaction and enzymatic browning affect the allergen from cherry (Prunus avium). J Agric Food Chem 52: 4002–4007.
22. Sancho AI, Rigby NM, Zuidmeer L, Asero R, Mistrello G, et al. (2005) The effect of thermal processing on the IgE reactivity of the non-specific lipid transfer protein from apple, Mal d 3. Allergy 60: 1262–1268.
23. Iwan M, Vissers YM, Fiedorowicz E, Kostyra H, Kostyra E, et al. (2011) Impact of Maillard reaction on immunoreactivity and allergenicity of the hazelnut allergen Cor a 11. J Agric Food Chem 59: 7163–7171.
24. Boulay A, Houghton J, Gancheva V, Sterk Y, Strada A, et al. (2008) A EuroPrevall review of factors affecting incidence of peanut allergy: priorities for research and policy. Allergy 63: 797–809.
25. Koppelman SJ, Bruijnzeel-Koomen CAFM, Hessing M, de Jongh HHJ (1999) Heat-induced conformational changes of Ara h 1, a major peanut allergen, do not affect its allergenic properties. J Biol Chem 274: 4770–4777.
26. Maleki SJ, Hurlbert BK (2004) Structural and functional alterations in major peanut allergens caused by thermal processing. J AOAC Int 87: 1475–1479.
27. Lehmann K, Schweimer K, Reese G, Randow S, Suhr M, et al. (2006) Structure and stability of 2S albumin-type peanut allergens: implications for the severity of peanut allergic reactions. Biochem J 395: 463–472.
28. Chung S-Y, Butts CL, Maleki SJ, Champagne ET (2003) Linking peanut allergenicity to the processes of maturation, curing, and roasting. J Agric Food Chem 51: 4273–4277.
29. Gruber P, Becker W-M, Hofmann T (2005) Influence of the Maillard reaction on the allergenicity of rAra h 2, a recombinant major allergen from peanut (Arachis hypogaea), its major epitopes, and peanut agglutinin. J Agric Food Chem 53: 2289–2296.
30. Li XM, Serebrisky D, Lee SY, Huang CK, Bardina L, et al. (2000) A murine model of peanut anaphylaxis: T- and B-cell responses to a major peanut allergen mimic human responses. J Allergy Clin Immunol 106: 150–158.
31. van Wijk F, Nierkens S, Hassing I, Feijen M, Koppelman SJ, et al. (2005) The effect of the food matrix on in vivo immune responses to purified peanut allergens. Toxicol Sci 86: 333–341.
32. Marsh J, Rigby N, Wellner K, Reese G, Knulst A, et al. (2008) Purification and characterisation of a panel of peanut allergens suitable for use in allergy diagnosis. Mol Nutr Food Res 52: 272–285.
33. Johnson PE, Van der Plancken I, Balasa A, Husband FA, Grauwet T, et al. (2010) High pressure, thermal and pulsed electric-field-induced structural changes in selected food allergens. Mol Nutr Food Res 54: 1701–1710.
34. Barkholt V, Jensen AL (1989) Amino acid analysis: Determination of cysteine plus half-cysteine in proteins after hydrochloric acid hydrolysis with a disulfide compound as additive. Anal Biochem 177: 318–322.
35. Kroghsbo S, Bøgh KL, Rigby NM, Mills ENC, Rogers A, et al. (2011) Sensitization with 7S globulins from peanut, hazelnut, soy or pea induces IgE with different biological activities which are modified by soy tolerance. Int Arch Allergy Immunol 155: 212–224.
36. Kroghsbo S, Madsen C, Poulsen M, Schrøder M, Kvist PH, et al. (2008) Immunotoxicological studies of genetically modified rice expressing PHA-E lectin or Bt toxin in Wistar rats. Toxicology 245: 24–34.
37. Schmitt DA, Nesbit JB, Hurlburt BK, Cheng H, Maleki SJ (2010) Processing can alter the properties of peanut extract preparations. J Agric Food Chem 58: 1138–1143.
38. Maleki SJ, Viguez O, Jacks T, Dodo H, Champagne ET, et al. (2003) The major peanut allergen Ara h 2, functions as a trypsin inhibitor, and roasting enhances this function. J Allergy Clin Immunol 112: 190–195.
39. Bøgh KL, Kroghsbo S, Dahl L, Rigby NM, Barkholt V, et al. (2009) Digested Ara h 1 has sensitizing capacity in Brown Norway rats. Clin Exp Allergy 39: 1611–1621.
40. Dyer S, Mack L, Cheng H, Maleki SJ (2008) Structural, chemical and immunogenic effects of roasting on Ara h 3, a major peanut allergen. J Allergy Clin Immunol 121: S183.
41. Westphal CD, Pereira MR, Raybourne RB, Williams KM (2004) Evaluation of extraction buffers using the current approach of detecting multiple allergenic and nonallergenic proteins in food. J AOAC Int 87: 1458–1465.
42. Poms RE, Capelletti C, Anklam E (2004) Effect of roasting history and buffer composition on peanut protein extraction efficiency. Mol Nutr Food Res 48: 459–464.
43. Blanc F, Adel-Patient K, Drumare MF, Paty E, Wal JM, et al. (2009) Capacity of purified peanut allergens to induce degranulation in a functional in vitro assay: Ara h 2 and Ara h 6 are the most efficient elicitors. Clin Exp Allergy 39: 1277–1285.

Is the Determination of Specific IgE against Components Using ISAC 112 a Reproducible Technique?

Rubén Martínez-Aranguren[1], María T. Lizaso[2], María J. Goikoetxea[1], Blanca E. García[2], Paula Cabrera-Freitag[1], Oswaldo Trellez[3], María L. Sanz[1]*

1 Department of Allergology and Clinical Immunology, Clínica Universidad de Navarra, Pamplona, Spain, **2** Allergology Service, Complejo Hospitalario de Navarra, Pamplona, Spain, **3** Department of Computer Architecture, Universidad de Málaga, Málaga, Spain

Abstract

Background: The ImmunoCAP ISAC 112 is a fluoro-immunoassay that allows detection of specific IgE to 112 molecular components from 51 allergenic sources. We studied the reliability of this technique intra- and inter- assay, as well as inter-batch- and inter-laboratory-assay.

Methods: Twenty samples were studied, nineteen sera from polysensitized allergic patients, and the technique calibrator provided by the manufacturer (CTR02). We measured the sIgE from CTR02 and three patients' sera ten times in the same and in different assays. Furthermore, all samples were tested in two laboratories and with two batches of ISAC kit. To evaluate the accuracy of ISAC 112, we contrasted the determinations of CTR02 calibrator with their expected values by T Student test. To analyse the precision, we calculated the coefficient of variation (CV) of the 15 allergens that generate the calibration curve, and to analyse the repeatability and the reproducibility, we calculated the intraclass coefficient correlation (ICC) to each allergen.

Results: The results obtained for CTR02 were similar to those expected in 7 of 15 allergens that generate the calibration curve, whereas in 8 allergens the results showed significant differences. The mean CV obtained in the CTR02 determinations was of 9.4%, and the variability of sera from patients was of 22.9%. The agreement in the intra- and inter-assay analysis was very good to 94 allergens and good to one. In the inter-batch analyse, we obtained a very good agreement to 82 allergens, good to 14, moderate to 5 allergens, poor to one, and bad to 1 allergen. In the inter-laboratory analyse, we obtained a very good agreement to 73 allergens, good to 22, moderate to 6 and poor to two allergens.

Conclusion: The allergen microarray immunoassay, ISAC 112, is a repeatable and reproducible in vitro diagnostic tool for determination of sIgE beyond the own laboratory.

Editor: Vladimir N. Uversky, University of South Florida College of Medicine, United States of America

Funding: RM is supported by a grant from the Spanish Research Network on Adverse Reactions to Allergens and Drugs (RIRAAF RD12 00130010: Red de Investigación de Reacciones Adversas a Alérgenos y Fármacos) of the Carlos III Health Institute, Madrid, Spain. All the authors (except PCF) belong to RIRAAF RD12 00130010. This study has been partly funded by a grant FIS 11/01634 from the Carlos III Health Institute. The funders had no role in study design, data collection and analysis, decision to publish, or preparation of the manuscript.

Competing Interests: Thermofisher supplies part of the material (ISAC CRD 112 kits) required for this study. This does not alter the authors' adherence to all the PLOS ONE policies on sharing data and materials.

* E-mail: mlsanzlar@unav.es

Introduction

Component-based allergological diagnosis has opened up a new era in the study of allergies. It allows the identification of specific sensitization against proteins or specific molecular components [1–4]. This new approach helps to clarify the molecular bases of primary sensitization and cross-reactivity phenomena [5–11]. It also helps to rationalize the indication for immunotherapy based on the administration of allergenic components [12–14] and constitutes a necessary tool in the choice of a diet free from allergens in food-allergic patients [12,15].

The technique of the commercially available protein microarray ImmunoCAP ISAC® specific IgE (sIgE) 112 offers the possibility of analyzing sIgE against 112 components of purified natural proteins and recombinant proteins from 51 different allergenic sources. Since its launch onto the market, this platform has generated great expectations [16–19], and its use is being introduced into clinical practice because, at least from the conceptual point of view, it could be an aid to the clinician in the diagnosis or treatment indication of certain patients, especially those polysensitized ones [6,20]. However, clinical and technical validations and comparative studies are still needed [21–23]. In fact, previous version of this platform (ISAC 103) showed high variability for certain allergens [21], and even low efficiency in diagnosing sensitizations to certain proteins [24]. Thus, data assessing reliability of this technique, now for version ISAC 112, are required even beyond each laboratory.

The objective of this study was to assess the accuracy, precision, repeatability and reproducibility of this platform. To this aim we carried out assays with the technique's calibrating sample and sera from polysensitized patients under different conditions including determinations performed both in the same assay and in different assays and considering as possible sources of additional variability the use of different batches of reagents and the performance of the technique in different laboratories.

Materials and Methods

Samples

A total of 20 samples were analyzed: the calibrator sample (CTR02), provided by the manufacturer and 19 sera from polysensitized patients. The research ethical committee from the Universidad de Navarra approved the study "Technical and clinical validation of the diagnostic capacity of microarrays of allergenic molecules in allergy to pollens and/or vegetable foods" in which this work has been done. Patients provided their written informed consent to participate in this study. After inclusion for this work, the data from the patients' sera were analyzed anonymously.

The CTR02 calibrator, according to information provided by the manufacturer, is composed of known amounts of chimeric monoclonal antibodies humanized against 15 molecular components (Amb a 1, Art v 1, Bet v 1, Can f 1, Can f 2, Can f 5, Der p 1, Der p 2, Fel d 1, Gal d 1, Gal d 2, Ole e 1, Phl p 1, Phl p 5, and Pru p 3). The antibodies against these 15 allergenic components are found in the calibrator in a range of 4 different concentrations expressed in ISAC Standardized Units (ISU) values for sIgE (1, 4, 15 and 50 ISU). This allows a calibration curve to be plotted from the 4 points of fluorescence intensity corresponding to the different ISU (figure 1).

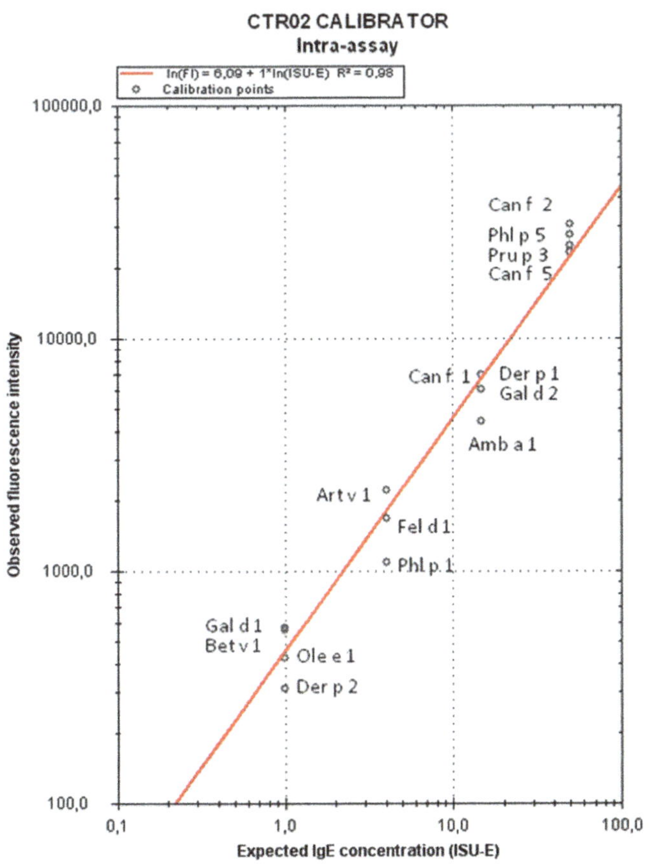

Figure 1. Calibration curve. Example of calibration curve used for the intra-assay analysis.

Of the 19 sera from the polysensitized patients, sera 1, 2, and 3, contained as a group detectable amounts of sIgE against the 15 allergens making up the calibration curve and against another 80 allergens (of the 112 represented in the microarray). Sixteen additional sera, numbered 4–19, showing a broad variety of sensitizations were also included in the study.

Patients' sera were frozen at −20°C after the blood collection until the immunoassays were performed and, among the different assays, samples were conserved at 4°C.

InmunoCAP ISAC 112 microarray

The microarray ISAC 112 (ThermoFisher, Uppsala, Sweden) is a solid phase fluoro immunoassay that detects IgE antibodies against the proteins fixed on ISAC surface. One slide contains 4 microarray and one kit 5 slides, 20 microarrays in total. The technique was performed following the manufacturer's instructions. Each microarray is incubated with a serum in order to label sIgE to each protein and subsequently it is incubated with a human anti IgE detection antibody conjugated with fluorescence.

Finally the fluorescence intensity of each microarray is measured by the scanner (LuxScan 10K/A, CapitalBio, Beijing, China) using following parameters: laser power (LP = 60) and photo-multiplier tube (PMT = 600).

The analysis of the digitalized images is performed with the software Phadia Microarray Image Analyzer (ThermoFisher). This software allows transforming the images fluorescence intensity in numerical data according to the calibration curve built with the calibrator CTR02 sample included in each assay, as previously described (figure 1). An acceptable calibration curve needs to show slope parameters (Y) between 5.5 and 6.8, and $R^2 > 0.85$ according to the information provided by ThermoFisher.

The sIgE values are expressed semiquantitatively as ISU. Results equal or greater than 0.30 ISU are considered positive, according to the indications of the manufacturer.

Intra-assay analysis

The repeatability of the ISAC 112 technique was assessed by analyzing the sIgE from the CTR02 calibrator and sera 1 to 3 obtained in 10 determinations performed in the same assay with 2 ISAC 112 kits from the same production batch. The calibration curve was obtained with the first determination of the CTR02 calibrator in the first kit in the first slide, first microarray.

Inter-assay analysis

The reproducibility of the technique was assessed by analyzing the sIgE results from the CTR02 calibrator and sera 1 to 3 obtained in 10 assays performed on 10 different days using 2 ISAC 112 kits from the same production batch. For each assay a calibration curve was plotted with the calibration curve performed in its own assay.

Inter-laboratory analysis

The reproducibility of the ISAC 112 technique was assessed by analyzing the levels of sIgE obtained from the 20 samples studied with 2 kits from the same batch. The analyses were performed in two different laboratories i.e.: Clínica Universidad de Navarra, and the Complejo Hospitalario de Navarra, both in Pamplona, Navarra, Spain. The reading of the chips was performed with the same conditions in each laboratory. The calibration curve was plotted with the determination of the CTR02 calibrator performed

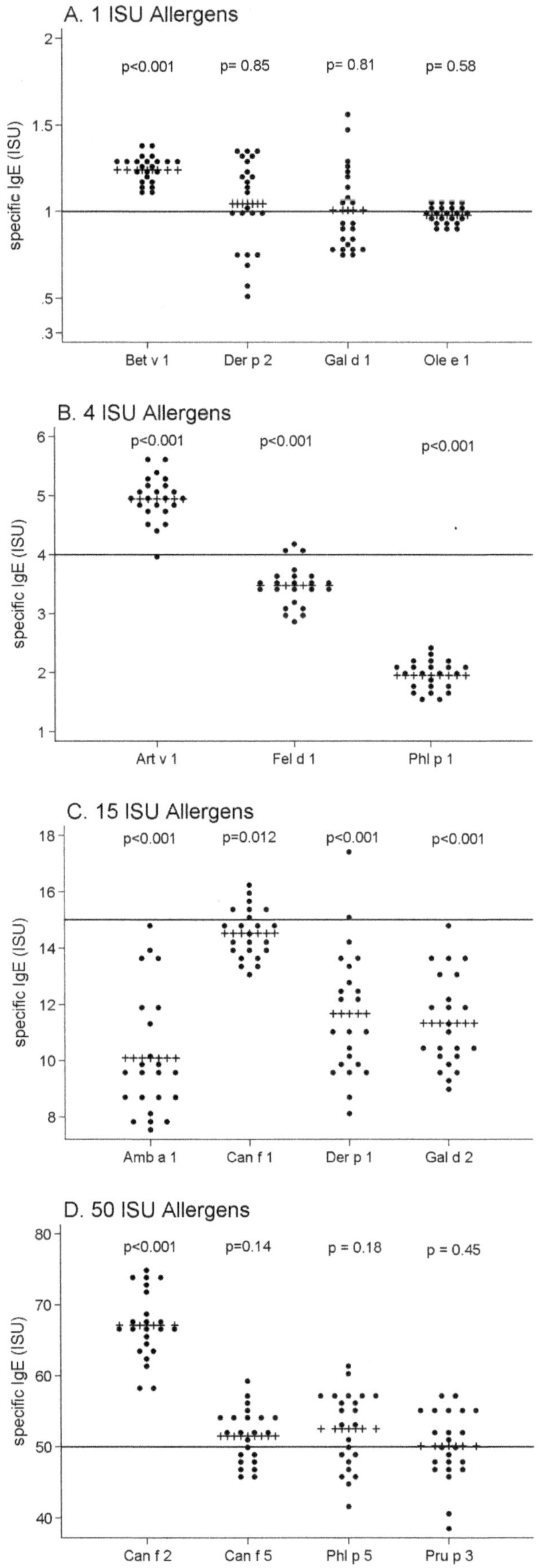

Figure 2. Accuracy of ISAC 112. Results obtained for the allergens that form the calibration curve with the intra-assay, inter-assay, inter-laboratory and inter-batch determinations performed with the calibrator CTR02, composed by chimeric antibodies. Expected ISU results are depicted by red line and the observed mean ISU results are depicted by red +++. Student T test was used for statistical analysis.

in each laboratory. Both scanners had been calibrated similarly by the same technician, the same day.

Inter-batch analysis

The reproducibility of the ISAC 112 technique was also assessed by analyzing sIgE levels from the 20 samples under study obtained from two kits from different production batch.

Statistical analysis of the data

We studied the *accuracy* of ISAC 112, understood as the similarity between the values obtained and those expected, and its *precision*, understood as the dispersion of the group of results obtained.

We evaluated the *accuracy* by the analysis of the determinations performed in all the assays with the sample CTR02, after comparison of the results expected and those obtained for each one of the 15 allergens that constitute the calibration curve by means of the Student's T test.

Furthermore, the *precision* of the allergens from the calibration curve was analyzed by calculating the coefficient of variation (CV) in all the assays, as the percentage of the standard deviation of the determinations divided by the mean. We calculated the CV from the results obtained from the CTR02 calibrator.

We analyzed the strength of agreement of the determinations under the same conditions, *repeatability*, and different conditions, *reproducibility*, of the results obtained in the different assays by calculating the intraclass coefficient correlation (ICC) for each allergen [25,26]. The level of agreement using the ICC was expressed using the classification of Fleiss [27] as: very good (ICC>0.90), good (0.71–0.90), moderate (0.51–070), mediocre (0.31–0.50) or poor (ICC<0.30).

Also, we analysed the *reliability* of the semiquantitative character of the technique comparing the number of allergens that modified the category of the IgE according to the range established by the manufacturer (<0.3 ISU, not detectable; ≥0.3–<1 ISU, low; ≥1–<15 moderated or high; and ≥15, very high), in the interassay determinations for each serum.

The Student's T test and the ICC for each allergen were performed using the statistical software package SPSS (Statistical Packaged for social science) for Windows, version 15.0 (Chicago, Illinois, USA). The CV was calculated using the program Excel version 12.0, Microsoft Office 2007.

Results

Accuracy

The average values obtained in the sIgE determinations against the allergens of the calibration curve Der p 2, Gal d 1, Ole e 1, Can f 1, Can f 5, Phl p 5 and Pru p 3 by ISAC resulted to be similar to those expected (figure 2). Nevertheless, the determinations of the remaining 8 allergens showed statistically significant differences ($p<0.05$) between the observed levels and those expected. Of these 8 allergens, six allergens (Art v 1, Fel d 1, Phl p 1, Amb a 1, Can f 1, Der p 1 and Gal d 2) are in the intermediate points of the calibration curve (4 and 15 ISU), whereas the Bet v 1 belongs to a 1 ISU calibration point and the

Can f 2 belongs to the 50 ISU calibration point. Despite these differences, all the calibrator CTR02 determinations gave place to a calibration curve within the slope parameters and R^2 considered by the manufacturer as acceptable (Y and R^2 maximum and minimum obtained at the assays 6.52–5.8 and 0.99–0.95, respectively)

Precision

When we analyzed the global variability in the results from the different determinations of the CTR02 calibrator, we obtained a mean CV of 9.42%.

The individual data of the calibrating sera allergens are expressed in figure 3.

Repeatability and reproducibility

Repeatability and reproducibility calculated using the ICC are summarised in table 1.

The analysis of the repeatability (intra-assay analysis) was very good for 94 of the 112 allergens represented in the microarray and good for the Bos d lactoferrin allergen. For the remaining 17 allergens the ICC could not be calculated as all the determinations were equal to 0 ISU.

The analysis of the inter-assay reproducibility was very good for 94 of the 112 allergens and good for the Pol d 5 allergen.

The reproducibility between the analyses of the determinations in two laboratories was very good for 73 allergens and good for 22 of the allergens represented in the microarray. The allergens Ara h 9, Art v 1, Bla g 5, Bos d 8, Bos d lactoferrin, and Phl p 12, showed a moderate agreement whereas in Jug r 2 and Alt a 6 agreement was mediocre. The ICC values could not be calculated for 9 allergens in inter-laboratories analysis because all the determinations for them were equal to 0 ISU.

Finally, in the analysis of the reproducibility between the two kits from different production batches we obtained a very good agreement for 82 allergens and good for 14 allergens. For the allergens Bos d 8, Lep d 2, Pen m 1, Ses i 1 and Ves v 5 we obtained a moderate ICC while for Bos d lactoferrin and Alt a 6 gave a mediocre and poor agreement respectively. The ICC values could not be calculated for 9 allergens in inter-batch analysis because all the determinations for them were equal to 0 ISU.

Disagreements in the IgE level

When analysing the number of disagreements in the interassay analysis determinations in patients' sera, we obtained the following results. The results of sIgE obtained modified from "not detectable" level to "low" level for 7 allergens when analysing sera 1 and 2, and for 9 allergens when analysing sera 3. The specific IgE levels modified from "low" to "moderate-high" for 7 allergens when analysing sera 1 and 2, and for 13 when analysing sera 3. The specific IgE level change from "moderate-high" to "very high" happened in 16 occasions when analysing sera 1, and in 15 occasions when analysing sera 2. Finally, the IgE level change from "not detectable" to "high" was observed for 4 and 5 allergens when using sera 1 and 2 respectively. This allergens were Act d 1, Asp f 1, Ara h 8, Ber e 1, Cor a 9, Mal d 1, Phl p 5, Phl p 12 and Pla l 1. The allergens that showed a greater number of disagreements were Jug r 2, Jug r 3 and Ses i 1, which had disagreements on the IgE level in the three sera studied.

Discussion

The technique of protein microarrays has been accepted as a useful method for the detection of sIgE against molecular components [28,29]. Thus, it has been shown its usefulness for the diagnosis of food allergies, to determine cross-reactivity phenomena or sensitization patterns in specific geographical areas [14,20]. Previously, several comparative studies between ISAC and other conventional techniques of sIgE detection, such as ImmunoCAP have been performed. These studies state that although the results obtained between both methods are not comparable, a good agreement between them was found [13,20,30].

However, few studies have been carried out into the variability and accuracy of this technique showing improvable results in previous versions of this microarray [17,21]. In the present study, we analyzed accuracy, variability and reproducibility in the new version, ImmunoCAP ISAC 112. The results obtained in the study show good reproducibility of the technique not only for one assay but even considering changes of the assays in different days, and using different batches and in different laboratories.

When analysing the accuracy of the technique, 8 of the 15 allergens that form the calibration curve showed statistically significant differences between the values obtained and those expected. Despite this fact, all the calibration lines were within

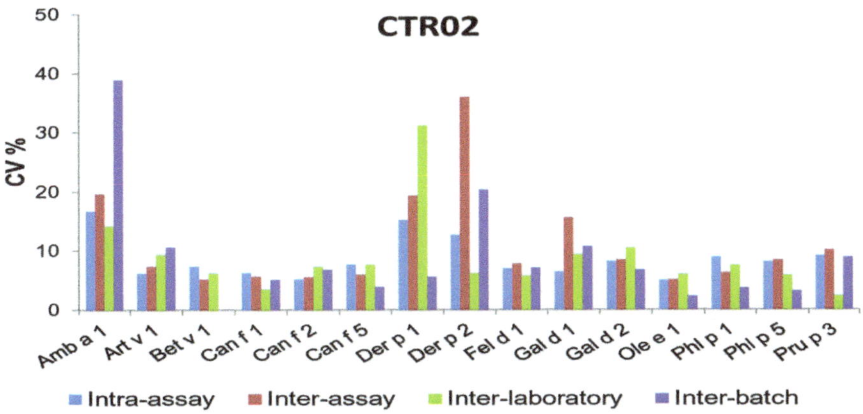

Figure 3. Variability of the ISAC 112 technique in the calibrator sample. Coefficient of Variation (CV) obtained to allergens of calibration curve. The results are the mean CV of 10 determinations intra- and inter-assay, and 2 determinations inter-laboratory and inter-batches of the calibrator sample.

Table 1. Intraclass Correlation Coefficient (ICC) of ISAC 112 results obtained from 10 determinations of 4 sera intra- and inter-assay and two determinations of 20 sera inter-laboratory and inter-batch.

ALLERGEN	INTRA-ASSAY	INTER-ASSAY	INTER-LAB	INTER-BATCH	ALLERGEN	INTRA-ASSAY	INTER-ASSAY	INTER-LAB	INTER-BATCH
Act d 1	0.983	0.978	0.950	0.995	Equ c 1	0.998	0.983	0.914	0.914
Act d 2	0.999	0.905	0.851	0.879	Equ c 3	0.999	0.996	0.948	0.954
Act d 5	0.978	0.955	0.834	*	Fag e 2	0.998	0.980	0.986	0.996
Act d 8	0.987	0.848	0.907	0.970	Fel d 1 †	0.994	0.987	0.981	0.993
Aln g 1	0.977	0.956	0.867	0.707	Fel d 2	0.996	0.996	0.987	0.775
Alt a 1	0.999	0.993	0.897	0.878	Fel d 4	0.997	0.966	0.970	0.925
Alt a 6	0.988	0.977	0.497	0.267	Gad c 1	0.999	0.986	0.995	0.988
Amb a 1 †	0.996	0.994	0.981	0.900	Gal d 1 †	1.000	0.918	0.970	0.993
Ana o 2	0.998	0.986	0.945	*	Gal d 2 †	0.998	0.969	0.987	0.986
Ani s 1	*	0.994	0.984	0.987	Gal d 3	1.000	0.993	0.998	0.999
Ani s 3	*	*	0.988	0.998	Gal d 5	0.998	0.986	0.997	0.922
Api g 1	0.998	0.978	0.986	0.980	Gly m 4	0.998	0.983	0.998	0.961
Api m 1	*	*	0.973	0.998	Gly m 5	0.997	0.990	0.838	0.944
Api m 4	*	*	*	*	Gly m 6	0.997	0.989	0.955	0.960
Ara h 1	0.997	0.990	0.979	0.963	Hev b 1	*	*	0.945	*
Ara h 2	0.997	0.993	0.937	0.991	Hev b 3	*	*	0.973	0.991
Ara h 3	*	*	0.991	0.928	Hev b 5	1.000	0.995	0.998	0.997
Ara h 6	0.990	0.983	0.868	0.960	Hev b 6.01	0.993	*	0.990	0.995
Ara h 8	0.994	0.980	0.853	0.850	Hev b 8	1.000	0.997	0.999	0.997
Ara h 9	0.997	0.971	0.680	0.992	Jug r 1	0.996	0.986	0.880	0.974
Art v 1†	1.000	0.996	0.703	0.997	Jug r 2	0.994	0.979	0.446	0.881
Art v 3	0.999	0.998	0.986	0.996	Jug r 3	0.999	0.984	0.921	0.983
Asp f 1	0.995	0.984	0.938	0.859	Lep d 2	0.999	0.977	0.941	0.697
Asp f 3	0.999	0.994	0.955	0.998	Mal d 1	0.998	0.994	0.992	0.998
Asp f 6	0.991	0.997	*	*	Mer a 1	1.000	0.996	0.991	0.984
Ber e 1	0.996	0.983	0.779	0.715	Mus m 1	0.992	0.994	0.813	0.997
Bet v 1†	0.999	0.994	0.984	0.973	MUXF3	1.000	0.989	0.923	0.998
Bet v 2	0.999	0.992	0.951	0.946	Ole e 1†	1.000	0.995	0.992	0.990
Bet v 4	0.998	0.990	0.885	0.846	Ole e 7	0.999	0.989	0.831	0.907
Bla g 1	*	*	*	*	Ole e 9	0.999	0.993	0.980	0.995
Bla g 2	*	*	*	*	Par j 2	0.998	0.985	0.998	0.996
Bla g 5	0.992	0.980	0.646	0.776	Pen m 1	*	*	0.994	0.663
Bla g 7	*	*	0.959	0.955	Pen m 2	*	*	*	*
Blo t 5	*	*	0.924	0.993	Pen m 4	0.999	0.995	0.911	0.973
Bos d 4	*	*	0.998	0.969	Phl p 1†	1.000	0.996	0.991	0.989
Bos d 5	0.998	0.995	0.882	0.883	Phl p 11	0.997	0.989	0.994	0.968
Bos d 6	0.999	0.986	0.988	0.983	Phl p 12	0.998	0.979	0.586	0.725
Bos d 8	0.996	0.966	0.566	0.670	Phl p 2	0.998	0.981	0.944	0.886
Bos d Lact	0.865	0.981	0.596	0.464	Phl p 4	0.997	0.993	0.891	0.969
Can f 1 †	0.998	0.993	0.973	0.983	Phl p 5†	1.000	0.992	0.952	0.990
Can f 2 †	1.000	0.999	0.977	0.998	Phl p 6	0.993	0.974	0.829	0.920
Can f 3	0.919	0.981	0.994	0.991	Phl p 7	0.999	0.987	0.784	0.995
Can f 5 †	0.999	0.998	0.996	0.999	Pla a 1	1.000	0.991	0.839	0.818
Che a 1	0.999	0.989	0.940	0.944	Pla a 2	1.000	0.988	0.733	0.904
Cla h 8	*	*	*	*	Pla a 3	0.986	0.964	0.821	0.984
Cor a 1.0101	0.998	0.991	0.998	0.988	Pla l 1	0.990	0.933	0.951	0.994
Cor a 1.0401	0.992	0.984	0.986	0.993	Pol d 5	0.983	0.891	0.996	0.998
Cor a 8	0.999	0.988	0.931	0.990	Pru p 1	0.994	0.944	0.972	0.969

Table 1. Cont.

ALLERGEN	INTRA-ASSAY	INTER-ASSAY	INTER-LAB	INTER-BATCH	ALLERGEN	INTRA-ASSAY	INTER-ASSAY	INTER-LAB	INTER-BATCH
Cor a 9	0.997	0.991	0.827	0.987	Pru p 3†	0.999	0.997	0.985	0.994
Cry j 1	1.000	0.988	0.751	0.839	Sal k 1	1.000	0.997	0.985	1.000
Cup a 1	0.999	0.990	0.981	0.990	Ses i 1	0.990	0.994	0.986	<u>0.533</u>
Cyn d 1	0.999	0.985	0.950	0.909	Tri a 14	0.999	0.993	0.985	0.993
Der f 1	0.999	0.997	0.988	0.944	Tri a 19.0101	1.000	0.994	1.000	0.999
Der f 2	0.991	0.989	0.951	0.955	Tri a aA_TI	0.999	0.994	0.979	0.995
Der p 1 †	0.997	0.994	0.931	0.983	Ves v 5	*	*	0.996	0.634
Der p 10	*	*	0.932	0.994					
Der p 2†	0.993	0.972	0.874	0.961					

*The ICC could not be calculated as all the determinations were equal to 0 ISU.
†Allergens detected by the calibration curve.
ICC ranges: very good (>0.9), good (0.71–0.90), moderate (0.51–0.70), mediocre (0.31–0.50) and poor (<0.30). Underlined are showed ICC values below 0.7.

acceptable limits of slope and R2 established by the technique's supplier. The fact that most allergens keep their category, even at low sIgE levels, supports the reliability of the results offered by the technique. Nevertheless, it should be highlighted that this is a semiquantitative technique and the IgE levels close to the cut off points between categories can fluctuate in different assays.

Regarding the technique's precision, the results obtained show a low variability when we analyse the determinations of the control sample CTR02, which is under 10% in most allergens. Also, the CV is similar both in the analysis performed in the same assay and in those performed in different assays. It is worth noting that the capacity of the allergen to attach itself to the surface of the ISAC array is lower than in quantitative techniques such as ImmunoCAP, in which the allergen is fixed under excess molarity conditions. This fact could make more clear differences in the allergen ability to bind to the microarray leading into differences in variability of specific IgE binding. Differences in reliability of some allergens from the microarray (like Amb a 1, Der p 1 or Der p 2) and considering that ISAC microarray is a semiquantitative technique suggest that ISAC 112 is not the best method to monitor sensitizations and patient's follow-up.

However, in our opinion these analyses demonstrated an evident improvement in the new version of the ISAC microarray. This improvement can be, among others, due to the calibration curve consisting in chimeric antibodies (sIgE) in contrast to the serum with known sIgE concentration from previous versions ISAC 103 [21]. This might be due to a good characterization of chimeric antibodies and the absence of other isotypes able to bind to the spotted allergens.

Finally, we studied the repeatability and reproducibility of the technique, analysing the ICC in the different assays. The results obtained in the intra-assay analysis show a good repeatability, obtaining good agreement strength for almost all the allergens present in microarray. Also, the reproducibility of the interassay analysis showed good concordance strength for these allergens. The reproducibility in the inter-laboratory and inter-batch analysis still has good agreement strength for most allergens. Nevertheless, this agreement strength was lower for 8 allergens in the inter-laboratory analysis and for 7 allergens in the inter-batch agreement. This slight decrease in the results' agreement strength could be due to the fact that only two determinations were performed in each analysis instead of 10 repetitions like in the interassay analysis. Also, the performance of analysis in different laboratories and with different batches means a greater source of variability.

In conclusion, ISAC 112 yields good reliability results taking into account that ISAC 112 gives semi-quantitative results. However, due to the low accuracy obtained in some of the studied allergens, the application of this semi-quantitative technique for diagnosis in clinical situations where results may have a major impact on the therapy prescribed may not be advisable. Even more, this study suggests that neither laboratory specific condition neither the change from one batch to another affect substantially microarray reliability.

Acknowledgments

All the authors of this article belong to the Research network in Adverse Reactions to Foods and Drugs (Red de Investigacion de Reacciones Adversas a Alimentos y Fármacos (RIRAAF)) RD12/0013/0010 at the Instituto Carlos III. ML Sanz and BE García belongs to the Committees of Immunology and Food Allergy of the Spanish Society of Allergy and Clinical Immunology (SEAIC).

Author Contributions

Conceived and designed the experiments: MTL MJG BEG MLS. Performed the experiments: RMMA MTL PCF. Analyzed the data: RMMA MTL MJG OT. Contributed reagents/materials/analysis tools: MTL BEG OT MLS. Wrote the paper: RMMA MJG BEG PCF MLS.

References

1. Valenta R, Lidholm J, Niederberger V, Hayek B, Kraft D, et al. (1999) The recombinant allergen-based concept of component-resolved diagnostics and immunotherapy (CRD and CRIT). Clin Exp Allergy 29: 896–904.
2. Asero R, Jimeno L, Barber D (2008) Component-resolved diagnosis of plant food allergy by SPT. Eur Ann Allergy Clin Immunol 40: 115–21.
3. Barber D, de la Torre F, Lombardero M, Antépara I, Colas C, et al. (2009) Component-resolved diagnosis of pollen allergy based on skin testing with profilin, polcalcin and lipid transfer protein pan-allergens. Clin Exp Allergy 39: 1764–73.

4. Lin J, Bardina L, Shreffler WG, Andreae DA, Ge Y, et al. (2009) Development of a novel peptide microarray for large-scale epitope mapping of food allergens. J Allergy Clin Immunol 124: 315–22.
5. Gamboa PM, Sanz ML, Lombardero M, Barber D, Sánchez-Monje R, et al. (2009) Component-resolved in vitro diagnosis in peach-allergic patients. J Investig Allergol Clin Immunol 19: 13–20.
6. Goikoetxea MJ, Cabrera-Freitag P, Sanz ML, Fernández-Benítez M (2010) The importance of in vitro component-resolved diagnosis in paediatric patients. Allergol Immunopathol 38: 37–40.
7. Palacin A, Quirce S, Armentia A, Fernández-Nieto M, Pacios LF, et al. (2007) Wheat lipid transfer protein is a major allergen associated with baker's asthma. J Allergy Clin Immunol 120. 1132–8.
8. Barber D, de la Torre F, Feo F, Florido F, Guardia P, et al. (2008) Understanding patient sensitization profiles in complex pollen areas: a molecular epidemiological study. Allergy 63: 1550–8.
9. Twardosz-Kropfmüller A, Singh MB, Niederberger V, Horak F, Kraft D, et al. (2010) Association of allergic patients' phenotypes with IgE reactivity to recombinant pollen marker allergens. Allergy 65: 296–303.
10. Díaz-Perales A, Lombardero M, Sánchez-Monge R, García-Selles FJ, Pernas M, et al. (2000) Lipid-transfer proteins as potential plant panallergens: cross-reactivity among proteins of Artemisia pollen, Castanea nut and Rosaceae fruits, with different IgE-binding capacities. Clin Exp Allergy 30: 1403–10.
11. Ebo DG, Bridts CH, Verweij MM, De Knop KJ, Hagendorens MM, et al. (2010) Sensitization profiles in birch pollen-allergic patients with and without oral allergy syndrome to apple: lessons from multiplexed component-resolved allergy diagnosis. Clin Exp Allergy 40: 339–47.
12. Ferrer M, Sanz ML, Sastre J, Bartra J, del Cuvillo A, et al. (2009) Molecular diagnosis in Allergology: application of the microarray tecnique J Investig Allergol Clin Immunol 19: 19–24.
13. Ott H, Baron JM, Heise R, Ocklenburg C, Stanzel S, et al. (2008) Clinical usefulness of microarray-based IgE detection in children with suspected food allergy. Allergy 63: 1521–8.
14. Sanz ML, Blázquez AB, Garcia BE (2011) Microarray of allergenic component-based diagnosis in food allergy. Curr Opin Allergy Clin Immunol 11: 204–9.
15. Renault NK, Mirotti L, Alcocer MJ (2007) Biotechnologies in new high-throughput food allergy tests: why we need them. Biotechnol Lett 29: 333–9.
16. Jahn-Schmid B, Harwanegg C, Hiller R, Bohle B, Ebner C, et al. (2003) Allergen microarray: Comparison of microarray using recombinant allergens with conventional diagnostic methods to detect allergen-specific serum immunoglobulin E. Clin Exp Allergy 33: 1443–9.
17. Mari A (2001) Multiple pollen sensitization: a molecular approach to the diagnosis. Int Arch Allergy Immunol 125: 57–65.
18. Scala E, Alessandri C, Bernardi ML, Ferrara R, Palazzo P, et al. (2010) Cross-sectional survey on immunoglobulin E reactivity in 23,077 subjects using an allergenic molecule-based microarray detection system. Clin Exp Allergy 40: 911–921
19. Wöhrl S, Vigl K, Zehetmayer S, Hiller R, Jarisch R, et al. (2006) The performance of a component-based allergen-microarray in clinical practice. Allergy 61: 633–9.
20. Sastre J, Landivar ME, Ruiz-García M, Andregnette-Rosigno MV, Mahillo I (2012) How molecular diagnosis can change allergen-specific immunotherapy prescription in a complex pollen area. Allergy 67: 709–11.
21. Cabrera-Freitag P, Goikoetxea MJ, Gamboa PM, Martínez-Aranguren R, Beorlegui C, et al. (2011) A study into the variability of the in vitro component-based microarray technique "ISAC CDR 103" J Invest Allergol Clin Immunol 21: 414–5.
22. Cabrera-Freitag P, Goikoetxea MJ, Beorlegui C, Gamboa PM, Gastaminza G, et al. (2011) Can component-based microarray replace fluorescent enzimoimmunoassay in the diagnosis of grass and cypress pollen allergy? Clin Exp Allergy 41: 1440–6.
23. Salcedo G, Díaz-Perales A (2010) Component-resolved diagnosis of allergy: more is better? Clin Exp Allergy 40: 836–8.
24. Villalta D, Asero R (2010) Is the detection of IgE to multiple Bet v 1-homologous food allergens by means of allergen microarray clinically useful? J Allergy Clin Immunol 125: 1158–61.
25. Prieto L, Lamarca L, Casado A (1998) La evaluación de la fiabilidad en las observaciones clínicas: el coeficiente de correlación intraclasse. Med Clin (Barc) 110: 142–45
26. Bravo G, Potvin L (1991) Estimating the reliability of continuos measures with Cronbach's alfa or the intraclass correlation coeficient: toward the integration of two traditions. J Clin Epidemiol 44: 381–390.
27. Fleiss JL (1986) Design and Analysis of Clinical Experiments. New York: John Wiley & Sons.
28. Hiller R, Laffer S, Harwanegg C, Huber M, Schmidt WM, et al. (2002) Microarrayed allergen molecules: diagnostics gatekeepers for allergy treatment. FASEB J 16: 414–6.
29. Canonica GW, Ansotegui IJ, Pawankar R, Schmid-Grendelmeier P, van Hage M, et al. (2013) A WAO - ARIA - GA2LEN consensus document on molecular-based allergy diagnostics. World Allergy Organ J 3; 6: 17.
30. Wang J, Godbold JH, Sampson HA (2008) Correlation of serum allergy (IgE) tests performed by different assay systems. J Allergy Clin Immunol 121: 1219–24.

Permissions

All chapters in this book were first published in PLOS ONE, by The Public Library of Science; hereby published with permission under the Creative Commons Attribution License or equivalent. Every chapter published in this book has been scrutinized by our experts. Their significance has been extensively debated. The topics covered herein carry significant findings which will fuel the growth of the discipline. They may even be implemented as practical applications or may be referred to as a beginning point for another development.

The contributors of this book come from diverse backgrounds, making this book a truly international effort. This book will bring forth new frontiers with its revolutionizing research information and detailed analysis of the nascent developments around the world.

We would like to thank all the contributing authors for lending their expertise to make the book truly unique. They have played a crucial role in the development of this book. Without their invaluable contributions this book wouldn't have been possible. They have made vital efforts to compile up to date information on the varied aspects of this subject to make this book a valuable addition to the collection of many professionals and students.

This book was conceptualized with the vision of imparting up-to-date information and advanced data in this field. To ensure the same, a matchless editorial board was set up. Every individual on the board went through rigorous rounds of assessment to prove their worth. After which they invested a large part of their time researching and compiling the most relevant data for our readers.

The editorial board has been involved in producing this book since its inception. They have spent rigorous hours researching and exploring the diverse topics which have resulted in the successful publishing of this book. They have passed on their knowledge of decades through this book. To expedite this challenging task, the publisher supported the team at every step. A small team of assistant editors was also appointed to further simplify the editing procedure and attain best results for the readers.

Apart from the editorial board, the designing team has also invested a significant amount of their time in understanding the subject and creating the most relevant covers. They scrutinized every image to scout for the most suitable representation of the subject and create an appropriate cover for the book.

The publishing team has been an ardent support to the editorial, designing and production team. Their endless efforts to recruit the best for this project, has resulted in the accomplishment of this book. They are a veteran in the field of academics and their pool of knowledge is as vast as their experience in printing. Their expertise and guidance has proved useful at every step. Their uncompromising quality standards have made this book an exceptional effort. Their encouragement from time to time has been an inspiration for everyone.

The publisher and the editorial board hope that this book will prove to be a valuable piece of knowledge for researchers, students, practitioners and scholars across the globe.

List of Contributors

Matthias Egger, Michael Wallner, Fatima Ferreira and Gabriele Gadermaier
Christian Doppler Laboratory for Allergy Diagnosis and Therapy, University of Salzburg, Salzburg, Austria

Claudia Alessandri, Danila Zennaro and Adriano Mari
Center for Molecular Allergology, IDI-IRCCS, Rome, Italy

Peter Briza
Department of Molecular Biology, University of Salzburg, Salzburg, Austria

Silvana Gaudieri
School of Anatomy and Human Biology, University of Western Australia, Nedlands, Australia
Centre for Forensic Science, University of Western Australia, Nedlands, Australia
Institute for Immunology and Infectious Diseases, Murdoch University, Murdoch, Australia

Hiba Albloushi
Centre for Forensic Science, University of Western Australia, Nedlands, Australia

Andrew Lucas and Elizabeth McKinnon
Institute for Immunology and Infectious Diseases, Murdoch University, Murdoch, Australia

Michaela Lucas
Institute for Immunology and Infectious Diseases, Murdoch University, Murdoch, Australia
PathWest and Laboratory Medicine, University of Western Australia, Nedlands, Australia

Andri Rauch
University Clinic of Infectious Diseases, University Hospital Bern and University of Bern, Bern, Switzerland

Julia di Iulio
Institute of Microbiology, University Hospital Centre and University of Lausanne, Lausanne, Switzerland

David Martino, Susan L. Prescott and Meri K. Tulic
School of Paediatrics and Child Health, University of Western Australia, Nedlands, Australia

Elisabeth Hoflehner, Karin Hufnagl, Irma Schabussova, Joanna Jasinska and Ursula Wiedermann
Institute of Specific Prophylaxis and Tropical Medicine, Center for Pathophysiology, Infectiology and Immunology, Medical University of Vienna, Vienna, Austria

Karin Hoffmann-Sommergruber and Barbara Bohle
Department of Pathophysiology and Allergy Research, Center for Pathophysiology, Infectiology and Immunology, Medical University of Vienna, Vienna, Austria

Rick M. Maizels
Institute of Immunology and Infection Research, University of Edinburgh, Edinburgh, United Kingdom

Huub F. J. Savelkoul
Cell Biology and Immunology Group, Wageningen University and Research Centre, Wageningen, The Netherlands

Yvonne M. Vissers
Cell Biology and Immunology Group, Wageningen University and Research Centre, Wageningen, The Netherlands
Food Chemistry Group, Wageningen University and Research Centre, Wageningen, The Netherlands

Fany Blanc, Laetitia Przybylski-Nicaise, Hervé Bernard, Jean-Michel Wal and Karine Adel-Patient
Unité d'Immuno-Allergie Alimentaire UR496, Département Alimentation Humaine, INRA, Jouy-en-Josas, France

Per Stahl Skov
RefLab ApS, Copenhagen, Denmark

Phil E. Johnson, Neil M. Rigby, Alan R. Mackie and Clare E. N. Mills
Institute of Food Research, Norwich Research Park, Colney, Norwich, United Kingdom

Barbara Ballmer-Weber
Allergy Unit, Department of Dermatology, University Hospital Zurich, Zurich, Switzerland

Laurian Zuidmeer-Jongejan
Laboratory of Allergy Research, Department of Experimental Immunology, Academic Medical Centre, University of Amsterdam, Amsterdam, The Netherlands

Zsolt Szépfalusi
Department of Pediatrics, Medical University of Vienna, Vienna, Austria

Janneke Ruinemans-Koerts
Department of Clinical Chemistry and Haematology, Rijnstate Hospital, Arnhem, The Netherlands

Ad P. H. Jansen
Department of Otorhinolaryngology, Radboud University Nijmegen Medical Centre, Nijmegen, The Netherlands

Harry J. Wichers
Cell Biology and Immunology Group, Wageningen University and Research Centre, Wageningen, The Netherlands
Food Chemistry Group, Wageningen University and Research Centre, Wageningen, The Netherlands
Food and Biobased Research, Wageningen University and Research Centre, Wageningen, The Netherlands

Philip R. Corlett, Jane R. Taylor and John H. Krystal
Department of Psychiatry, Ribicoff Research Facility, Yale University, New Haven, Connecticut, United States of America

Victoria Cambridge, Fernando Sergio Arana, Hannah L. Morgan and Naresh Subramanian
Brain Mapping Unit, Department of Psychiatry, University of Cambridge, School of Clinical Medicine, Addenbrooke's Hospital, Cambridge, United Kingdom

Jennifer M. Gardner and Jennifer S. Piggot
University of Cambridge, School of Clinical Medicine, Addenbrooke's Hospital, Cambridge, United Kingdom

Danielle C. Turner, Jessica C. Everitt, Amy L. Milton, Michael R. F. Aitken, Anthony Dickinson and Barry J. Everitt
Department of Psychology, University of Cambridge, Cambridge, United Kingdom

Jonathan L. Lee
University of Birmingham, School of Psychology, Edgbaston, Birmingham, United Kingdom

Anthony R. Absalom
Department of Anesthesiology, University Medical Center Groningen, Groningen University, Groningen, The Netherlands

Ram Adapa
Division of Anaesthesia, School of Clinical Medicine, University of Cambridge, Addenbrooke's Hospital, Cambridge, United Kingdom

Paul C. Fletcher
Brain Mapping Unit, Department of Psychiatry, University of Cambridge, School of Clinical Medicine, Addenbrooke's Hospital, Cambridge, United Kingdom
Cambridgeshire and Peterborough NHS Foundation Trust, Elizabeth House, Fulbourn Hospital, Cambridge, United Kingdom

Jenn-Ren Hsiao, Chun-Yen Ou, Hung-I Lo, Cheng-Chih Huang, Wei-Ting Lee, Sen-Tien Tsai and Fang-Ting Wang
Department of Otolaryngology, National Cheng Kung University Hospital, College of Medicine, National Cheng Kung University, Tainan, Taiwan

Jehn-Shyun Huang, Ken-Chung Chen and Tung-Yiu Wong
Department of Stomatology, National Cheng Kung University Hospital, College of Medicine, National Cheng Kung University, Tainan, Taiwan

Chia-Jui Yen and Shang-Yin Wu
Division of Hematology/Oncology, Department of Internal Medicine, National Cheng Kung University Hospital, College of Medicine, National Cheng Kung University, Tainan, Taiwan

Yuan-Hua Wu, Wei-Ting Hsueh and Ming-Wei Yang
Department of Radiation Oncology, National Cheng Kung University Hospital, College of Medicine, National Cheng Kung University, Tainan, Taiwan

Yi-Hui Wang, Ya-Ling Weng, Han-Chien Yang and Jeffrey S. Chang
National Institute of Cancer Research, National Health Research Institutes, Tainan, Taiwan

Jang-Yang Chang and Kwang-Yu Chang
Division of Hematology/Oncology, Department of Internal Medicine, National Cheng Kung University Hospital, College of Medicine, National Cheng Kung University, Tainan, Taiwan
National Institute of Cancer Research, National Health Research Institutes, Tainan, Taiwan

Chen-Lin Lin
Department of Nursing, National Cheng Kung University Hospital, College of Medicine, National Cheng Kung University, Tainan, Taiwan

Susanne Glaumann and Caroline Nilsson
Department of Clinical Science and Education, Södersjukhuset, Centre for Allergy Research, Karolinska Institutet, Stockholm, Sweden
Sach's Children's Hospital, Södersjukhuset, Stockholm, Sweden

Anna Nopp and S. G. O. Johansson
Department of Medicine, Clinical Immunology and Allergy Unit, Karolinska Institutet, Stockholm, Sweden

Magnus P. Borres
Thermo Fisher Scientific, Uppsala, Sweden
Department of Pediatrics, Institute for Clinical Sciences, The Sahlgrenska Academy at the University of Gothenburg, Sweden

Stefano Alessandri
CERM, Centro di Ricerca di Risonanze Magnetiche and Department of Agricultural Biotechnology, University of Florence, Florence, Italy

Ana Sancho, Clare E. N. Mills and Neil Rigby
Institute of Food Research, Norwich, United Kingdom

Stefan Vieths
Paul-Ehrlich-Institut, Langen, Germany

Jean-Michel Wal
INRA, UR496 Immuno-Allergie Alimentaire, CEA/iBiTeC-S/SPI, CEA de Saclay, Gif sur Yvette, France

Peter R. Shewry
Rothamsted Research, Harpenden, United Kingdom

Karin Hoffmann-Sommergruber
Department of Pathophysiology and Allergy Research, Medical University of Vienna, Vienna, Austria

Renata Curciarello, Angela M. Candreva and Guillermo H. Docena
Laboratorio de Investigaciones del Sistema Inmune-LISIN, Departamento de Ciencias Biológicas, Facultad de Ciencias Exactas, Universidad Nacional de La Plata, La Plata, Buenos Aires, Argentina
Centro de Investigaciones y Desarrollo en Criotecnología de Alimentos-CIDCA, Facultad de Ciencias Exactas, Universidad Nacional de La Plata, La Plata, Buenos Aires, Argentina

Paola L. Smaldini and Carlos A. Fossati
Laboratorio de Investigaciones del Sistema Inmune-LISIN, Departamento de Ciencias Biológicas, Facultad de Ciencias Exactas, Universidad Nacional de La Plata, La Plata, Buenos Aires, Argentina

Virginia González and Gustavo Parisi
Centro de Estudios e Investigaciones, Departamento de Ciencias y Tecnología Universidad Nacional de Quilmes, Quilmes, Buenos Aires, Argentina

Ana Cauerhff
Centro de Investigación y Desarrollo en Fermentaciones Industriales, CINDEFI (UNLP y CONICET) and Instituto de Investigaciones Bioquímicas de Buenos Aires (IIBBA-CONICET), Fundación Instituto Leloir, Buenos Aires, Argentina

Ivana Barrios and Luis Bruno Blanch
Cátedra de Química Medicinal, Departamento de Ciencias Biológicas, Facultad de Ciencias Exactas, Universidad Nacional de La Plata, La Plata, Buenos Aires, Argentina

Silvana Petruccelli
Centro de Investigaciones y Desarrollo en Criotecnología de Alimentos-CIDCA, Facultad de Ciencias Exactas, Universidad Nacional de La Plata, La Plata, Buenos Aires, Argentina

Ramkrashan Kasera and Naveen Arora
Allergy and Immunology Section, CSIR-Institute of Genomics and Integrative Biology, Delhi, India
University of Pune, Ganeshkhind, Pune, India

Anand Bahadur Singh
Allergy and Immunology Section, CSIR-Institute of Genomics and Integrative Biology, Delhi, India
Shakuntala Lavasa
USLavasa Medical and Research Center, Chandigarh, India

Komarla Nagendra
Bengaluru Allergy Centre, Bangalore, India

Anna Maria Riccio, Anthi Rogkakou, Giorgio Walter Canonica and Giovanni Passalacqua
Allergy and Respiratory Diseases, Department of Internal Medicine, University of Genoa, Genoa, Italy

Daniele Saverino
Section of Human Anatomy, Department of Experimental Medicine, University of Genoa, Genoa, Italy

Giampaola Pesce and Marcello Bagnasco
Medical and Radiomethabolic Therapy, Department of Internal Medicine, University of Genoa, Genoa, Italy

Maurizio Severino
Allergy Unit, Ospedale San Giovanni di Dio, Florence, Italy

Patrizia Bonadonna
Allergy Service, Verona General Hospital, Verona, Italy

Erminia Ridolo
Experimental and Internal Medicine, University of Parma, Parma, Italy

Marina Mauro
Allergy Unit, Sant'Anna Hospital, Como, Italy

Chih-Yung Chiu
Department of Pediatrics, Chang Gung Memorial Hospital, Keelung, Taiwan
Community Medicine Research Centre, Chang Gung Memorial Hospital, Keelung, Taiwan
Division of Pediatric Pulmonology, Chang Gung Memorial Hospital, College of Medicine, Chang Gung University, Taoyuan, Taiwan

Yu-Lin Huang, Yu-Ling Tu, Tsung-Chieh Yao, Kuo-Wei Yeh and Jing-Long Huang
Community Medicine Research Centre, Chang Gung Memorial Hospital, Keelung, Taiwan
Division of Allergy, Asthma, and Rheumatology, Department of Pediatrics, Chang Gung Memorial Hospital, and Chang Gung University College of Medicine, Taoyuan, Taiwan

Ming-Han Tsai and Man-Chin Hua
Department of Pediatrics, Chang Gung Memorial Hospital, Keelung, Taiwan
Community Medicine Research Centre, Chang Gung Memorial Hospital, Keelung, Taiwan

Min-Hye Kim
Department of Internal Medicine, Division of Allergy and Clinical Immunology, Seoul National University Hospital, Seoul, Republic of Korea
Institute of Allergy and Clinical Immunology, Seoul National University Medical Research Center, Seoul, Republic of Korea
Seoul National University Hospital Regional Pharmacovigilance Center, Seoul, Republic of Korea
Department of Internal Medicine, Ewha Womans University School of Medicine, Seoul, Republic of Korea

Suh-Young Lee and Seung-Eun Lee
Department of Internal Medicine, Division of Allergy and Clinical Immunology, Seoul National University Hospital, Seoul, Republic of Korea
Institute of Allergy and Clinical Immunology, Seoul National University Medical Research Center, Seoul, Republic of Korea

Sang-Heon Cho and Hye-Ryun Kang
Department of Internal Medicine, Division of Allergy and Clinical Immunology, Seoul National University Hospital, Seoul, Republic of Korea
Institute of Allergy and Clinical Immunology, Seoul National University Medical Research Center, Seoul, Republic of Korea
Seoul National University Hospital Regional Pharmacovigilance Center, Seoul, Republic of Korea

Min-Suk Yang
Department of Internal Medicine, Division of Allergy and Clinical Immunology, Seoul National University Hospital, Seoul, Republic of Korea
Institute of Allergy and Clinical Immunology, Seoul National University Medical Research Center, Seoul, Republic of Korea
Department of Internal Medicine, SMG-SNU Boramae Medical Center, Seoul, Republic of Korea

Jae-Woo Jung
Institute of Allergy and Clinical Immunology, Seoul National University Medical Research Center, Seoul, Republic of Korea
Department of Internal Medicine, Chung-Ang University College of Medicine, Seoul, Republic of Korea

Chang Min Park and Whal Lee
Department of Radiology and Institute of Radiation Medicine, Seoul National University College of Medicine, Seoul, Republic of Korea

Lise Moussu, Virginie Panayotopoulos, Flore Amat and Jocelyne Just
Allergology department, Centre de l'Asthme et des Allergies, Hôpital d'Enfants Armand-Trousseau (Assistance Publique Hôpitaux de Paris) - Université Pierre et Marie Curie, Paris, France

Philippe Saint-Pierre
Laboratoire de Statistiques Théoriques et Appliquées, Université Pierre et Marie Curie, Paris, France

Rémy Couderc
Service de Biochimie et Biologie Moléculaire, Hôpital d'Enfants Armand-Trousseau (Assistance Publique Hôpitaux de Paris), Paris, France

Marie Ekbäck, Irene Devenney and Karin Fälth-Magnusson
Division of Pediatrics, Department of Clinical and Experimental Medicine, Faculty of Health Sciences, Linköping University and Department of Pediatrics, County Council of Östergötland, Linköping, Sweden

Michaela Tedner
Pediatric Clinic, Täby, Stockholm, Sweden

Göran Oldaeus
Pediatric Clinic, County Hospital Ryhov, Jönköping, Sweden

Gunilla Norrman
Pediatric Clinic, Hudiksvall, Sweden

Leif Strömberg
Department of Pediatrics in Norrköping, County Council of Östergötland, Norrköping, Sweden

Natalia Deus-de-Oliveira, Shayany P. Felix, Camila Carrielo-Gama, Keysson V. Fernandes and Olga L. T. Machado
Laboratório de Química e Função de Proteínas e Peptídeos/Centro de Biociências e Biotecnologia, Universidade Estadual do Norte Fluminense - Darcy Ribeiro, Campos dos Goytacazes, Rio de Janeiro, Brazil

Renato Augusto Da Matta
Laboratório de Biologia Celular e Tecidual/Centro de Biociências e Biotecnologia, Universidade Estadual do Norte Fluminense - Darcy Ribeiro, Campos dos Goytacazes, Rio de Janeiro, Brazil

Monica Vasudev., Dorothy S. Cheung., Hannah Pincsak, Shun-Hwa Li, Ke Yan, Pippa Simpson,
Trivikram Dasu and Mitchell H. Grayson
Department of Pediatrics, Medical College of Wisconsin, Milwaukee, Wisconsin, United States of America

Sara Pereira Menezes, Thyago Hermylly Santana Cardoso and Carlos Priminho Pirovani
UESC, Centro de Biotecnologia e Genética, Ilhéus, Bahia, Brasil

Jane Lima dos Santos
UESC, Centro de Microscopia Eletrônica, Ilhéus, Bahia, Brasil

Fabienne Micheli
UESC, Centro de Biotecnologia e Genética, Ilhéus, Bahia, Brasil
CIRAD, UMAR AGAP, Montpellier, France

Fátima Soares Motta Noronha, Andréa Catão Alves and Ana Maria Caetano Faria
UFMG, Instituto de Ciências Biológicas, Pampulha, Belo Horizonte, Minas Gerais, Brasil

Abelmon da Silva Gesteira
Embrapa Mandioca e Fruticultura, Cruz das Almas, Bahia, Brasil

Rosa Anna Iorio and Stefano Del Duca
Department of Biological, Earth and Environmental Sciences, University of Bologna, Bologna, Italy

Elisabetta Calamelli, Chiara Pula, Andrea Pession and Giampaolo Ricci
Department of Pediatric Allergology of the Women's, Children's and Adolescents' Health Gozzadini Children's Hospital Sant'Orsola-Malpighi, University of Bologna, Bologna, Italy

Magda Lodolini and Fortuna Scamardella
Laboratory Analysis Unit. Maggiore Hospital, Bologna, Italy

Jaroslav Golias, Miloslav Kverka, Klara Klimesova, Petr Sotkovsky, Lenka Palova-Jelinkova and Ludmila Tuckova
Department of Immunology and Gnotobiology, Institute of Microbiology, v.v.i., Academy of Sciences of the Czech Republic, Prague, Czech Republic

Martin Schwarzer, Hana Kozakova and Dagmar Srutkova
Department of Immunology and Gnotobiology, Institute of Microbiology, v.v.i., Academy of Sciences of the Czech Republic, Novy Hradek, Czech Republic

Michael Wallner and Fatima Ferreira
Christian Doppler Laboratory for Allergy Diagnosis and Therapy, Department of Molecular Biology, University of Salzburg, Salzburg, Austria

Antonios Patelis, Maria Gunnbjörnsdottir and Christer Janson
Department of Medical Sciences: Respiratory Medicine and Allergology, Uppsala University, Uppsala, Sweden

Magnus P. Borres
Immunodiagnostics, Thermo Fischer Scientific, Uppsala, Sweden

Thorarinn Gislason
University of Iceland, Medical Faculty and Department of Respiratory Medicine and Sleep, Landspitali University Hospital, Reykjavik, Iceland

Kjell Torén
Section of Occupational and Environmental Medicine, Institute of Medicine, University of Gothenburg, Gothenburg, Sweden

Bertil Forsberg
Division of Occupational and Environmental Medicine, Umeå University, Umeå, Sweden

Kjell Alving
Department of Women's and Children's Health, Uppsala University, Uppsala, Sweden

Peter Burney
Respiratory Epidemiology and Public Health, Imperial College, London, United Kingdom

Andrei Malinovschi
Department of Medical Sciences: Clinical Physiology, Uppsala University, Uppsala, Sweden

Takeshi Yamamoto, Toshihisa Kodama, Jaemin Lee, Naho Utsunomiya, Shusaku Hayashi and Makoto Kadowaki
Division of Gastrointestinal Pathophysiology, Institute of Natural Medicine, University of Toyama, Toyama, Toyama, Japan

Hiroshi Sakamoto
Department of Physical Therapy, Health Science University, Fujikawaguchiko, Yamanashi, Japan

Hirofumi Kuramoto
Department of Applied Biology, Kyoto Institute of Technology, Kyoto, Kyoto, Japan

Stine Kroghsbo, Katrine L. Bøgh and Charlotte B. Madsen
National Food Institute, Technical University of Denmark, Søborg, Denmark

Neil M. Rigby, Philip E. Johnson, Louise J. Salt and E. N. Clare Mills
Institute of Food Research, Norwich Research Park, Colney, Norwich, United Kingdom

Karine Adel-Patient
INRA, UR496, Unité d'Immuno-Allergie Alimentaire, Jouy-en-Josas, France

Rubén Martínez-Aranguren, María J. Goikoetxea, Paula Cabrera-Freitag and María L. Sanz
Department of Allergology and Clinical Immunology, Clínica Universidad de Navarra, Pamplona, Spain

María T. Lizaso and Blanca E. García
Allergology Service, Complejo Hospitalario de Navarra, Pamplona, Spain

Oswaldo Trellez
Department of Computer Architecture, Universidad de Málaga, Málaga, Spain

Index

M

N

O

P

R

S

T

U

V